BOIES FUNDAMENTALS OF OTOLARYNGOLOGY

A TEXTBOOK OF EAR, NOSE, AND THROAT DISEASES

GEORGE L. ADAMS, M.D.
Department of Otolaryngology,
University of Minnesota Hospital and Clinic,
Minneapolis, Minnesota

LAWRENCE R. BOIES, Jr., M.D.
Chief of Otolaryngology, St Paul-Ramsey
Medical Center, St. Paul, Minnesota;
Department of Otolaryngology,
University of Minnesota Hospital and Clinic,
Minneapolis, Minnesota

PETER A. HILGER, M.D.
Staff, Department of Otolaryngology,
St. Paul-Ramsey Medical Center,
St. Paul, Minnesota;
Department of Otolaryngology,
University of Minnesota Hospital and Clinic,
Minneapolis, Minnesota

Sixth Edition

1989
W. B. SAUNDERS COMPANY
Harcourt Brace Jovanovich, Inc.

Philadelphia, London, Toronto, Montreal, Sydney, Tokyo

W. B. SAUNDERS COMPANY
Harcourt Brace Jovanovich, Inc.

The Curtis Center
Independence Square West
Philadelphia, PA 19106

Library of Congress Cataloging-in-Publication Data

Fundamentals of otolaryngology.
 Boies fundamentals of otolaryngology: a textbook of ear, nose, and throat disease.—6th ed./George L. Adams, Lawrence R. Boies, Jr., Peter A. Hilger.
  p. cm.
 Rev. ed. of: Boies's fundamentals of otolaryngology. 5th ed. 1978.
 Includes bibliographies and index.

 1. Otolaryngology. I. Boies, Lawrence R., 1898–1987. II. Adams, George L. (George Linton), 1941– . III. Boies, Lawrence R., 1932– . IV. Hilger, Peter A., 1948– . V. Title.
  [DNLM: 1. Otorhinolaryngologic Diseases. WV 100 F981]
 RF46.F96 1989
 617'.51—dc19
 DNLM/DLC
 for Library of Congress   88–39685
                                                                           CIP

Editor: Lisette Bralow
Manuscript Editor: Donna Walker
Production Manager: Frank Polizzano
Indexer: Roger Wall

FUNDAMENTALS OF OTOLARYNGOLOGY   ISBN 0-7216-3102-9

Copyright © 1989, 1978, 1964, 1959, 1954, 1949 by W. B. Saunders Company.

All rights reserved. No part of this publication may be reproduced or transmitted in any form or by any means, electronic or mechanical, including photocopying, recording, or any information storage and retrieval system, without written permission from the publisher.

Printed in the United States of America.

Last digit is the print number: 9   8   7   6   5   4   3   2   1

CONTRIBUTORS

GEORGE L. ADAMS, M.D.
Associate Head and Associate Professor, Department of Otolaryngology, University of Minnesota Medical School. Staff, Veterans Administration Medical Center, Minneapolis, Minnesota.
Diseases of the Middle Ear and Mastoid; Disorders of the Salivary Glands; Diseases of the Nasopharynx and Oropharynx; Malignant Tumors of the Head and Neck

JOHN H. ANDERSON, M.D., PH.D.
Assistant Professor, Department of Otolaryngology and Physiology, University of Minnesota Medical School, Minneapolis, Minnesota.
The Vestibular System

JOHN D. BANOVETZ, M.D.
Clinical Associate Professor, Department of Otolaryngology, University of Minnesota Medical School. Staff, Abbott Northwestern Hospital, Minneapolis Childrens Medical Center, North Memorial Medical Center, Riverside Medical Center, Unity Medical Center, Minneapolis, Minnesota.
Benign Laryngeal Disorders

NORMAN T. BERLINGER, M.D., PH.D.
Staff, Minneapolis Childrens Medical Center, North Memorial Medical Center, Minneapolis, Minnesota.
Infections in the Immunocompromised Host

MALCOLM N. BLUMENTHAL, M.D.
Clinical Professor, University of Minnesota Medical School. Director, Section of Allergy, University of Minnesota Hospital, Minneapolis, Minnesota.
Allergic Conditions in Otolaryngology Patients

LAWRENCE R. BOIES, JR., M.D.
Associate Professor, Department of Otolaryngology, University of Minnesota Medical School, Minneapolis. Chief of Otolaryngology, St. Paul-Ramsey Medical Center, St. Paul, Minnesota.
Diseases of the External Ear; Facial Pain, Headache, and Otalgia

JAMES I. COHEN, M.D., PH.D.
Assistant Professor of Otolaryngology/Head and Neck Surgery, Oregon Health Sciences University (OHSU). Attending Staff, Oregon Health Sciences University, Veterans Administration Medical Center, Portland, Oregon.
Anatomy and Physiology of the Larynx; Benign Neck Masses

CONTRIBUTORS

ARNDT J. DUVALL, III, M.D.
Professor, Department of Otolaryngology/Head and Neck Surgery, University of Minnesota Medical School. Staff, University of Minnesota Hospital, Minneapolis, Minnesota.
Embryology, Anatomy, and Physiology of the Ear

MEREDITH GERDIN, M.A., C.C.C.
Speech and Language Pathologist, University of Minnesota Hospital and Clinic, Minneapolis, Minnesota.
Speech and Language Disorders

ROBERT J. GORLIN, D.D.S., M.S., D.Sc (Athens)
Professor, Oral Pathology and Genetics, University of Minnesota School of Dentistry; Professor, Departments of Pathology, Dermatology, Pediatrics, Obstetrics-Gynecology, and Otolaryngology, University of Minnesota Hospitals. Consultant, Veterans Administration, Mt. Sinai Hospital, Hennepin County Medical Center, Minneapolis Children's Hospital, Minneapolis; Ramsey County General Hospital, Gillette State Hospital for Crippled Children, St. Paul Children's Hospital, St. Paul, Minnesota.
Diseases of the Oral Cavity

DONNA G. GREENFIELD, M.S.
Research Assistant, Department of Communication Disorders, University of Minnesota Medical School, Minneapolis, Minnesota.
Audiology

PETER A. HILGER, M.D., M.S.
Assistant Professor, Department of Otolaryngology, University of Minnesota Medical School, Minneapolis. Staff, St. Paul-Ramsey Medical Center, St. Paul, Minnesota.
Applied Anatomy and Physiology of the Nose; Diseases of the Nose; Diseases of the Paranasal Sinuses; Facial Plastic Surgery

FRANK M. LASSMAN, Ph.D.
Professor of Audiology, Departments of Otolaryngology, Physical Medicine, and Communication Disorders, University of Minnesota Medical School, Minneapolis, Minnesota.
Audiology; Speech and Language Disorders

SAMUEL C. LEVINE, M.D.
Assistant Professor, Department of Otolaryngology, University of Minnesota Medical School. Staff, Veterans Administration Medical Center, Minneapolis, Minnesota.
The Vestibular System; Audiology; Diseases of the Middle Ear and Mastoid; Diseases of the Inner Ear; Disorders of the Facial Nerve

STEPHEN L. LISTON, F.R.A.C.S., F.R.C.S., F.A.C.S.
Clinical Associate Professor, Department of Otolaryngology, University of Minnesota Medical School, Minneapolis. Staff Otolaryngologist, United and Children's Hospital, St. Joseph's Hospital, St. John's Hospital, Midway Hospital, Divine Redeemer Hospital, St. Paul, Minnesota.
Embryology, Anatomy, and Physiology of the Ear; Embryology, Anatomy, and Physiology of the Oral Cavity, Pharynx, Esophagus, and Neck

ROBERT H. MAISEL, M.D.

Associate Professor, Department of Otolaryngology, University of Minnesota Medical School. Chief, Department of Otolaryngology, Hennepin County Medical Center, Minneapolis, Minnesota.

Disorders of the Facial Nerve; Tracheostomy

MICHAEL M. PAPARELLA, M.D.

Clinical Professor, Department of Otolaryngology, University of Minnesota Medical School. Secretary, International Hearing Foundation, Director, Otopathology Laboratory, University of Minnesota, Minneapolis, Minnesota.

Diseases of the Middle Ear and Mastoid

LEIGHTON G. SIEGEL, M.D.

Clinical Associate Professor, Department of Otolaryngology/Head and Neck Surgery, University of Minnesota Medical School, Minneapolis. Staff, Childrens Hospital, Minneapolis; United Hospital, St. Joseph's Hospital, University Hospital, St. Paul, Minnesota.

The Head and Neck History and Examination; Diseases of the Lower Air Passages, Esophagus, and Mediastinum: Endoscopic Considerations

VIRGINIA WIGGINTON, M.A., C.C.C.

Speech and Language Pathologist, University of Minnesota Hospital and Clinic, Minneapolis, Minnesota.

Speech and Language Disorders

KENT S. WILSON, M.D.

Clinical Assistant Professor, University of Minnesota Medical School, Minneapolis. Staff, Health East, United Hospital, Children's Hospital, St. Paul, Minnesota.

Maxillofacial Trauma

PREFACE

Eleven years have passed since publication of the Fifth Edition of *Boies Fundamentals of Otolaryngology*. The original text, printed more than 40 years ago, provided clinical information on the management and care of patients with otolaryngology disorders. Each subsequent edition has included more basic science information. We recognize that there are now three- and four-volume texts available in the field of otolaryngology–head and neck surgery, and we have endeavored to limit this text to the basic principles of diagnosis, recognition of causative factors, and management of the more common problems. The new Sixth Edition stresses basic science principles of anatomy, embryology, and physiology and correlates this information with the clinical findings to assist in understanding the management of disorders of the ears, nose, throat, head, and neck. The textbook, in a sense, has been entirely rewritten and not just updated. The illustrations, for the most part, have been replaced with better quality artwork. The textbook has been expanded to keep pace with the expanding scope of our specialty. The added sections on wound healing and wound repair provide basic information for repair of minor defects.

The current authors are teachers at the University of Minnesota who lecture to the sophomore class sessions in otolaryngology. Chapters outside the normal scope of otolaryngology have been written by experts in those areas in order to provide a more thorough presentation of the material. While the text is aimed primarily at medical students at the beginning of their clinical years, the material will be of value to family physicians and first-year residents in family practice and otolaryngology. Those who plan to specialize in head and neck surgery are provided with references in which more complex procedures are described in greater detail.

The format for the Sixth Edition has changed significantly to comply with today's medical school curricula. Besides the emphasis on pathophysiology, there is a greater emphasis on basic principles. In the margins of each chapter, specific major points are highlighted or re-emphasized. This method indexes important facts for the student to recall. The editors of the Sixth Edition have tried to provide the basic information necessary in the most concise, easily understood manner for a medical student on a busy otolaryngology–head and neck surgery rotation.

The current editors wish to acknowledge material originally prepared by authors of the Fifth Edition whose chapters have been expanded and revised by the current faculty. Special thanks for past contributions to Doctors Mary Jayne Capps, Anderson C. Hilding, Robert H. Mathog, Kurt Pollak, Cedric A. Quick, Melvin E. Sigel, Ms. Carol Berman, Mr. Richard L. Hoel, and Ms. Elaine LaBenz.

GEORGE L. ADAMS
LAWRENCE R. BOIES, JR.
PETER A. HILGER

CONTENTS

PART ONE

HISTORY AND EXAMINATION

1
The Head and Neck History and Examination 3
Leighton G. Siegel

PART TWO

THE EAR

2
Embryology, Anatomy, and Physiology of the Ear 27
Stephen L. Liston and Arndt J. Duvall, III

3
The Vestibular System 39
John H. Anderson and Samuel C. Levine

4
Audiology 46
Frank M. Lassman, Samuel C. Levine, and Donna G. Greenfield

5
Diseases of the External Ear 77
Lawrence R. Boies, Jr.

6
Diseases of the Middle Ear and Mastoid 90
Michael M. Paparella, George L. Adams, and Samuel C. Levine

7
Diseases of the Inner Ear 123
Samuel C. Levine

8
Disorders of the Facial Nerve 142
Robert H. Maisel and Samuel C. Levine

9
Facial Pain, Headache, and Otalgia 157
Lawrence R. Boies, Jr.

PART THREE

THE NOSE AND PARANASAL SINUSES

10
Applied Anatomy and Physiology of the Nose 177
Peter A. Hilger

11
Allergic Conditions in Otolaryngology Patients 196
Malcolm N. Blumenthal

12
Diseases of the Nose 206
Peter A. Hilger

13
Diseases of the Paranasal Sinuses 249
Peter A. Hilger

PART FOUR

THE ORAL CAVITY AND PHARYNX

14
Embryology, Anatomy, and Physiology of the Oral Cavity,
Pharynx, Esophagus, and Neck 273
Stephen L. Liston

15
Diseases of the Oral Cavity 282
Robert J. Gorlin

16
Disorders of the Salivary Glands 317
George L. Adams

17
Diseases of the Nasopharynx and Oropharynx 332
George L. Adams

18
Infections in the Immunocompromised Host 370
Norman T. Berlinger

PART FIVE

THE LARYNX

19
Anatomy and Physiology of the Larynx 383
James I. Cohen

20
Benign Laryngeal Disorders 392
    John D. Banovetz

21
Speech and Language Disorders 412
    Virginia Wigginton, Meredith Gerdin, and Frank M. Lassman

PART SIX

NEOPLASMS OF THE HEAD AND NECK

22
Benign Neck Masses 429
    James I. Cohen

23
Malignant Tumors of the Head and Neck 443
    George L. Adams

PART SEVEN

DISEASES OF THE TRACHEA AND CERVICAL ESOPHAGUS

24
Diseases of the Lower Air Passages, Esophagus, and Mediastinum: Endoscopic Considerations 471
    Leighton G. Siegel

25
Tracheostomy 490
    Robert H. Maisel

PART EIGHT

PLASTIC AND RECONSTRUCTIVE SURGERY

26
Facial Plastic Surgery 505
    Peter A. Hilger

27
Maxillofacial Trauma 526
    Kent S. Wilson

Index 541

PART ONE

HISTORY AND EXAMINATION

1

THE HEAD AND NECK HISTORY AND EXAMINATION

by Leighton G. Siegel, M.D.

The skills required to obtain a medical history and perform a physical examination of the head and neck are fundamental, require little time of the examiner, and yet are so clinically rewarding that they should be included in every general examination. Systemic disorders commonly produce symptoms and signs within the head and neck. A general history and examination are thus part of every head and neck evaluation.

Additional details regarding the history and examination are found in the chapters dealing with specific areas and problems.

BASIC EQUIPMENT AND TECHNIQUE FOR A HEAD AND NECK EXAMINATION

Head Mirror, Light Source, and Position. This description of the light source, head mirror, and positioning of the patient and the examiner is applicable throughout the entire otolaryngologic examination.

The examiner may stand or sit but should be comfortable. A good examination cannot be made when one must bend and stoop. The patient is seated, with the head slightly higher than the examiner's head. The patient should lean forward slightly, keeping his back straight, with feet on the floor and legs uncrossed. For examination of the ear, the patient is turned to the right or the left.

The light source should be a point source if possible. It can be a simple unfrosted 100-watt or stronger light bulb, situated on a gooseneck stand without a reflector. Lights designed specifically for this purpose are optimal. The light is positioned slightly behind and just to the right of the patient's head.

There is no adequate substitute for a proper head mirror and light source when examining the cavities of the head and neck. Indeed, a good part of the examination cannot be done in any other manner. The most useful size head mirror has a 3½-inch diameter with a ½-inch hole in the center and focal length of about 14 inches. The head mirror is positioned over the physician's left eye so that it is possible to see the patient and the focused spot of light through the hole in the center of the mirror as well as with the other eye. At the same time the mirror shades both eyes from the direct glare of the light source. The mirror should be as close to the physician's face as possible to provide a wide angle of view. The examiner then directs the area of the patient to be examined into the field of view and avoids repositioning himself. A focusable light on a headband may be substituted for the described head mirror and light source.

A head mirror or light leaves both of the examiner's hands free for the examination.

The Ear

Patient History

The minimal history should include an inquiry about hearing impairment, head noises (tinnitus), dizziness (vertigo) or imbalance, discharge from the ear, and earache. If any of these complaints are found, they should be characterized in detail. The following outline is a practical guide for inquiry into these complaints.

Hearing Impairment

Typical complaints produced by hearing loss are: "I can hear when there is one person but not when I am with a group of people or when it's noisy." "Everyone mumbles nowadays." "My child only hears what he wants to hear." "My child is over one year old and isn't talking." "My wife (for some reason it's frequently a wife) says I am not paying attention and she wants my hearing checked."

Specific questions that might be asked include:

1. Was onset sudden or gradual? Duration?
2. Which ear is affected, or are both involved?
3. Does the hearing get alternately better and worse?
4. Do things merely sound quiet, or is understanding also a problem and under what circumstances?
5. Was the onset associated with other illness, trauma, noise exposure, or the use of medication, including aspirin?
6. Is there a family history of hearing impairment?
7. Was there any prenatal or postnatal difficulty or disease or difficulty with delivery?
8. Has there been any past ear disease or surgery?
9. Was there occupational, military, recreational, or other noise exposure?
10. Is there a history of measles, mumps, influenza, meningitis, syphilis, severe viral illness, or use of ototoxic drugs such as kanamycin, streptomycin, gentamicin, or certain diuretics?
11. What social, occupational, or educational handicap does the hearing loss produce?

Head Noises

1. What is the nature of the noise? Can it be described as ringing, high-pitched, roaring, humming, hissing (sound of escaping steam), or pulsating (synchronous with pulse)?
2. Is the noise heard all the time or only in a very quiet room?
3. Is it heard after noise exposure at work or elsewhere?

Dizziness

1. Does the patient describe the symptom as lightheadedness, imbalance, spinning, or a tendency to fall? Toward which direction? Is the dizziness affected by head position? Is it present when lying down? Is onset related to getting up quickly?
2. What are the frequency and duration of attacks?
3. Is the dizziness continuous or episodic?
4. Have the patient describe the first attack. How long is the interval between episodes?

5. What other symptoms occur simultaneously? Do they include nausea, vomiting, tinnitus, a feeling of fullness in the ear, weakness, fluctuation in hearing, or loss of consciousness?
6. Is there a history of ear infections, perforations, head injury, or ear surgery?
7. Is there a history of any generalized diseases, such as diabetes mellitus, neurologic disorders, arteriosclerosis, hypertension, thyroid disorders, syphilis, anemia, malignancies, or heart or lung disease?
8. Is there a history of any allergic disorders?

Discharge from the Ear

1. Is it associated with itching or pain?
2. Is the drainage bloody or purulent? Is there an odor?
3. Duration? Has there been previous drainage?
4. Is it preceded by an upper respiratory infection or getting the ear wet?

Earache

1. Characterize the pain.
2. Is this a recurrent problem? If so, how often does it occur?
3. Is the pain just in the ear or does it spread to or come from another place?
4. Does anything seem to trigger the pain such as chewing, biting down, coughing, or swallowing. (Many locations in the head and neck will refer pain to the ear.)
5. Are there any other head or neck symptoms?

Examining the Ear

Examination should begin with inspection and palpation of the pinna and tissues around the ear. The external ear canal should also be examined, initially without a speculum prior to visualization of the tympanic membrane. Remember that the external ear canal is not straight. To straighten it for

Retract the ear up and back in adults and down in infants.

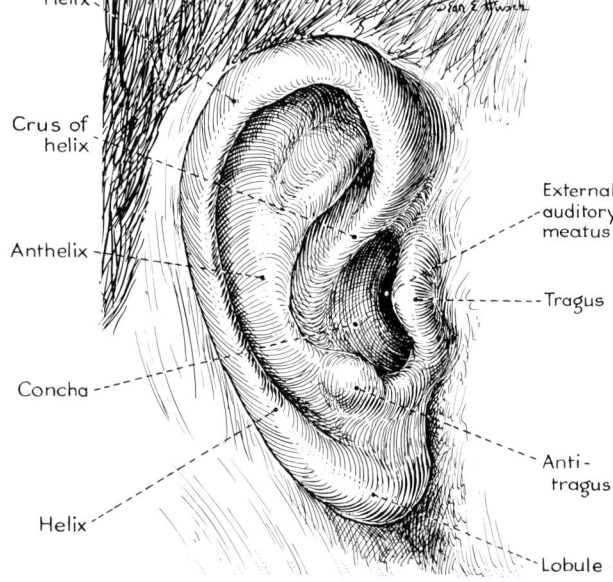

FIGURE 1–1. The auricle and external auditory meatus. The names of the external markings of the auricle are useful to locate lesions accurately when descriptions are made.

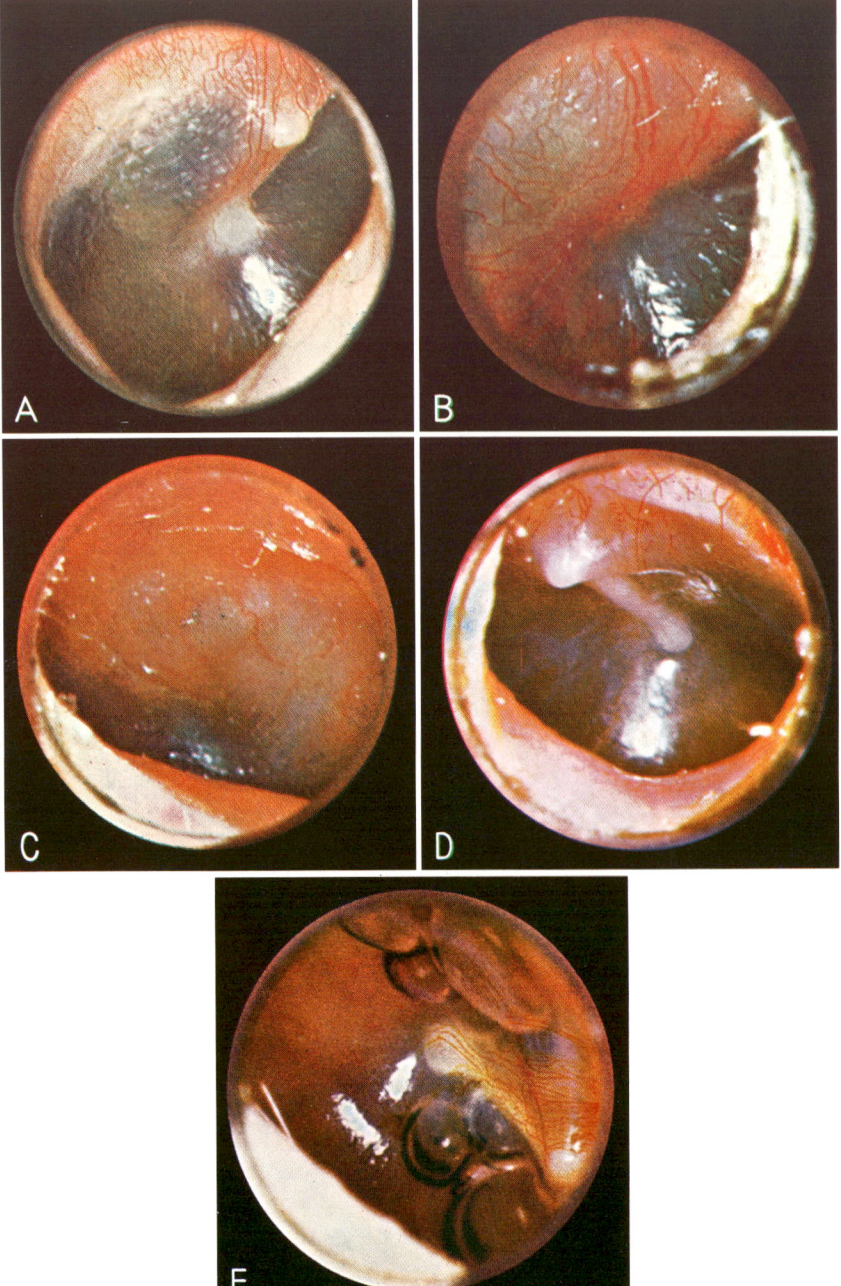

FIGURE 1–2. *A*, Normal tympanic membrane. *B*, Early stage of acute purulent otitis media. *C*, Later stage of acute otitis media. *D*, Serous otitis media. *E*, Bubbles in the middle ear are seen in serous otitis media after inflammation. (Courtesy of Dr. Richard A. Buckingham and Dr. George E. Shambaugh, Jr.)

examination, grasp the pinna and retract it backward and upward in adults and downward in infants. The appearance of the normal ear and right tympanic membrane is illustrated in Figures 1–1 and 1–2.

The **hand-held aural speculum** is used in conjunction with a head mirror and light source. It is thin-walled and funnel-shaped, should have a nonreflective surface, and is available in a selection of sizes (Fig. 1–3). The

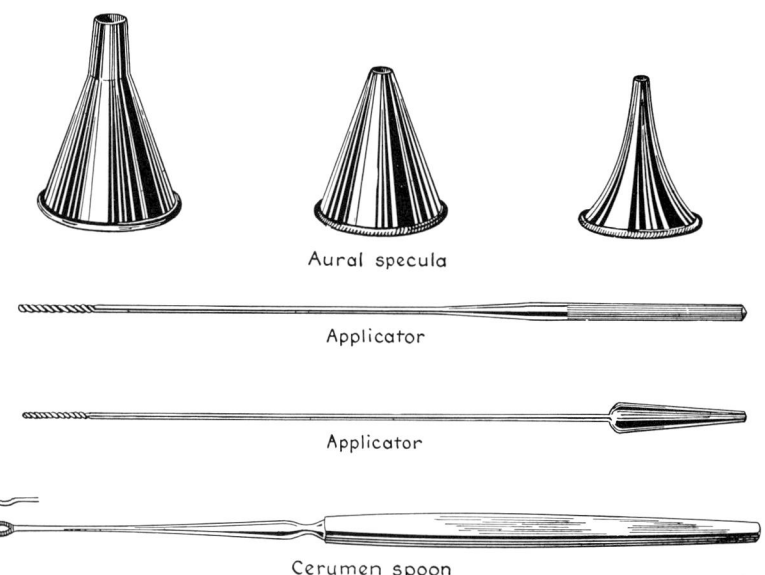

FIGURE 1–3. The largest aural speculum that will fit into the external meatus should be employed. Applicators should be thin and malleable. Some physicians prefer to bend the shaft of an applicator at an angle so that the fingers that grasp and manipulate the applicator will be out of the line of vision. The cerumen spoons in several sizes may be obtained with a fenestrated tip in the form of a loop. This tip should be thin, serrated, without sharp edges, and bent at about a 30 degree angle.

examiner chooses the largest one that comfortably fits the external ear canal. Since the opening is small, the speculum must be swiveled within the ear canal to visualize the entire tympanic membrane. All specula are held in the left hand so that the right, or dominant, hand is free to position the patient or manipulate instruments. Left-handed examiners may make compensatory adjustments. The hand-held speculum is best when manipulations, such as wax removal, need to be done (Fig. 1–4).

Battery-powered otoscopes are commonly used. The most useful of these have fiberoptic illumination, give a magnified view of the tympanic membrane, and are provided with a sealed head and pneumatic bulb attachment. Manipulation (as in removing wax) is much more difficult than with a head mirror and hand-held speculum (Fig. 1–5). An "operating" or open head is also available for the battery-powered otoscope. Manipulation through the open operating head is somewhat easier than with a sealed head, but unfortunately the great advantage of pneumatic inspection is not possible. As with the hand-held speculum, the largest size fitting the ear canal is used and must be swiveled within the ear canal to visualize the entire tympanic

Only part of the ear is seen through a speculum.

It must be moved to scan the entire ear.

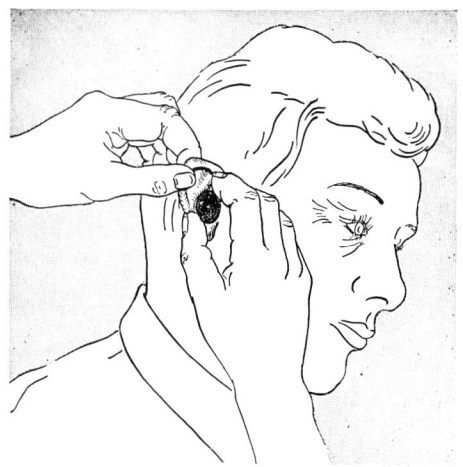

FIGURE 1–4. The technique of examining the external auditory canal and the drumhead through a speculum is as follows: Grasp the auricle with the thumb and index finger of the free hand and gently pull it backward and slightly upward. The speculum held between the thumb and index finger of the other hand is then inserted gently into the external meatus. As the light from the head mirror is reflected through the speculum, the direction in which the speculum points needs to be altered slightly so as to visualize the margins of the canal and the entire drumhead.

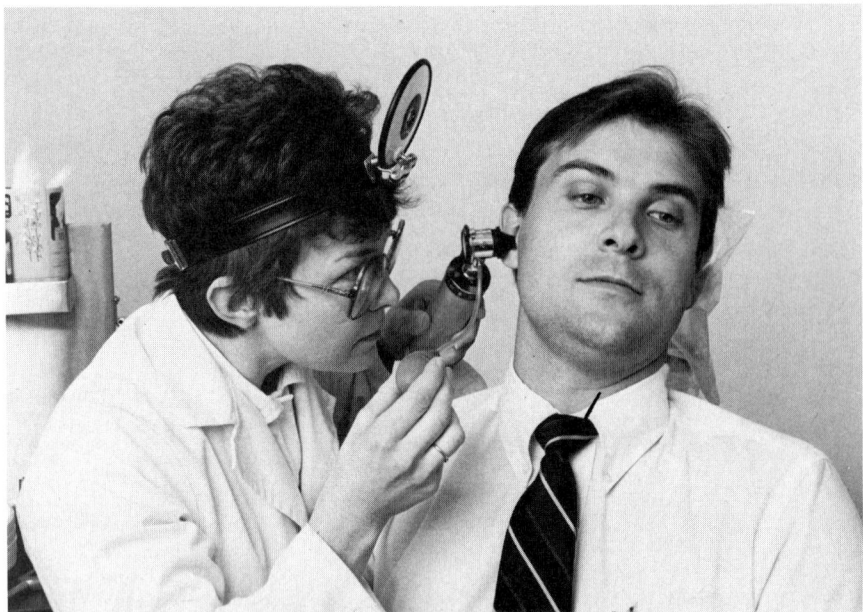

FIGURE 1–5. A hand-held battery-powered otoscope with a sealed system allows for pneumatic otoscopy. Only gentle pressure is required to move a normal tympanic membrane.

membrane. Inspection of the external ear canal must not be neglected in an effort to view the tympanic membrane.

Pneumatic otoscopy will readily detect the presence of a perforation of the tympanic membrane or fluid in the middle ear. This technique should be a part of every pediatric ear examination and is often needed for adults. The principle is that of increasing and decreasing air pressure within the external ear canal while visualizing the movement of the tympanic membrane in response to the pressure changes. The aural speculum is attached to a sealed chamber with a glass viewing window for the examiner. The speculum should have a bulbous flare at the end to provide a good seal when inserted into the ear canal (Fig. 1–6). A rubber bulb is attached to the sealed chamber using a short piece of flexible tubing. The bulb is squeezed in order to apply

Valsalva's maneuver (ask the patient to pinch the nose and blow) may also reveal tympanic membrane motion.

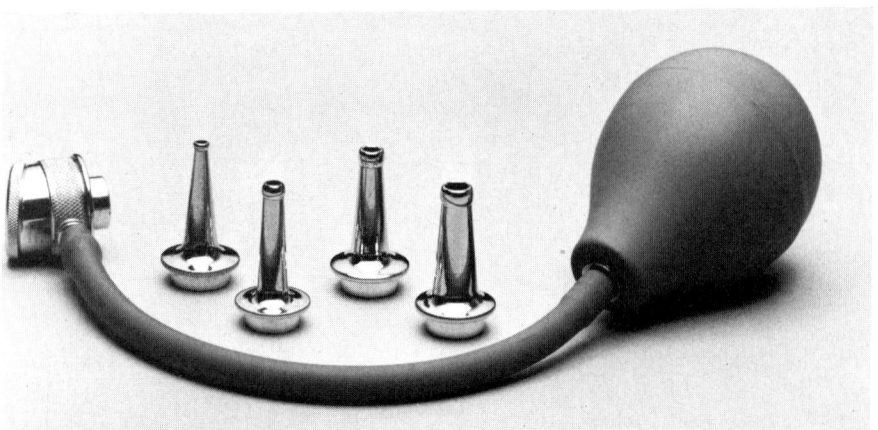

FIGURE 1–6. The Siegle pneumatic otoscope permits determination of tympanic membrane mobility. The special speculum allow a tight seal of the external ear canal.

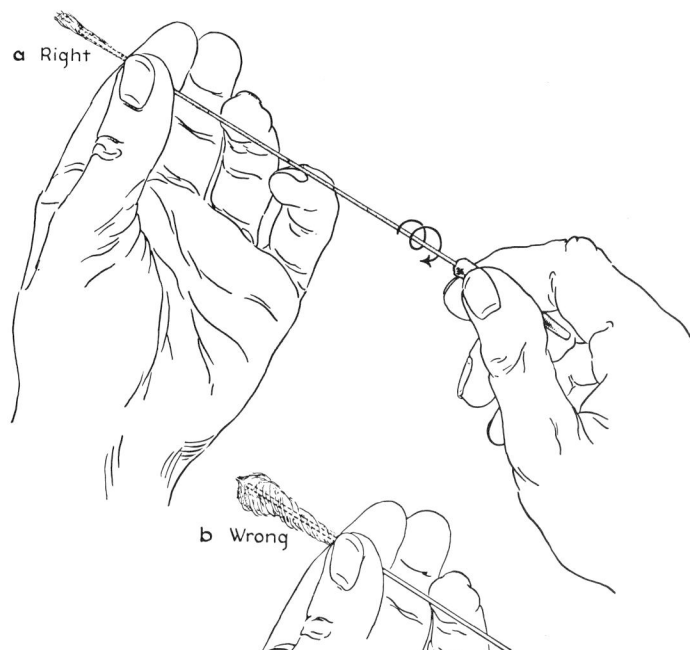

FIGURE 1–7. Winding a cotton applicator is easily done by twisting the wire, not the cotton.

a small amount of pressure in the external ear canal while observing the tympanic membrane. If a perforation is present, the tympanic membrane will have no movement. Movement will be abnormal in the presence of fluid. A shifting meniscus will distinguish an air-filled level in the middle ear from a scar on the tympanic membrane.

Cleansing of the External Ear Canal. The external ear canal may be blocked with cerumen or a purulent discharge. Cleansing of the ear canal should be done gently, causing the patient little or no pain. Wax may be removed through the aural speculum with a cerumen spoon or with an alligator forceps. If there is moisture in the external ear canal, a suction or cotton-tipped metal applicator may be used for cleaning (Fig. 1–7). If the tympanic membrane has no perforation, the ear may also be cleaned by irrigation with water that is approximately body temperature. If other temperatures are used, vertigo and/or discomfort will be produced (Fig. 1–8).

To remove wax or foreign material, try to get behind it. Poking it may drive it deeper.

Clinical Hearing Tests

Clinical hearing testing requires the use of tuning forks. The best single fork is the Riverbank 512 cycle fork. Higher frequency tuning forks may not sustain a tone long enough to allow adequate testing, and lower frequency tuning forks stimulate vibratory sensation in bone, which is sometimes difficult to distinguish from low tone hearing. Basic tuning fork tests are the Weber and Rinne tests, which are described in Figures 1–9 and 1–10. Another hearing test is the Schwabach test, in which the bone conduction of the examiner is compared with that of the patient. The heel of the fork is held against the patient's mastoid bone until the patient no longer can hear the tone. It is then placed against the mastoid bone of the examiner, who attempts to hear it. Of course, the examiner must have no hearing loss to properly judge this test.

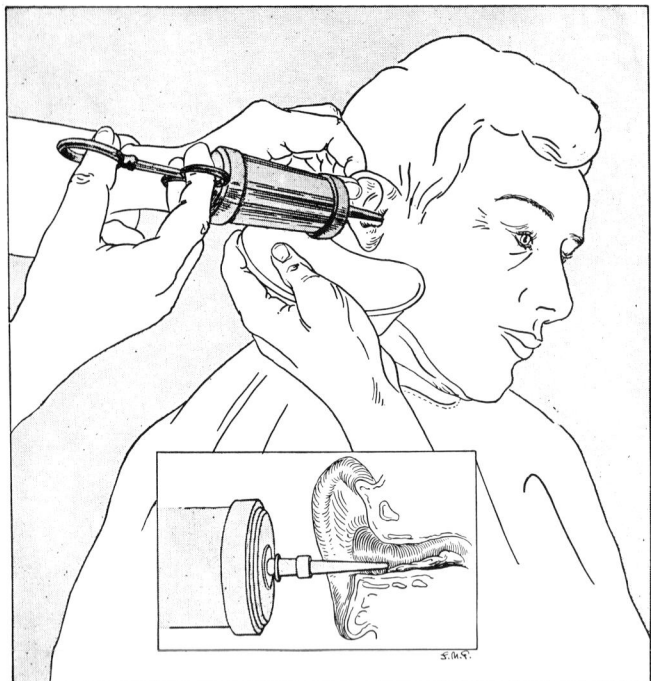

FIGURE 1–8. The use of the irrigating syringe. When the external canal is irrigated, it is important to protect the patient with a light waterproof apron that can be fastened snugly over a folded towel around his neck. A basin curved so that it can be easily pressed against the side of the neck just below the auricle receives the irrigating fluid and the material washed out. The irrigating tip is placed just within the meatus and pointed along the floor of the canal.

Screening audiometric testing and vestibular testing are essential for the evaluation of ear and vestibular disorders and should be available in the primary care setting. These subjects are discussed in detail in Chapter 2.

The Nose and Sinuses

There is little doubt that the nose and the sinuses are the most commonly diseased organs in the human body, and patients who suffer from disorders of these areas occupy a considerable portion of the physician's time. Most diseases of the nose and sinuses are amenable to definitive therapy. A

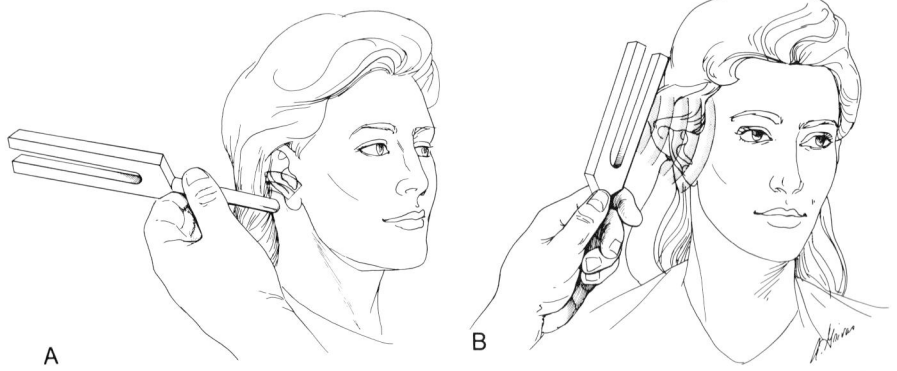

FIGURE 1–9. Rinne test. This test is used to compare the duration of bone conduction with that of air conduction for the ear being tested. A fork of 512 Hz struck a moderate blow and is held by the stem firmly against the mastoid bone (*A*). When the patient signals that he no longer hears the vibrating fork, the duration of bone conduction is noted and the fork is immediately transferred to position (*B*) so that the prongs are about one-half inch away and broadside to the external auditory meatus. When the patient no longer hears by air the sound of the vibrating fork, note the air conduction. In a normal ear, the fork is heard approximately twice as long by air conduction as by bone.

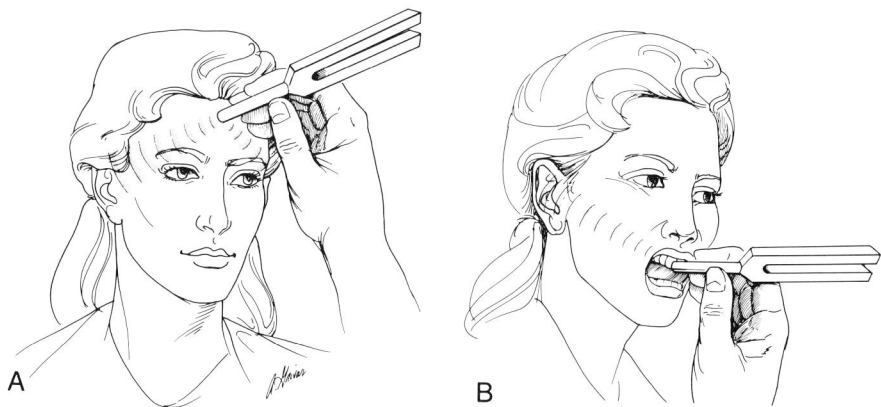

FIGURE 1-10. Weber test. This test determines whether monaural impairment is of conductive or neural origin by comparing the bone conduction of both ears. A 512 Hz tuning fork can be placed on the forehead or the teeth. *A*, Normal response. *B*, The fork is heard on the right side. If the right ear is the diseased ear, then the loss is of the conductive type. If the left ear is the diseased ear, then the hearing loss is of the sensorineural type.

majority of patients with nasal or sinus disease have one or more of the following symptoms: discharge, nasal obstruction, colds, headache or other pain, epistaxis, sneezing attacks, occasional external swelling, loss of or change in smell, and allergy. If any of these complaints are found, they should be characterized in detail. The following is a practical guide for inquiry into these complaints. Further information to be considered in the history can be found in the chapters dealing with the nose and paranasal sinuses.

Only a small percentage of patients with sinus complaints will have sinusitis. Look for other causes of their symptoms.

Patient History

Discharge

1. Is one side or are both sides involved?
2. Duration? Continual or intermittent, and how so? Age at onset?
3. Is the discharge watery or thick? Purulent or bloody?
4. Does it occur with environmental or seasonal changes?

Obstruction

1. Is one side or are both sides involved?
2. Duration? Continual or intermittent, and how so? Age at onset?
3. Is there a history of injury?
4. Is there a history of nasal or other otolaryngologic surgery?
5. Is there a history of allergic disorders, especially those associated with seasonal variation? If suggestive, a complete allergic history is indicated.
6. Does the patient use nasal sprays or medications?

Bleeding

1. What is the duration? Frequency? How long ago was the last episode?
2. Is the bleeding unilateral or bilateral?
3. Does bleeding originate from the anterior or posterior nares or both?
4. Does it occur only in winter?
5. Is there a history of trauma?
6. Does the patient have a bleeding tendency?
7. Does the patient use any medications?
8. Is hypertension present?

Loss or Change of Smell (Anosmia)

1. Is the loss associated with trauma, upper respiratory infection, systemic illness?
2. Is the loss or change of smell partial or complete?
3. Is there any history of sinus or nasal disease?
4. Are there other systemic symptoms?

The Normal Nose

The appearance of the external nose and face often gives a clue to the patient's symptoms. A thin, narrow nose that looks attractive often functions poorly. Inspection of the columella may show evidence of a deviated septum. Crepitation may result from a nasal fracture, or tenderness may be found in infection. Edema or "bags" under the eyes in children may indicate allergy.

A good light source is imperative in nasal examination.

Interior rhinoscopy allows visualization of the inferior and middle turbinates as well as the nasal septum. The mucosa should not be swollen or congested and should be slightly pink. Remember that the nasolacrimal duct exits into the inferior meatus. The anterior ethmoid sinuses, the maxillary sinus, and the frontal sinus drain into the middle meatus. The posterior ethmoid sinus drains into the superior meatus and the sphenoid into the high posterior nasal cavity (Fig. 1–11).

Equipment and Techniques

The positions of the patient, examiner, and light source are as described earlier under basic techniques. Here the patient sits directly facing the examiner. As in the examination of the ear, the speculum is held in the left hand, leaving the right (dominant) hand free to position the patient's head and to manipulate instruments. Left-handed examiners may make compensatory adjustments.

The nasal speculum should be used without causing discomfort to the patient. Often the nasal speculum will have an undesirable stiff spring built into the handle. It is best to have a very soft spring or no spring at all in

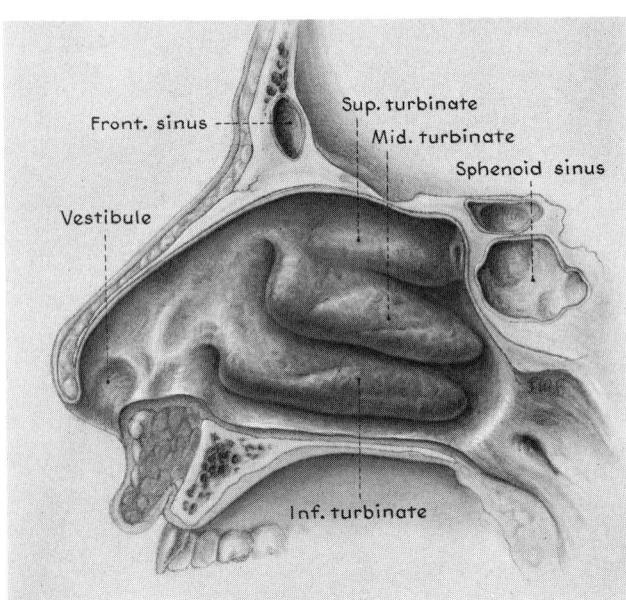

FIGURE 1–11. The shape, position, and relationship of the turbinates on the lateral nasal wall.

order to better judge the pressure being applied to the nose. The examiner's right hand is placed on top of the patient's head so that it can be tilted and moved. The left forefinger is stabilized on the side of the patient's nose and the speculum opened in an up-and-down direction in the nasal vestibule. It is often helpful to gently grasp the ala of the nose between the forefinger and the speculum and apply slight traction toward the examiner. This avoids discomfort and provides the best view. The speculum remains in the same hand when inspecting the opposite nasal cavity.

The intranasal examination begins with inspection of the nasal vestibule. Folliculitis of the vibrissae may occur in this area. The nasal mucosa is examined, and the septum is visualized as well as inspected carefully for purulent discharge or polyps that may be coming from the sinuses. Topical vasoconstrictors, such as 0.5 per cent phenylephrine (Neo-Synephrine), applied in a spray or on cotton placed intranasally, will decongest the mucosa to improve the view in patients with obstructive mucosal swelling. The floor of the nose should be seen all the way back to the soft palate. The patient is asked to say "k k k k," and if no obstruction is present, the soft palate is seen to rise with each vocalization.

A battery-powered otoscope is frequently used to examine the interior of the nose at the bedside. This examination is inadequate and of limited usefulness.

Other Methods of Nasal and Sinus Examination. Palpation and percussion over the frontal and maxillary sinuses or the teeth may produce pain in some cases of sinusitis. Transillumination is useful but is not a substitute for radiographs in the evaluation of sinus disease. Cultures and sensitivity tests are needed when infection is present, and smears for eosinophils are indicated in cases of allergy. Endoscopic techniques using flexible and rigid instruments are of increasing usefulness in evaluating pathology in portions of the nasal cavity and nasopharynx that are difficult to visualize with traditional methods.

Paranasal sinus radiographs are required to fully evaluate the absence or presence and extent of sinus disease. Indeed, only a presumptive diagnosis of sinus disease can be made without them. The four most useful views are the lateral, Waters, Caldwell, and base of the skull.

Mouth, Pharynx, and Salivary Glands

Patient History

Patients with *disorders of the mouth* usually will have one or more of the following symptoms: pain, bleeding, the presence of a mass or lump, difficulty in eating or speaking, discharge, and disturbance in taste. If any of these symptoms are present, detailed inquiry should be made into their characteristics, as in the following list, for example:

1. Are the symptoms acute or chronic?
2. Which areas are involved?
3. Are there associated local or systemic symptoms or disease?
4. Has there been recent trauma or dental work?

The most frequent pharyngeal complaints are sore throat; a discharge in the throat; a sense of a lump, fullness, or swelling; and difficulty in swallowing (dysphagia). The following lists can be used as a practical guide for inquiry into these complaints. Further information to be included in the history will be suggested in the chapters dealing with these disorders.

Sore Throat

1. Frequency?
2. What is the duration of each episode?
3. Is the sore throat accompanied by fever, discharge, expectoration, difficulty in swallowing, difficulty breathing, voice change, or cough?
4. Location and duration of external swelling?
5. Is there any referred pain, such as earache? If so, which side?
6. What treatment has been given in the past?
7. Has the patient been a smoker? How much?

Discharge in the Throat

1. Duration of discharge?
2. Is the discharge mucoid, purulent, or blood-stained?
3. Is the amount profuse or scanty?
4. Is it coughed or spit up?
5. Is it worse on arising in the morning?

Difficulty in Swallowing (Dysphagia)

1. Duration (weeks, months, or years)?
2. Is the difficulty increasing?
3. Does the patient have any pain with swallowing or without, including heartburn?
4. How well can the patient swallow ordinary food? Does the obstruction increase when swallowing liquids or solid food?
5. Where does the obstruction seem to be? (Have patient indicate level.)
6. Is there any regurgitation? Does it have any odor?
7. Has the patient lost weight? If so, what amount?

Nasopharyngeal symptoms may include drainage or obstruction of nasal breathing. The eustachian tube orifice may be blocked, producing a hearing loss. Any adult with persistent unilateral middle ear fluid should have the nasopharynx carefully examined for neoplasm.

Patients with salivary gland disease will usually complain of one or more of the following symptoms: swelling of the cheek or beneath the jaw, which may or may not be related to eating; pain in these areas, which may or may not be related to eating; dryness of the mouth; and discharge into the mouth. As with disorders of the mouth, symptoms of salivary disease should be characterized in detail:

1. Are symptoms acute or chronic?
2. Is one or are several glands involved?
3. Are there associated systemic or local symptoms or disease?
4. Has the patient experienced any trauma or had any dental extractions recently?

The Normal Mouth, Pharynx, Nasopharynx, and Salivary Glands

Oral findings are generally more important than changes in pharyngeal mucosa.

All too frequently the examiner looks through, rather than at, the oral cavity in a rush to see the pharynx or larynx. An adequate examination of the mouth, pharynx, nasopharynx, and salivary glands can best be done in a systematic manner. The normal appearances and textures of these structures are difficult to illustrate and should be learned through experience by conscientious examination of patients.

Equipment and Technique

Head Mirror and Light Source. The positions of the patient, light source, and head mirror are exactly as described earlier under basic techniques. Of course, in this case the patient sits facing the examiner. The flashlight or otoscope may be used as an emergency light source at the bedside but is inadequate for a proper examination of these structures.

The Tongue Depressor. A wooden tongue depressor is commonly used for the oral examination. If firmer retraction of the tongue is required, two wooden depressors may be used together or a metal tongue depressor may help (Fig. 1–12). The tongue depressor is grasped near its midportion. The patient is not asked to stick out the tongue for the oral and pharyngeal examination, since this tends only to obscure the view.

Suboptimal instructions—"Stick your tongue out and say 'ahh.'"

The tongue blade is first used to retract the cheek and lips for complete inspection of the buccal mucosa, teeth, and gingiva. The floor of the mouth and associated salivary ducts are then inspected. By drying the mouth with a swab of cotton, saliva can be seen, expressed from Stensen's and Wharton's ducts. The lateral and posterolateral aspects of the tongue and floor of the mouth are then carefully examined. The tongue must be retracted medially to visualize the trigone areas posterior to the molar teeth. These are common sites for otherwise asymptomatic carcinoma. The under and upper surfaces of the tongue are then visualized, as well as the hard and soft palates. The tonsils and pharynx can be seen by depressing the middle third of the tongue and pulling it forward while pressing down. Avoid touching the back of the tongue, as this stimulates gagging. The tonsils and tonsillar fossa, anterior and posterior pillars, lateral and posterior pharyngeal walls, a portion of the base of the tongue, and occasionally the tip of the epiglottis may be seen directly in this manner.

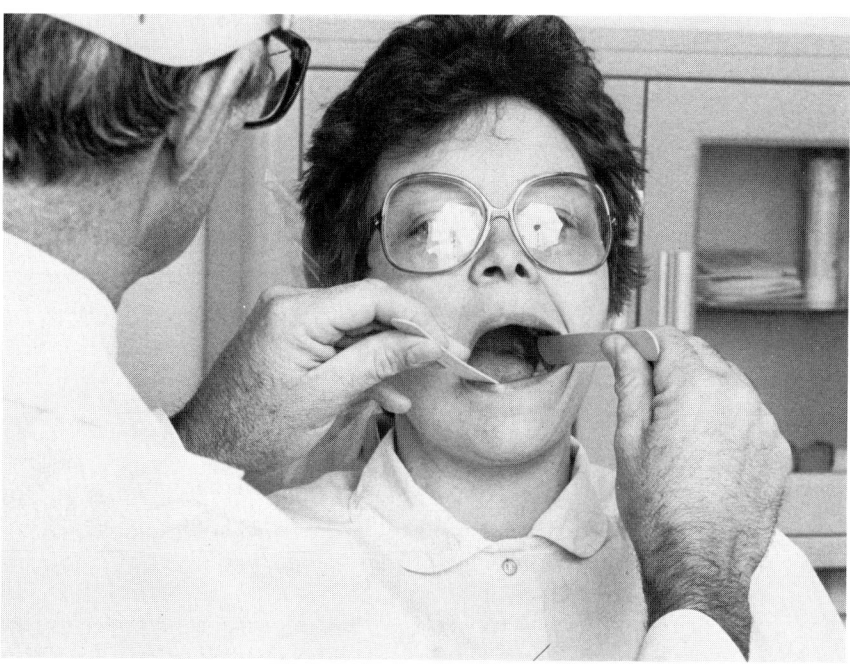

FIGURE 1–12. The use of two tongue depressors and the head light allows one tongue blade to push the lip to the side and the second tongue blade to push the tongue aside. This permits adequate visualization of the retromolar trigone, gingiva, and floor of the mouth.

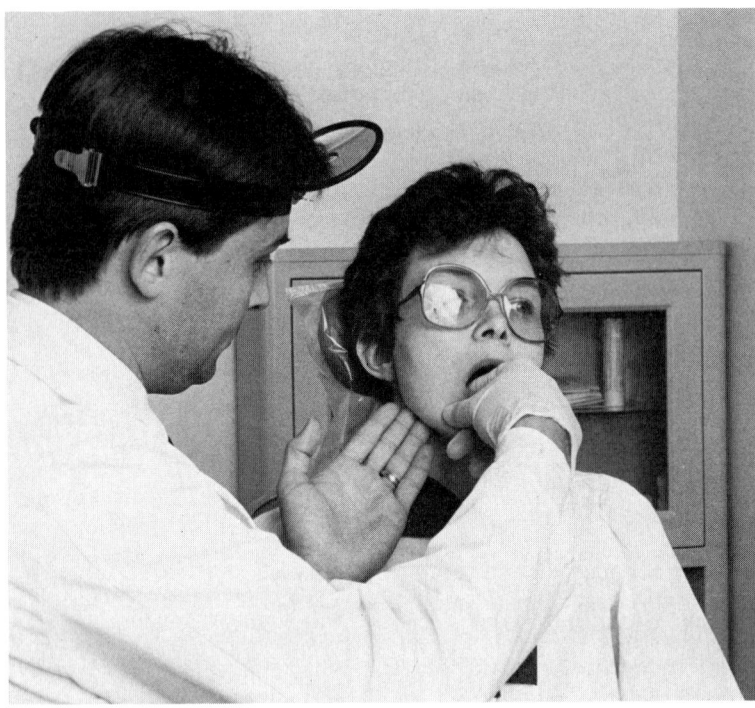

FIGURE 1–13. By combining intraoral palpation of the neck, the extent of a lesion is better defined.

Bimanual palpation is very useful.

Palpation. All areas in the oral cavity and pharynx appearing unusual or producing symptoms must be palpated. Tumors and cysts lying deep within oral tissues can be found only by palpation. Calculi in the submaxillary ducts can frequently be detected in this manner (Fig. 1–13). Salivary glands, except for ptotic submaxillary glands in the elderly, are normally not palpable. The temporomandibular joints can easily be palpated by placing the fingertips in the external ear canals and asking the patient to open and close the mouth.

The Nasopharynx

The nasopharynx can often partially be seen directly through the nares when the interior of the nose is examined. A more complete examination of the nasopharynx is done with the No. 0 nasopharyngeal mirror (Fig. 1–14). The mirror is warmed, usually over an alcohol lamp, so that the patient's breath will not fog it and obscure the view. The examiner checks the temperature of the mirror by placing it against the back of the hand before inserting it into the patient's mouth. The tongue is depressed as for the pharyngeal examination, and the mirror is positioned in the pharynx. The posterior third of the tongue should not be touched to reduce the likelihood of stimulating the gag reflex. The posterior pharyngeal wall is less sensitive than the tongue, and the soft palate is least sensitive. While the mirror is in the oropharynx, the patient is told, "Think about breathing through your nose." The soft palate will then drop, and the nasopharynx can be scanned with the mirror (Fig. 1–15).

Only a small portion of the nasopharynx can be seen at one time. The examiner must mentally put the images together while rotating the mirror to view the entire area (Fig. 1–16). It is generally easiest to orient initially the posterior margin of the nasal septum and choana. The mirror then can

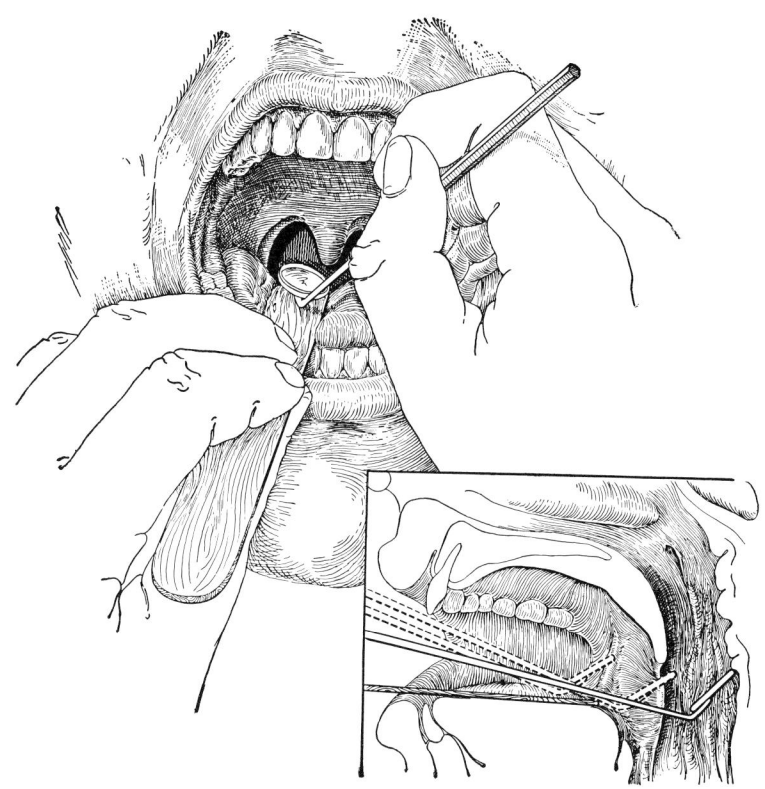

FIGURE 1–14. Examination of the nasopharynx by means of a mirror introduced through the mouth. Inset shows the various positions in succeeding portions of the examination. A tongue blade is gently introduced and the tongue pushed downward. The mirror is slipped along the tongue blade and in many cases does not even touch the tongue itself. The mirror is held exactly as one holds a pen during writing. The handle is lowered as the mirror is introduced into the mouth until light is reflected from the mirror into the nasopharynx. This light returns to the mirror and to the observer's eye. The mirror is rotated by moving the thumb on the handle so that the handle turns on its long axis. This permits a panoramic view of the nasopharynx.

be rotated laterally to reveal the superior and middle turbinates, the torus, and the eustachian tube orifices.

The nasopharynx can also be examined with a nasal endoscope. This is a telescope-like device that gives a magnified view of the nasopharynx. It is introduced through the nose after the area has been anesthetized. The nasopharynx can be directly visualized through the mouth by retracting the soft palate. Several mechanical devices are available for this. One simple way consists of passing a soft catheter through the nose until it can be seen in the pharynx. A hemostat is used to grasp this end and pull it out the mouth. Pulling gently on both ends of the catheter will retract the soft palate and allow direct visualization of the nasopharynx. Even better visualization can be obtained by simultaneously using two catheters, one through each nostril. Adequate topical anesthesia should be used during this manipulation.

It is possible to palpate the nasopharynx.

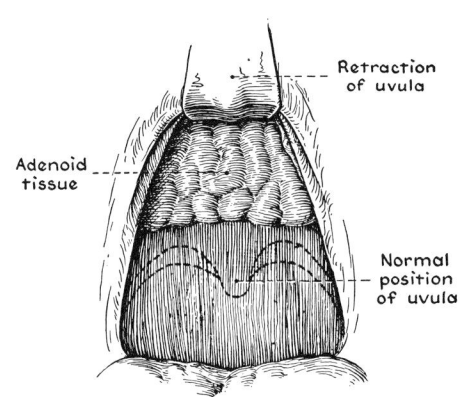

FIGURE 1–15. Adenoid mass as seen at operation and drawn directly from life. A retractor is shown pulling the soft palate and uvula upward to expose the lower portion of the adenoid vegetations. Note the sharp inferior margin of the adenoid mass.

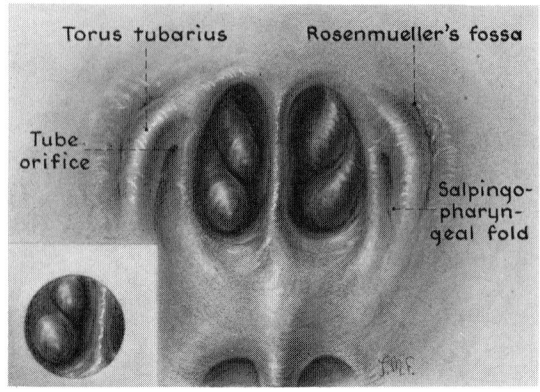

FIGURE 1–16. Nasopharynx as viewed through nasopharyngeal mirror inserted into the throat through the mouth. The amount of the nasopharynx seen in the mirror at one time is indicated in the small inset, but by moving the mirror the entire nasopharynx can be examined, and information on all parts of nasopharynx shown in larger figure can be obtained.

The Larynx and Hypopharynx

Patient History

Patients with diseases involving the hypopharynx or larynx often complain of one or more of the following symptoms: hoarseness, cough, difficulty in swallowing (dysphagia), and the sensation of a lump, fullness, swelling, or foreign body. The following lists can be used as a guide to detailed inquiry into the specific symptoms. Indications for further inquiry are discussed in the chapters relating to laryngopharyngeal, tracheobronchial, and esophageal diseases.

Sense of Lump, Fullness, or Swelling

1. Duration?
2. Site?
3. Is the sensation intermittent or constant?
4. Is it painful or painless? If painful, is there any referred pain, such as earache?
5. Is there any actual difficulty in swallowing or breathing?
6. Is the patient nervous or worried about cancer?

Difficulty in Swallowing (Dysphagia)

1. Duration (weeks, months, or years)?
2. Is the difficulty increasing?
3. Does the patient have any pain?
4. How well can the patient swallow ordinary food? Does the obstruction increase when swallowing liquids or solid food?
5. Where does the obstruction seem to be? (Have patient indicate level.)
6. Is there any regurgitation? If so, is there any odor?
7. Has the patient lost weight? If so, what amount?

Hoarseness

1. Duration (weeks, months, or years)?
2. Was the onset sudden or gradual?
3. Was the voice completely gone at any time? If so, for how long?
4. Has the patient ever been hoarse before? If so, when and how often?
5. Was the hoarseness preceded by a head cold or sore throat?
6. Is there any discomfort in the region of the larynx?
7. Does the patient cough? Can the patient raise much phlegm?

8. Is there any pain related to the use of the voice? Is there discomfort in breathing?
9. Is there a history of excessive alcohol ingestion or smoking?

Cough

1. Duration (weeks, months, or years)?
2. In what part of the throat does the cough seem to start?
3. What is coughed up?
4. Are there situations in which the cough is worse, such as during exposure to cold air, smoke, dust, or other irritants? Is it worse at night when lying down or during exercising?
5. Has the patient lost weight? If so, how much?
6. Is there any loss of appetite or strength?
7. Is hemoptysis present?
8. Is there a history of smoking?

The Normal Larynx and Hypopharynx

The appearance of the normal larynx and hypopharynx is illustrated in Figure 1–17. There should be no pooling of secretions in the vallecula or piriform sinuses. Normally, pharyngeal walls move symmetrically with gagging and the vocal cords move symmetrically with phonation. The upper trachea can be inspected through the vocal cords when using the laryngeal mirror.

Equipment and Technique

Head Mirror and Light Source. The positions of the light source, head mirror, examiner, and patient are similar to those described under general techniques with the patient facing the examiner. The patient should be sitting upright and leaning slightly forward, with the neck slightly flexed on the thorax and the head extended on the neck, as if pushing the chin toward the examiner (Fig. 1–18). The patient is then told to open the mouth and stick out the tongue. The tongue is grasped by the fingers of the left hand using a gauze sponge and held in place. It is seldom helpful to pull the tongue out further than the patient presents it, although a firm grip may be needed to hold it there. Attempts to pull it out further are usually quite

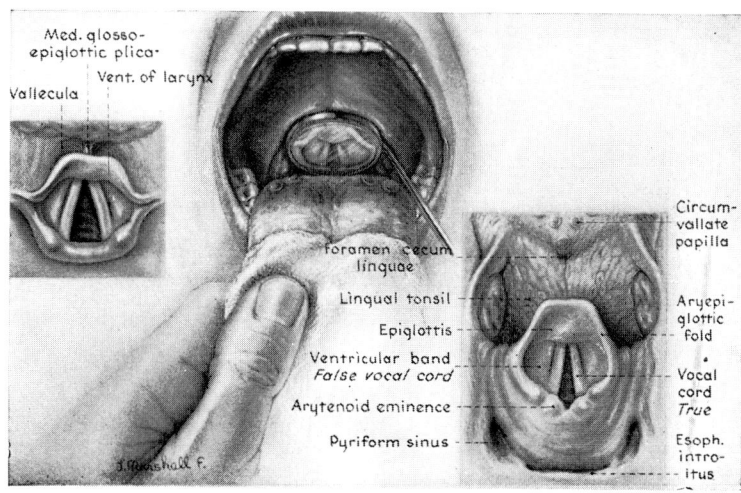

FIGURE 1–17. Indirect laryngoscopy requires a mirror of the proper size warmed so that it will not steam on the patient's exhalation. Gentle tension should be made on the patient's tongue, using a strip of gauze to grasp the tongue and gently pull it out. The under surface should be protected against the patient's lower incisor teeth. Carelessness on this point is often a source of considerable discomfort to the patient and makes it difficult for him to cooperate successfully.

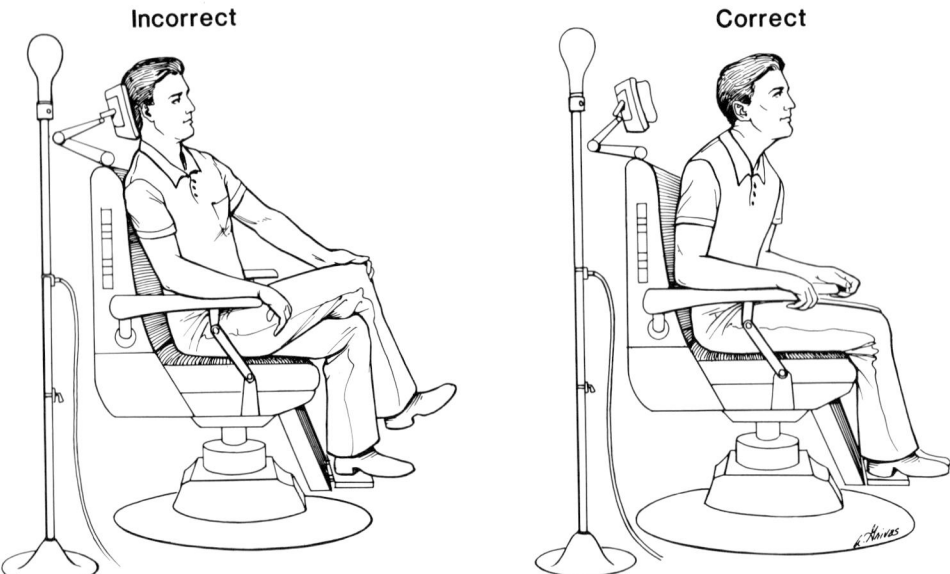

FIGURE 1–18. Proper positioning for examination of the larynx, pharynx, oral cavity, and neck. The patient sits upright, bent forward at the waist with the head slightly projected. Note that the light source is at the same level as the patient's eyes.

Transnasal fiberoptic laryngoscopy offers a more complete assessment than mirror examination.

uncomfortable for patients. Take care to avoid traumatizing the tongue on the lower incisor teeth.

The back of a No. 4 laryngeal mirror is warmed over the alcohol lamp or other device. Its temperature is checked on the back of the examiner's hand prior to use. If the patient is a child or seems worried about the flame and heat, the examiner should place the mirror against the patient's hand or arm to demonstrate that it won't burn, after checking the mirror temperature on the back of his own hand. Antifogging liquid may be used as an alternative to warming the mirror. Children as young as three years of age may have a laryngeal examination if they are not frightened.

The mirror is then placed against the soft palate, which is gently raised upward by the mirror. This allows visualization of the hypopharynx and larynx. Raising the mirror upward will avoid touching the tongue or posterior pharynx and activating the gag reflex. Ask the patient to pant if gagging becomes a problem. The examination cannot be rushed and should be done in a systematic manner beginning with the base of the tongue and working downward. Every structure should be seen. The patient is asked to say "eeee" and then to take a deep breath. This may be repeated several times to allow visualization and evaluation of the motion of the vocal cords and arytenoid cartilages (see Fig. 1–17). Methods of managing a "gag reflex" or otherwise difficult patients are discussed at the end of this chapter.

The Neck and Face

Patients with disease of the neck and face may have many and varied symptoms. Pain, weakness of muscles or muscle groups, dysesthesia, swelling or masses, deformities, and changes in the appearance of the skin are the more common complaints. These should be characterized as to their exact location, time of onset, duration, and any associated symptoms (both local and systemic). The examiner should be aware that different types of light (incandescent, fluorescent, or daylight) will each give the skin a slightly different color. Percussion over the sinuses and teeth may elicit pain or tenderness. Auscultation of the neck will help evaluate the carotid arteries and over the skull will help identify vascular tumors or arteriovenous malformations or shunts.

Cranial nerve and otoneurologic testing can easily be done as part of the otolaryngologic examination. Much is automatically done, such as observing vocal cord and pharyngeal motion as an indication of the function of cranial nerves IX and X. A brief outline of specific functions follows.

The olfactory nerve is checked by presenting familiar odors such as chocolate or vanilla to one nostril while the other is held closed. Standard scratch and sniff odors may be used.

The optic nerve can be roughly checked with visual acuity and visual field tests. The fundus should be inspected as part of every general examination.

Oculomotor, trochlear, and abducens nerves are evaluated when pupillary reflexes are elicited and range of motion of the eyes is checked. The examiner should ask specifically about diplopia.

The trigeminal nerve supplies sensation to the face which is easily evaluated. Absence of the corneal reflex is often found with enlarging acoustic neuromas. Blinking occurs when the cornea is touched with a wisp of cotton but not when the sclera is touched.

The facial nerve controls the muscles of facial expression which are easily observed during the neck and face examination. Facial paralysis is an interesting and important topic, which is covered in detail in Chapter 8 in this text.

The cochleovestibular nerve mediates hearing and balance. These functions are discussed in detail throughout this text. A gross assessment of hearing followed by tuning fork and audiometric testing will evaluate hearing function. The evaluation of vestibular function and vertigo is discussed in Chapter 3. Nystagmus, past-pointing, gait, Romberg, and tandem standing abnormalities often occur with vestibular disorders and should be checked. Central nervous system diseases that produce changes in proprioception and coordination may mimic vestibular disease. These functions should be evaluated, since they are not affected by primary vestibular disease.

The glossopharyngeal nerve supplies sensation to the pharynx and is responsible for the gag reflex. The gag reflex should be checked on both sides of the pharynx with the tongue blade when the pharynx is inspected.

The vagus nerve innervates the muscles of the palate, pharynx, and larynx. Symmetrical motion of these structures is observed normally as part of the pharyngeal and laryngeal examination.

The accessory nerve is tested by having the patient shrug both shoulders against resistance, and the sternocleidomastoid is palpated while the head is turned against resistance.

The hypoglossal nerve supplies motor innervation to the tongue. Unilateral atrophy or fasciculation or the inability to protrude the tongue in the midline indicates a hypoglossal lesion.

This is only a brief sketch of basic neurologic evaluation as related to otolaryngology. Malignancies arising in the pharynx and nasopharynx have direct access to the foramina in the base of the skull and can present as cranial nerve palsy mimicking neurologic disease. The differential diagnosis of sensorineural hearing loss, particularly when unilateral, and of all patients

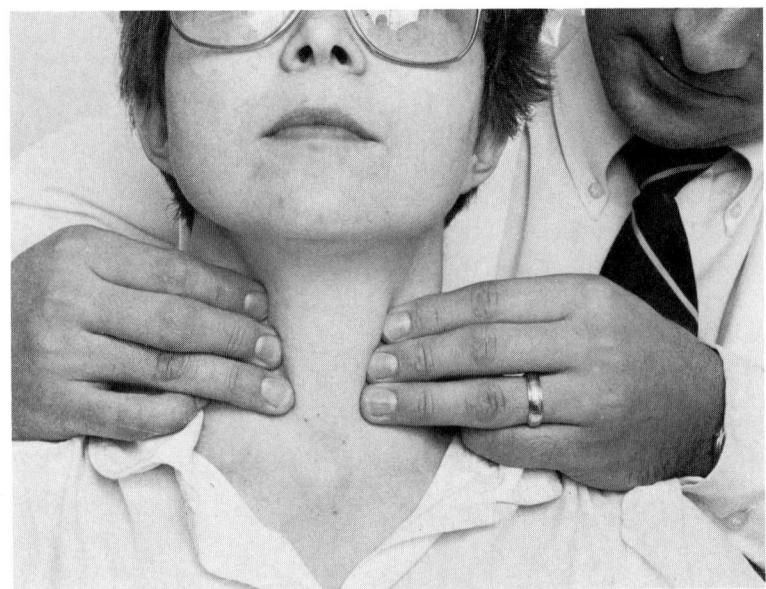

FIGURE 1–19. Examination of the neck while standing allows the examiner to compare both sides of the anterior triangles of the neck. This is the preferred method for examining the thyroid gland and for anterior cervical adenopathy.

with vertigo must include a systematic and thorough cranial nerve and general neurologic evaluation.

Palpation of the neck and face should be done in a systematic manner. Cervical and metastatic nodes are often located in the anterior triangle of the neck. This area must be carefully inspected, particularly deep to the sternocleidomastoid muscle and along the course of the carotid sheath. Structures that normally can and should be palpated are the hyoid bone, the thyroid and cricoid cartilages and the thyrohyoid and cricothyroid spaces, tracheal rings, the sternocleidomastoid muscle, the carotid arteries, and the clavicles and supraclavicular spaces. Crepitation of the thyroid cartilage against the cervical vertebrae is normally present. All the soft tissues of the neck can be examined and described by anatomic triangles (Fig. 1–19).

Develop a routine or mental checklist for palpating the neck.

The thyroid gland is normally not palpable. Examination is easiest when standing behind the patient with the thumb behind the fingers in front of the lower portion of the sternocleidomastoid muscle. The patient is asked to swallow while this area is palpated. Thyroglossal duct cysts occur on or near the midline in the upper half of the neck. They slide upward when the tongue is protruded. Branchial cleft cysts may be beneath the anterior portion of the sternocleidomastoid muscle anywhere along its course. A node over the cricothyroid membrane is often metastatic from the larynx or thyroid gland. The trachea may deviate from the midline in the presence of mediastinal or pulmonary disease. Subcutaneous emphysema usually indicates a ruptured esophagus or airway. This is, of course, only a small list of possible findings.

MISCELLANEOUS PROBLEMS AND SPECIALIZED TECHNIQUES

Anesthesia, Sedation, and Restraint

The otolaryngologic examination can nearly always be completed without the use of topical anesthesia, sedation, or restraint. The gag reflex is rarely a problem to an experienced examiner. The use of sedation or topical anesthesia may help in the examination of the patient with a difficult gag reflex. These drugs, however, carry a risk factor and should not be used unless the examiner is completely familiar with the maximum safe dosage of these drugs and the side effects and toxic symptoms that may appear. The examiner must know precisely what measures to take if such problems do occur and should have available emergency equipment and drugs to deal with them. Restraint of young children is occasionally needed. This can usually be done by the mother who is seated and holding the child, also seated, in her lap.

A child may feel more secure when seated in his mother's lap for an examination.

Biopsy

The examiner should not hesitate to perform a biopsy of any nonvascular mucosal or cutaneous lesion for which the diagnosis is not immediately apparent. Biopsy of deeper structures should be made only after a thorough examination fails to reveal their origin or nature. Do not biopsy nasal polyps in young males, as the highly vascular angiofibroma may have the appearance of a polyp.

Special Studies

Specimens are easily obtained for cytologic studies from all mucosal surfaces, both directly and via endoscopy. Culture, sensitivity tests, and smears are indicated when infection is present in these areas. Endoscopic procedures, including nasopharyngoscopy, direct laryngoscopy, bronchoscopy, and esophagoscopy, are extremely useful in the diagnosis of head and neck, tracheobronchial, or esophageal disease. Other useful special techniques and studies are described in appropriate chapters of this text.

Fine needle biopsy is generally a safe and rewarding evaluation technique.

PART TWO

THE EAR

2
EMBRYOLOGY, ANATOMY, AND PHYSIOLOGY OF THE EAR

by Stephen L. Liston, M.D., and Arndt J. Duvall, III, M.D.

The embryology, anatomy, and physiology of the ear are the means to understand function, and, therefore, pathology and treatment. To correlate the basic knowledge within these disciplines is to better understand ultimately the treatment of problems in hearing and balance. Our equilibrium is more basic, and more important, than hearing. An organism can exist without hearing but cannot exist without being in balance with its environment. Therefore, the vestibular mechanism, as a part of the organism's orientation to its environment, phylogenetically arose before hearing. The ear contains the vestibular portion of balance, but our orientation to the environment is also determined by our eyes and by our deep tendon sense. The ear is the organ of hearing and of balance.

Anatomically, the ear is divided into three parts—the external, middle, and inner ear. The external and middle ear develop from the branchial apparatus. The inner ear develops entirely separately from the otic placode. Thus a congenital abnormality can occur in one part, while the other parts may develop normally.

The external canal is one-half cartilaginous and two-thirds bony.

DEVELOPMENT OF THE EAR

External Ear

The external ear canal is derived from the ectodermal first branchial cleft. The tympanic membrane represents the closing membrane of the first branchial cleft. During one stage of its development, the external ear canal actually is closed completely by a meatal plug of tissue but reopens again, and this may be a factor in some cases of atresia or stenosis of this structure. The pinna is derived from the margins of the first branchial cleft and the first and second branchial arches. The pinna is supplied by the auriculotemporal branch of the mandibular nerve and by the lesser occipital and greater auricular nerves, which are branches of the cervical plexus.

Sensation from the posterosuperior portion of the external canal is transmitted by the seventh cranial nerve.

Middle Ear

The middle ear cavity is derived from the endodermal first branchial cleft. This air-containing structure expands into the tubotympanic recess (Fig. 2–1), which continues to expand around the bones and nerves of the middle ear (Fig. 2–2) and extends more or less into the mastoid region. The ossicles are derived from the cartilage of the branchial arches. To simplify this

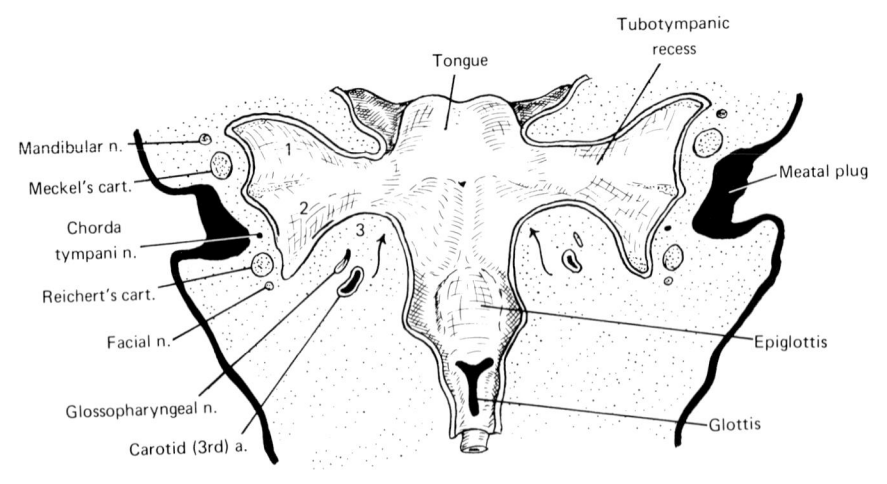

FIGURE 2–1. Floor of the pharynx of an embryo showing the formation of the tubotympanic recess. The recess arises as a lateral expansion of the pharyngeal lumen at the level of the first three internal pharyngeal grooves and pouches. The external auditory meatus is shown as a solid "meatal plug" of ectoderm growing deeply into the mesoderm from the upper end of the first external pharyngeal groove to make contact with the tubotympanic recess, the "drum" being formed at the area of contact. (From Davies J: In Paparella MM, Shumrick DA (eds): Otolaryngology. Vol 1: Basic Sciences and Related Disciplines. Philadelphia, WB Saunders Co, 1973, p 172.)

Jacobson's nerve traverses vertically across the promontory of the middle ear.

concept, the malleus can be considered to derive from the cartilage of the first branchial arch (Meckel's cartilage), while the incus and stapes derive from the cartilage of the second branchial arch (Reichert's cartilage). The chorda tympani nerve runs from the second arch (facial) to the nerve of the first arch (mandibular-lingual). The tympanic nerve (of Jacobson) runs from the nerve of the third arch (glossopharyngeal) to the facial nerve. Both of these nerves lie in the middle ear cavity. The muscles of the middle ear derive from the muscles of the branchial arches. The tensor tympani, which attaches to the malleus, derives from the first arch and is supplied by the mandibular nerve (cranial nerve V). The stapedius muscle, a derivative of the second arch, is supplied by a division of the seventh nerve.

Inner Ear

The ectodermal otic placode is located on the lateral surface of the head of the embryo. This placode sinks to form an otic pit and is eventually

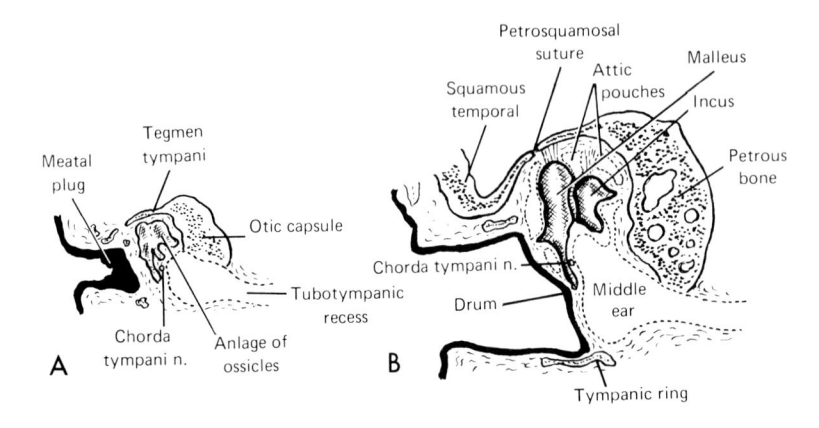

FIGURE 2–2. Two longitudinal sections of the external and middle ear showing the progressive dorsal extension of the mesenchyme ("epitympanic tissue") by which the attic recesses are formed and the ossicles become surrounded by mucous membrane. (From Davies J: In Paparella MM, Shumrick DA (eds): Otolaryngology. Vol 1: Basic Sciences and Related Disciplines. Philadelphia, WB Saunders Co, 1973, p 175.)

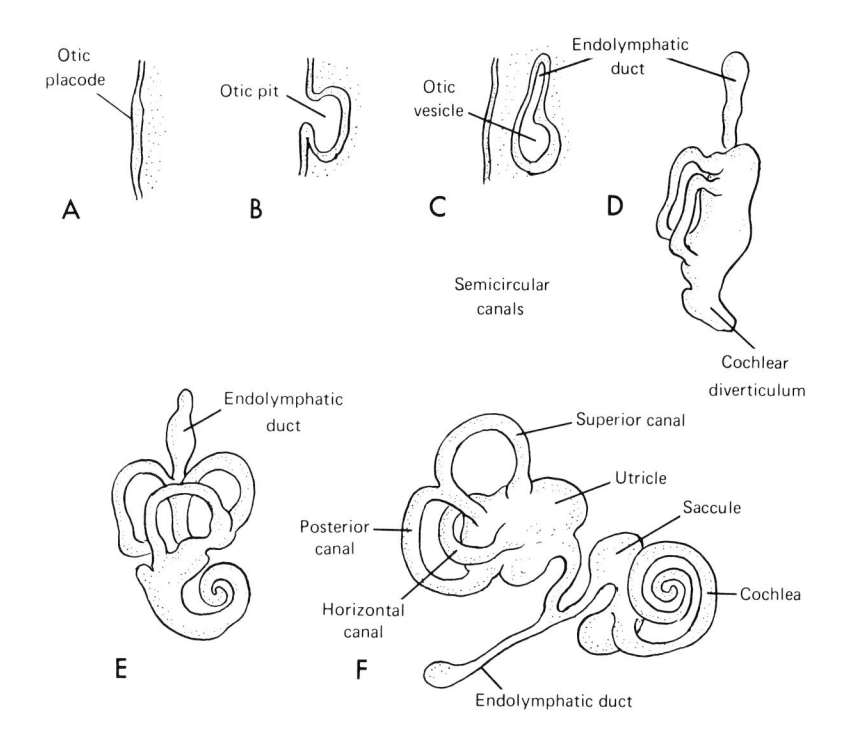

FIGURE 2–3. Stages in the development of the otocyst. *A*, As an ectodermal placode; *B*, as a pit; *C*, as an elongated vesicle isolated from the surface ectoderm; *D* to *F*, the events leading to the formation of the membranous labyrinth. (Modified from Streeter; from Davies J: *In* Paparella MM, Shumrick DA (eds): Otolaryngology. Vol 1: Basic Sciences and Related Disciplines. Philadelphia, WB Saunders Co, 1973, p 176.)

buried beneath the surface as the otic vesicle (Fig. 2–3). This vesicle comes to lie close to the developing hindbrain and to a collection of neurons known as the acousticofacial ganglion. This ganglion is important in the development of the facial, acoustic, and vestibular nerves. The auditory vesicle forms a diverticulum that comes to lie close to the developing neural tube and that will become the endolymphatic duct. Then the otic vesicle constricts, forming a superior utricle and inferior saccule. Three flange-like projections develop from the utricle. The membranous lining away from the periphery of these flanges resorbs, leaving three semicircular canals at the periphery of the flanges. The saccule gives off a spiral cochlear duct. Specialized end-organs phylogenetically derived from the naked neuromast develop in the semicircular canals to form cristae, in the utricle and saccule to form maculae, and in the cochlea to form the organ of Corti. These end-organs come into connection with the neurons of the acousticofacial ganglion. These neurons form the ganglia of the vestibular nerve and the spiral ganglia of the cochlear nerve.

The mesenchyme around the otic ganglion condenses into a cartilaginous capsule around the membranous derivatives of the otic vesicle. This cartilage resorbs in certain areas around what is now the membranous labyrinth, leaving a space that communicates via the cochlear aqueduct with the space containing CSF and forms the perilymphatic spaces of the bony labyrinth. The membranous labyrinth contains endolymph. The bone derived from the cartilaginous capsule of the otic vesicle is a special type of bone known as endochondral bone.

The Temporal Bone

The temporal bone, which contains the ear, is derived from four separate parts (Fig. 2–4). The bony external ear canal is derived from the tympanic

FIGURE 2–4. The temporal bone at birth and in the adult.

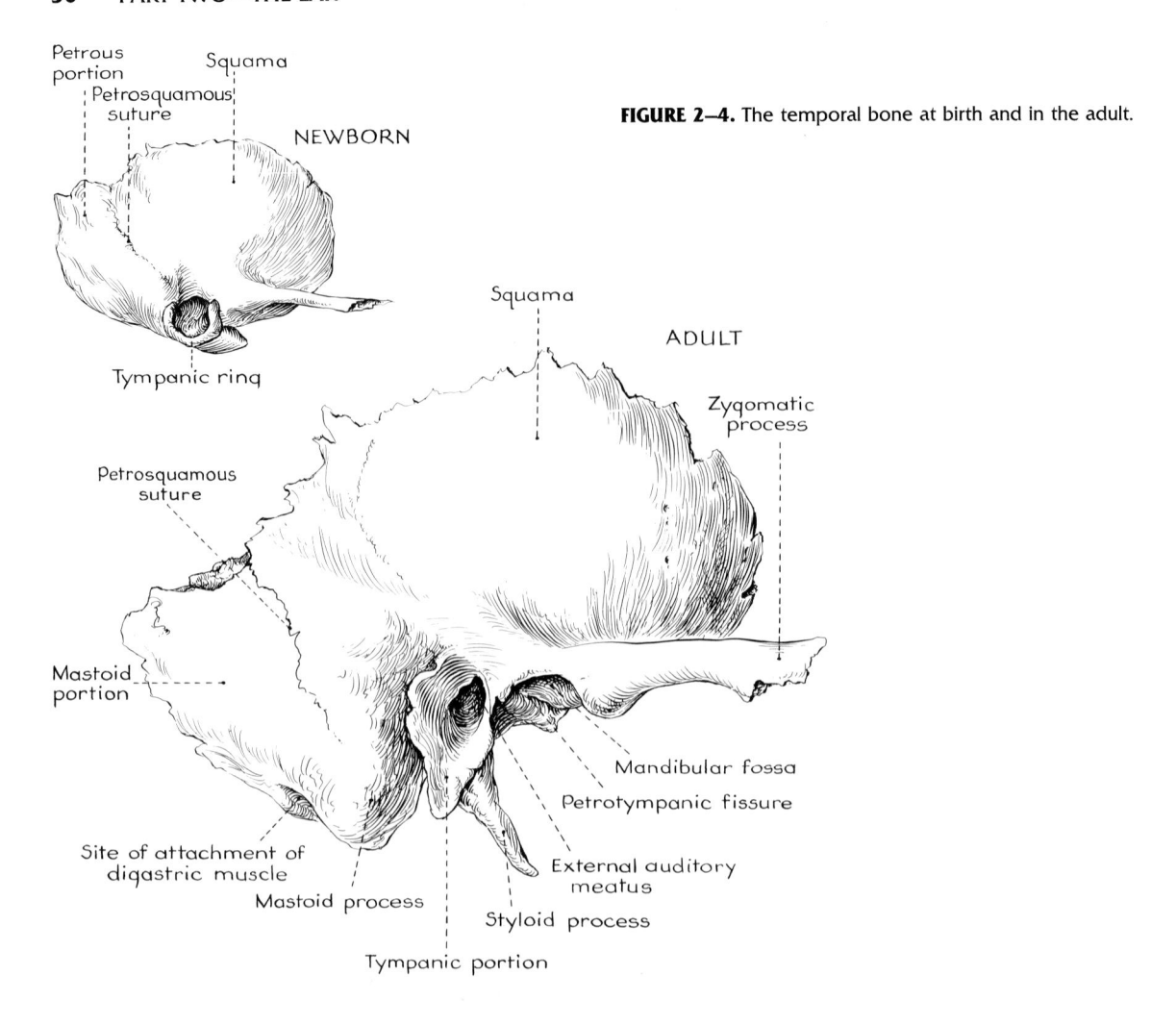

The facial nerve of an infant is not as protected by the mastoid process.

ring. The styloid process is derived from the second branchial cartilage. The squamous portion develops in cartilage. The petrous portion is derived from the cartilaginous capsule of otic vesicle. There are suture lines between these various portions visible on the definitive temporal bone. The mastoid (breastlike) process is not present at birth, and this means that the infant's facial nerve is very superficial. The air-containing derivatives of the tubotympanic recess extend from the middle ear via the aditus to the antrum, an air-containing region in the mastoid bone. However, how far the pneumatization of the rest of the mastoid process extends varies. Some bones are poorly pneumatized or sclerotic, some are moderately pneumatized or diploic, while frequently the mastoid and much of the petrous and even squamous temporal bone is filled by air cells (Fig. 2–5).

ANATOMY OF THE EAR

The external ear, or pinna, is composed of cartilage covered by skin. The shape of the cartilage is unique and in treating injuries to the external ear

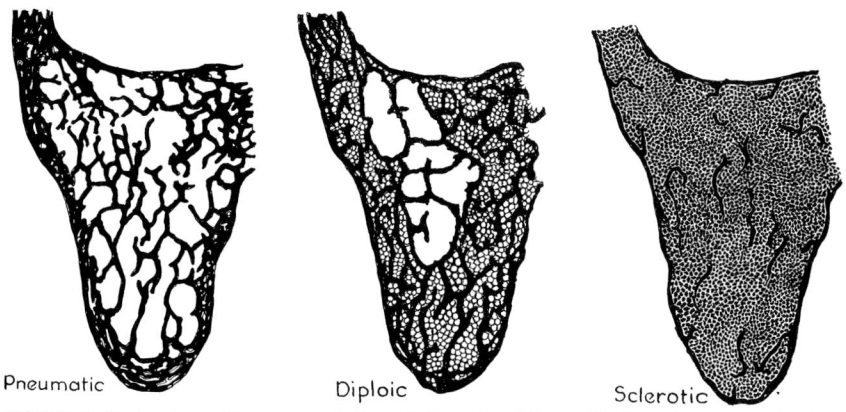

FIGURE 2–5. A schematic representation of the role of the epithelium in pneumatization and the types of mastoid development. (In part, after Fowler.)

every effort should be made to preserve this structure. The skin can be stripped off the underlying cartilage by hematoma or pus and the necrosis of the underlying cartilage leads to a cosmetic deformity of the pinna (cauliflower ear).

The external ear canal is cartilaginous laterally but bony medially. There is often a narrowing of the external ear canal at the bone-cartilage junction. The temporomandibular joint and parotid gland are anterior to the external ear canal, while the mastoid process is posterior to the ear canal. The facial nerve exits the stylomastoid foramen and passes lateral to the styloid process posteroinferior to the external ear canal and then runs beneath the external ear canal to enter the parotid gland. The cartilage of the external ear canal is one of the surgical landmarks used to find the facial nerve; the tympanomastoid suture is another such landmark.

The skin of the external canal lies directly over bone. Even slight inflammation is very tender for there is no room for expansion.

The Tympanic Membrane

The tympanic membrane, or eardrum, is a conical structure with the point of the cone, the umbo, directed medially. The tympanic membrane is generally round. It is important to realize that part of the middle ear cavity, the epitympanum, which contains the bodies of the malleus and incus, extends above the upper limit of the tympanic membrane, and that there is a hypotympanic part of the middle ear cavity extending below the tympanic membrane. The tympanic membrane is composed of an outer epidermal layer, a middle fibrous layer in which the handle of the malleus is embedded, and an inner mucosal layer. The fibrous layer is missing above the lateral process of the malleus, and this causes that part of the membrane, called Shrapnell's membrane, to be flaccid. The appearance of the tympanic membrane on clinical examination is shown in Figure 2–6.

The Middle Ear

The air-containing middle ear can be conceptualized as a box with six sides. The posterior wall is wider than the anterior wall, so the box is wedge-shaped. The promontory of the medial wall extends laterally toward the umbo of the tympanic membrane, so the box is narrower in the middle (Fig. 2–7).

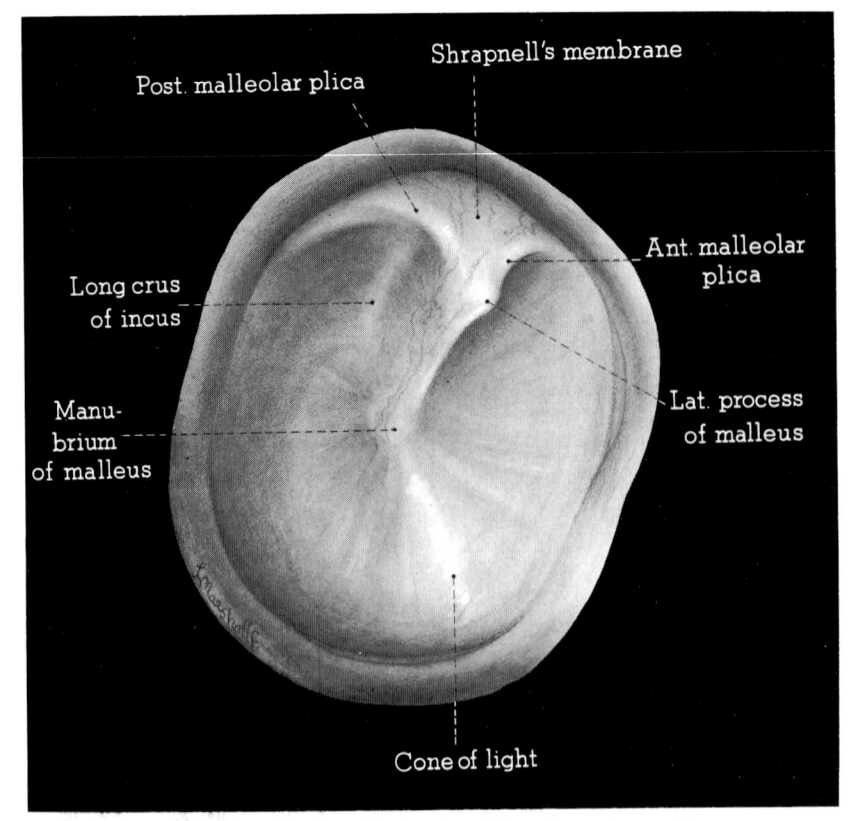

FIGURE 2–6. The right drumhead (membrana tympani).

The superior wall of the middle ear abuts the floor of the middle cranial fossa. The posterior wall superiorly contains the aditus to the antrum of the mastoid, and below this is the facial nerve. The stapedius muscle arises in the region of the facial nerve, and the tendon passes through a bony pyramid to the neck of the stapes. The chorda tympani nerve arises from the facial nerve below the stapedius and passes forward lateral to the incus but medial to the malleus to exit the middle ear via the petrotympanic suture. The chorda tympani nerve joins the lingual nerve and carries secretomotor fibers to the submandibular ganglion and taste fibers from the anterior two thirds of the tongue.

The floor of the middle ear is the roof of the jugular bulb, which superolaterally is the sigmoid sinus and then more centrally the transverse sinus. This is the major venous outflow of the cranial cavity. The auricular branch of the vagus nerve enters the middle ear via the floor. The anterior wall inferiorly is the wall of the carotid canal. Above this the eustachian tube opens and the tensor tympani muscle occupies the area superior to the eustachian tube and passes back to hook around the cochleariform process and insert into the neck of the malleus.

The lateral wall of the middle ear is the bony wall of the epitympanum above, the tympanic membrane, and the bony wall of the hypotympanum below.

The most prominent feature of the medial wall is the bony promontory

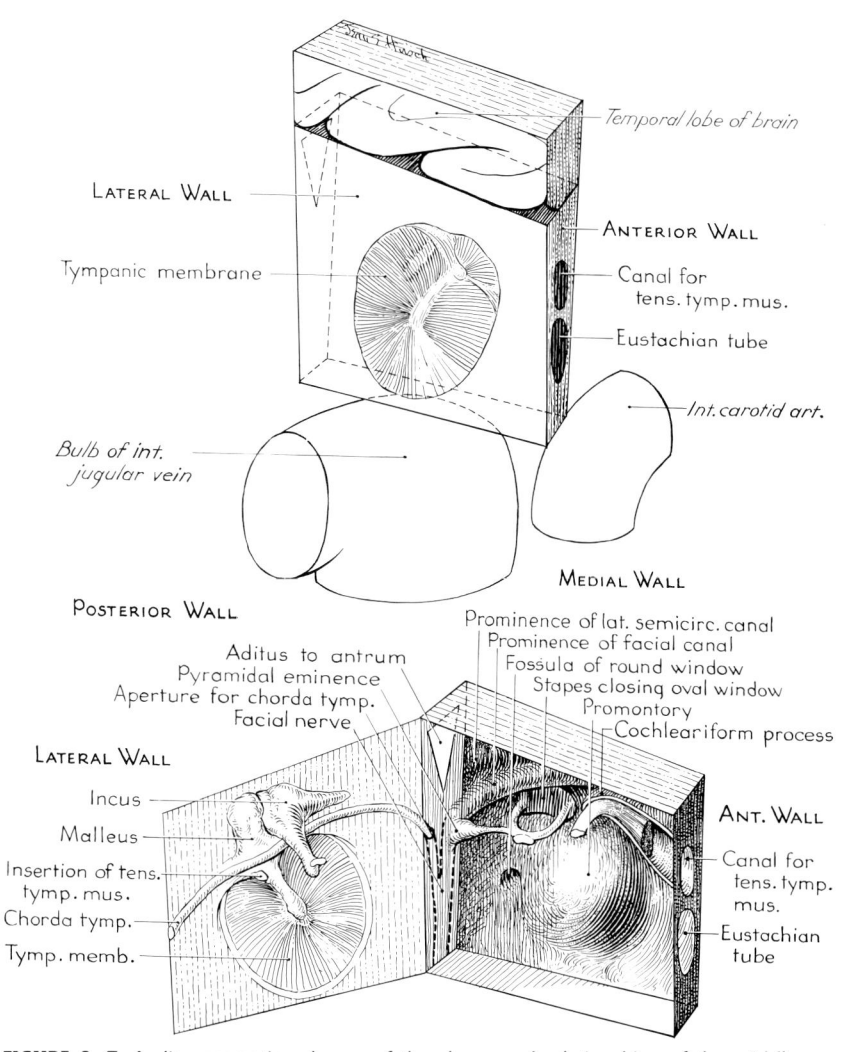

FIGURE 2–7. A diagrammatic scheme of the shape and relationships of the middle ear structures.

covering the first turn of the cochlea. The tympanic nerve runs across the promontory. The opening of the round window is located posteroinferior to the promontory. The footplate of the stapes is located in the oval window on the posterosuperior margin of the promontory. The bony fallopian canal containing the facial nerve runs above the oval window from the cochleariform process anteriorly to the stapedial pyramid posteriorly.

The mastoid cavity is shaped like a three-sided pyramid, the apex pointed caudally. The roof of the mastoid is the middle cranial fossa. The medial wall is the lateral wall of the posterior cranial fossa. The sigmoid sinus flows beneath the dura mater of this region. The anterior wall contains the aditus and antrum. The bulge of the lateral semicircular canal projects into the antrum. Below these two landmarks, the facial nerve runs in its bony canal to exit the temporal bone at the stylomastoid foramen, which is located at the anterior end of a ridge formed by the insertion of the digastric muscle. The lateral wall of the mastoid is subcutaneous bone easily palpable posterior to the pinna.

The Eustachian Tube

The eustachian tube (Fig. 2-8) connects the middle ear cavity with the nasopharynx. The lateral part of the eustachian tube is bony, while the medial two thirds is cartilaginous. The origin of the tensor tympani is located in the superior bony portion, while the carotid canal is inferior to the bony portion. The cartilaginous portion runs across the base of the skull to enter the pharynx above the superior constrictor. This portion is normally closed, but is opened by contractions of the levator palati and tensor palati innervated by the pharyngeal plexus and mandibular nerve, respectively. The eustachian tube serves to equalize the air pressure on both sides of the tympanic membrane.

The eustachian tube is horizontal at birth and inclines medially at 45° in the adult.

The Inner Ear

The inner ear has such a convoluted shape that it is referred to as the labyrinth. The derivatives of the otic vesicle form a closed cavity, the membranous labyrinth, filled with endolymph, the only extracellular fluid in the body that is high in potassium and low in sodium. This is surrounded by the fluid perilymph (high in sodium and low in potassium), which in turn is encased in the bony otic capsule. The membranous and bony labyrinths have vestibular and cochlear portions. The vestibular portion (pars superior) is concerned with balance, while the cochlear portion (pars inferior) is our organ of hearing.

The cochlea (Fig. 2-8) is coiled like a snail's shell or horn of plenty for two and one-half turns. The axis of the spiral is called the modiolus and contains the nerve bundles and arterial supply from the vertebral artery.

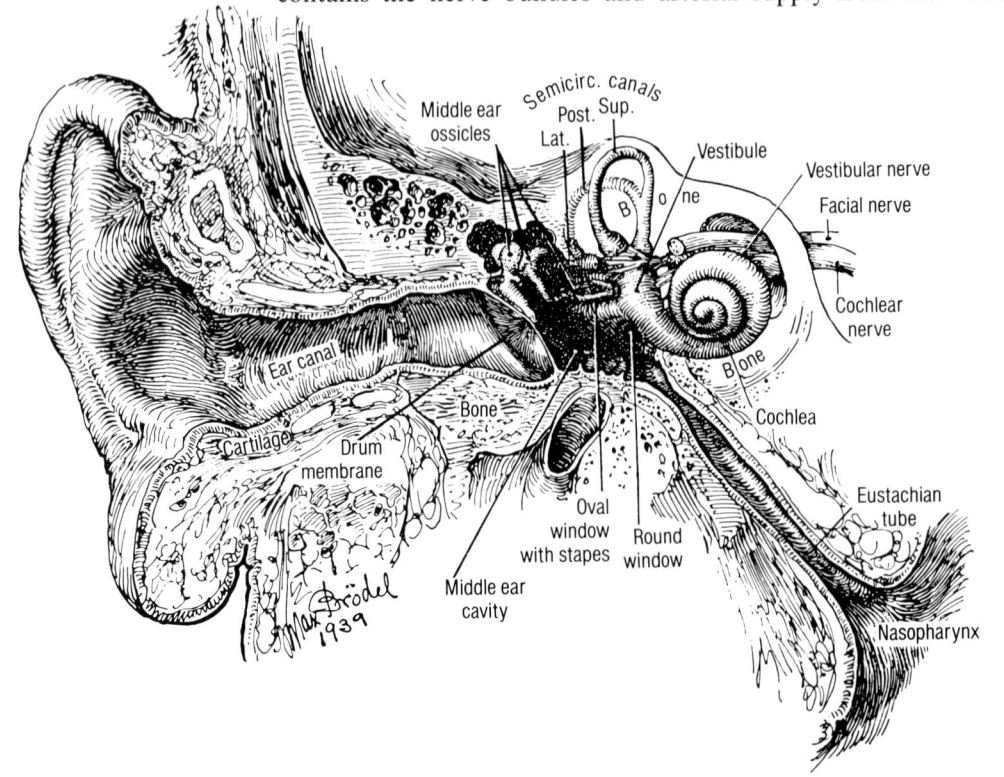

FIGURE 2–8. The relative size and the topography of the eustachian tube are depicted in this drawing by Brödel.

FIGURE 2–9. Cross-section of lower second cochlear turn. RM, Reissner's membrane; L, spiral limbus; TM, tectorial membrane; HS, Hensen's stripe; TH, auditory teeth of Huschke; TC, interdental ("T") cells; BM, basilar membrane; MN, myelinated nerves; HP, habenulae perforatae; PC, pillar cells; DC, Deiters' cells; OHC, outer hair cells; IHC, inner hair cells; SC, Schuknecht's channels; ISC, inner sulcus cells; OSC, outer sulcus (Claudius) cells; HC, Hensen's cells; BC, Böttcher's cells; ESC, external sulcus cells; SP, spiral prominence; SV, stria vascularis; SL, spiral ligament. (From Duvall AJ, III, Klinkner A: Macromolecular tracers in the mammalian cochlea. Am J Otolaryngol 4(6):400–410, 1983.)

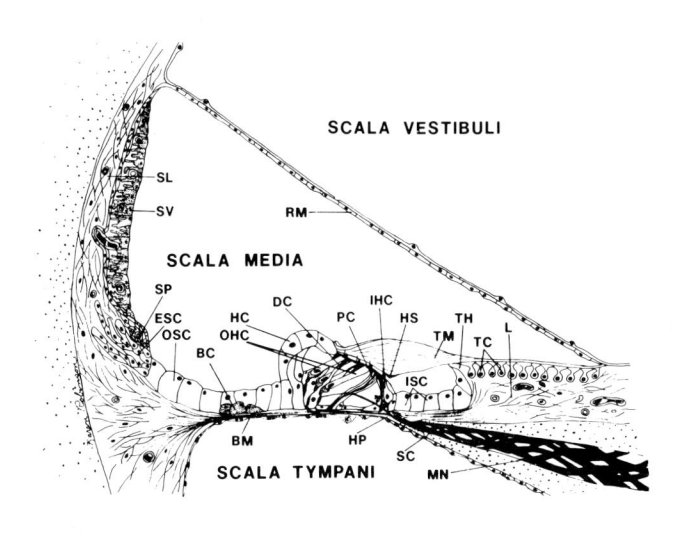

The nerve fibers then run through a bony shelf, the osseous spiral lamina, to reach the sensory cells of the organ of Corti (Fig. 2–9). The bony cavity of the cochlea is divided into three portions by the endolymph-containing, 35 mm long cochlear duct. The upper scala vestibuli contains perilymph and is divided from the cochlear duct by the thin Reissner's membrane. The lower scala tympani contains perilymph and is divided from the cochlear duct by the osseous spiral lamina and the basilar membrane. The perilymph of these two scalae communicates at the apex of the spiral cochlea past the blind end of the cochlear duct, through a small opening called the helicotrema. The basilar membrane is narrow at the base (high tones) and wide at the apex (low tones).

Sitting upon the basilar membrane, from the base to the apex, is the organ of Corti, which contains the essential organelles of the peripheral neural mechanism of hearing. The organ of Corti contains one row of inner hair cells (3,000) and three rows of outer hair cells (12,000). They are suspended through holes on the horizontal arm of a teeter-totter formed by supporting cells (Fig. 2–10). Afferent and efferent nerve-ending boutons attach to the lower ends of the hair cells. From the superior surface of the hair cells project stereocilia that are attached to a gelatinous, acellular, overlying, rather flat mantle called the tectorial membrane. This tectorial membrane is secreted and supported by a medially placed platform called the limbus.

The vestibular part of the inner ear is made up of the saccule, utricle, and semicircular canals. The utricle and saccule both contain a macula that is

FIGURE 2–10. The organ of Corti. The hair cells are suspended from the horizontal portion of a rigid teeter-totter formed by the reticular lamina and the inner and outer pillars. (Schematic drawing by Arndt J. Duvall, III, M.D.)

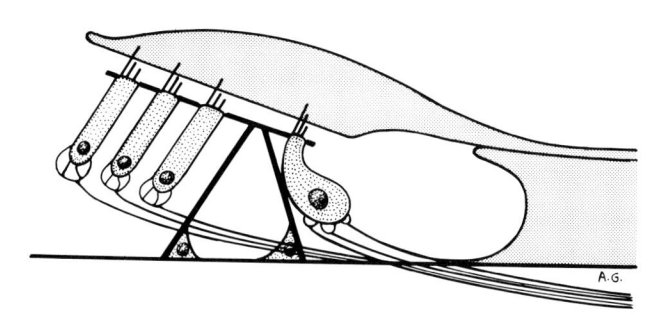

covered with hair cells. Overlying these hair cells is a gelatinous layer into which the cilia project, and within this gelatinous layer are calcium-containing otoliths, which have a heavier density than the endolymph. These otoliths are pulled on by gravity, and this shearing force bends the cilia of the hair cells and stimulates the receptors.

The saccule communicates with the utricle via a narrow duct that is also the passage leading to the endolymphatic sac. The utricular macula is on a plane perpendicular to the saccular macula. The three semicircular canals open into the utricle. Each semicircular canal has one end which is dilated into an ampulla that contains the hair cells of the crista. The hair cells project into a gelatinous cupula. Movements of the endolymph within the semicircular canal will move the cupula, which will bend the cilia of the hair cells of the crista and stimulate the receptors (see Chapter 3).

FUNCTION OF THE EAR

The pinna is, to some extent, a "collector" of sound. The external auditory canal, because of its shape and dimension, greatly amplifies the sounds in the region of 2 to 4 kHz; it will amplify these frequencies by 10 to 15 dB. Thus, sounds in this frequency range are most hazardous from the standpoint of acoustic trauma.

The middle ear contains the malleus, incus, and stapes (Fig. 2–11). The handle of the malleus is embedded in the tympanic membrane. The tensor tympani muscle inserts into the neck of the malleus. The head of the malleus articulates with the anterior surface of the body of the incus within the epitympanum. The incus has a short process that projects backwards and a long process that passes down to articulate with the head of the stapes.

The natural axis of rotation of the malleus and incus is along a line from the short process of the incus to the region of the neck of the malleus. The stapes is a stirrup-shaped bone. The contractions of the stapedius muscle can be measured by using impedance audiometry, and these measurements are an important clinical tool. The middle ear is an impedance-matching device between air (our environment) and liquid (inner ear). When sound waves transmitted through air reach fluid, 99.9 per cent of the energy is reflected. Only 0.1 per cent is transmitted (a loss of 30 dB). The middle ear compensates for the loss primarily because the tympanic membrane has an area 17 times greater than that of the stapedial footplate. The ossicular chain contributes a levered gain of 1.2/1. Thus, a middle ear is unnecessary in creatures that live in water.

The vibrations of sound are transmitted through the external auditory canal and middle ear to the inner ear via the stapes, causing a travelling wave to be created along the basilar membrane and its organ of Corti. The peak of the travelling wave along the 35 mm long basilar membrane is determined by the frequency of the sound wave. This results in bending of the stereocilia by shearing action with the tectorial membrane, thus depolarizing the hair cells and creating action potentials in the attached auditory nerve fibers. It is here that the mechanical sound waves are converted to the electrochemical energy for transmission through the eighth cranial nerve. At least some frequency analysis occurs at the organ of Corti level. The electrical event in the organ of Corti can be measured and is called the cochlear

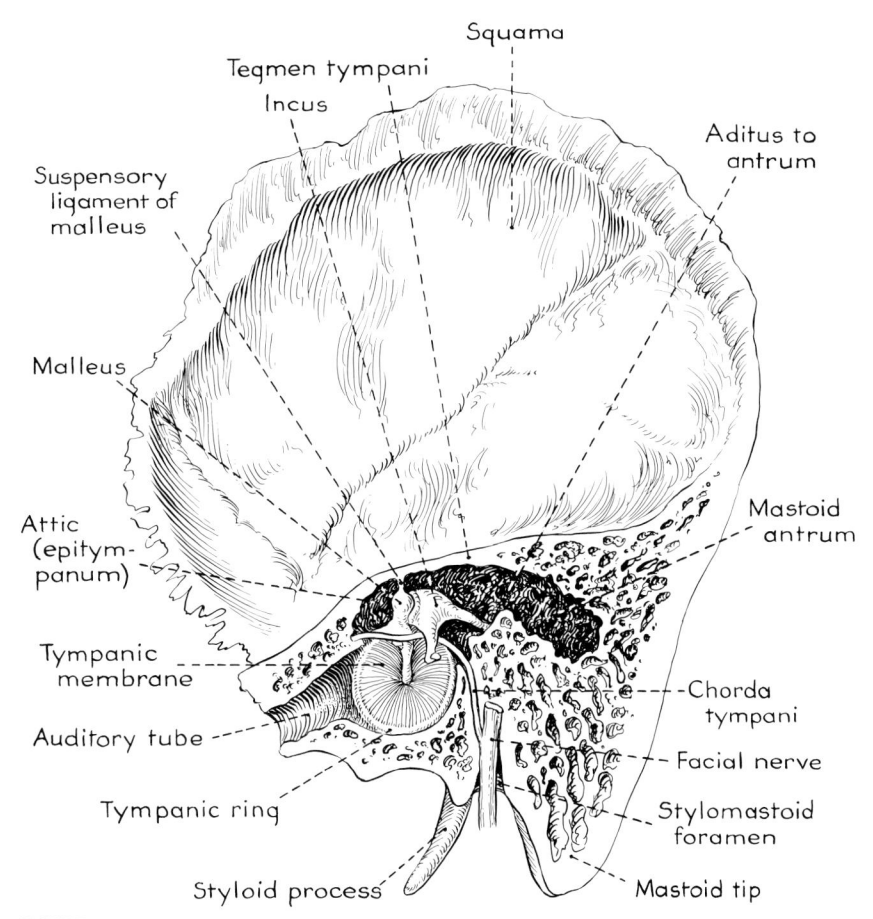

FIGURE 2–11. A drawing (after Fowler) from a section through the mastoid, antrum, and middle ear, looking outward from behind the drumhead.

microphonic. The electrical events occurring in the neurons also can be measured and are called the action potential.

The spiral ligament is on the lateral bony wall of the cochlear duct. It is the lateral anchor of the basilar membrane and contains the stria vascularis, the only vascularized epithelium in the body. Two of the three types of cells in the stria vascularis are rich in mitochondria and have very large surface areas in relation to their volume. Thus, the stria is uniquely constructed as a fluid and electrolyte transport system. It is thought to play a large role in the maintenance of the electrolyte composition of the endolymph (high in potassium, low in sodium) and to act as a second battery for the organ of Corti. It is the source of the scala media direct current potential (80 millivolts). As the basic nutrient supply of cells in the body is blood and its flow creates noise, the stria vascularis is the unique adaptation to provide nutrients to the organ of Corti while keeping the vascular supply at a distance, thus improving the signal-to-noice ratio at the organ of Corti.

There are about 30,000 afferent neurons that innervate the 15,000 hair cells in each cochlea. Each inner hair cell is innervated by many neurons. Only a small percentage (about 10 per cent) of the afferent neurons innervate the outer hair cells, but there is considerable branching, such that each afferent

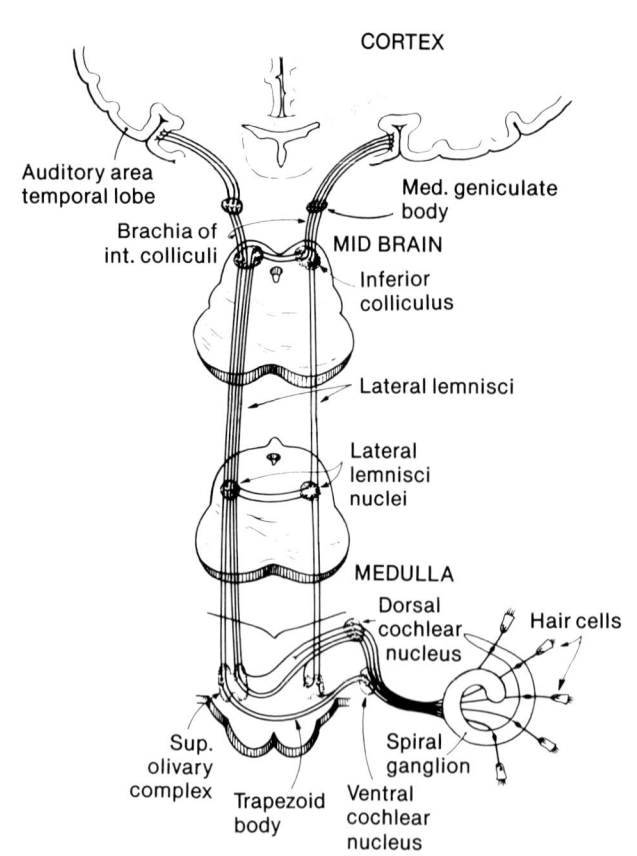

FIGURE 2–12. Diagram of central auditory connections as deduced from animal experiments and some human pathologic material (after Lang). (From A Guide to the Care of Adults with Hearing Loss published by the American Academy of Ophthalmology and Otolaryngology.)

neuron derives from many outer hair cells and each outer hair cell is innervated from many different afferent neurons.

There are also about 500 efferent nerve fibers reaching each cochlea. These also branch extensively, such that each outer hair cell has many efferent nerve endings. Any one outer hair cell's efferent nerve endings are not all derived from one efferent neural fiber.

The neural fibers of the cochlear nerve (Fig. 2–12) pass to the dorsal and ventral cochlear nuclei. Most fibers from the nuclei cross the midline and ascend to the contralateral inferior colliculus, but some ascend ipsilaterally. There are further crossovers at the nuclei of the lateral lemniscus and inferior colliculi. From the inferior colliculi, the auditory pathway runs to the medial geniculate body and then to the auditory cortex of the temporal lobe. Because of the frequent crossing over of nerve fibers, central lesions of the auditory pathways almost never cause a unilateral hearing loss.

The neural fibers of the vestibular nerve pass to one of the four vestibular nuclei and from there are widely distributed, with pathways to the spinal cord, cerebellum, and other parts of the central nervous system.

References

Anson BJ, Donaldson JA: Surgical Anatomy of the Temporal Bone and Ear. Philadelphia, WB Saunders, 1981.

Schuknecht HF, Gulya AJ: Anatomy of the Temporal Bone with Surgical Implications. Philadelphia, Lea & Febiger, 1986.

Shambaugh GE, Glasscock ME: Surgery of the Ear. Philadelphia, WB Saunders, 1980.

3

THE VESTIBULAR SYSTEM

by John H. Anderson, M.D., Ph.D., and Samuel C. Levine, M.D.

PHYSIOLOGY

Sensory signals coming from the inner ear, the retina of the eye, and the musculoskeletal system are integrated in the central nervous system (CNS) in order to control gaze and the position and movement of the body in space. In this section we briefly describe the equilibrium receptors and discuss their role. When we refer to the "vestibular system," we mean not only the receptors but also the pathways in the CNS which are involved in processing the afferent signals and which activate motoneurons.

Adequate stimulus: acceleration, a change in velocity per unit of time.

The receptors are hair cells located in the cristae of the semicircular canals and the maculae of the otolith organs. Functionally there are two types. Those of the semicircular canals are sensitive to rotation, specifically to angular acceleration (which is a change in angular velocity), and those of the otolith organs are sensitive to linear motion, specifically to linear acceleration, and to changes in head position relative to gravity. This difference in sensitivity to linear versus angular acceleration is due to the geometry of the canals and otolith organs and the physical characteristics of the structures overlying the hair cells.

Hair Cells. Morphologically, the individual hair cells of the canals and otolith organs are very similar. Each has a structural polarization that is defined by the positions of the stereocilia relative to the kinocilium (see Fig. 3–1). Corresponding to this, there is a functional polarization in the response of the hair cells (see Fig. 3–2). If a movement causes the stereocilia to be bent toward the kinocilium, then the hair cells are excited. If the movement is in the opposite direction and causes a bending away from the kinocilium, then the hair cells are inhibited. In the absence of any movement, there is some release of transmitter from the hair cells which causes the afferent nerve fibers to have a spontaneous or resting firing rate. This makes it possible for the afferents to be either excited or inhibited, depending on the direction of the movement.

Polarization of hair cells: structural and functional.

Semicircular Canals. In any one canal the polarization is the same for all the hair cells, and during a rotation they are all either excited or inhibited. The three canals are approximately perpendicular to each other, and each canal of one ear is approximately coplanar with a canal from the other ear. Thus, there are three pairs: left horizontal–right horizontal, left anterior–right posterior, and left posterior–right anterior. During a rotation one canal of a pair will be excited while the other will be inhibited. For example, if the head is in a normal, upright position and there is an acceleration in the horizontal plane causing a rotation to the right, then the afferents of the right horizontal canal will be excited and those of the left canal will be inhibited. If the rotation is in the vertical plane, causing a forward rotation,

Canal pairs: excitation and inhibition.

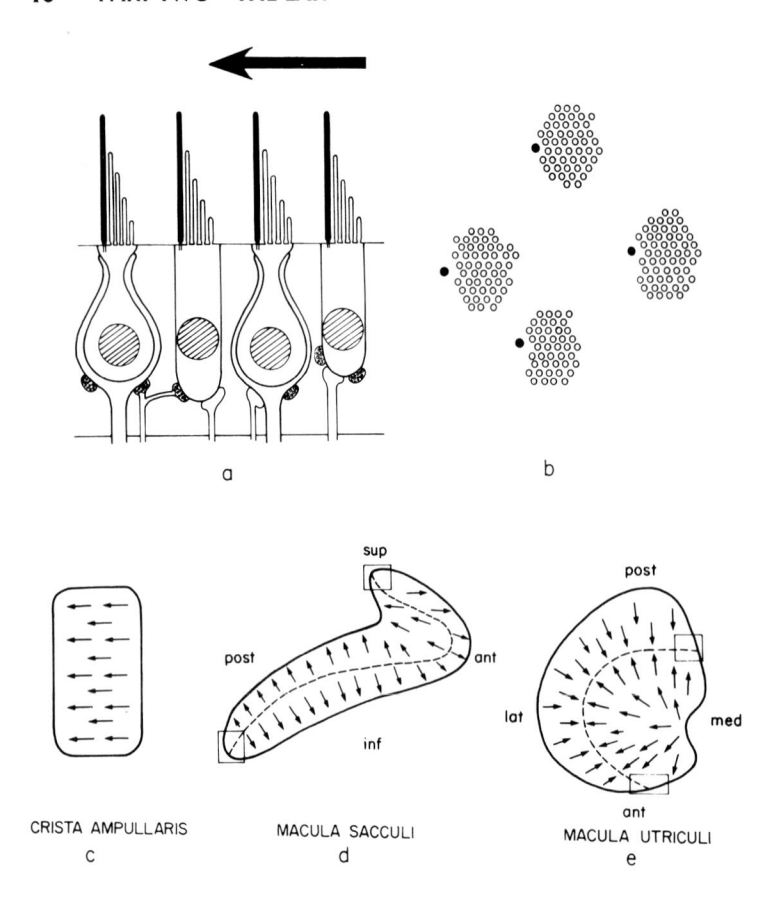

FIGURE 3–1. Diagram of morphologic polarization of the sensory cells and the polarization pattern of the vestibular sensory epithelia. Morphologic polarization *(arrow)* of a sensory cell is determined by the position of the kinocilium in relation to the stereocilia. *a,* Section perpendicular to the epithelium. Note increasing length of stereocilia toward the kinocilium. *b,* Section parallel to the epithelial surface. *c,* The sensory cells on the crista ampullaris are polarized in the same direction. *d,* Macula sacculi and *(e)* macula utriculi are divided by an arbitrary curved line into two areas, the pars interna and the pars externa, with opposite morphologic polarization. On the macula sacculi the sensory cells are polarized away from the dividing line; on the macula utriculi they are polarized toward the line. Constant irregularities in the polarization pattern are found in areas corresponding to the continuation of the striola peripherally (rectangles in *d* and *e*). (From Lindeman HH: Studies on the morphology of the sensory regions of the vestibular apparatus. *In* Advances in Anatomy, Embryology and Cell Biology. New York, Springer-Verlag, 1969, p 59.)

Canal stimulus: angular acceleration.

then the anterior canals of both sides will be excited and the posterior canals inhibited.

It should be noted that angular acceleration is the adequate stimulus for the semicircular canal afferents. A constant velocity rotation will not excite them. Of course, in order to reach a given velocity, there must be an acceleration and the effects of this will decay to zero over time, up to a few

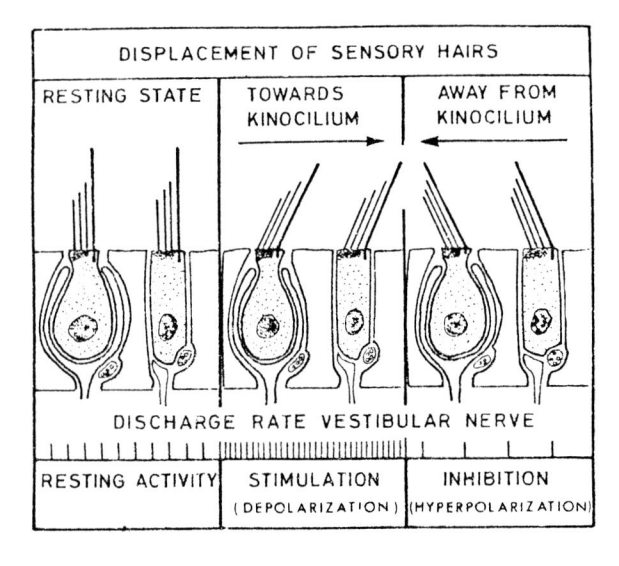

FIGURE 3–2. Electrical discharge rate of the hair cells as a function of displacement of the sensory hairs. (From Wersall J, Lundquist P-G: Morphological polarization of the mechanoreceptors of the vestibular and acoustic systems. *In* Second Symposium on the Role of the Vestibular Organs in Space Exploration, January 25–27, 1966, Fig 27, p 68. Published by NASA.)

minutes. This time lag is due to CNS processing of the afferent activity and to the inertia of the cupula and the viscosity of the endolymph, which cause the displacement of the cupula to lag behind the change in the angular velocity of the head. For example, consider the effect of suddenly coming to a stop after rotating to the right, in a clockwise direction. This deceleration to zero velocity is equivalent to an acceleration in the opposite direction, to the left. Therefore, the afferents of the left canal will be excited and those of the right inhibited. If this is done in complete darkness, then the subject will have the perception that he is rotating to the left. As the cupula of each canal returns to its resting position, the subject will perceive that he comes to a stop.

Otolith Organs. There are two otolith organs: the utriculus, which is located approximately in the horizontal plane of the head, and the sacculus, which is located approximately in the vertical plane. In contrast to the semicircular canals, the hair cells of a given otolith organ do not all have the same polarization. In the utricular macula, the kinocilium is located on the side of the hair cell located closest to the central region, the striola. Thus, during a given head tilt or linear acceleration, some of the afferents will be excited and others will be inhibited. However, this does not mean that there will be a cancellation of the responses in the CNS. The afferents with a given polarization may project to different neurons in the vestibular nuclei and may subserve different functions. Also, because there are different polarizations within each macula, the CNS has information about linear motion in three dimensions, even though there are only two maculae.

Otolith stimulus: linear acceleration and gravity.

Vestibular Reflexes. The afferents go the CNS and synapse on neurons in the vestibular nuclei in the brain stem. Neurons in the vestibular nuclei then project to other parts of the brain; some go directly to the motoneurons innervating the extraocular muscles and to spinal motoneurons and others go to the brain stem reticular formation, cerebellum, and other structures.

Direct connections between the vestibular nuclei and the extraocular motoneurons constitute one important pathway by which eye movements and the vestibulo-ocular reflex (VOR) are controlled. The VOR is an eye movement that has a "slow" component opposite to the head rotation and a "fast" component in the same direction as the head rotation. The slow component compensates for the head movement and serves to stabilize an image on the retina. The fast component serves to redirect gaze to another part of the visual field. This alteration in the direction of the eye movement during vestibular stimulation is one example of a normal nystagmus.

Nystagmus: slow phase (compensatory) alternating with fast phase (in opposite direction).

EVALUATION OF VESTIBULAR FUNCTION

A number of clinical tests can be performed to determine whether or not the vestibular system is functioning normally and, if not, where the problem might be. Some are designed to stimulate a particular end-organ, such as one pair of semicircular canals or the otolith organs during whole body rotation in the dark. Other tests are designed to look at the interaction among several sensory inputs, such as muscle proprioceptive, visual, and vestibular inputs, which can all be present during changes in body or head posture.

One important objective for the otolaryngologist is to determine whether or not the cause for vertigo (the sensation that the world is moving relative to the subject) is due to a problem in the inner ear and/or the eighth nerve

Differential diagnosis: inner ear and central nervous system.

or in the central nervous system. Examples of central disorders include multiple sclerosis and other demyelinating diseases, tumors, vascular disease and stroke, and drug toxicity. Examples of peripheral disorders include Meniere's disease, labyrinthitis, ototoxicity due to antibiotics, and acoustic neuromas.

Eye movements (VOR responses) are measured in many tests of vestibular function. In these cases it is therefore necessary to first evaluate the oculomotor system. This is done by examining spontaneous eye movements in the light and dark and movements to visual targets, saccades, and pursuit tracking.

For some vestibular tests it is necessary to prevent visual fixation and optokinetic stimulation (movement of the visual surround relative to the subject). For this purpose the stimulus can be applied in complete darkness, with the eyes closed, or with the subject wearing +20 diopter lenses (Frenzel glasses). In the latter two situations, however, the gain of the VOR is reduced; complete darkness with the eyes open is the optimum condition.

The eye movements can be measured with electrodes placed on the outer canthus of each eye for horizontal movements and above and below the eyes for vertical movements (Fig. 3–3). There is an electrical potential difference between the retina and cornea of each eye, which thus acts as an electric dipole. Movement of the eye changes the orientation of the dipole, and this changes the potential difference between the two electrodes on the surface of the skin.

Caloric Stimulation. In this test the subject is placed with the plane of one semicircular canal (usually the horizontal) aligned with a plane vertical to the earth. Then a fluid that is either warmer or colder than body temperature is placed in the external ear canal. Consequent to this there is a transfer of heat to or from the inner ear, which results in a convection current in the endolymph. This causes a deflection of the cupula in the canal which is aligned with gravity and stimulation of its afferents. The maximum velocity of the slow component and the time course of the nystagmus are measured when there is no vision present.

Calorics: 1) Stimulate horizontal canal in one ear; 2) Similar to low frequency rotation.

The standard position is with the head tilted backward approximately 60 degrees so that the horizontal canal is in the vertical plane. A cold fluid applied to the right ear causes a nystagmus with the slow phase to the right and a warm fluid causes a slow phase to the left. The response typically lasts two to three minutes. A significantly reduced response to stimulation of one ear compared to the other is evidence for a peripheral deficit on that side. However, the complete absence of a response to caloric stimulation does not necessarily mean that there is no canal function on that side. The stimulus is roughly equivalent to slowly moving the head in one direction (although only one ear is stimulated) and is analogous to giving a single, low-frequency, pure tone for evaluating hearing. A complete vestibular examination should also evaluate the response to rapid head movements.

Passive, whole-body rotation.

Rotation. There are two forms of rotation testing. One involves placing the subject on a chair that is centered on the axis of rotation of a torque motor. When the subject is seated upright and tilts his head approximately 30 degrees downward, the horizontal canals can be maximally stimulated. Neck movement is prevented so that rotation will move the body and head together. Rotation may be unidirectional with constant angular acceleration in one direction for a short time period (e.g., 18 seconds) or oscillatory (e.g., sinusoidal). The amplitude and time course of the response are

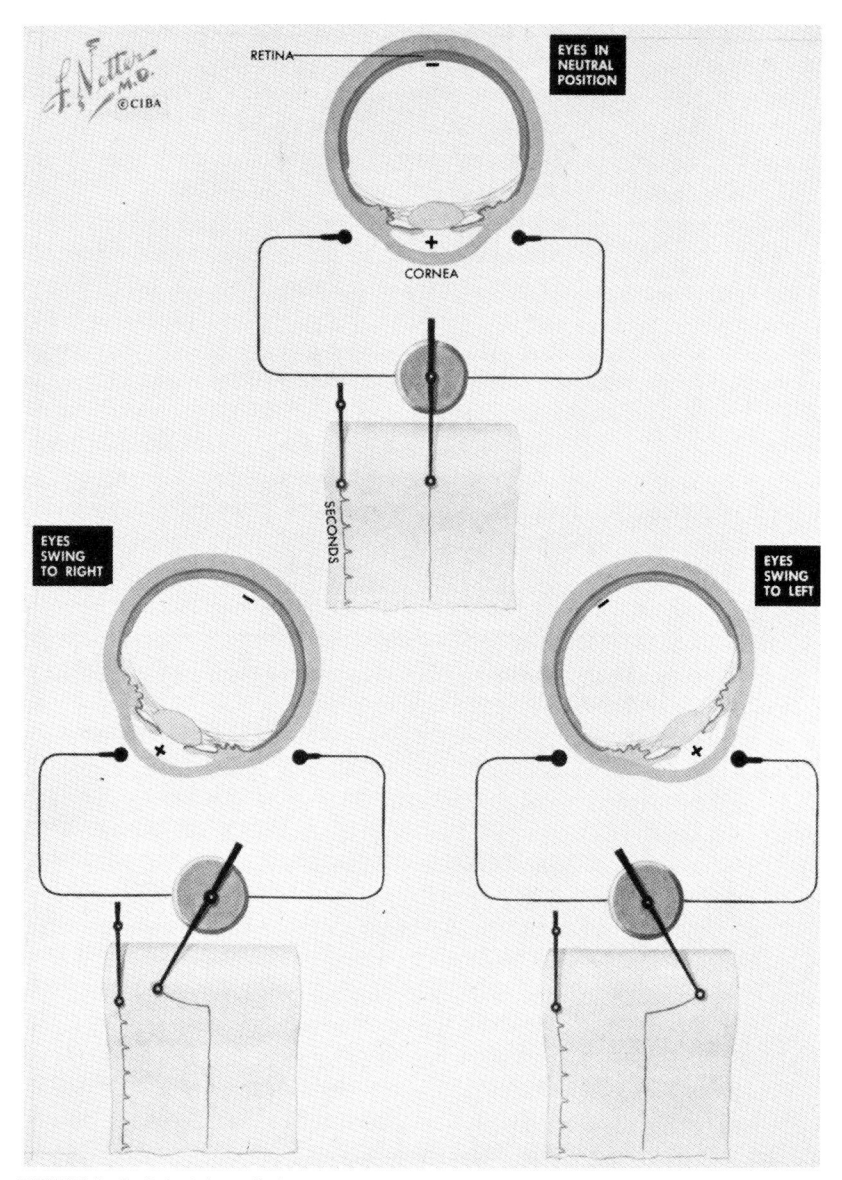

FIGURE 3–3. Principles of electronystagmography. A diagrammatic explanation of the correctional potential and amplification of changes in electrical activity by differential electrodes. The motion of the eyes is recorded on paper and represented by upward and downward pen deflection. (From CIBA Symposia.)

measured for constant accelerations, and the phase and gain are measured for sinusoidal rotations.

Another paradigm involves the subject himself moving his head back and forth. In this case there is stimulation of both the vestibular receptors and the receptors in the neck muscles. The latter may play an important role in compensating for the loss of vestibular function. Although this is a complicating factor, the paradigm has the advantage that very rapid head movements with large amplitudes can be attained so that the vestibular labyrinth (together with the neck muscle receptors) can be very strongly

Active head movement and high frequency stimulation.

stimulated in a natural manner. This complements the lower frequency, whole body rotation. Together these two tests can provide a quantitative description of the vestibular system over a wide range of stimulus frequencies.

Compared to caloric stimulation, the rotation tests offer several advantages: (1) The stimulus (i.e., acceleration of the head) can be controlled and precisely measured, and this allows a quantitative analysis of input/output relations to be made. (2) The system can be tested over a wide range of stimulus parameters (e.g., many frequencies of head movement). (3) Information about the integrity of both the peripheral labyrinth and the CNS can be obtained. (4) Because of the quantitative methods of analysis, it might be possible to more accurately measure vestibular function over time in order to monitor the progression of a disease or the effectiveness of a treatment.

Advantages of rotation: 1) Quantitate the stimulus; 2) Vary stimulus parameters; 3) Information about both inner ear and CNS.

The response to caloric stimulation, on the other hand, is more variable from subject to subject. This is due, in part, to the fact that there is considerable variability in the actual stimulus to the receptors. There is variation in the time course over which the fluid is applied to the ear canal and in the transfer of heat between the fluid and the labyrinth. The latter depends upon the amount of tissue between the external ear canal and the labyrinth and the blood flow through it, neither of which can be controlled or measured. Thus, the time course and magnitude of the actual stimulus to the semicircular canal are not known.

Positional Testing. At present there is no well-defined protocol for quantitatively testing otolith function or for testing the effect of gravity on the vestibular receptors. However, by placing the head in different positions relative to gravity and at the same time measuring the eye movements, some information can be gained. One condition that can be diagnosed is benign paroxysmal positional vertigo (BPPV). In this case the vertigo is associated with a rapid change in head position. It is sudden in onset and is of short duration. The condition is believed to result from a structural alteration of the cupula of the posterior semicircular canal, which makes it sensitive to gravity.

A test for BPPV is the following: The patient is seated on an examining table in a completely dark room (or wearing Frenzel glasses). Then the patient is suddenly placed in a prone position with the head turned sharply backward and to one side. When the affected side is down, there will be a nystagmus (usually with a vertical or rotatory component) that is delayed in onset (3 to 10 sec) and that lasts for only about 30 sec. Upon repeated testing, the nystagmus will diminish and then disappear. It is fatigable. When the nystagmus does not have a latent period and is not fatigable, CNS disease must be considered as a possible cause.

Posturography. Recently a new technique has become available for testing upright posture. Subjects stand on a platform that measures the force exerted by each foot, and the positions of the head and hips are measured. Several different conditions are used: normal vision with a fixed platform to stand on, no vision (complete darkness), no ankle movement (the platform moves with the subject to keep the ankle angle constant and to thereby prevent stimulation of muscle and joint receptors), and visual conflict (the visual field or drum that surrounds the subject moves with the subject as he sways back and forth). Subjects who have impaired vestibular function have the greatest difficulty when the platform and the visual field both move with the subject. In this condition there is a sensory conflict: Vision and proprioceptive

Sensory conflict: vestibular system provides an inertial reference.

inputs detect no motion while in fact the body is swaying back and forth. In normal subjects, the vestibular system provides an inertial reference to resolve this conflict and posture is maintained. The vestibular-deficient subjects, however, cannot do this.

SUMMARY

The test paradigms discussed above illustrate some of the interactions among visual, muscle proprioceptive, and the different vestibular sensory signals, canal and otolith. In real-life situations all the sensory inputs contribute to maintaining posture and gaze and adapting to a sensory, motor, or CNS deficit. When evaluating the function of the vestibular system, it is important to realize this and to use appropriate test stimuli under different experimental conditions. There is no single test for vestibular function which can answer all questions.

References

Black FO: Vestibulospinal function assessment by moving platform posturography. Am J Otolaryngol 6:39–46, 1985.

Fineberg R, O'Leary DP, Davis LL: Use of active head movements for computerized vestibular testing. Arch Otolaryngol Head Neck Surg 113:1063–1065, 1987.

Honrubia V, Baloh RW, Yee RD, Jenkins HA: Identification of the location of vestibular lesions on the basis of vestibulo-ocular reflex measurements. Am J Otolaryngol 1(4):291–301, 1980.

Honrubia V, Jenkins HA, Baloh RW, et al: Vestibulo-ocular reflexes in peripheral labyrinthine lesions: I. Unilateral dysfunction. Am J Otolaryngol 5:15–26, 1984.

Hudspeth AJ: Transduction and tuning by vertebrate hair cells. Trends Neurosci, Sept 1983, pp 366–369.

Leigh RJ, Zee DS: The Neurology of Eye Movement. Philadelphia, FA Davis, 1983.

Miles FA, Lisberger SG: Plasticity in the vestibulo-ocular reflex: A new hypothesis. Annu Rev Neurosci 4:273–300, 1981.

Robinson DA: The use of control systems analysis in the neurophysiology of eye movements. Annu Rev Neurosci 4:463–503, 1981.

Takahashi M, Uemura T, Fuyishiro T: Compensatory eye movement and gaze fixation during active head rotation in patients with labyrinthine disorders. Ann Otol 90:241–245, 1981.

4

AUDIOLOGY

by Frank M. Lassman, Ph.D., Samuel C. Levine, M.D., and Donna G. Greenfield, M.S.

Purposes of Audiology

Audiology, which is the science of hearing, involves the evaluation of hearing and the rehabilitation of individuals with communication problems related to hearing impairment. There are two reasons for evaluation: (1) medical diagnosis of the location and type of disease and (2) assessment of the impact of hearing impairment upon learning, social interaction, and vocation.

Hearing measurements can add precision to diagnose the locus of pathologic involvement and specific disease entities. Patients with different diseases within the same area (e.g., noise deafness and Meniere's syndrome both involve the cochlea) report very different hearing experiences and will have potentially different audiometric findings. Likewise, the qualities of the impaired hearing experience will limit attention skills, language development, speech precision, and general communication effectiveness in ways specific to the degree and type of impairment. Plans for special education and rehabilitation should be influenced and guided by the hearing measurement along with other important variables such as intelligence, motivation, and family support. The physician is forced to look at the integrity of the middle ear somewhat indirectly and is totally unable to examine the cochlea and the auditory nervous system except by studying the way they function in response to sound.

Types of Hearing Evaluation

The patient's ability to hear can be determined in ways ranging from informal procedures to highly standardized and precise measurements requiring special equipment. The more frequent and routine hearing testing becomes in the office, the greater skill the examiner will develop in its use and practical application. The following types of hearing tests will be discussed in this chapter: tuning fork tests, pure tone audiometry, speech audiometry, special tests, and pediatric audiometry. It is important that they be viewed as an aggregate with supplementary and complementary purposes generating a test battery.

Types of Hearing Impairment

Three general types of hearing impairment are identified by hearing tests: conductive, sensorineural, and combined or mixed. Conductive hearing problems are due to disorders of the external or middle ear. Sensorineural hearing problems are secondary to disturbance of the cochlea, eighth nerve, or central auditory channels. Earlier terms such as "nerve" loss and "perceptive" loss have been discarded because most so-called nerve diseases were found in or had originated in the cochlea, whereas "perceptive" suggested a psychological dynamic. The distinction between "cochlear" and "retrocochlear" is considered by some to be useful when the test battery is sufficiently sophisticated. Mixed or combined hearing loss involves disturbances of both conductive and sensorineural mechanisms.

Types of hearing impairment: (1) conductive, (2) sensorineural (cochlear and retrocochlear), (3) mixed.

Testing Models

Air conduction (AC) utilizes the external and middle ear in the transmission of sound to the cochlea and beyond. It is thought to be the usual avenue of sound transmission. In **bone conduction** (BC), the skull is set into vibration by direct contact with a periodically oscillating body, such as a tuning fork. The bone-conducted stimulus is thought to set the cochlear fluids into motion, bypassing the external and middle ear. Bekesy (1932) has shown that the vibrating patterns of the cochlea are the same regardless of whether sound has been introduced by air conduction or bone conduction.

The bone conduction test has been traditionally treated as a measure of the integrity of the cochlea and beyond. Normal bone conduction hearing strongly suggests normal cochlear, nerve, and brain stem function. If the sensorineural component (BC) is normal, while the total system (AC) is impaired (BC>AC), the impairment is judged to have resulted from damage to the remaining portion of the system, i.e., the middle ear and/or external ear, not measured by the normal bone conduction finding. On the other hand, if the bone conduction measurement is no more sensitive than the air conduction (BC≤AC), the total impairment is judged to have resulted from damage or change in the cochlear or retrocochlear mechanism. But many investigators led by Tonndorf have challenged this traditional interpretation of the absent air/bone gap. They demonstrate some elevation of bone conduction threshold secondary to middle ear disturbances.

TUNING FORK TESTS

A set of tuning forks sampling the auditory range from low to high frequencies makes a survey of hearing sensitivity easy for the physician. The usual set samples some of the C notes of the musical scale, i.e., 128, 256, 512, 1024, 2048, 4096, and 8192 Hz. Hz is the abbreviation for hertz, which is the contemporary designation for "cycles per second," the unit of frequency. The higher the frequency, the higher the pitch. Limiting the survey to the so-called speech frequencies—512, 1024, and 2048 Hz—is usually sufficient.

Threshold

The tuning fork is held by the stem, and one of the tines is struck against a firm but resilient surface, such as the heel of the hand or the elbow. Care should be taken not to strike the fork against the edge of a table or some other unyielding object that will produce overtones, some of which are audible at some distance from the fork, and may even cause permanent alteration in the vibratory pattern of the fork. The fork is held close to the ear, and the patient is asked to report when the sound is no longer audible. At that report, the fork is placed next to the examiner's ear and the interval between that time and the time at which the sound is no longer audible to the examiner is measured. The procedure not only provides a rough estimate of relative hearing sensitivity but, if forks are available in various frequencies, offers a pitch sensitivity pattern.

With care, forks can provide important diagnostic information.

Schwabach Test

The Schwabach test compares the patient's bone conduction to that of the examiner. While the stem of the vibrating fork is held against the mastoid, the patient reports when the sound becomes inaudible. At that moment, the examiner applies the fork stem to his own mastoid and measures the time (in seconds) the examiner can still perceive the sound.

Schwabach: mastoid to mastoid.

A **normal Schwabach** is obtained when the patient and examiner have approximately equal bone conduction. A **prolonged or increased Schwabach** is assigned when the patient's bone conduction is appreciably longer than the examiner's, as in the instance of conductive hearing impairment. When the examiner can hear the fork well after the patient, suggesting a sensorineural hearing impairment, the term **diminished Schwabach** is applied. The interpretations of the Schwabach test are shown in Table 4–1.

Rinne Test

The Rinne test compares the patient's hearing by bone conduction against that by air conduction. The hilt of the vibrating fork is held against the patient's mastoid (bone conduction) until sound is no longer heard; the tines are then placed close to the same ear (air conduction). The normal ear will resume hearing the fork by air conduction, a finding called the **positive Rinne** (AC>BC). These results are explained by an impedance mismatch.

Rinne: compares bone conduction to air conduction

The patient with sensorineural hearing impairment will also yield a positive Rinne, if the fork is audible at all, since the sensorineural disturbance should affect both air conduction and bone conduction routes equally (AC>BC).

The term **negative Rinne** is applied when the patient cannot resume hearing by air conduction after the fork is no longer audible by bone conduction (AC<BC). Rinne test interpretations are summarized in Table 4–2.

TABLE 4–1. SCHWABACH TEST RESULTS, TYPE OF HEARING IMPAIRMENT, AND LOCATION OF EAR DISORDER

SCHWABACH TEST RESULT	HEARING STATUS	LOCUS
Normal	Normal	None
Prolonged	Conductive loss	External and/or middle ear
Diminished	Sensorineural loss	Cochlear and/or retrocochlear

TABLE 4–2. RINNE TEST RESULTS, TYPE OF HEARING IMPAIRMENT, AND LOCATION OF EAR DISORDER

RINNE TEST RESULT		HEARING STATUS	LOCUS
Positive	AC ≥ BC	Normal or sensorineural impairment	None or cochlear-retrocochlear
Negative	AC < BC	Conductive impairment	External or middle ears

Weber Test

The Weber test extends the familiar experience of hearing one's own voice louder when an ear is blocked. The stem of the vibrating fork is held to the midline of the forehead, and the patient is asked to report whether the sound is heard in the left, right, or both ears.

In general, the patient perceives the sound of the fork in the ear with better bone conduction or greater conductive component. If the tone is heard in the reportedly poorer ear, a conductive hearing loss should be suspected for that ear. If heard in the better ear, sensorineural loss is suspected for the poorer ear. The fact that the patient lateralizes the perception to the conduction-impaired ear rather than to the better ear may seem incongruous to the patient and sometimes to the examiner.

The Weber test is most useful in instances of unilateral impairment, but ambiguity may develop when one ear has both conductive and sensorineural (combined) involvement or when a tuning fork of only one frequency is available. The clinician should use the Weber test only in conjunction with other tests and should not interpret the test by itself.

Bing Test

The Bing test is an application of the so-called occlusion effect, in which the fork is heard louder as the normal ear is occluded. If the auditory meatus is alternately occluded and left open, as the vibrating fork is held to the mastoid, an increase and decrease in loudness will be perceived by the normal ear (positive Bing). A similar result will occur with sensorineural hearing impairment, but the patient in whom the conductive mechanism is already modified, as in otitis media or otosclerosis, should not notice any loudness changes (negative Bing).

Reliability and Validity

With repeated careful administration of tuning fork tests, the examiner develops skill in their use. Problems of reliability (repeatability) ensue from judgment errors of both patient and examiner regarding the "moment of inaudibility" as the tonal experience decays into silence. The tests are more difficult to accomplish with children and patients with a limited attention span.

Reliability refers to the repeatability of test results. Validity here refers to the extent of testing what you think you are testing. It is possible to have very reliable and yet totally invalid results.

The clinician should avoid the use of low-frequency (128 and 256 Hz) forks, since they require control of background noise, as in a special sound-conditioned room, which is usually unavailable to the average practitioner. For physical reasons, a 500 Hz fork, rather than 1000 Hz and 2000 Hz forks, is better able to provide useful Bing test results.

A common error in the Rinne and Schwabach tests arises from the nature of bone conduction. A vibrating fork applied to the right mastoid vibrates not only the right temporal bone but the entire head; thus, the left ear is being stimulated simultaneously. Attenuation across the head is minimal. In the Rinne test the response to a bone-conducted stimulus will reflect the ear with better bone conduction, regardless of which ear it may be. Hence, it is possible to obtain the bone conduction response of the left ear when testing the right ear. And if bone conduction is greater than air conduction, the result is a **false-negative Rinne.**

Similarly, an **increased or prolonged Schwabach** for the right ear may actually be a response of the left ear in which bone conduction is better than in the right ear. The incidence of the **false-negative Rinne** and the **false increased Schwabach** may be reduced by a request for localization from the patient. It may also be controlled by the introduction of a masking noise into the nontested ear from a masking device such as a "Barany buzzer." This should be done with some caution, since the high-intensity masking noise may itself be lateralized across the skull and back to the tested ear.

But diagnostic "power" will increase when forks are coupled with the other audiometric tests in the diagnostic battery.

Because of these problems of validity and reliability, it is wise to use a battery of tuning fork tests, affording an opportunity for comparison among test indications, rather than to depend upon one test. This also partly accounts for the development of electrical audiometry.

PURE TONE AUDIOMETRY

Instruments called **audiometers,** which were developed in the early 1920's, sample the octave series of the C scale in the tradition of tuning forks. Tonal intensity could be maintained at a fixed level rather than one that immediately began a steady decay, as with tuning forks. The tone could be interrupted as desired, or the intensity could be attenuated at fixed intervals with arrays of electrical impedance—hence an opportunity to quantify the intensity of the sound. It remained only to apply a unit of intensity, a decibel notation, to the continuum of intensity, and the era of modern pure tone audiometry was born. The decibel (dB) is a very convenient unit that is the logarithmic ratio of two powers or pressures.

Pure Tone Audiometers

The "basics" of pure-tone audiometry.

The pure tone audiometer is an electronic device which produces sounds that are relatively free of noise or sound energy in overtones, hence "pure" tones. A selection of tones approximately preserving the C scale octave relations is available: 125, 250, 500, 1000, 2000, 4000, and 8000 Hz. Tones at half-octave intervals (750, 1500, 3000, and 6000 Hz) are also provided. The audiometer has three essential parts: a variable frequency oscillator to produce these sounds, an attenuator to permit variations of intensity (typically in 5 dB steps), and a transducer (either earphones or a bone vibrator and sometimes a loudspeaker) to convert electrical to acoustic energy.

Air Conduction and Bone Conduction

There are two sources of sound, conventionally. One is from earphones held snugly against the ears by a headband. Each ear is tested separately, and the results are graphed as the **air conduction** audiogram. The second source of sound is a bone conduction oscillator or vibrator held snugly against the mastoid (or forehead) by a headband. The vibrator sets the skull into oscillation with associated disturbance of the fluids of the cochlea. The results, graphed as the **bone conduction** audiogram, are usually interpreted as bypassing the middle ear, being a measure of "cochlear reserve" and reflecting the status of the auditory nervous system. We will see later how the latter interpretation is not entirely accurate but is generally useful.

Threshold

The objective of the measurement is to determine the lowest intensity level in decibels that can be heard for each frequency and thus the **threshold** of audibility for that sound.

Audiometric Zero and Intensity Range

The threshold hearing level derived for a patient is compared against audiometric "zero." This is the median average threshold of a large sample of young adults with no hearing complaints, no history of ear disease, and no recent colds. Each frequency has its separate zero with zero-calibrated values built into the audiometer output. Since "zero" represents an average value of threshold sensitivity, there must be lesser intensities available to measure even more sensitive hearing. The same scale has not always been used. Older test results may vary from current tests only because of the different standards.

All patients are compared to a group of young adults with normal hearing.

Audiometer intensities may range from -10 dB to as high as 110 dB. If a patient requires 45 dB of intensity above the normal to perceive a particular sound, his hearing threshold level is 45 dB; if his sensitivity is closer to the normal and he requires an increase of only 20 dB above normal, his threshold is a 20 dB hearing level. If it is indeed 10 dB *more* sensitive than the average, his hearing threshold level is designated as a negative value, or -10 dB.

Audiogram Notation for Air Conduction and Bone Conduction

The audiogram is a graph of the patient's hearing sensitivity for various frequencies. Measures are recorded for each ear separately, with frequency displayed on the abscissa and intensity on the ordinate. Standard symbols for air conduction and bone conduction are shown in the audiogram key in Figure 4–1. Air conduction symbols are connected by a solid line as illustrated on the audiogram. Bone conduction symbols are connected by a broken line when an air-bone gap exists; otherwise, they are not connected. Color coding is not necessary for identifying sidedness in this symbol system. However, if color is employed, red should be used for the right ear symbols and connecting lines and blue for the left ear. Graphing the right and left ears on separate audiograms has been used to avoid audiogram clutter.

Procedures for Threshold Determination

Patient Preparation

1. The patient should be seated so that he cannot see the control panel or the examiner. Many examiners prefer seeing the patient's profile.

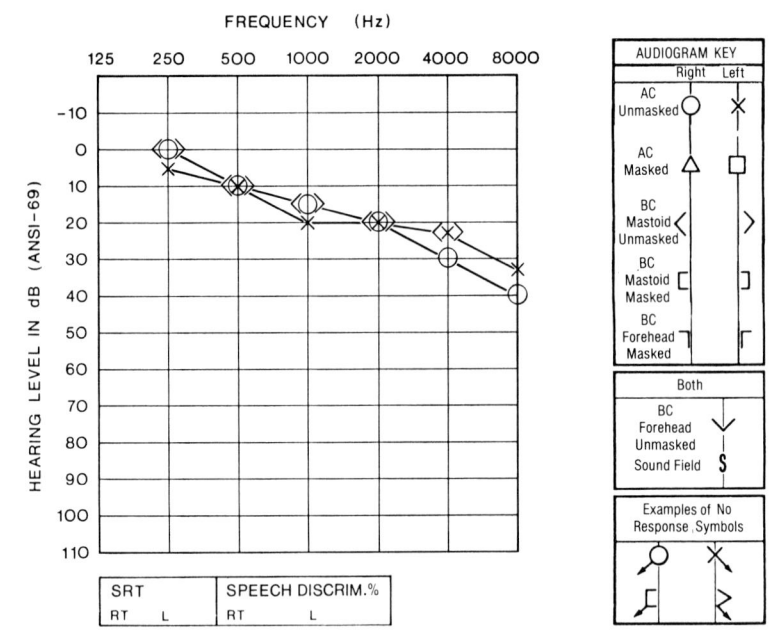

FIGURE 4–1. Audiogram and key showing standard symbols.

2. Items that might prevent proper fitting of the earphones or might otherwise affect the measurement results should be removed. Examples include earrings, glasses, hats, some wigs, chewing gum, and cotton in the external auditory canal. At this time the examiner might check for collapsing external auditory canal by observing the movement of the canal walls as he exerts pressure on the pinna and the tragus. Air-bone gaps of as much as 15 to 30 dB have been reported from collapsing canals. This problem can be dealt with by holding the earphones loosely against the pinna, presenting the test stimuli in a sound field while the opposite ear is muffed or masked, using circumaural earphone cushions, or inserting an earmold into the canal to maintain an air passage to the drumhead.
3. Instructions should be clear and concise. It is important that the patient know what to listen for and what response behavior is expected. He must be encouraged to respond to the faintest sound he can detect.
4. The opening in the earphone cushion is placed over the opening of the auditory canal.

Simply raising the hand or finger or depressing a button that activates a signal light is used as a response. The patient should be instructed to continue to respond as long as he detects the test signal. This allows the examiner to exert more control over the response behavior by varying not only the interstimulus interval but also the duration of the signal itself. This is particularly important when the patient gives numerous false-positive responses.

Threshold Determination

1. Test the better ear first utilizing the following sequence of frequency presentation: 1000 Hz, 2000 Hz, 4000 Hz, 8000 Hz, 1000 Hz (repeat), 500 Hz, 250 Hz. With the exception of the 1000 Hz repetition, the

same sequence can be used on the other ear. If a threshold difference of 15 dB or more exists in any octave interval, the half-octave frequency should be tested.
2. From a starting intensity of 0 dB hearing level (HL), the tone should be presented in ascending 10 dB increments using a tonal duration of one to two seconds until the patient responds. Hearing level is the intensity in decibels necessary for a response from the patient compared to the "zero" standard of the clinical audiometer.
3. The tone should be increased 5 dB, and if the patient responds, the tone should be decreased in 10 dB steps until it is inaudible.
4. Successive ascents using 5 dB increments should continue until a mode or typical response is obtained. This seldom requires more than three ascents.
5. After establishing a threshold for the initial test frequency, enter the appropriate symbol on the audiogram.
6. Proceed to the next frequency in the sequence. Initiate the tone at a level 15 to 20 dB below the threshold of the previously tested frequency. For example, if the threshold at 1000 Hz is 50 dB, begin testing at 30 or 35 dB at 2000 Hz.
7. This technique can be applied to establishing bone conduction thresholds as well as air conduction thresholds. In bone conduction threshold audiometry, 6000 and 8000 Hz are usually not available.

Validity

Comparison of air conduction and bone conduction thresholds continues to be an important determinant in the decision-making process related to medical and surgical management of otologic diseases. The difference between the air and bone thresholds is called the air-bone gap.

Interaural Attenuation and Cross Hearing

Interaural attenuation is the reduction of a signal's intensity as it is transmitted from one ear to the other. For example, a 1000 Hz tone presented to one ear at 65 dB (re audiometric zero) may be subjected to 55 dB interaural attenuation before it reaches the other ear as a 10 dB signal, which will be perceived only if the cochlea receiving it is sensitive to 10 dB signals. The terms *cross hearing* and *shadow curve* are commonly applied when the listener responds to the test signal in the nontest ear. Cross hearing most likely occurs through the skull via bone conduction even though the signal is presented through air conduction receivers.

It appears that 45 dB is a reasonable estimate of the minimum interaural attenuation that occurs before cross hearing results for the frequency range from 250 Hz through 8000 Hz. Therefore, whenever there are air conduction interaural threshold differences of 45 dB or more, the validity of the results obtained for the poorer ear should be questioned.

Large sensitivity differences between ears merit close attention.

Interaural attenuation for a signal presented by bone conduction is negligible. Placing the bone vibrator on either the mastoid or the frontal bone will produce vibrations throughout the entire skull. This provides a potential for essentially equal stimulation of both cochleas. The absence of significant interaural attenuation for bone conduction signals often creates problems in correctly identifying air-bone relationship in the test ear. For example, when an air conduction threshold difference exists between ears, the bone conduction threshold can, theoretically, be at least as good as the air conduction threshold of the better ear. Is the air-bone gap on the test ear a true gap or is it being cross-heard by the nontest ear?

In order to validate measurement results, it is necessary to exclude the nontest ear by means of an efficient masker so that responses obtained from the patient can be related to the test ear. Interaural attenuation data can be applied to "rules" regarding when to mask. In air conduction testing, whenever the presentation level of the test signal exceeds the bone conduction threshold of the nontest ear by 45 dB or more, masking should be used. In bone conduction testing, the nontest ear should be masked whenever an air-bone gap exists on the test ear.

Masking

Masking is the obscuring of one sound by another, or the elevation in the threshold of one signal produced by the introduction of a second signal. Although the most efficient masker of a pure tone is another tone of the same frequency, there is an obvious problem in differentiating the masked signal from the masker. Narrow band noise is the most efficient masker of pure tones. This consists of energy in a limited band of frequencies whose center frequency is the same as the pure tone signal being tested. Getting just the right level of masking is difficult. Too little masking results in hearing in the nontest ear. Too much will give a wrong threshold.

Hood (1962) outlined the fundamental methods of masking:

1. Establish the air conduction audiogram of both ears in the normal way of masking, if necessary, of the nontest ear, i.e., when the difference in the hearing loss between the two ears exceeds 50 dB.
2. Find the bone conduction threshold with the bone conductor applied to the mastoid of the test ear without masking of the nontest ear.
3. Apply the masking of the appropriate band to the nontest ear by means of an insert receiver and find a bone conduction threshold reading.
4. Apply the "shadowing" procedure thus: Increase the level of the masking noise by 10 dB above threshold and retest the bone conduction threshold. If the bone conduction threshold is raised by 10 dB, increase the masking intensity by another 10 dB and repeat. Continue this procedure until the point is reached at which the bone conduction remains constant with further additional incremented steps of 10 dB of the masking noise. This is the "change over" point and gives the true bone conduction threshold of the test ear.

Since masking signals follow the same rules of interaural attenuation as other air-conducted stimuli being presented through the same type of transducer, overmasking can occur when the level of the masker exceeds the level of the bone conduction threshold of the test ear by 45 dB or more. The linear relationship described previously will again be evidenced as overmasking occurs. The "plateau" method described here is graphically illustrated in Figure 4–2.

Speech signals follow the same general "rules" of interaural attenuation and cross hearing as those assigned to pure tone signals. Thus, the same

FIGURE 4–2. The "plateau" method of masking. Line AB illustrates the linear relationships between signal and masking noise when the tone is cross-heard on the masked ear. B is the change-over point, and line BC is the plateau. Note that as the masking level is increased, no changes in the threshold occur until point C is reached. At this level, the noise reaches the tested ear, and both ears are being masked (overmasking). The linear relationship, line CD, again exists between tone and masking signal.

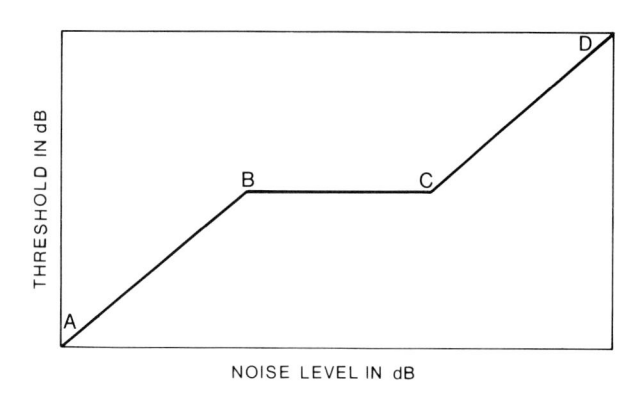

criterion regarding when to mask for pure tone testing is applicable when doing speech audiometry; i.e., when presentation level of the signal exceeds the bone conduction threshold of the nontest ear by 45 dB, masking should be used. The examiner must pay particular attention to this relationship when testing for speech discrimination, since the words are being presented at suprathreshold levels.

Although narrow bands of noise are preferred when masking pure tones, their frequency responses are too limited to mask the broad spectrum of speech. The preferred maskers are either white noise or speech noise, which is a white noise shaped by filters to resemble the frequency spectrum of speech.

Regardless of which noise is utilized, effective masking levels must be established for the particular audiometer being used. This can be accomplished by averaging the effective levels at 500, 1000, and 2000 Hz or through measurements on a group of individuals with normal hearing. The noise and speech can be mixed into the same earphone and speech thresholds determined when several noise levels are used. This tells the examiner the dial setting required to obtain the desired threshold shift in the masked ear.

Classic Interpretation

Audiograms may be interpreted according to degree of loss, configuration or pattern of loss, and air conduction–bone conduction relationships.

Audiogram interpretation and the air/bone gap.

A "pure" conductive loss may show any degree of impairment up to approximately 70 dB hearing level (HL). Losses greater than 70 dB HL must include some sensorineural component. Sensorineural losses may be of any degree, from the mildest to the most profound.

By far the most important contribution to audiogram interpretation is found in the relationships between air conduction and bone conduction thresholds, that is, the presence or absence of the air-bone gap. These relationships may be described generally as follows:

1. When bone conduction thresholds are better (more sensitive) than air conduction thresholds by 10 dB or more and are normal, the loss is **conductive** (Fig. 4–3).
2. When bone conduction thresholds are the same as air conduction thresholds and neither is normal, the loss is **sensorineural** (Fig. 4–4).
3. When bone conduction thresholds are reduced but are still better than air conductions by 10 dB or more, the loss is **mixed** or **combined** (Fig. 4–5).

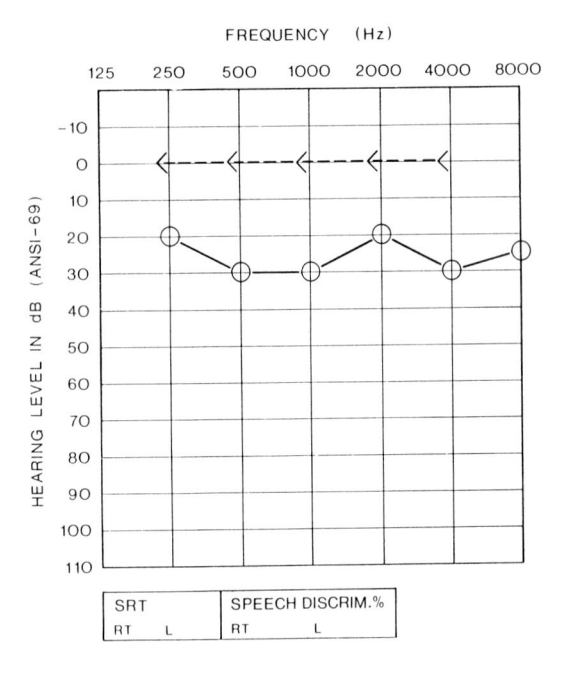

FIGURE 4–3. The reduced air conduction and normal bone conduction (air-bone gap) thresholds typical of a conductive hearing impairment.

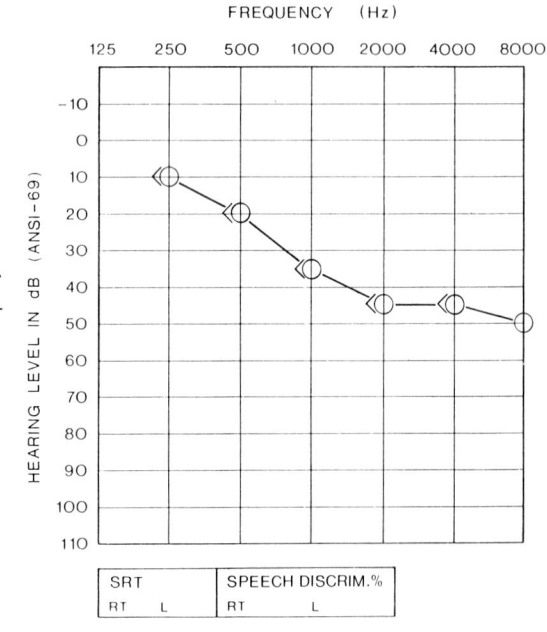

FIGURE 4–4. Equally reduced air and bone conduction thresholds typical of a sensorineural hearing impairment.

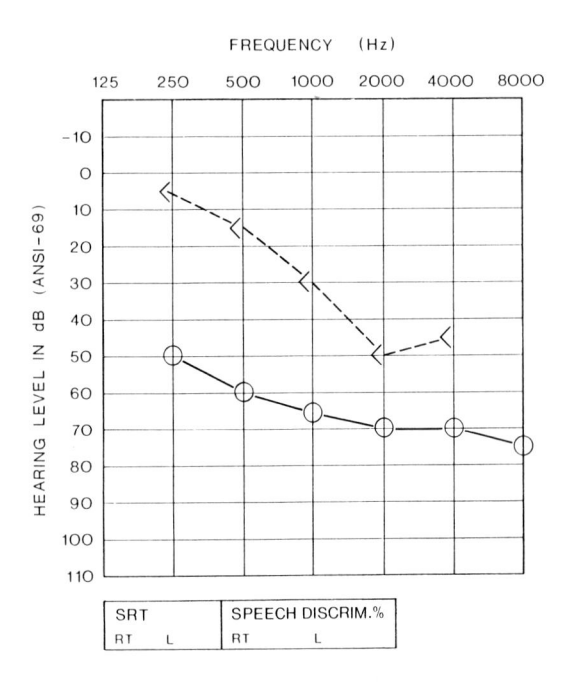

FIGURE 4–5. Unequally reduced air and bone conduction thresholds with retention of air-bone gap typical of mixed or combined hearing impairment.

When the air/bone gap is present there is some alteration of the conductive-transforming mechanism of the external or middle ear. An absent air-bone gap is seen as an index of sensorineural involvement. But the "Carhart notch" in otosclerosis is recognized as a bone conduction threshold elevation by a middle ear pathology, and others see a high frequency loss of bone conduction secondary to otitis media. So caution should be exercised with a strict interpretation of the absent air/bone gap.

More examples of typical audiograms are shown on pp 64–66.

IMPEDANCE AUDIOMETRY AND ACOUSTIC IMMITTANCE

Tympanometry

Impedance audiometry has assumed an increasingly important role in the audiologic assessment battery. Tympanometry is an **indirect** measure of the compliance (mobility) of the tympanic membrane and ossicular system under conditions of positive, normal, and negative pressure. High acoustic energy is introduced into the ear by a probe tube; some is absorbed, and the remainder is reflected back out the canal and collected by a second channel of the probe tube. In the normal ear, a measuring device shows the reflected energy to be less than the incident energy. On the other hand, when the ear is filled with fluid, the drum is thickened, or the ossicular system is stiffened, the energy reflected is greater than that in the normal ear. The amount of reflected energy is more equivalent to the incident energy. This relationship is used as a measure of **compliance.**

The tympanogram is a graphic representation of relative compliance in the tympano-ossicular system while air pressure changes are produced in the external meatus. Maximum compliance will be obtained at normal air pressure, while compliance is reduced as air pressure is increased or decreased from normal. Persons with normal hearing and with sensorineural hearing impairments will demonstrate a normal tympano-ossicular system.

Liden (1969) and Jerger (1970) developed a classification of tympanograms. The classification types, which are illustrated in Figure 4–6, are as follows:

Tympanogram types

Type A (Normal Tympanogram). Maximum compliance occurs at or near ambient air pressure, suggesting normal middle ear pressure.

Type A_S. Maximum compliance occurs at or near ambient air pressure, but compliance is lower than in type A. Fixation or stiffening of the ossicular system is often associated with type A_S.

Type A_D. Very high maximum compliance occurs at ambient pressure, with extremely rapid increase in compliance as pressures are reduced toward normal ambient pressure. Type A_D is associated with ossicular discontinuity or a monomeric tympanic membrane.

Type B. The tympanogram is relatively "flat" or "dome shaped," showing little change in the reflective quality of the tympano-ossicular system as air pressures change in the external canal. The type B tympanogram is associated with middle ear fluid, thickened drum, or impacted cerumen. The impedance characteristics of the tympano-ossicular system are dominated by the incompressible nature of the abnormality present. Small pressure changes have little effect.

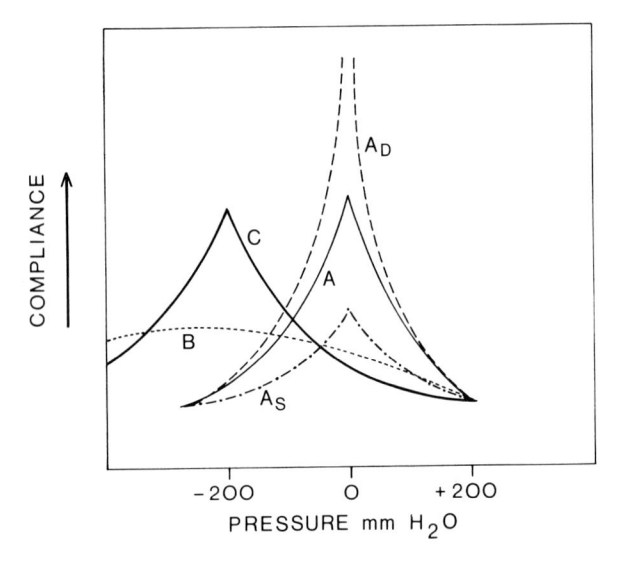

FIGURE 4–6. One system of tympanogram classification. A = normal; A_S = stiffened tympano-ossicular system; A_D = disarticulation; B = fluid, tympanosclerosis, or impacted cerumen; C = negative middle ear pressure.

Type C. Maximum compliance occurs with negative equivalent pressure in excess of 100 mm H_2O in the external canal. Otoscopic examination usually reveals a retracted tympanic membrane and may show some fluid in the middle ear.

A W-shaped tympanogram associated with an atrophic scar of the tympanic membrane or adhesion of the middle ear is discernible but usually requires a higher frequency probe tone before it can be demonstrated.

Acoustic Immittance

Acoustic immittance measurements have developed with appropriate technology to quantify the ease with which acoustic energy enters the ear. In addition or in place of patterns A, A_S, A_D, B, and C, acoustic immittance describes and quantifies primary physical parameters of those patterns. These include: (1) static admittance or tympanogram peak height; (2) equivalent canal volume or acoustic admittance with +200 decapascals of ear canal pressure; (3) tympanometric peak pressure (TPP), or the pressure at which maximum admittance obtains; and (4) the gradient (GR) or tympanometric width where there is 50 per cent reduction in the maximum admittance. Whether immittance introduces new fundamentals or is a more precise expression of the Jerger/Liden graphics may be argued. Nevertheless, a clearer separation of measures may be correlated with ear disorders. The advantage of a tympanogram type (A, etc.) is its broad-stroked description, which can be eye-balled and communicated easily among professionals. The admittance parameters have the potential for greater differentiation with a profile of three to four parameters rather than any single measure.

Table 4–3 shows means and 90 per cent ranges for four admittance parameters derived with the Welch Allyn Microtymp by Margolis and Heller (1987) for children and adults. The parameters include peak admittance for 226 Hz (Peak Ya), equivalent ear canal volume (+200 Vec), tympanometric peak pressure (TPP), and tympanometric gradient (GR).

The future direction for immittance testing exploits the differential ballistics and diaphragm physics made available by using Luscher frequency stimuli. The potential here is to expose the presence of eardrum calcified

TABLE 4–3. NORMATIVE VALUES FOR FOUR TYMPANOMETRIC PARAMETERS*

	CHILDREN		ADULTS	
	Mean	Range	Mean	Range
Peak Ya	.50	.22–.81	.72	.27–1.38
(mmhos)	.74	.42–.97	1.05	.63–1.46
+200 Vec (cc)	−30.4	−139–+11	−18	−33–0
TPP (daPa)	100	59–151	77	51–115
GR (daPa)				

*Derived by Margolis and Heller (1987) using a 226 Hz stimulus; parameters include peak eardrum admittance (Peak Ya), equivalent ear canal volume (+200 Vec), tympanometric peak pressure (TPP), and gradient (GR) or tympanogram width.

plaques, adhesions of the drum and ossicles, stapedial fixation, and other middle ear aberrations not presently discernible with the conventional 220 Hz stimulus.

Acoustic Reflex

The acoustic reflex arc contains a direct pathway of three to four neurons. It connects the auditory nerve to both stapedial motor neurons. The reflex occurs bilaterally even though the eliciting signal is introduced to only one ear. Contraction of the stapedial muscle, inserting in the head of the stapes, produces a stiffening effect on the tympano-ossicular system. The result is increased impedance, which manifests itself as an increase of the reflected energy of the tone being presented to the probe tube ear. Signal strength to elicit the reflex in subjects with normal hearing ranges from 70 to 90 dB HL with a pure tone stimulus.

A mild to moderate unilateral conductive hearing loss (30 to 40 dB HL) can elevate the acoustic reflex threshold by the amount of the conductive component when the stimulus is presented to the impaired ear. Elevated reflex thresholds have also been noted when cochlear losses exceed 60 to 65 dB HL on the stimulated ear.

The absence of the acoustic reflex can be attributed to various factors, including a significant sensorineural hearing loss in the ear being stimulated, a retrocochlear lesion in the stimulated ear, facial nerve involvement on the probe ear side, congenital absence of the stapedius muscle, surgical removal of the stapes, and a moderate or greater conductive hearing loss in the stimulated ear.

The acoustic reflex may occur but not be a recordable event. For example, the slight increase in tension caused by the contraction of the stapedius will not significantly change the existing stiffness of the tympano-ossicular discontinuity, since the contraction of the stapedius muscle cannot affect the stiffness of the system.

Elevated acoustic reflex thresholds occur when stimulating the affected ears of patients with extra-axial brain stem lesions and patients with multiple sclerosis. In both classes of patients, there tends to be a high incidence of acoustic reflex decay (continuous stimulation 10 seconds) with a reflex half-life as short as 3 seconds in some individuals. Abnormal reflex decay can be a sign of an eighth nerve tumor. The acoustic reflex is of value in assessing peripheral facial nerve function. The acoustic reflex can be used in assessing the hearing of neonates and other children too young to cooperate and as a part of a test battery for functional hearing loss. Its accuracy is sufficient for

TABLE 4–4. CONDITIONS CONTRIBUTING TO NORMAL, ELEVATED, AND ABSENT ACOUSTIC REFLEXES

Normal reflex (70 to 90 dB HL)
  Normal hearing
  Cochlear (recruiting) 60 dB HL
Elevated reflex (90 to 125 dB HL)
  Unilateral conductive hearing impairment
    (normal tympanogram, probe ear)
  Cochlear (80 to 100 dB HL)
  Retrocochlear hearing impairment
Absent reflex (125 dB HL)
  Eighth nerve lesions
  Unilateral conductive, probe ear
  Bilateral conductive
  Disarticulation, probe ear
  Facial paralysis, probe side
  Stapes fixation, probe ear

a rough estimate of the degree of loss. Table 4–4 summarizes conditions contributing to normal, elevated, and absent acoustic reflexes.

SPEECH AUDIOMETRY

Pure tone testing provides information regarding degree of hearing loss, audiometric configurations, and type of hearing loss, i.e., conductive or sensorineural. Although inferences are drawn and speculations are made from pure tone thresholds regarding the ability to hear and understand speech, pure tone audiometry is not a *direct* measure of those abilities and is subject to error. The need to assess the communication aspect of hearing led to the development of tests that utilized speech itself as the stimulus material. The development proceeded in two rather broad directions, namely, measures of sensitivity (speech reception threshold) and measures of understanding (word discrimination score).

Speech Reception (Recognition) Threshold

The speech reception threshold (SRT), which some refer to as the recognition threshold or speech threshold (ST), is the faintest presentation level in decibels at which the patient is able to correctly identify 50 per cent of the test words. An efficient test utilizing spondee (two syllable, equal stress) words has been developed which relates well with the threshold for sentences and continuous discourse. The speech reception threshold test utilizing spondee words is the conventional method of measuring sensitivity for the understanding of speech.

The test can be administered using either recorded words or live voice monitored with a VU meter. Better test-retest reliability is achieved when recorded stimuli are used. The usual response required of the patient is a verbal repetition of the words.

The spondee threshold agrees closely with the pure tone average of 500, 1000, and 2000 Hz or with the average of 500 and 1000 Hz when the hearing drops sharply through the middle frequencies. This relationship can serve as a means of assessing the reliability of the pure tone threshold data obtained for a specific patient. The examiner should question a difference of 15 dB or more between the SRT and the pure tone average. The patient may misunderstand the directions, become uncooperative, or sometimes exaggerate a hearing loss for personal gain.

Speech Discrimination

The assessment of a patient's ability to recognize speech provides much information. It is useful in diagnosis and treatment. A number of lists have been developed which are phonetically balanced, i.e., reflecting the relative incidence of the various speech sounds in the English language. Lists are also balanced for vocabulary familiarity. The word lists are presented to the patient at a level 30 dB or 40 dB above his SRT. The patient responds verbally. The speech discrimination score is a percentage based on the number of words the patient repeats correctly.

Retrocochlear lesions may be identified on discrimination tests.

The maximum speech discrimination score can generally be achieved when the word lists are presented at 35 to 40 dB above the SRT of patients with normal hearing, with conductive hearing loss, and frequently with mild sensorineural losses. The expected score presented at this level may approach 94 to 100 per cent. For severe hearing impairments, in which threshold approaches the output limits of the audiometer, test of discrimination is often accomplished at the patient's most comfortable level of loudness.

It may be necessary to present the word lists at several intensity levels in order to demonstrate the top score. For some of these patients the max may be no better than 50 to 60 per cent, and instead of a better score resulting from greater intensity of the stimulus words, the score may actually deteriorate. This phenomenon is called "rollover." The most dramatic speech discrimination losses occur when the patient has an eighth nerve lesion, such as an acoustic neuroma; scores of 20 per cent or less can occur even with relatively mild hearing levels.

The diagnostic power of discrimination tests may be enhanced by degrading the stimulus or its environment. For example, word lists with filtering of information above 500 Hz may be difficult to recognize through the ear opposite the temporal lobe tumor or the temporal lobe epileptic focus. Competing messages in the same ear with word lists will degrade performance in the ear with the "bottleneck" problem of the acoustic tumor.

Problems

The nature of the recorded word lists will determine the discrimination score. Variables such as precision of articulation, syllabic rate, and familiarity are standardized within a given set of word lists but not among the sets. Different sets yield different scores on the same ear.

AUDITORY BRAIN STEM EVOKED RESPONSE TESTS (ABR)

Electrical potentials evoked by sound from the brain (scalp) have been the subject of study by clinicians for three-quarters of this century. Various response components including late responses, middle latency responses, electrocochleography, and fast responses have attracted attention. Auditory brain stem evoked response testing (ABR) has become more important over the last 20 years and its clinical use has become widespread. ABR as we know it was not really performed until 1968. Testing equipment was advanced rapidly, and by 1971, Jewett had established definitive descriptions of what the ABR looked like. Advancing this technology has been the rapid decline in price and size of computer components that are essential to the operation of ABR measurement apparatus.

Technique

ABR's represent the electrical response of the eighth nerve and some portion of the brain stem which occurs in the first 10 to 12 msec after an auditory stimulus is sensed by the inner ear. By presenting a series of clicks to the ear, synchronous firing from high frequency auditory fibers is elicited. Unfortunately, it is difficult to read a single electrical response. In order to clearly see this pattern, an averaging scheme must be used to make each of the waves or stimulation sites apparent. Current standards present a click stimulus at 75 dB or 80 dB above the threshold. This click repeats at a fixed repetition rate, e.g., 11/sec or 33/sec, until 1500 or 2000 click responses have been "averaged." Electrodes placed over the mastoids are compared with the midforehead, creating an EEG. By averaging these waves of the EEG, a pattern emerges. These wave forms, which were described by Jewett in 1971, are labelled I through VII. It is clear now that waves I and II arise from the area of the eighth cranial nerve and that later waves are generated higher in the brain stem (Fig. 4–7).

Variables concerning the intensity and polarity of the click can be controlled. Patient conditions such as body temperature and medications can affect the recording, but under most circumstances they are not a significant problem in obtaining a reliable wave pattern.

The results of this test are then mapped out showing the relative time of waves I through V. This time period is referred to as the latency of each wave and the inter-wave latency intervals. It is also possible to describe amplitudes and a general morphology.

Clinical Use

Clinically, the ABR is useful in several situations. First, it is helpful in the diagnosis of cerebellopontine angle tumors. Second, it may be helpful in

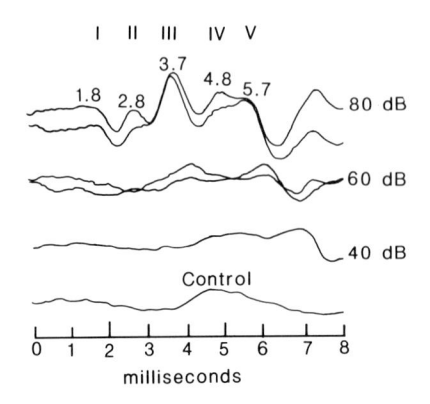

FIGURE 4–7. Jewett peaks are labeled with roman numerals. Each time 2000 clicks are averaged a new line is drawn. The lines are all reproducible. As the sound level approaches threshold, wave V appears to move to the right and other waves are less distinct.

FIGURE 4–8. The peaks are harder to see and occur at a later time. The wave form is difficult to reproduce on successive trials. This patient had a 1.5 cm acoustic neuroma.

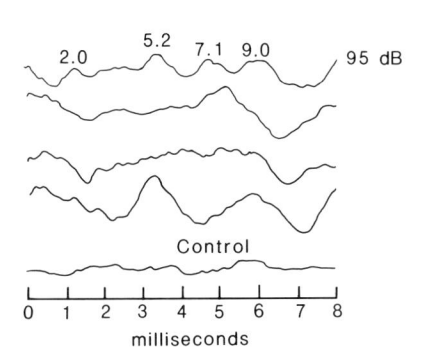

Meniere's disease and non-Meniere's dizziness. Third, it is helpful in establishing a hearing threshold for infants and difficult-to-test patients. Finally, it may have value in evaluating auditory processing disorders.

ABR testing became a prominent method for the diagnosis of acoustic neuromas. Selters and Brackmann reported very high predictive validity (approximately 95 per cent) for this testing method. Specifically, the test is better than any other audiologic test previously used. ABR measurements are obtained using the latency between waves I and V. As this wave I to III latency increases, the likelihood of a diagnosis of cerebellopontine tumor increases. This is true even when lesions are extremely small and other tests may be unrevealing. As the mass becomes larger and damage to hearing becomes more severe, the wave forms may become indistinct and may even disappear entirely (Fig. 4–8).

Meniere's Disease

In evaluating patients with Meniere's disease, it is important to look for retrocochlear causes of pathology, such as acoustic tumors. Additionally, it is important to ascertain that the problem is in fact in the cochlea itself. ABR is an accurate indicator of this process. Apparently, cochlear lesions have little effect on the latencies and conduction times in the pathway once the cochlear delay has been removed. As the intensity of the stimulus increases, the delay declines dramatically. This decline is nonlinear and is indicative of the loudness recruitment seen in Meniere's disease.

Threshold Evaluation

Patients who are uncooperative, or patients who cannot cooperate because of age or mental status, can have their hearing evaluated using ABR. It is difficult to obtain an absolute threshold, but it is possible to get close to a threshold using ABR. It is often used in neonatal intensive care situations, in which infants are particularly prone to sensorineural hearing loss. ABR thresholds with clicks correlate well with pure tone thresholds of 2 KHz and 4 KHz. They correlate less well with 500 Hz, although recent work with special filters and other strategies may help with this problem.

Brain Stem Disorders

Dysfunction of the brain stem can be evaluated using the ABR. The test has been found to be helpful in the diagnosis of multiple sclerosis. MS patients have ABR's that are difficult to reproduce. They have frequently changing ABR patterns that can be normal at one time and unrecognizable or distorted the next. It provides a way of documenting and, in some cases, diagnosing multiple sclerosis.

Coupled with the electric responses of later time frames to form an electric response battery, the ABR can help to describe the integrity of the entire auditory nervous system and address such considerations as auditory processing disorders and attention deficits.

PEDIATRIC AUDIOMETRY

The normal development of speech and language communication, personal and family relationships, and intellectual and educational achievement depends upon intact hearing. It therefore becomes incumbent upon the physician either to develop some skill in evaluating the hearing of young patients or to identify available resources to accomplish this objective.

It is now clear that the early years are especially important for the acquisition of language skills. Early identification is critical if the hearing-impaired infant is to have the necessary rehabilitative and educational assistance and if the family is to have the appropriate support. A child who is not learning to talk by the age of 12 to 18 months naturally causes parental anxiety; this condition should also signal to the family physician a high risk for hearing impairment and the necessity for hearing evaluation.

The hearing of all infants and children can be evaluated. The hearing measurement of children can be subdivided into four categories: (1) behavioral observation audiometry, (2) play audiometry, (3) speech audiometry, and (4) "objective" audiometry, usually requiring special technology. The physician should be able to perform selected tests from each of these categories.

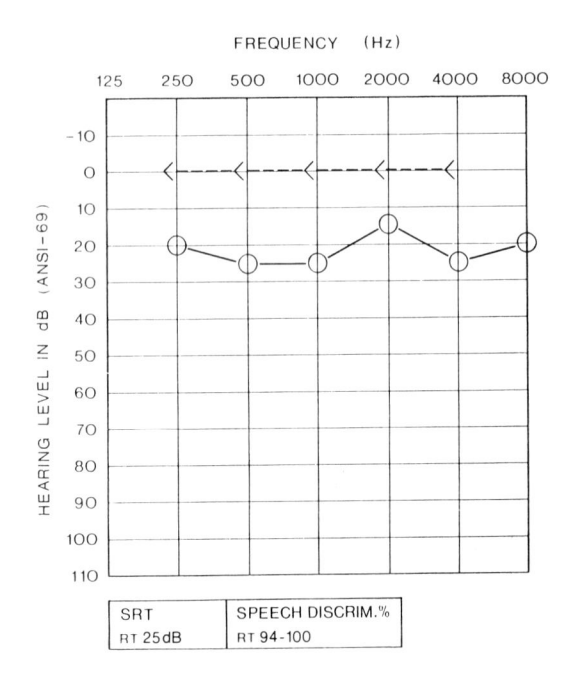

FIGURE 4–9. The most common conductive type audiogram is that for **serous otitis media.** Its air conduction audiogram is relatively flat, with a mild to moderate degree of impairment and an air-bone gap usually at all frequencies. Screening audiometry programs that ignore losses less than 20 dB HL are likely to miss the mild serous otitis shown here.

FIGURE 4–10. The increased impedance of acute purulent otitis media, tympanosclerosis, or ossicular disarticulation results in a larger air-bone gap and conductive impairment. But note that the discrimination score remains high despite the greater air conduction threshold loss.

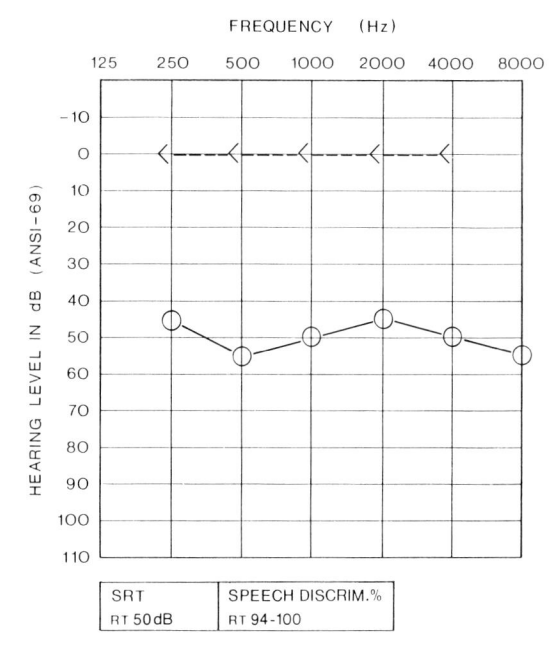

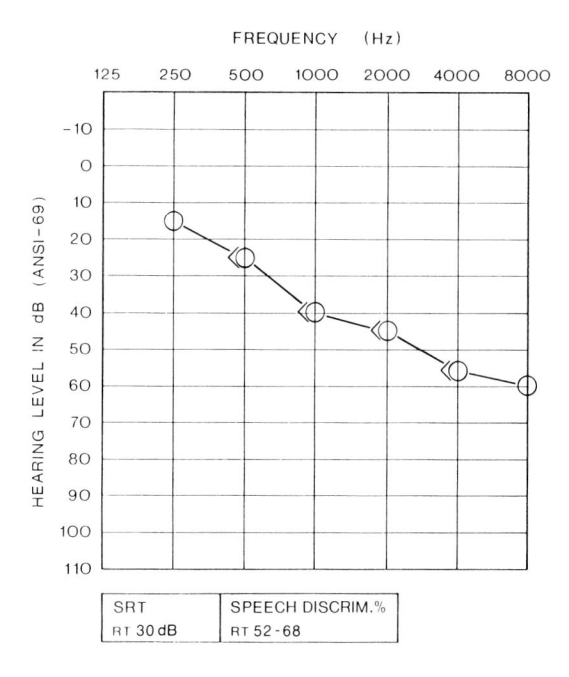

SRT	SPEECH DISCRIM.%
RT 50 dB	RT 94–100

FIGURE 4–11. The possibility that the aging process is general and not confined to one aspect of the auditory system should make the audiogram of presbycusis less predictable. Metabolic, vascular, atherosclerotic, cochlear-mechanical, sensory (organ of Corti), and neural degenerative changes have been suggested. A separate audiogram for each of these changes seems reasonable, but statistically a "typical" audiogram does emerge showing hearing impairment, greater for the high frequencies, with no air-bone gap. Speech discrimination is reduced, often beyond the prediction from the purely filtering model of the audiogram. This latter failure in discrimination, greater than would be expected from the audiogram, has earned the special name "phonemic regression" and is thought to be suggestive of neural and/or central factors.

SRT	SPEECH DISCRIM.%
RT 30 dB	RT 52–68

FIGURE 4–12. The average air conduction audiograms for successive age intervals found at the Wisconsin State Fair in 1954. The average audiogram of several 80-year-old patients is shown with the average speech audiometric findings. (Data from Hearing Levels of Adults by Age and Sex, United States, 1960–1962. Public Health Service Publication No 1000, Ser 11, No 11; recalculated by H Davis to ISO reference level for Chapter IV in Davis H, Silverman SR: Hearing and Deafness. New York, Holt, Rinehart and Winston, 1970.)

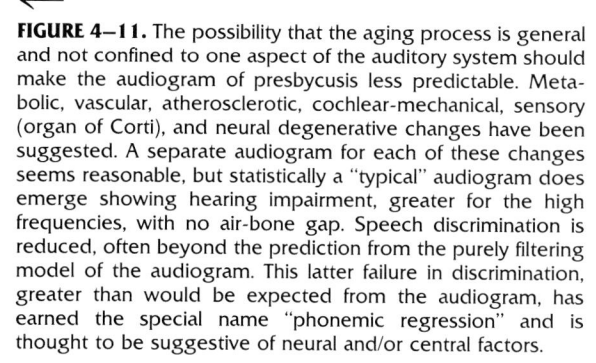

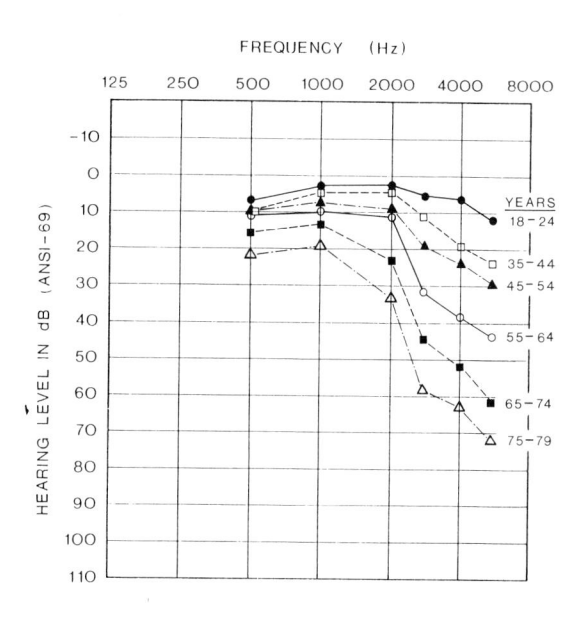

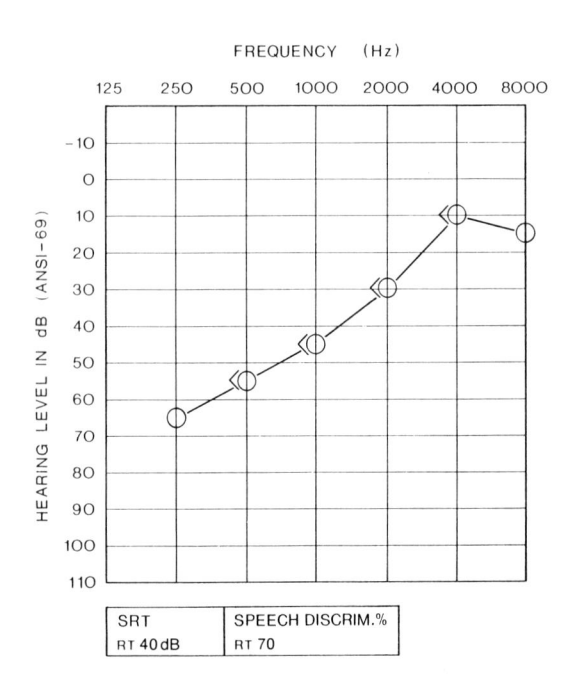

FIGURE 4–13. The characteristic notch at 4000 Hz (3000 to 6000 Hz) secondary to continuous noise exposure is seen. The notch deepens and widens with continuing exposure, lack of recovery time, and increase of intensity, especially for certain patients. Discrimination for speech is eventually compromised as the loss broadens to involve first 2000 Hz and then 1000 Hz.

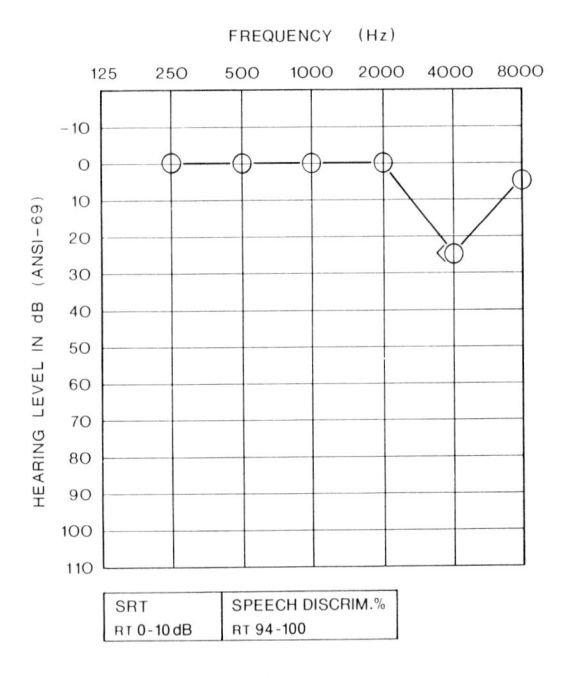

FIGURE 4–14. The progressive nature of otosclerosis requires at least two or three audiograms before the complete audiometric signature is manifest. The first audiogram shows a low-frequency compression resulting from the tightened ossicular chain (ankylosis). The notch in the bone conduction at 2000 Hz is called the "Carhart notch." The audiogram flattens in the next stage with air-bone gaps leveling. In the third stage, bone conduction worsens and there is a high-frequency sensorineural hearing loss, suggesting cochlear otosclerosis.

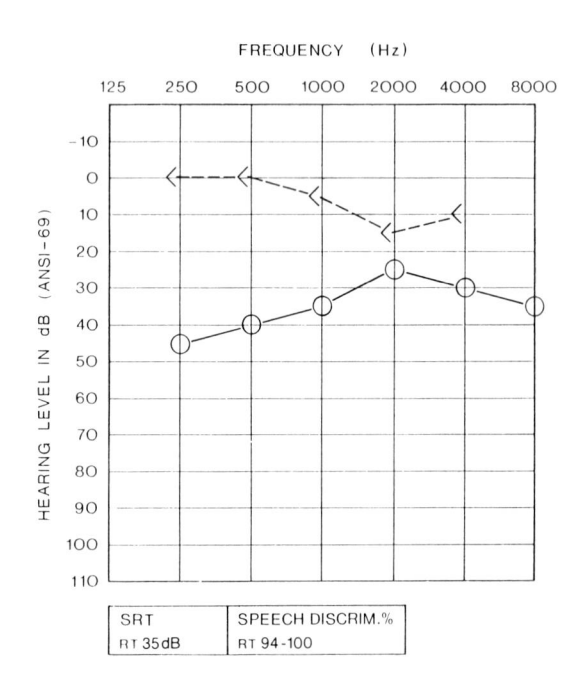

FIGURE 4–15. Another fluctuant hearing impairment meriting serial audiometry is exemplified by endolymphatic hydrops. This disease often shows a low-frequency sensorineural hearing loss. The degree of impairment may vary sometimes as much as 30 to 40 dB from day to day. Discrimination scores will vary with the degree of loss and can be very poor, especially in later or mature stages of the disorder.

Newborn to 24 Months

A number of clinical tests have given way to ABR testing in this area. Behavioral tests were often difficult to evaluate, were sometimes inconsistent, and required more experienced examiners. Most neonatal units use ABR to screen any child thought to be at risk for hearing loss. Current recommendations include:

1. Family history of deafness
2. Maternal rubella
3. Any child with anomalies of the head and neck
4. Bilirubin of 20 mg/dl or higher
5. Birth weight of 1500 gm or less

In "older" children, sedation with chloral hydrate may be necessary in order to limit their activity. This does not interfere with the test results. Rarely, only general anesthesia will settle a hyperactive child. While this is not desirable, it can be used successfully.

Instrumental or Operant Conditioning (Play Audiometry)

Two to Four Years

Instrumental or operant conditioning, known familiarly as "play audiometry," is remarkably successful with children two to four years of age. If the child will accept the headphones, and most will with proper inducements, this method will produce an audiogram for each ear separately, including an air-bone comparison.

The child is taught (conditioned) to put an object in a specific place (e.g., put a marble in the box, cow in the barnyard, a ring on the post, or the piece in the form board) when he hears the sound. Enthusiasm or praise is usually sufficient reinforcement. Threshold finding method is similar to that for adults. If those methods fail, an ABR may be useful.

Speech Audiometry

Using speech to measure hearing has impressive face validity. When the child can repeat words, point to the proper object, or perform the requested action, the examiner has sampled a considerable portion of the nervous system, but there are problems. The language chosen must be appropriate for the child's age and cultural environment. The intrinsic limitation on language development imposed by the hearing impairment will limit the range of vocabulary, sentence complexity, and so on. Nevertheless, certain practices in speech audiometry are useful.

Three-year-old and some two-year-old children can be taught to repeat familiar words or point to familiar objects. A speech reception threshold can be obtained if these words are spoken or played through a calibrated speech audiometer.

Discrimination scores can be accomplished with single syllable word lists at a kindergarten level (PB-K). A number of auditory discrimination tests (the DIP, the WIPI, and the G-F-W) have been standardized as picture identification tasks for young children.

For the child who is adventitiously hearing impaired, the physician ought to be able to obtain speech reception thresholds and discrimination estimates similar to those obtained in adults, but the language restrictions of the congenitally hearing impaired child will seriously limit applications without considerable listening training.

NONORGANIC HEARING IMPAIRMENT

A "functional" or "nonorganic" hearing impairment suggests that there is no otologic disorder to account for hearing loss behavior. It is partly a diagnosis by exclusion, yet many patients with this diagnosis exaggerate an existing organic hearing problem (functional overlay), making this criterion difficult to maintain.

An operational definition of some popularity relies on the identification of audiometric inconsistencies. The "nonorganic" component is the discrepancy itself. The rationale continues that if "nonorganic" is dependent upon audiometric discrepancy, then the confirmation of organic involvement is found in audiometric findings that are internally consistent. The more sensitive thresholds, especially the best speech thresholds and discrimination scores, are favored as organic measures when consistency has been demonstrated.

The identification of nonorganic hearing impairment depends upon the observation and measurement of inconsistent behaviors, primarily audiometric. These behavioral categories include the following:

1. Inconsistent communicative and social behaviors
2. Inconsistent audiometric behavior
3. Audiometric test-retest inconsistency
4. Audiometric intertest inconsistency
5. Special behavioral tests
6. Special "objective" tests

Special Behavioral Tests and Objective Tests

The **Stenger test** is usually an effective verification of unilateral deafness. A louder sound in one ear will mask the presence of the same sound at low sensation level in the other. If a tone is introduced into the good ear at 5 to 10 dB above threshold, it will be reported as audible. If the same tone is introduced simultaneously into the opposite ear at a higher loudness experience, it will be audible only in the second ear. If the second ear is truly hearing impaired, the patient will report hearing (good ear). But if deafness is feigned for the second ear, the patient will not report detection because awareness is controlled by the masking from the opposite ("deaf") ear. When sound is extinguished from the second ear, the patient will again report hearing from the first ear.

The **modified Stenger test,** or **speech Stenger,** is especially useful when the patient experiences diplacusis, a different pitch experience in the right versus left ear for the same objective pure tone stimulus. Diplacusis, often seen with cochlear disorders, will enable the awareness of sounds in both ears during the Stenger test. The Stenger test can then be accomplished with a speech stimulus in the same intensity relationships as the pure tone Stenger test.

The **Doerfler Stewart test** of either monaural or binaural impairment exploits the ability of those with normal hearing and conductive and sensorineural hearing impairments to recognize speech when background noise is 10 to 25 dB more intense than speech. The nonorganic impairment often shows a "noise interference level" at an intensity level **equal** to the speech intensity level.

Another test of the effect on speech is the "delayed feedback" or "delayed side tone" test. As the patient reads aloud, his speech is recorded and played back to him with a 0.2 second delay time through earphones. Changes in fluency, rate, and intensity level, sometimes rather dramatic, will occur when delayed speech reaches an interfering intensity level. It is most effective with claims of profound unilateral (good ear masked) or bilateral impairment. Those with valid hearing impairment will demonstrate no disturbance.

Objective tests cited earlier are useful with the problem. The patient is betrayed by a normal acoustic reflex threshold while feigning total deafness. The ABR threshold is obviously useful and is instructive in describing a functional component superimposed on an organic loss.

HEARING CONSERVATION IN INDUSTRY

Although some industries have had effective hearing conservation programs for many years, proliferation of such programs did not occur until the passage of the federal Occupational Safety and Health Act (OSHA), which mandated efforts to protect the hearing of employees working in areas of high noise levels. The act specifies noise measurement techniques, provides guidelines for noise control, suggests allowable exposure durations for various noise levels, and outlines a hearing conservation program.

To determine the effect of the noise on hearing, it is necessary to establish pre-employment or pre-exposure baseline hearing data. This serves several functions: (1) it establishes a base line against which subsequent hearing test results can be compared; (2) it identifies hearing loss that existed prior to placement in an environment with potentially damaging noise levels; and (3) it helps to establish the employer compensation liability.

Although personal ear protective devices (ear plugs or muffs) serve to reduce the level of noise reaching the ear, the most effective means of employee protection is reduction and control of the environmental noise level itself. Assessment of the effectiveness of the protective measures can be accomplished by periodic monitoring of the employees' hearing as well as the noise levels of the environment.

HEARING AIDS

Anyone who has trouble hearing and understanding speech should be considered for amplification. Fitting a hearing aid is a complicated process involving not only the severity and type of loss, but also ear differences, discrimination skills, and other psychoacoustic variables. It must also address cosmetic considerations, family and social pressures, sensorimotor skills, and independence. The Food and Drug Administration regulations mandate a 30-day trial for the new hearing aid user, a time to explore whether the instrument is appropriate and effective.

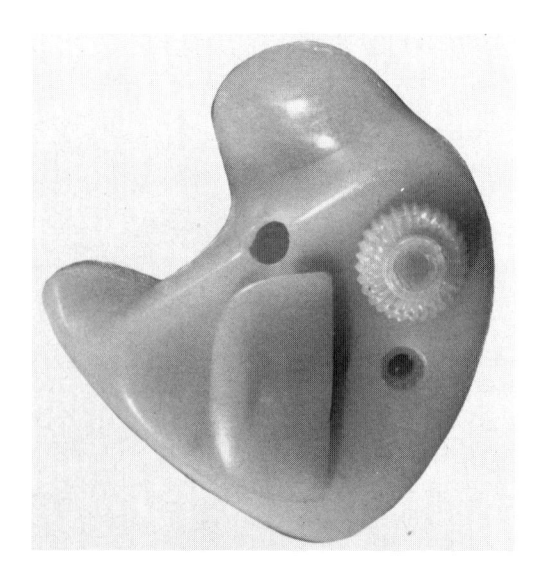

FIGURE 4–16. "In-the-ear" (ITE) hearing aid.

Amplification Features

A hearing aid is a miniature public address system. It has a microphone, an amplifier, a loudspeaker, and a battery as power source. It is further adapted with gain control, tone control, and maximum power control. Recently, automatic signal processing devices have been added in an effort to improve the signal-to-noise ratio in background noise. These components are "packaged" for wearing in the ear (ITE) (Fig. 4–16) behind the ear (BTE) (Fig. 4–17), and on the body (Fig. 4–18). The smallest of the ITE type are the "canal" aids with some components set deeper in the canal and closer to the eardrum.

Hearing Aid Selection

Once it has been determined that an individual would benefit from hearing aid use, the specifications for that aid must be selected. A number of methods and formulas have been developed to accomplish this objective. Generally, each selection procedure requires audiometric information consisting of (1) the hearing thresholds, (2) the most comfortable level (MCL) and (3) the loudness discomfort level (LDL). The various formulas are

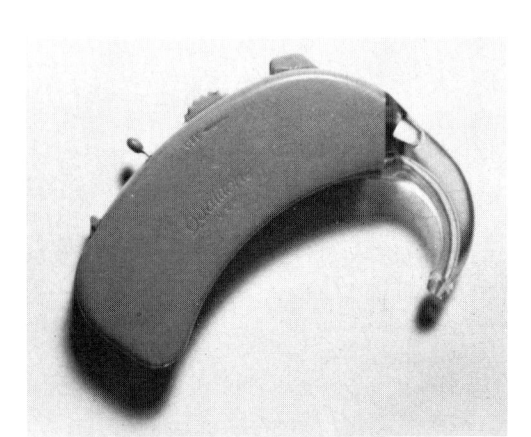

FIGURE 4–17. A "behind-the-ear" (postauricular) hearing aid.

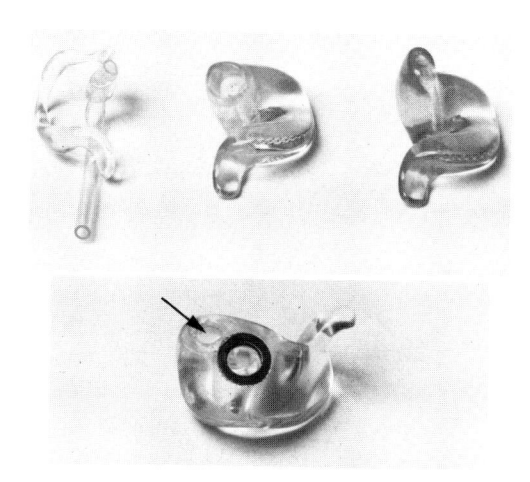

FIGURE 4–18. Earmold types. *Above,* From left to right are a nonoccluding earmold with tube held by a retainer, an earmold with a short and hollowed bore, and a standard earmold. *Below,* Earmold with vent indicated by arrow.

similar in that they prescribe the amplification needed to optimize speech discrimination without reaching the loudness discomfort level. Usually, the threshold of each frequency is multiplied by a factor that may range from approximately 0.33 to 0.50 depending on frequency.

These formulas do not propose that the hearing loss will be completely compensated by the hearing aid. Indeed, a person with a 60 dB sensorineural hearing loss would find 60 dB of gain intolerable and would prefer a gain of 30 dB to 40 dB.

Behind the Ear (BTE) and in the Ear (ITE)

The choice between BTE and ITE style of hearing aid depends upon severity of hearing loss and patient preference. With advances in hearing aid technology, ITE hearing aids can be used with hearing losses of up to 70 to 80 dB hearing level. ITE aids, with large vents or the so-called IROS fitting, can be effective with precipitous hearing losses of higher frequencies.

The canal style hearing aid, popular because of cosmetic appeal, provides benefit for mild-to-moderate hearing losses. However, it has less flexibility in frequency response and available gain compared with the BTE or ITE hearing aids. Canal fittings are further handicapped in small ears where venting is difficult, and the user experiences a "down-the-barrel" enclosure effect.

Ear Selection

Binaural hearing is strongly recommended whenever possible. The advantages of binaural amplification may include (1) improved speech discrimination in background noise; (2) binaural summation, which results in a loudness advantage compared with the loudness when listening to the same signal monaurally; (3) the "squelch effect," or suppression of background noise when attending to a primary signal; (4) elimination of the head shadow effect; (5) localization; and (6) judgments of naturalness.

For personal or for audiologic reasons, some patients may not be candidates for binaural amplification. Therefore, it becomes necessary to select the one ear that can benefit most from amplification. Generally speaking, the ear chosen is the ear with the better speech discrimination and widest dynamic range. The dynamic range is the difference between the hearing threshold level and the threshold of discomfort.

Unilateral Hearing Loss. If the unilateral hearing loss does not exceed 60 to 70 dB hearing loss, if speech discrimination is relatively good, and if amplified sound is tolerated well, amplification can be used in the impaired ear. This arrangement will provide the user with some binaural cues and will minimize the head shadow effect.

If the impaired ear does not meet these criteria, a CROS (Contralateral Routing of Signals) hearing aid can be used. The microphone is housed in one hearing aid, and the amplifier and receiver are located in the second hearing aid. This arrangement also can be built into eye glasses. The signal, therefore, is delivered from the impaired ear to the ear with normal hearing. A radio frequency circuit may be used to transmit sound from one side to the other. Although the CROS hearing aid does little to improve localization, it does occasionally prove helpful in certain noise listening conditions and also minimizes the head shadow effect.

Variations of the CROS, namely, the Bi-CROS or the Multi-CROS, can be used when a significant hearing loss exists in the better ear, and the poorer ear is not deemed suitable for amplification. The Bi-CROS has a microphone in each hearing aid and a single amplifier feeding sound into the better ear.

Hearing Aids for Children

Amplification for hearing-impaired children should be recommended as early as possible. As soon as hearing measurements indicate the presence of a hearing loss sufficient to cause a delay in the child's speech and language development and medical evaluation indicates the loss is not reversible, hearing aid usage should be initiated.

For obvious reasons, the hearing-impaired infant is unable to provide the audiologist with much information regarding how the aid sounds or with data regarding speech discrimination function with various aids. The choice of hearing aid is usually based not on direct psychoacoustic measures of aided hearing performance but on the electroacoustic characteristics of several suitable instruments and an extrapolation of data obtained when those aids were used by older children and adults. Any error in fitting an aid to a very young child should be in the direction of underfitting rather than overfitting the loss, avoiding high acoustic gain and excessive maximum power.

Cochlear Implants

Some individuals receive little benefit from hearing aid use. Indeed, the hearing aid may provide the individual with only vibrotactile stimulation and not with improvement in speech discrimination.

For some of these individuals, the cochlear implant has been recommended. The cochlear implant is designed for patients with profound sensorineural deafness. The functioning of the sensory hair cells is impaired in these individuals, whereas the auditory nerve may still function adequately. Several kinds of cochlear implants have been developed. All the devices have four features in common: a microphone for picking up the sound, a microelectronic processor for converting the sound into electrical signals, a transmission system for relaying the signals to the implanted components, and a long, slender electrode that the surgeon inserts into the scala tympani to the inner reaches of the cochlea. This electrode is intended to deliver electrical stimuli directly to the fibers of the auditory nerve in one or more places. Some devices developed have only single-channel electrodes, whereas others have multichannel electrodes.

Depending on the type of cochlear implant, it may provide information regarding intensity, segmental features such as voiced/voiceless, consonants, tempo and rhythm, intonation, and word stress. These auditory cues in conjunction with lipreading may significantly improve speech discrimination abilities. The multichannel devices seem to be assisting lipreading and, in a few patients, seem to improve discrimination without lipreading. Work in this area continues to be experimental, and clinical decisions should remain conservative and realistic.

AURAL REHABILITATION

Aural Rehabilitation for Adults

The goal of aural rehabilitation should be to improve the patient's effectiveness in everyday communications. Developing a rehabilitation program to achieve this goal is dependent on a comprehensive assessment of the individual patient's communication problem and social and vocational communication needs. Participation by the patient depends on his motivation; therefore, it is important that he understand his communication problem and be informed regarding ways therapy can assist him in resolving or minimizing some facets of that problem. Since communication is a dynamic process occurring between two or more persons, inclusion of the patient's family or close friends during specific segments of therapy may prove beneficial.

Lipreading, or speechreading, and auditory training are traditional components of aural rehabilitation. The patient should be helped to make maximal use of visual clues while recognizing some of the limitations of speechreading. During auditory training, the therapist may have the patient practice auditory discrimination by having him listen to monosyllabic words in quiet and noisy surroundings. Additional work might center on localization, telephone use, means of improving the signal-to-noise ratio, and care and maintenance of the aid.

Patients may be seen on an individual basis and in group sessions. Counseling and specific tasks can often be accomplished most effectively on a one-to-one basis. Group sessions allow an opportunity to structure various types of communication situations that might be considered normal, everyday situations for demonstration and teaching purposes.

The patient should be assisted in developing an awareness of environmental cues and how those cues can supplement his reduced auditory information. How language structure imposes certain restraints on the speaker should be demonstrated. Environmental clues, facial expression, body movement, and natural gesture tend to complement the spoken message. When the auditory information necessary for comprehension is incomplete, the environmental clues serve to fill in the gaps. All aspects of aural rehabilitation should help the patient to interact more effectively with his environment.

Education of the Hearing-Impaired Child

The importance of preschool training for hearing-impaired children cannot be stressed too strongly. Infants before the age of six months have been observed to grossly discriminate speech patterns. First words generally emerge between 12 and 16 months of age, and children between one and five years of age are most responsive to learning language. When diagnosis, hearing aid usage, and language training are initiated early, maximum stimulation can be provided during that critical period for language acquisition. The increasing number of schools and rehabilitation centers providing training for the hearing-impaired child reflects this concern for early educational and language training opportunities. Many programs do not have a minimum age for enrollment; the only requisite for admission is identification of the hearing loss, regardless of age.

Preschool Programs

Because of the influence of the parents' language input on the child's early linguistic maturation, parents are encouraged to assume a more active role in the education and language training of their hearing-impaired preschoolers. Many preschool programs offer descriptions and demonstrations of techniques that the parents can use at home to assist the child in developing lipreading and listening skills. The parents also receive instruction regarding hearing loss, language development, communication problems, hearing aid maintenance, and child management. During the first three years, the parents are the primary source of language stimulation. Most educators feel that as the parents' knowledge about communication increases, their effectiveness as teachers will likewise increase.

When the child is enrolled in a nursery school program, the teacher assumes a more dominant role in language training. The parents' participation, while not diminishing, is more closely related to the teacher's lesson plans in order to supplement and expand classroom activities at home. The emphasis of the nursery school program is on language development, expansion of vocabulary, improved communication skills, and socialization with peers.

As a child prepares to leave the preschool program, placement recommendations are made based on his language and communication skills, social maturity, and academic readiness. Placement options include a self-contained class for hearing impaired in a day school setting, residential school for hearing impaired, or full- or part-time integration (mainstreaming) in a normal hearing class.

Integration (Mainstreaming)

Children who are integrated into normal classes generally have developed good aural/oral communication skills. However, children whose primary method of communication is sign language may attend normal classes with the help of an interpreter.

Efforts should be made to provide the necessary adaptations and services to maintain the child in the regular classroom. The ambient noise level and reverberation characteristics of typical classrooms tend to create difficulties for the hearing-impaired student. Preferential seating near the teacher, acoustic treatment of the classroom (drapes, carpet, acoustic tiles), or the use of an auditory trainer can alleviate the problem significantly. Academic tutoring with emphasis on previewing and reviewing new vocabulary and new concepts can serve to fill in what the child misses in the classroom.

Methodology

The form of communication one should teach the hearing-impaired child has been a matter of controversy for many years. Initially, the methods were reduced to oralism vs. manualism (sign language), with many advocates and variations on each theme.

There are several different methods used to develop oral language/speech skills by deaf children. They emphasize lipreading and hearing in various combinations from the extreme of amplified hearing exclusively and without lipreading to almost the same emphasis on lipreading. As hearing aids of greater strength and fidelity were developed, the child's residual hearing became a more important determinant of the educational method. The development of auditory training devices with the teacher wearing a microphone/transmitter at a constant distance from her mouth afforded greater speech precision and better speech/background noise relationships.

American Sign Language (Ameslan) is a system of handsigns in general use in this country. Each gesture signifies a word, a phrase, or a concept. Abstractions tend to be communicated in concrete terms. The main criticism of Ameslan is its crude grammar. The syntactical structure does not mirror spoken or written English nor are there markers for past tense or plurals. The various shadings and subtle differences in words may come blurred in Ameslan communication.

Finger spelling is a finger alphabet. It is usually used to augment rather than replace Ameslan. Finger spelling is important when exact names and numbers need to be communicated in an otherwise almost totally Ameslan system. Ameslan and finger spelling were developed into variants, such as Seeing Essential English (SEE), which answered some of the criticism of Ameslan alone. The "combined approach" and the "Rochester method" joined manual communication with speech.

More recently, *Total Communication* has emerged to become a leading educational philosophy and practice. Its basic tenet is that every possible means should be used to communicate with the hearing-impaired child. The child is exposed to sign language, finger spelling, natural gestures, facial expressions, lipreading, bodily movement, speech heard through a hearing aid, and auditory training. Some critics question whether multimodal or even bimodal stimulation can be facilitative or just confusing. Many believe that the teacher's bias determines the child's eventual choice of communication modality.

Whatever approach is best suited for the hearing-impaired child depends upon a number of factors such as age of onset and of identification, severity and type of hearing loss, auditory processing skills, home environment and parental involvement, and age of hearing aid usage. In an enlightened program, advocacy of a method does not occur. The unique talents and needs of the individual child are considered by the professional along with the family, and the educational method or approach is tailored to meet those needs.

References

Bekesy GV: Zur theorie des hörens bei der Schallaufnahme durch Knochenleitung. Ann Physik 13:111–136, 1932.

Carhart R: Clinical application of bone conduction audiometry. Arch Otolaryngol 51:798–807, 1950.

Glasscock ME, Jackson CG, Josey AF: The ABR Handbook. 2nd ed. New York, Thieme Publishers, 1987.

Hood JD: Bone conduction: A review of the present position with special reference to the contributions of Dr. Georg von Bekesy. J Acoust Soc Am 24:1325–1332, 1962.

Jerger J: Clinical experience with impedance audiometry. Arch Otolaryngol 92:311–324, 1970.

Jewett DL, Williston JS: Auditory evoked far fields averaged from the scalp of humans. Brain 94:681–696, 1971.

Katz J: Handbook of Clinical Audiology. 3rd ed. Baltimore, Williams & Wilkins, 1985.

Liden G: The scope and application of current audiometric tests. J Laryngol Otol 83:507–520, 1969.

Margolis RH, Heller JW: Screening tympanometry criteria for medical referral. Audiology 26:197–208, 1987.

Paparella MM, Brady DR, Hoel R: Sensorineural hearing loss in chronic otitis media and mastoiditis. Trans Am Acad Ophthalmol Otolaryngol 14:108–115, 1970.

Selters WA, Brackmann DE: Acoustic tumor detection with brainstem electric response audiometry. Arch Otolaryngol 103:151–124, 1977.

Tonndorf J: Bone conduction: Studies in experimental animals. Acta Otolaryngol Suppl 213:1–132, 1966.

5

DISEASES OF THE EXTERNAL EAR

by Lawrence R. Boies, Jr., M.D.

The external ear includes the auricle, or pinna, and the external auditory canal. The canal has both a cartilaginous and a bony portion. As noted in Chapter 2, the tympanic membrane divides the middle ear from the external ear.

The external ear serves to collect and funnel sound waves to the middle ear structures. Because of the unique anatomy of the auricle and the curved, or spiral, configuration of the canal, the external ear protects the tympanic membrane from injury, foreign bodies, and thermal effects (see Fig. 1–1).

The external ear affords protection to the tympanic membrane.

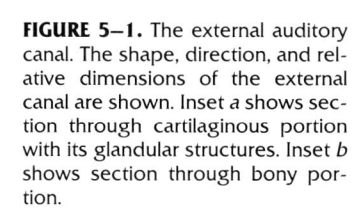

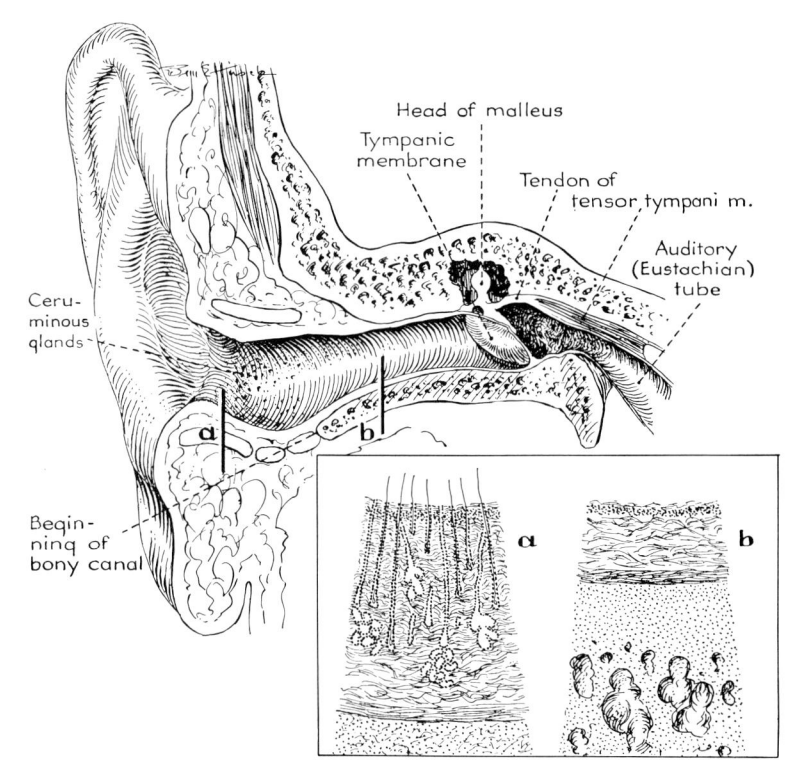

The external auditory canal is roughly 2.5 cm long, extending from the anterior lip of the concha to the tympanic membrane. The outer one third is referred to as cartilaginous, while the inner two thirds is the bony portion (Fig. 5–1). The narrowest area of the canal is near the bone-cartilage

FIGURE 5–1. The external auditory canal. The shape, direction, and relative dimensions of the external canal are shown. Inset *a* shows section through cartilaginous portion with its glandular structures. Inset *b* shows section through bony portion.

77

junction. Only the outer one third, or cartilaginous portion, is mobile. When one inserts an otoscope, the auricle normally must be pulled posterolaterally in order to view the bony canal and tympanic membrane. Together with the outer layer of the tympanic membrane, the canal forms an epithelium-lined pouch that can trap moisture, making this area susceptible to infections under certain conditions.

The auricle is pulled posterolaterally to insert an otoscope.

The skin lining the cartilaginous portion is thicker than that lining the bony portion and contains hair follicles, the number of which varies among individuals but which help afford a barrier in the canal. The anatomy of the bony external auditory canal is unique in that it is the only place in the body where there is skin directly overlying bone with no subcutaneous tissue. Thus, this area is extremely sensitive and any swelling is very painful, as there is no room for expansion.

One way the external ear provides protection is through the formation of cerumen, or ear wax. Most of the glandular structures, the sebaceous and apocrine glands that produce cerumen, are located in the cartilaginous portion of the canal. The exfoliated cells of the stratum corneum also contribute to the formation of this unusual substance, which provides a protective, water-repellent coating to the canal wall. The pH of the combined ingredients is around 6, an additional factor that acts to prevent infection. Furthermore, migration of desquamated epithelial cells provides a self-cleansing mechanism from the tympanic membrane outward.

Cerumen has protective qualities.

Infection and inflammation of the external ear canal are among the most common otolaryngologic problems, especially during warm, humid weather. The more common presenting symptoms of conditions involving the auricle and external auditory canal may include the following: pain (otalgia), itching, swelling, bleeding, and a blocked sensation.

Ear canal infections are more common in a warm, humid environment.

A careful examination of the ear and surrounding region will usually reveal a specific problem. The importance of the remainder of the otolaryngologic examination should be stressed. Points of interest in the patient's history might include past external ear infections, recent swimming, other skin problems, allergies, trauma, and the use of ear jewelry, especially items containing nickel.

CERUMEN

Cerumen is the product of both sebaceous and apocrine glands, which are located in the cartilaginous portion of the external auditory canal. There are two basic types, "wet" and "dry." Their autosomal pattern of inheritance was not widely recognized until 1962 when it was reported by Matsunaga. The wet type is dominant. Caucasians have a greater than 80 per cent probability of having a wet, sticky, honey-colored ear wax that may darken on exposure to the elements. Blacks have an even greater predisposition toward this type. In the Mongoloid races, including the American Indian, the dry, scaly, "rice brand" phenotype is more frequently seen. Neither variant has a clear association with inflammatory conditions involving the external canal.

Cerumen is known to have protective qualities. It acts as a vehicle for the removal of epithelial debris and contaminants away from the tympanic membrane. It provides lubrication and prevents desiccation of the epidermis with its associated fissuring. Studies have demonstrated that wet and dry cerumen have quite similar bactericidal effects. Although these studies were carried out in vitro, it is probable that in vivo results would be comparable.

Cerumen has bactericidal properties.

It is the fatty acids, lysozyme, and immunoglobulin components of cerumen that are believed to be inhibitory or bactericidal.

Excessive cerumen accumulation is not a disease. Some people produce an unusual amount just as some perspire more easily than others. In some individuals, the cerumen can cake and form a solid plug; in others, a large amount of cerumen with a buttery consistency blocks the canal. The patient may experience a sense of blockage or pressure. When a solid plug of cerumen becomes moistened, such as following bathing, it may swell and cause temporary hearing impairment.

There is a general tendency for cerumen to be drier in older individuals because of physiologic atrophy of the apocrine glands with subsequent lessening of the sweat component of the cerumen. Also, in older patients in particular, canal blockage may be due not to wax but to a build-up of epithelial debris. Because the normal external canal is narrowest at the midportion, use of cotton swabs can push the cerumen deep to the narrow isthmus against the drumhead, making removal difficult and painful.

Cerumen tends to be drier in older individuals.

Removal of cerumen is most commonly done with a curette under direct visualization. One should emphasize here the importance of adequate visualization and exposure. In most cases this is best accomplished with head mirror illumination and a simple speculum. Water irrigation by special metal syringe is another common method. Some physicians recently have preferred the use of a dental-type irrigating device. While the pinna is elevated superiorly and posteriorly to straighten the canal, body temperature water is administered in a posterosuperior direction to allow the water to pass between the mass of cerumen and the posterior wall of the canal. In a fair number of cases, however, after several irrigations the patient will still complain of blockage, and examination reveals a large plug still present. At this point suction is occasionally employed. The Hartmann type of alligator forceps is also useful in removing hard plugs. In using irrigating devices one must take great care not to damage the tympanic membrane. If there is any question of a prior tympanic membrane perforation, irrigation should be avoided.

Several methods are available for cerumen removal.

Avoid irrigation if a tympanic membrane perforation may exist.

Occasionally the patient is sent home and instructed to use an appropriate ear drop for a brief period of time. Such preparations include mineral oil, hydrogen peroxide, Debrox, and Cerumenex. Long-term or improper use of some commercial preparations may cause skin irritations or even contact dermatitis.

KERATOSIS OBTURANS AND CHOLESTEATOMA OF THE EXTERNAL AUDITORY CANAL

Two distinct entities, keratosis obturans and cholesteatoma of the external auditory canal, may present as a keratin plug occluding the external auditory canal. Keratosis obturans is usually bilateral and may be associated with bronchiectasis and chronic sinusitis. The patient presents with pain and hearing loss. Although widening of the external canal and hyperplasia and inflammation of the epithelium and subepithelium are observed, there is no bony erosion. Both an overproduction of squamous epithelium and squamous plugs and a faulty migration of the epithelium have been postulated to cause this condition. Plug removal and treatment of the inflammatory process are the recommended therapy.

Cholesteatoma of the external auditory canal is usually unilateral. The patient presents with dull pain and intermittent otorrhea due to bony erosion and secondary infection. Circumscribed periostitis and faulty epithelial migration have been postulated as causes. Treatment consists of debridement of the bone, or canalplasty and tympanomastoidectomy where appropriate, to prevent the progression of bony erosion.

EXTERNAL OTITIS

The term external otitis has long been used to describe a variety of conditions. The spectrum of infections and inflammations includes both acute and chronic forms. Under infections one must consider bacterial, fungal, and viral agents. Noninfectious inflammations include the dermatoses, some of which are primary conditions directly involving the external ear. Shapiro has pointed out that the distinction between an external otitis that is primarily a dermatosis and that which is of infectious origin is not always clear. A dermatosis may become infected after a time, while a skin infection may develop an eczematous reaction to the causal organism. Again, a careful history and examination often will give a clue to the primary condition.

Emphasis here will be on the infections and inflammatory conditions of the external ear which most frequently confront the physician.

Infections may occur as a result of certain predisposing factors, such as the following:

1. Change from the normally acid pH of the canal skin to an alkaline pH
2. Environmental changes, especially the combination of increased temperature and humidity
3. A mild trauma, frequently due to excessive swimming or cleaning of the ear

Principles in management which apply generally to all types of "external otitis" include the following:

1. Careful cleaning of the canal by suction or cotton wipes
2. Evaluation of discharge, canal wall edema, and tympanic membrane, if possible; decision whether to use a wick to apply medication
3. Selection of local medication

Acute Infections and Inflammations

Furunculosis (Otitis Externa Circumscripta)

This common condition is confined to the fibrocartilaginous portion of the external auditory meatus (Fig. 5–2). If the examiner passes a speculum into the canal without first retracting the pinna to observe the ear, this infection could be missed. Furunculosis begins in a pilosebaceous follicle and is usually caused by *Staphylococcus aureus* or *S. albus*. In more severe cases, surrounding cellulitis may extend beyond this area. Pain may be quite marked because of limited room for expanding edema in this anatomic area. Eventually, abscess formation occurs and a "point" may form, at which time drainage can be established by needle. Otherwise, treatment will depend on furuncle size and the surrounding reaction. Systemic treatment may be advisable. Topical medications (Table 5–1), heat, and an analgesic are generally prescribed.

Furunculosis begins in a pilosebaceous follicle.

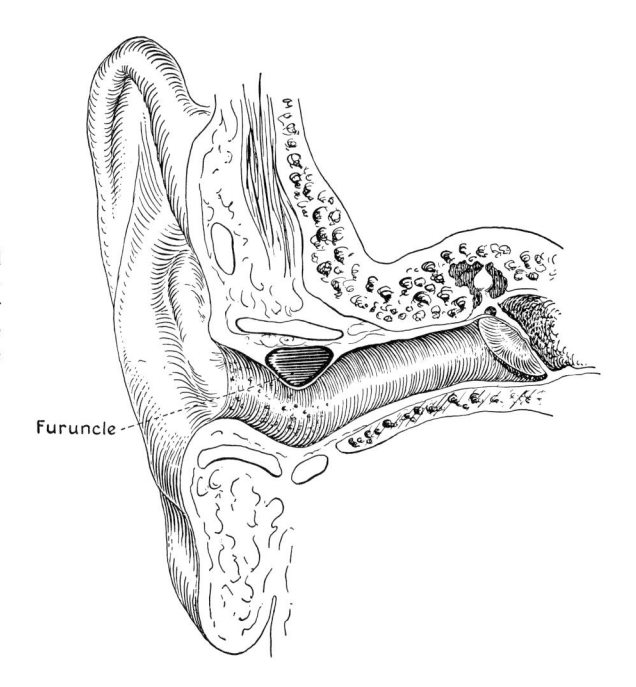

FIGURE 5–2. A furuncle in the external auditory canal may be extremely painful because it develops in a membranocartilaginous area where there is little room for expansion. Invariably this cause of pain in the area of the ear is suspected when passive movements of the auricle cause discomfort.

Diffuse Otitis Externa

This type of infection is otherwise known as "swimmer's ear." Occurring during hot, humid weather, it is caused predominantly by the *Pseudomonas* group and, less often, by *Staphylococcus albus, Escherichia coli,* and *Enter-*

Swimmer's ear is common during hot, humid weather.

TABLE 5–1. TOPICAL DRUGS FOR TREATMENT OF EXTERNAL OTITIS

DRUGS	SPECTRUM OF ORGANISMS
Colistin	*Pseudomonas aeruginosa*
	Klebsiella-Enterobacter group
	Escherichia coli
Polymyxin B	*Pseudomonas aeruginosa*
	Klebsiella-Enterobacter group
	Escherichia coli
Neomycin	*Staphylococcus aureus* and *S. albus*
	Escherichia coli
	Proteus group
Chloramphenicol	*Staphylococcus aureus* and *S. albus*
	Klebsiella-Enterobacter group
	Escherichia coli
	Proteus group
Nystatin Clotrimazole Miconazole Tolnaftate Carbol-fuchsin (Castellani's paint)	Fungal organisms
Thymol/alcohol Salicylic acid/alcohol Boric acid/alcohol Acetic acid/alcohol	Mainly fungal organisms—may also be effective against bacterial infections by lowering pH of canal skin
M-cresyl acetate Aqueous merthiolate	Generally antiseptic

obacter aerogenes. Lakes, oceans, and private pools are all potential sources of this type of infection. Diagnostic features include:

1. Tragal tenderness
2. Severe pain
3. Canal wall swelling involving most of the canal
4. Scanty discharge
5. Normal or slightly diminished hearing
6. Absence of obvious fungal particles
7. Possible presence of tender regional adenopathy

Diffuse otitis externa usually is very painful.

The stroma overlying the bone of the inner third of the canal is very thin, allowing minimal room for swelling. Thus, the subjective discomfort the patient experiences is often out of proportion to the extent of the disease visualized.

Use of an ear wick may be indicated.

Because of the degree of circumferential canal wall edema often seen, a wick may be required to bring medication into contact with most of the canal wall. A short strip of gauze packing may be used for this purpose; however, specially designed products, such as the Pope Otowick, are now widely available and are generally preferred. An alligator-type ear forceps is ideal for introduction of ear wicks, with the wick then kept saturated with the selected otic solution. One has the choice of several different otic medications for the treatment of diffuse external otitis (see Table 5–1). Frequently used otic drops include Cortisporin (polymyxin B, neomycin, hydrocortisone), Coly-Mycin S (colistin, neomycin, hydrocortisone), Pyocidin (polymyxin B, hydrocortisone), VoSol HC (acetic acid—nonaqueous 2 per cent, hydrocortisone), and Chloromycetin (chloramphenicol).

Only in severe cases should systemic drugs be considered; bacterial sensitivity studies are recommended. Systemic antibiotics are required especially if perichondritis or chondritis of the ear cartilage is suspected. Diffuse external otitis secondary to acute or chronic otitis media may be encountered. Treatment then must be aimed primarily toward the middle ear involvement in these cases.

Fungal Infections (Otomycosis)

Several fungi may cause inflammatory reactions in the external auditory canal. The two most common fungi found there are *Pityrosporum* and *Aspergillus (A. niger, A. flavus).* The *Pityrosporum* organism may cause only a superficial scaling similar to dandruff of the scalp, may be associated with an inflammatory seborrheic dermatitis, or may form the basis on which more uncomfortable infections develop, such as furuncles or eczematous changes. The same is true of the *Aspergillus* organism. It is sometimes found in the canal in the absence of any symptoms except for a sense of blockage, or it may be involved in an inflammatory process, invading the epithelium of the canal or drumhead and causing acute symptoms. Occasionally, *Candida albicans* is encountered.

Fungal infections are much more common in the southeastern United States and in the tropics. Also, it should be noted that there has been a tendency in lay terminology to attribute most external ear infections to "a fungus." This obviously is not the case.

Treatment again involves careful cleansing of the canal by wiping, suctioning, and, at times, even gentle irrigation followed by drying. Available otic solutions such as VoSol (acetic acid—nonaqueous 2 per cent), Cresylate (m-cresyl acetate), and Otic Domeboro (acetic acid 2 per cent) are of value in most cases. Recently, there has been increasing acceptance of specific topical fungicides such as nystatin-containing preparations (Mycostatin, Mycolog) and clotrimazole (Lotrimin), which are not available solely as otic preparations.

Herpes Zoster Oticus (Ramsay Hunt Disease)

The onset of facial paralysis, when accompanied by otalgia and a herpetic eruption involving portions of the external ear, is considered to be caused by a viral infection involving the geniculate ganglion. The vesicular skin involvement may be limited to the specific area of the external canal innervated by a small sensory branch of the seventh cranial nerve, extend to the auricle, or have faded by the time the patient is seen. Other combinations of symptoms may exist owing to progressive involvement of vestibular and acoustic fibers of the eighth cranial nerve. Treatment is mainly symptomatic, although systemic steroids are not infrequently prescribed for the facial paralysis, depending on results of nerve function testing.

Perichondritis

This condition develops when trauma or inflammation causes an effusion of serum or pus between the layer of perichondrium and the cartilage of the external ear. In most cases of trauma, the injury is in the form of a laceration or is the result of incidental damage during surgery on the ear. Occasionally, it follows simple bruising without hematoma. An inadequately treated furuncle provides a ready source of a potent causative agent, such as a virulent type of micrococcus (*Staphylococcus*), streptococcus, or *Pseudomonas aeruginosa*. The diagnosis is simple; the involved part of the auricle swells, becomes reddened, feels warm, and is very tender upon palpation (Fig. 5–3).

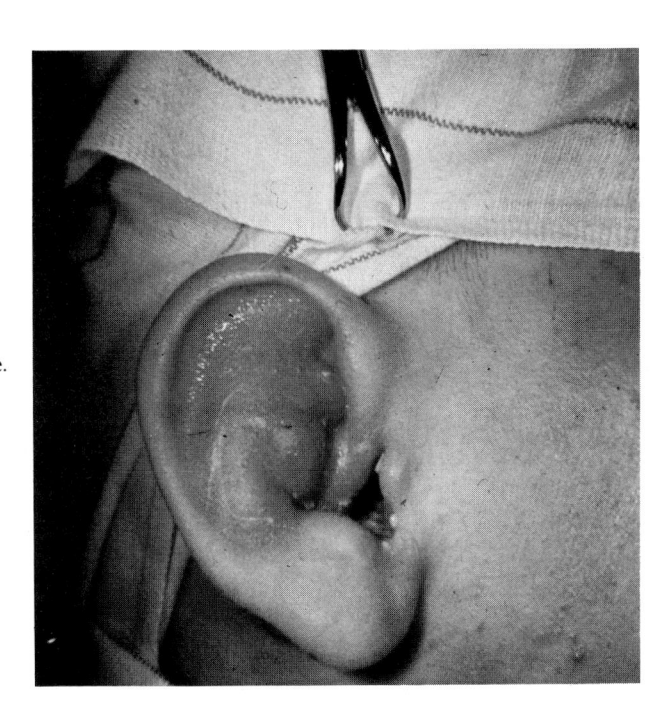

FIGURE 5–3. Perichondritis of the auricle.

A parenteral antibiotic is indicated as well as topical treatment of any associated canal infection. Choice of preferable drug is based on culture results or other indications of the organism involved. If the condition seems to be spreading and there is evidence of fluid under the perichondrium, incision for the evacuation of fluid is indicated. Because cartilage has no direct blood supply, when the perichondrium is separated, cartilage necrosis may ensue. Necrotic cartilage, therefore, should be excised and drainage maintained. Gross permanent deformity of an auricle can result from perichondritis.

Incision and drainage of fluid or pus under the perichondrium is usually indicated.

Eczematous Dermatitis

The practicing otolaryngologist not infrequently encounters a lesion that involves the external canal and adjacent portions of the meatus and concha and is characterized by redness, itching, swelling, and a stage of watery exudation followed by crusting. As implied earlier, the differentiation between primary dermatosis and infection may be difficult. A seborrheic dermatitis or a skin reaction related to neomycin sensitivity may present in this fashion. The label of eczematous dermatitis is often used because of the characteristic appearance of the lesion.

Differentiation between a primary dermatosis and infection may be difficult.

When a considerable portion of the auricle is involved and the lesion seems to be spreading, wet dressings using a solution such as Burow's may be advisable for 24 to 48 hours, at which time fluorinated steroid ointment and solution are employed. Naturally, if an infection is suspected, topical antibiotics may be required.

If the acute stage is not controlled, chronic changes characterized by thickening of the skin, and even stenosis of the external canal, may develop. The chronic stage may be troublesome because of periods of uncomfortable itching and the tendency of the patient to resort to scratching, thus causing further irritation. In such cases consultation with a dermatologist may be beneficial.

Chronic Infections and Inflammations

Bacterial infections of the external auditory canal wall may become chronic owing to lack of treatment, inadequate treatment, recurrent trauma, the presence of a foreign body such as a hearing aid mold, or a draining otitis media. Management involves identification of the organism and factors contributing to the chronicity.

Long-standing cases may cause gradual stenosis of the canal due to fibrotic thickening of the wall (Fig. 5–4). A surgical procedure involving resection of the thickened canal tissue and grafting has been devised and has been successful in alleviating an otherwise irreversible condition.

Chronic fungal infections may occur in mastoid cavities in need of cleaning.

The most common chronic fungal ear infections seen by the otolaryngologist are those infesting mastoid cavities in need of cleaning. Following removal of infection debris, such cavities may be treated with antifungal drops or powdered with a combination of neomycin and boric acid.

Another frequently seen chronic condition might be termed the "chronic itchy ear" for want of a better term. In most cases this condition would best be classified as a primary noninfectious dermatosis. There may have been a history of an acute external otitis. On examination the canal skin appears dry, with absence of cerumen and occasional signs of excoriation. No exudate or discharge is present. Treatment is directed toward control of itching.

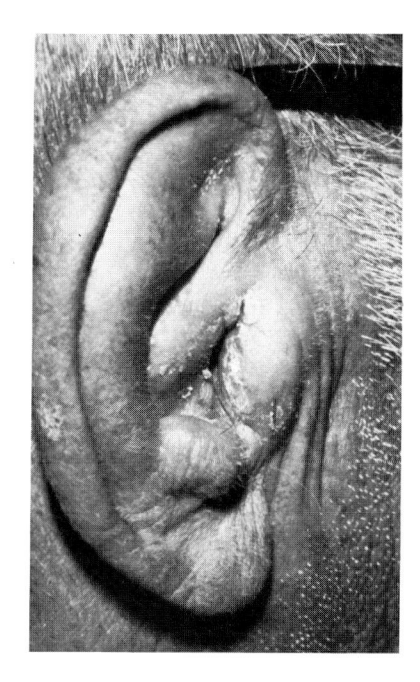

FIGURE 5–4. Stenosis of the external auditory canal caused by fibrotic thickening of the walls due to chronic infection.

Usually long-term application of hydrocortisone cream is required. In some cases psychiatric help may be indicated.

Necrotizing External Otitis

In treating external otitis in the elderly person, one should always bear in mind the possibility of necrotizing external otitis, a severe infection involving the temporal bone and soft tissue of the ear. Caused by *Pseudomonas aeruginosa*, it is generally found in elderly diabetics and is considered more common in warm climates.

Necrotizing external otitis is more commonly seen in elderly diabetics living in a warm environment.

Patients with recalcitrant external otitis of more than two weeks' duration should be evaluated carefully for other symptoms indicating necrotizing external otitis. In some cases patients have presented with seventh cranial nerve dysfunction and normal ear examination. Comprehensive diagnostic imaging, including CT, bone scan, and gallium scans, can be helpful to determine the presence of this disease. Routine bone scans alone are not sufficient to differentiate between severe external otitis and necrotizing external otitis.

Although extended mastoidectomy was the favored mode of treatment, with the advent of *Pseudomonas*-specific antibiotics, systemic antibiotic intervention is currently the first line of therapy. It has been postulated that invasive surgery without antibiotic coverage will encourage the spread of infection in these already debilitated patients. It is therefore recommended that surgery be limited to the removal of sequestra, drainage of abscesses, and local debridement of granulation tissue. The recommended drug therapy is an aminoglycoside plus an anti-*Pseudomonas* beta-lactam antibiotic.

Systemic antibiotic intervention is currently the first line of therapy.

It must be emphasized that even though the patient may appear to be cured, prolonged therapy of at least six weeks is recommended, therapy that is now possible on an out-patient basis owing to the advances in home health care.

Prolonged therapy is recommended.

Relapsing Polychondritis

This disease of unknown etiology leads to inflammation and destruction of cartilage. While this is a generalized disorder of cartilage, involvement of the nose and ears is seen in 80 to 90 per cent of cases. The auricular deformity resembles an acute infectious perichondritis or an inflamed cauliflower ear. The loss of cartilage may lead to "floppy" ears and saddle-nose deformities. Alternation of the inflammation between the two ears (without predisposing cause) or the presence of fever suggests this disorder. Tinnitus and vertigo may be encountered as well as hearing loss due to collapse of the external auditory meatus. When the larynx, trachea, and bronchi are involved, hoarseness and even death due to collapse of laryngotracheal and bronchial walls may result.

Involvement of both nasal and aural cartilage is seen in up to 90 per cent of cases.

Disease activity fluctuates, and the disorder has an unpredictable prognosis. There may be a single occurrence or multiple recurrences over many years. Treatment includes salicylates or corticosteroids for an acute attack, although some controversy surrounds the use of the latter. Dapsone has been used to prevent recurrent attacks. Affected structures should be protected from trauma.

TRAUMA

Lacerations

The most common lacerations of the ear occur as a result of the patient digging in an ear with a finger or using an instrument such as a hairpin or paper clip. A laceration of the canal wall may result in transient bleeding, thus worrying the patient, who will usually then consult a physician. No treatment other than keeping the ear dry is normally required. The patient is reassured following examination to rule out tympanic membrane perforation.

Severe lacerations involving the auricle should be explored for cartilaginous damage. The cartilage should be approximated carefully before plastic repair of the skin is done. Such wounds should be observed closely for the development of infections of the perichondrium. Prophylactic antibiotics are given if there has been gross contamination of the wound or exposed cartilage.

Frostbite

Frostbite of the auricle can occur rapidly in environments with a low temperature and a high wind chill factor. Because it is insidious, it is not painful until rewarming occurs. Outcome depends on the depth of injury and the duration of exposure. Injury is thought to occur by direct cellular damage and by microvascular insult leading to local ischemia.

Rapid rewarming in water between 100 and 108°F is recommended for frostbite.

Rapid rewarming is the current therapeutic recommendation. The affected ear should be bathed in water at a temperature between 100 and 108°F until there is objective evidence that thawing has occurred. Analgesia will be required. The full extent of injury may not be apparent for several days, so the patient who is sent home must be followed carefully.

Surgical debridement should be delayed. Clinically apparent infection should be treated with antibiotics. Patients with very stiff cartilage of the pinna probably had prior frostbite.

Hematoma

This condition is most frequently seen in wrestlers and boxers. Untreated, it may result in the so-called cauliflower ear. Simple needle aspiration of the hematoma has been used in the past, but most physicians now recommend more vigorous treatment by incision and drainage of collected blood under sterile conditions, followed by the application of a pressure dressing, particularly in the conchal area. Localized pressure is better obtained by using through and through sutures over dental rolls or other similar materials. Treatment is best accomplished as soon as practical following injury, before organization of the hematoma begins. Wrestlers should be reminded about wearing protective headgear, even during practice.

MALFORMATIONS

A variety of congenital abnormalities involving the external ear and canal result from maldevelopment in both the first and second branchial arches. The auricular deformities are the most prominent, of which the most common is the lop-ear deformity in which the ears protrude excessively. Several plastic procedures have been devised for the correction of this condition. Further discussion of this topic is included in Chapter 27.

Other malformations of the auricle include an abnormally large or small pinna (macrotia and microtia). Congenital defects such as rudimentary ear appendages and even total absence of the ear are occasionally encountered and may be associated with partial or complete stenosis of the canal. Such conditions may involve both soft tissue and bone. In select cases surgical procedures can correct hearing loss resulting from canal stenosis.

Another, rarely seen, developmental defect of the ear involves first branchial cleft abnormalities. These present as cysts or sinus tracts involving the pinna and external auditory canal. There are two types of first branchial cleft abnormalities. Type I anomalies contain ectodermal tissue only, are

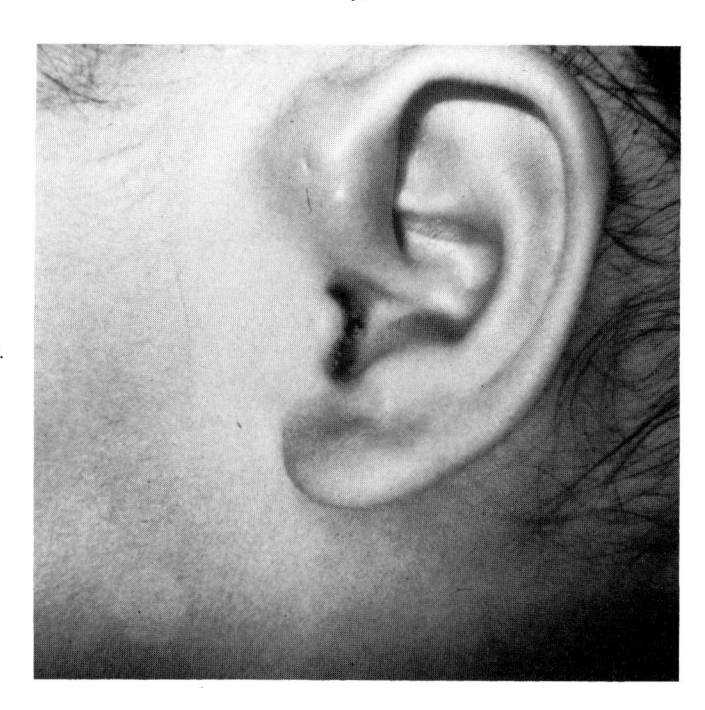

FIGURE 5–5. Infected preauricular sinus.

free of cartilage, and are of first cleft origin only. Type II abnormalities contain both epithelium of first cleft origin and cartilage from the first and second arches. The sinus tract may be observed to drain intermittently and occasionally become infected (Fig. 5–5). Usually a tract can be identified by methylene blue injection and excised. In some patients, these tracts may pass medially or lateral to the facial nerve; thus, the facial nerve must be identified during the dissection.

NEOPLASMS

A variety of skin lesions, including neoplasms, may be encountered on the auricle and in the external canal (Fig. 5–6). Few are peculiar to this anatomic region. Somewhat unusual from the standpoint of appearance is the osteoma, a benign tumor of the external canal wall which presents as a single, firm, rounded growth attached by a smaller bony pedicle to the inner third (or bony portion) of the canal wall. This tumor should be differentiated from an exostosis, which is more common and which consists of a rounded protuberance of hypertrophic canal bone (usually multiple and bilateral). The cause of exostoses is not completely clear; it has been stated that these growths occur more frequently in people who do a great deal of swimming in cold waters. Exostoses usually require no treatment, although they may result in more frequent canal blockage by cerumen in some individuals. Osteomas are carefully chiseled from the canal wall with the aid of the operating microscope. Benign polyps from the middle ear present in the external canal. Careful removal under the operating microscope is indicated if they are not responsive to medical treatment; in such cases they should be examined histologically.

Squamous cell carcinoma, the most common malignancy of the external auditory canal, is amenable to cure if diagnosed early and properly treated. Chronic discharge, often serosanguinous, and free bleeding, pain, and

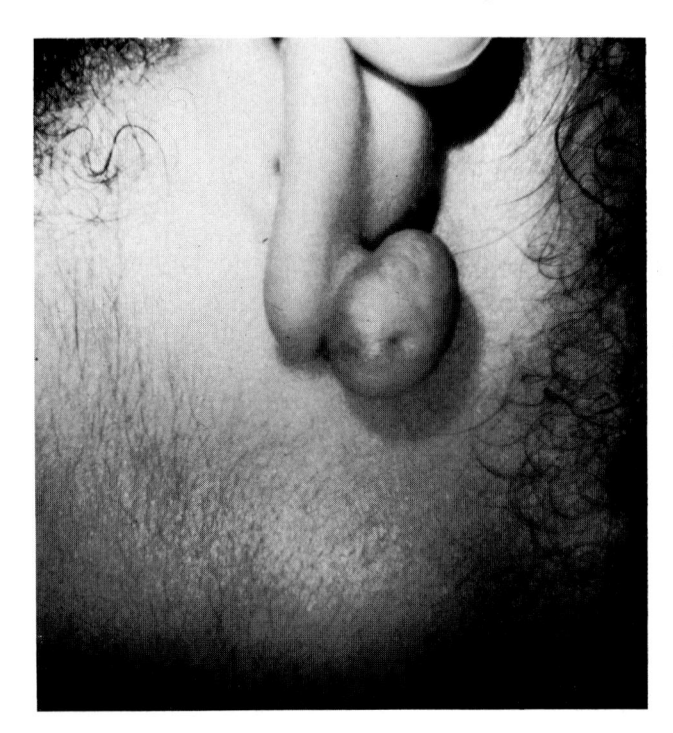

FIGURE 5–6. Keloid of lobule following ear piercing.

swelling within the canal are manifestations that, singly or in combination, should suggest the possibility of a new growth. A chronic external otitis that does not respond to the preceding recommendations requires a biopsy. Facial paralysis is a late development.

Malignant tumors involving the pinna are much more common than those seen in the canal itself. The two main types seen are squamous cell and basal cell carcinomas. The preferred initial treatment is surgical excision. Regional node dissection may be indicated with the squamous cell variety.

MISCELLANEOUS

Sebaceous cysts occur in the postauricular fold and are often multiple. Large cysts may become inflamed intermittently and are more likely to be cured by complete excision than by drainage alone.

Nodules involving the helix may represent localized areas of chondritis, known as chondrodermatitis nodularis chronicis helicis (painful nodule). They are more common in men and occur most often on the superior helix or anthelix. While steroid injection is sometimes adequate treatment, local excision provides both a cure and a pathologic diagnosis.

Gouty tophi may occur in the subcutaneous tissue or cartilage of the auricle as whitish-yellow nodules containing urate or sodium biurate cystals. Unsightly tophi may be excised.

Pain in the area of the auricle and external canal in the absence of physical findings certainly deserves investigation. The subject of otalgia will be discussed in Chapter 9.

References

Chai T-J, Chai TC: Bactericidal activity of cerumen. Antimicrob Agents Chemother 18:638–641, 1980.
Chander JR: Malignant external otitis. Laryngoscope 78:1257–1294, 1968.
Corey JP, Levandowski RA, Panwalker AP: Prognostic implications of therapy for necrotizing external otitis. Am J Otol 6:353–358, 1985.
Fairbanks DN (ed): Antimicrobial Therapy in Otolaryngology—Head and Neck Surgery. 4th ed. Washington, DC, American Academy of Otolaryngology, 1987.
Goodman WS, Middleton WC: The management of chronic external otitis. J Otolaryngol 13:183–186, 1984.
Hyslop NE: Ear wax and host defense. N Engl J Med 284:1099–1100, 1971.
Lucente FE, Parisier SC, Som PM, Arnold LM: Malignant external otitis: A dangerous misnomer? Otolaryngol Head Neck Surg 90:266–269, 1982.
Matsunaga E: The dimorphism in human normal cerumen. Ann Hum Genet 25:273–286, 1962.
Meyers BR, Mendelson MH, Parisier SC, Hirschman SZ: Malignant external otitis. Arch Otolaryngol Head Neck Surg 113:974–978, 1987.
Naiberg J, Berger G, Hawke M: The pathologic features of keratosis obturans and cholesteatoma of the external auditory canal. Arch Otolaryngol 110:690–693, 1984.
Neal GD, Gates GA: Invasive *Pseudomonas* osteitis of the temporal bone. Am J Otol 4:332–337, 1983.
Senturia BH, Morris MD, Lucente FE: Diseases of the External Ear. 2nd ed. New York, Grune & Stratton, Inc, 1980.
Sessions DG: Frostbite of the ear. Laryngoscope 81:1220–1232, 1971.
Shapiro SL: Some remarks on otitis externa. Eye Ear Nose Throat Mon., 52:61–68, 1973.
Shire JR, Donegan JO: Cholesteatoma of the external auditory canal and keratosis obturans. Am J Otol 7:361–364, 1986.
Sismanis A, Huang CE, Adedi E, Williams GH: External ear canal cholesteatoma. Am J Otol 7:126–129, 1986.
Stone M, Fulghum RS: Bactericidal activity of wet cerumen. Ann Otol Rhinol Laryngol 93:183–186, 1984.
Uri N, Kitzes R, Meyer W, Schuchman G: Necrotizing external otitis. The importance of prolonged drug therapy. J Laryngol Otol 98:1083–1085, 1984.

6

DISEASES OF THE MIDDLE EAR AND MASTOID

by Michael M. Paparella, M.D., George L. Adams, M.D., and Samuel C. Levine, M.D.

Diseases of the middle ear and mastoid are common throughout the United States and the world. For example, excluding the common cold, several studies indicate otitis media to be the next most common problem seen in a pediatric office. Inflammation of the middle ear cleft (eustachian tube, middle ear, and mastoid) is especially prevalent in children and in underserved areas such as ghettos, Indian reservations, and certain areas of Alaska. It is also likely that genetics plays a role, as there is often a history of ear disease in parents and siblings. Since the widespread use of antibiotics for otitis media and mastoiditis in the mid-1930's, the rates of mortality and serious complications resulting from otitis media have been greatly reduced. However, today, middle ear disease often presents in a chronic or insidious form causing hearing loss and drainage. Morbidity usually means hearing loss, which interferes with educational, social, or professional functions. In school-age children middle ear fluid problems (for example, serous otitis media) are quite common; the child may demonstrate a poor performance in school until the problem is detected through screening and is then diagnosed and treated.

DISEASES OF THE TYMPANIC MEMBRANE

Diseases of the tympanic membrane are usually associated with pathologic changes of the middle ear and mastoid. These tympanic membrane changes seen during otoscopic examination provide important information for diagnosing underlying disorders, such as active or inactive otitis media and mastoiditis. Occasionally diseases are primarily localized in the tympanic membrane (see Fig. 1–2 A).

Tympanic membrane diseases accompanied by underlying pathologic processes can result in the following physical features. The tympanic membrane may become thickened owing to inflammation. It may contain white thick patches or even become entirely white and thick owing to deposition of hyalinized collagen in its middle layer as a result of previous inflammation (tympanosclerosis). The tympanic membrane may become thinner from loss of its middle layers (membrana propria); this is almost always due to eustachian tube ventilation dysfunction. In such cases of ventilation dysfunction, the eustachian tube either may provide inadequate ventilation or may remain open all the time, allowing air to move in and out of the middle ear with respiration, resulting in ischemia and necrosis of the fibrous (middle) layer. The tympanic membrane may be retracted if there is a vacuum in the middle ear, or it may bulge when fluid, infection, or a tissue mass such as a tumor is present in the middle ear. Most commonly a perforation may exist in the tympanic membrane. Perforations can result from trauma and may or may not be accompanied by an underlying problem such as an ossicular chain disruption. Chronic otitis media with drainage is always accompanied by a perforation of the tympanic membrane. Such perforations may be extremely small and difficult to see or quite large and obvious. These perforations can be classified as four types, based on the site of pathologic involvement: tubal, central, marginal, and pars flaccida. The first two are generally safe; the last two usually are more serious (Fig. 6–1).

Chronic otitis media implies a tympanic membrane perforation with intermittent or persistent discharge.

Myringitis refers to an inflammation of the tympanic membrane. As has been indicated, inflammation of the tympanic membrane can accompany middle ear inflammation or be associated with external otitis. However, myringitis specifically pertains to inflammation in which the tympanic membrane is primarily involved. In hemorrhagic, or bullous, myringitis the most notable finding is bleb formations (bullae) on the tympanic membrane and adjacent canal wall. This clinical appearance can occur in children, in whom it is associated with the common bacteria that cause acute suppurative otitis media. These bullae contain serous fluid, blood, or both, and appear red or purple. Differential diagnosis includes external otitis and herpes zoster oticus (Ramsay Hunt syndrome). In adults hemorrhagic myringitis is usually a self-

FIGURE 6–1. *A,* Tubal perforation near the tympanic mouth of the eustachian tube. The disease is essentially an inflammation of the mucosa of the eustachian tube and middle ear. *B,* This large, central perforation may be accompanied by necrosis of the ossicles, granulations, and polyp formation. *C,* This marginal perforation or *(D)* this small perforation through pars flaccida is often accompanied by cholesteatoma.

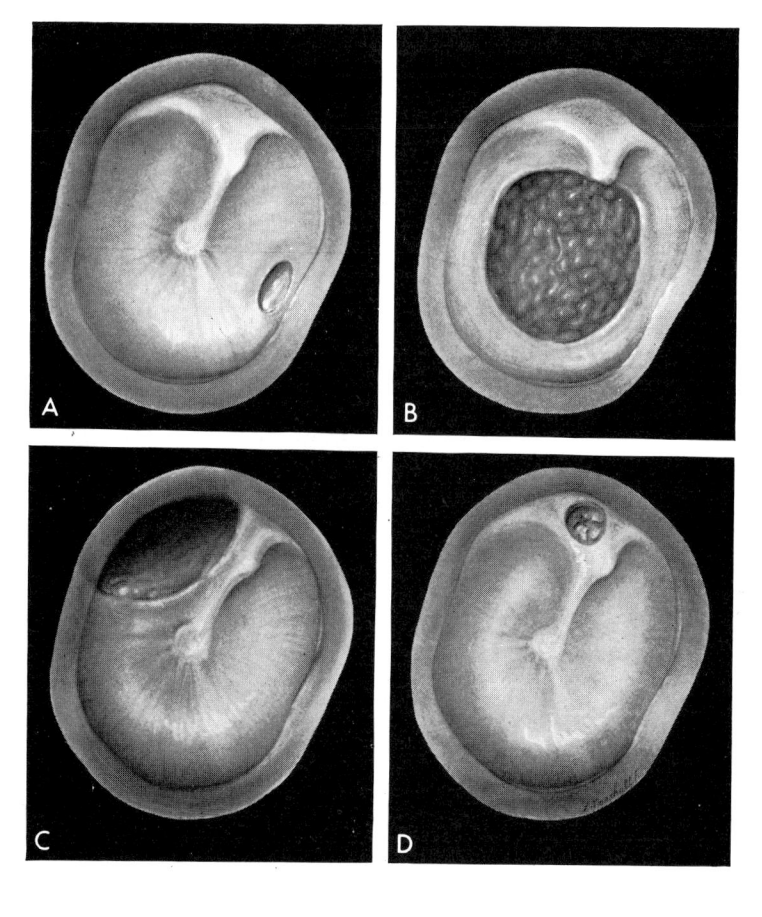

limited disease and is associated with infections caused by *Mycoplasma pneumoniae*. Sensorineural hearing loss has been reported as a result of this infection. When there are systemic manifestations, erythromycin is the drug of choice. For relief of pain the blebs or vesicles can be disrupted with a fine needle or myringotomy knife.

DISORDERS OF THE EUSTACHIAN TUBE

The eustachian tube connects the middle ear cavity with the nasopharynx and is intimately related to diseases of both. The lateral third as it enters the middle ear is bony, whereas the medial two thirds is fibrocartilaginous. The infant eustachian tube differs from that of the adult. In the infant it is short, wide, and horizontal in location, and this is one reason why inflammation of the eustachian tube is so common in infants, especially during the period of bottle feeding. As the child grows, the eustachian tube elongates, narrows, and develops a downward course medially. The tube is normally closed and opens by active muscular contraction of the tensor veli palatini muscle during swallowing and certain other times such as yawning or opening of the jaws. Functions of the eustachian tube are (1) ventilation, (2) drainage, and (3) protection of the middle ear from contamination by nasopharyngeal secretions. Ventilation provides equalization of atmospheric pressure on both sides of the tympanic membrane. The tube opens by muscular activity when the pressure differential is 20 to 40 mm Hg. An intact tensor veli palatini muscle is essential for this function.

Tensor veli palatini muscle function is essential for proper eustachian tubal activity.

Eustachian tube ventilation can be assessed in the office by looking for lateral displacement of the tympanic membrane with an otoscope or, in the presence of a perforation, listening through an auscultation tube while the patient squeezes the nostrils and swallows (Toynbee maneuver) or squeezes the nose and blows hard against the occluded nostrils, with a closed mouth, allowing his ears to "pop" (Valsalva maneuver). The middle ear can also be inflated by politzerization, during which air is forced through the nose while the nasopharynx is closed as the patient swallows. The air is introduced through the nose with a Politzer bag with an olive tip. Direct eustachian tube catheterization was a common procedure in the past but is seldom performed today.

Secretions formed in the middle ear will drain into the nasopharynx through a normally functioning eustachian tube. A vacuum will develop in the middle ear during periods of eustachian tube obstruction. Prolonged obstruction can lead to increased fluid production, perpetuating the problem. When not relieved by medical management, the vacuum has to be interrupted by myringotomy. Then drainage of the fluid can occur via the eustachian tube.

Being normally closed, the eustachian tube protects the middle ear from contaminated nasopharyngeal secretions and pathogenic organisms. The normal protection can be interfered with by heavy nose blowing or continual exaggerated sniffling, thus allowing passage of organisms into the middle ear.

Disorders affecting the eustachian tube include an abnormally patent tube, palatal myoclonus, obstruction, and cleft palate.

Abnormally Patent Eustachian Tube

An abnormally patent eustachian tube is open all the time so that air enters the middle ear with respirations. The patient's history usually reveals a significant weight loss which leads to loss of adipose tissue around the eustachian tube orifice. Other chronic illnesses and certain muscular disorders have an association with this condition. A significant number of women on birth control pills and men taking estrogens have been observed to have a patent eustachian tube. The condition can produce autophony (hearing one's respiration), a sensation of fullness, or a "plugged-up" feeling in the ear. During otoscopic examination, the patient is asked to breathe heavily through the nose while the mouth is closed. The tympanic membrane in this patient will be atrophic and thin and will move in and out with respiration, a telltale diagnostic sign. A variety of procedures can be employed to obstruct the eustachian tube at its pharyngeal end. A simple and effective method that has been used to correct this problem is to insert a ventilation tube through the tympanic membrane in order to decrease the disturbing effects.

Autophony results from an abnormally patent eustachian tube.

Palatal Myoclonus

Palatal myoclonus is a fairly rare condition in which the palatal muscles undergo periodic rhythmic contractions. This results in a clicking sound in the ear of the patient and may be heard by the examiner's ear. Although the exact cause of palatal myoclonus is unknown, it has been associated with vascular lesions, multiple sclerosis, aneurysms of the vertebral artery, tumors, and various other lesions of the brain stem or cerebellum. Usually no treatment is needed; rarely, incision of the tensor tympani muscle of the middle ear can be considered.

Eustachian Tube Obstruction

Eustachian tube obstruction can result from a variety of conditions, including inflammation such as nasopharyngitis or adenoiditis. When a nasopharyngeal tumor obstructs the eustachian tube, the first clinical finding can be fluid in the middle ear. As such, in any adult patient with chronic unilateral serous otitis media the possibility of nasopharyngeal carcinoma must be considered. Obstruction may also be caused by a foreign body, such as a posterior pack for nasal epistaxis, or mechanical trauma from aggressive adenoidectomy resulting in scarring and closure of the tube. Operative procedures that interfere with the tensor veli palatini also can cause permanent eustachian tube dysfunction, although not actual obstruction. Such procedures include aggressive operative procedures for surgical removal of tumors in the vicinity of the pterygoid plates.

Cleft Palate

Cleft palate deformity results in eustachian tube dysfunction due to lack of anchorage of the tensor palatini muscle. In the unrepaired cleft palate, this prevents the muscle from exerting sufficient contraction on the eustachian tube orifice to open it during swallowing. This inability of the tube to open results in inadequate ventilation of the middle ear, and inflammation ensues. Thus, the incidence of middle ear disease in children with cleft palate is extremely high, varying from recurrent serous otitis media to tympanosclerosis to chronic suppurative otitis media. The incidence of middle ear abnormality is almost 100 per cent in the first three months of life. By mid teen age, there is a less frequent incidence of serous otitis media, but many adolescents have a conductive hearing impairment and an abnormal appearing tympanic membrane. Otologic management requires early treatment of aural disease. Surgical repair of the cleft palate is undertaken as soon as possible for functional purposes. Many children require frequent placement of ventilation tubes, and often a long-lasting type tube is inserted. Adenoidectomy in cleft palate patients or patients with a submucous cleft is avoided, since this can produce palatal dysfunctions, nasality of voice, and regurgitation of liquids into the nasopharynx.

Barotrauma*

Boyle's Law: volume of a gas varies inversely to pressure.

Barotrauma is damage to tissues caused by changes in barometric pressure which occur during diving or flying. Boyle's Law states that a decrease or increase in environmental pressure will expand or compress, respectively, a given enclosed volume of a gas. If the gas is contained within a flexible structure, that structure can be damaged by this expansion or compression. Barotrauma can occur whenever the gas-filled spaces in the body (middle ear, sinus, lung) become enclosed spaces through blockage of normal venting pathways.

The middle ear is the most common site of barotrauma, primarily because of the complexity of eustachian tube function. The eustachian tube is normally closed but opens with swallowing, chewing, yawning, and the Valsalva maneuver. Colds, allergic rhinitis, and individual anatomic variation all predispose to eustachian tube dysfunction. Increasing pressure requires a "clearing" action as described above to equalize pressure, but decreasing pressure can usually be equalized passively. As environmental pressure decreases, the air in the middle ear will expand and passively vent through the eustachian tube. As environmental pressure increases, the air in the middle ear and within the eustachian tube is compressed. This tends to collapse the eustachian tube. Once the pressure difference between the environment and the middle ear space becomes too great (about 90 to 100 mm Hg), the cartilaginous portion of the eustachian tube will firmly collapse. If more air cannot be added through the eustachian tube to restore the middle ear volume, structures of the middle ear and adjacent tissue can be damaged as the pressure difference continues to grow. A predictable sequence of injury occurs as the relative vacuum develops within the middle ear space. First the tympanic membrane is retracted inward. This stretches the eardrum and causes rupture of small vessels to produce an injected appearance and hemorrhagic blebs within the drum. As the pressure builds, small vessels within the middle ear mucosa also dilate and rupture, causing a hemotympanum. Occasionally the pressure will rupture the tympanic membrane.

Middle ear barotrauma can occur in underwater diving or flying. The change in pressure in the first 17 feet of water is equal to the pressure change

---

*The section on Barotrauma was written by Rick Odlund, M.D., former Navy Diving Medical officer.

in the first 18,000 feet of altitude. Therefore, changes in environmental pressure occur much more quickly in diving than in flying. This explains the higher relative incidence of middle ear barotrauma in divers. Middle ear barotrauma can occur with compressed air diving (SCUBA) or breathhold diving. It most commonly occurs at depths of 10 to 20 feet. Although the relative incidence is higher in diving, more people fly than dive. Commercial aircrafts are pressurized, but only to 8000 feet. The potential for barotrauma is clearly present, but not at the incidence level caused by diving.

Symptoms of middle ear barotrauma include pain, a feeling of fullness, and decreased hearing. The diagnosis is confirmed by otoscopy. The eardrum will be injected and may exhibit hemorrhagic blebs within the drum or blood behind the drum. Occasionally, the tympanic membrane will perforate. There may be a mild conductive hearing loss. The treatment consists of decongestants and cessation of diving or flying until the patient can equilibrate middle ear pressures again. Severe cases may take as long as four to six weeks to resolve, but most resolve in two to three days. Antibiotics are not indicated unless a perforation has also occurred in dirty water. Prevention can be accomplished by avoiding flying or diving with colds and using proper clearing technique. Once pain is present, the eustachian tube has probably collapsed. When diving the best action at this point is to abort the dive or ascend a few feet and try equalizing the pressure again. When flying in commercial aircraft this is not possible, so it is very important to prevent collapse of the eustachian tube. The best method is to begin gentle clearing maneuvers several minutes before the scheduled arrival time. If the person must fly with a cold, decongestant nasal spray or oral decongestants should be utilized.

It should be emphasized that persistent tinnitus, vertigo, and sensorineural hearing loss are symptoms of inner ear damage. Infrequently, middle ear barotrauma will result in damage of the inner ear. Inner ear damage is a serious problem and may require surgical treatment to prevent permanent hearing loss. All persons complaining of hearing loss with barotrauma should have a tuning fork test battery done to be sure the hearing loss is conductive and not sensorineural. Brief episodes of vertigo that occur while ascending or descending are called alternobaric vertigo. This is a common complaint, usually associated with middle ear barotrauma. As long as the vertigo stops within a few seconds, no treatment or further evaluation is necessary.

DISORDERS OF THE OSSICULAR CHAIN

The importance of the transmission of sound from the intact tympanic membrane to the oval window by the intact ossicular chain was discussed in Chapter 2. Disruption of this chain or fixation, whether by disease, trauma, or a congenital process, will be discussed here.

Congenital Problems

The ossicles can be congenitally deformed, disrupted, or fixed. Since they derive from the first and second branchial arches, other developmental anomalies of these arches (syndromes) often occur as well, such as Treacher Collins syndrome, which is congenital stenosis of the ear plus maxillofacial dysostoses. Ossicular deformities can also occur in isolation. Common deformities include a missing portion of the incus and fixation of the stapes. There are a variety of forms of congenital stenosis. These children may be born without a pinna or with only a rudimentary one (microtia). The deformity of the pinna can, in a general way, be correlated with the amount of deformity to be expected below in the middle ear and tympanic membrane. There can be complete lack of development of the external auditory canal, or it can appear with a blind end or develop with a concentric narrowing. The functional aspects of this problem (deafness) should be corrected before consideration is paid to cosmetic repair of the pinna. Children with congenital hearing loss require early identification and treatment. Hearing aids should be used at the earliest possible time. Cosmetic correction of a microtia is recommended before first grade to reduce peer pressure. Bone-anchored hearing aids may assist the surgical aplasia procedures. Isolated ossicular deformities are usually correctable through surgery. If the stapes is fixed, a stapedectomy and prosthesis replacement will re-establish hearing.

As mentioned before, the ossicles can become fixed owing to tympanosclerosis in patients who have previously had otitis media.

Otosclerosis

Otosclerosis is an autosomal dominant trait.

A common cause of conductive hearing loss in adults is otosclerosis. Otosclerosis is an autosomal dominant disorder, seen in both men and women, that begins to cause progressive conductive deafness in early adulthood. The patient develops symptoms in the late teens and early twenties. While usually bilateral, it can occur unilaterally. Histologically, otosclerosis is quite common, occurring in as much as 10 per cent of the population. However, only a small percentage develop the clinical manifestations of hearing loss. This is a disease of the bony labyrinth, in which an area of otospongiosis (soft bone) forms, especially in front of and adjacent to the footplate, causing fixation of the footplate. Although conductive deafness is the main problem, in time sensorineural hearing loss due to cochlear otosclerosis can develop as well.

The patient usually complains of a hearing loss when a level of 40 dB or greater is reached. The primary care physician's most important diagnostic tool is the 512 Hz tuning fork to demonstrate a negative Rinne test. Bone conduction is heard louder than air conduction by the patient. The Weber test is helpful and will be positive in the involved ear if unilateral otosclerosis is present or in the ear with the greater conductive hearing loss. The tympanic membrane is usually normal in appearance but occasionally will have a pink or orange discoloration due to the vascular otospongiosis in the middle ear as seen through the tympanic membrane (positive Schwartze's sign). Surgical procedures offer an excellent chance for restoring hearing, depending mainly on cochlear function. The major postoperative complication is sensorineural hearing loss, with an incidence of 2 to 3 per cent in experienced hands. Patients must be assessed very carefully through audiologic as well as otologic examination (Fig. 6–2).

Middle Ear Trauma

Perforation of the tympanic membrane can be caused by sudden changes in pressure—barotrauma, blast injuries—or by foreign objects in the ear

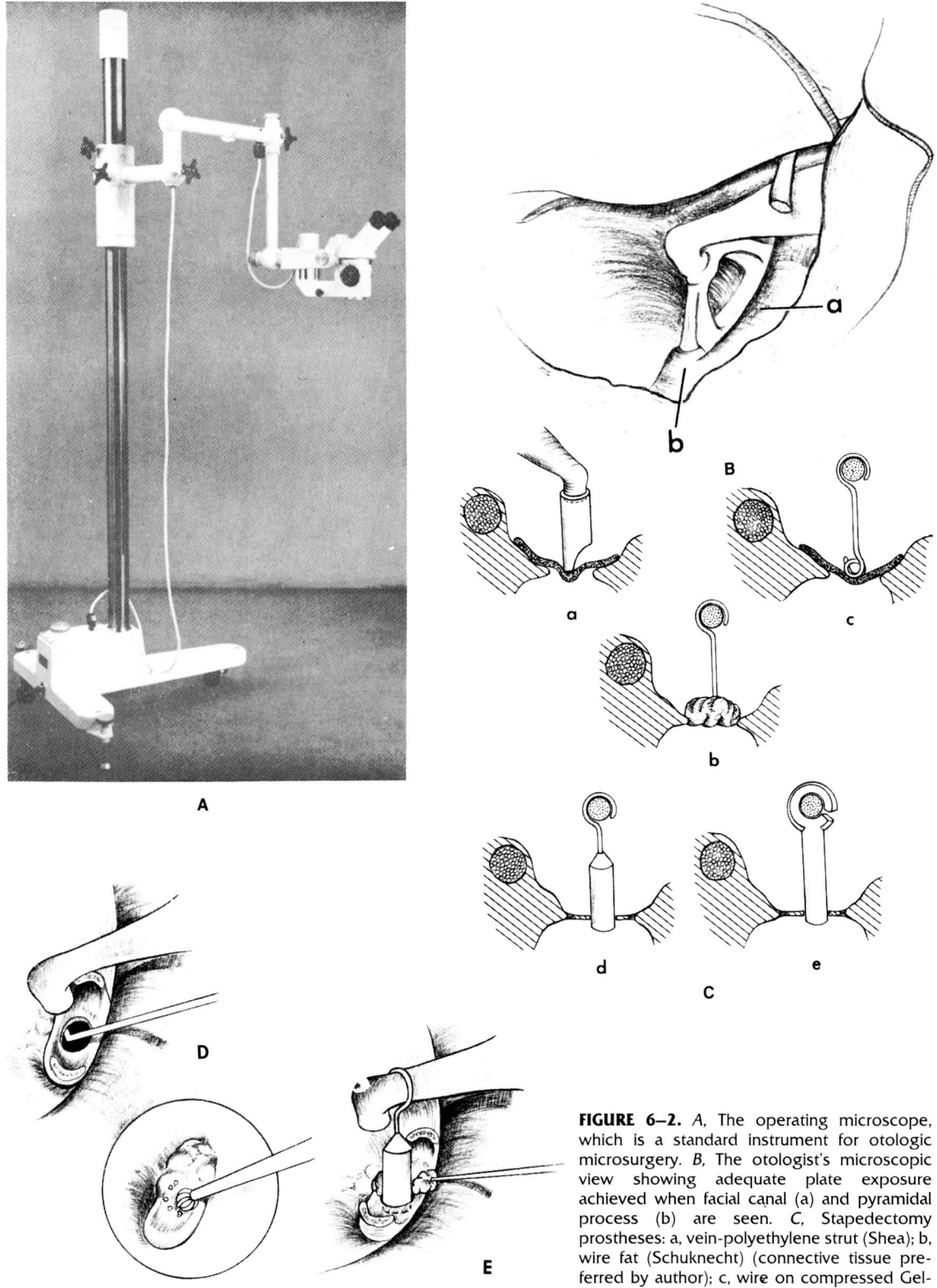

FIGURE 6–2. *A,* The operating microscope, which is a standard instrument for otologic microsurgery. *B,* The otologist's microscopic view showing adequate plate exposure achieved when facial canal (a) and pyramidal process (b) are seen. *C,* Stapedectomy prostheses: a, vein-polyethylene strut (Shea); b, wire fat (Schuknecht) (connective tissue preferred by author); c, wire on compressed Gelfoam (House); d, wire Teflon piston; e, Teflon piston (Shea). In some cases there is obliterative otosclerosis so that *(D)* the very thick footplate is thinned with a microscopic drill and a large (at least 1 mm) opening is made. *E,* The piston prosthesis is secured into position by Gelfoam or connective tissue over the footplate. (*B* to *E* from Paparella MM, Shumrick DA (eds): Otolaryngology, Vol 2. Philadelphia, WB Saunders Co., 1973, p 305.)

canal (cotton-tipped applicators, pen tips, paper clips, etc.). Symptoms include pain, bloody drainage, and hearing impairment ("it sounds like I'm in a barrel").

Perforations occurring during water sports require systemic antibiotics.

Clean, traumatic perforations are treated by protecting the ear from water and administering systemic antibiotics if there is pain or inflammation. Most clean, uncomplicated perforations will heal spontaneously. When spontaneous healing does not occur, repair can usually be done in the office setting and requires unrolling the edges of the perforation and applying one of many materials suitable for "patching." When not effective, a more formal myringoplasty will be required.

Contaminated perforations, such as those that occur from a fall while water skiing, are treated with antibiotic ear drops as well as systemic antibiotics because infection with drainage invariably occurs. No attempt at closure is made until the infection resolves.

Perforations caused by hot slag, as can occur in welders, are particularly painful and difficult to close by usual means. The heat cauterization of the adjacent tissues which occurs prevents spontaneous closure.

Of greatest concern are perforations resulting in injury to the ossicular chain. This injury is suspected when significant hearing loss (>25 dB) and vertigo, rather than pain and a hollow sensation of sounds, are present. The perforation may be in the posterior superior quadrant. The presence of vertigo and hearing loss is a true otologic emergency, and immediate exploration of the middle ear and ossicular chain is necessary. A displaced or subluxed stapes may be encountered. Retrieval of the stapes from the oval window or even a stapedectomy may be necessary. The vertigo will be controlled, but hearing recovery cannot be assured.

Vertigo and/or sensorineural hearing loss occurring with a traumatic perforation represents an otologic emergency.

Blast injuries from close proximity to an explosion are particularly prone to long-term sequelae. Rather than discrete ruptures of the tympanic membrane, particles of squamous epithelium are scattered throughout the middle ear. The ossicles can be displaced an incredible distance. Ultimate results are dependent upon the extent of injury, but prolonged drainage and possible later cholesteatoma formation are possible.

ACUTE PURULENT OTITIS MEDIA

Hippocrates said, "Acute pain of the ear with continued strong fever is to be dreaded for there is danger that the man may become delirious and die." Acute otitis media and mastoiditis were major problems prior to the introduction of antibiotic therapy in the mid 1930's. Today patients with uncomplicated acute otitis media are treated successfully by the pediatrician or the family physician.

The middle ear is usually sterile, which is remarkable considering the flora of organisms which exists in the nasopharynx and pharynx. The combined physiologic action of cilia and mucus-secreting enzymes (for example, muramidase) and antibodies acts as a defense mechanism when these microbial contaminants are exposed to the middle ear space during the act of swallowing. Acute otitis media results when this physiologic mechanism is disrupted. In addition to the surface defense mechanism, an important subepithelial capillary network provides humoral factors, polymorphonuclear leukocytes, and other phagocytic cells. Obstruction of the eustachian tube is a basic causative factor in acute otitis media. Thus, a major barrier against bacterial

TABLE 6–1. PATHOGENIC BACTERIA IN CHILDREN WITH ACUTE OTITIS MEDIA

Streptococcus pneumoniae
Haemophilus influenzae (nontypeable)
Streptococcus Group A
Branhamella catarrhalis
Staphylococcus aureus
Staphylococcus epidermidis
Infants
Chlamydia trachomatis
Escherichia coli
Klebsiella species

invasion is lost, and bacterial species that may not ordinarily be pathogenic are able to colonize the middle ear, invade tissue, and cause infection. Although the majority of respiratory infections are caused by viral agents, most acute otitis media infections are caused by pyogenic bacteria. The most frequently recovered bacteria include *Streptococcus pneumoniae, Haemophilus influenzae,* and beta-hemolytic streptococci (Table 6–1). *Streptococcus pneumoniae* is by far the most common organism in all age groups. *H. influenzae* is a frequent pathogen recovered from children under five years of age, although it remains a significant pathogen in adolescents as well.

Classic symptoms of acute purulent otitis media include pain, fever, malaise, and sometimes headache in addition to earache; in children particularly, anorexia and sometimes nausea and vomiting are present. Fever may be quite high in small children but can be absent in 30 per cent of cases. The tympanic membrane typically is red and bulging either in part or in its entirety (Fig. 6–3), and the vessels over the tympanic membrane and malleus handle become injected and therefore more prominent. In short, there is an abscess of the middle ear.

Because of the increasing incidence of ampicillin resistance, antibiotics are combined with clavulanic acid and are effective against beta-lactamase formers. Either a cephalosporin or ampicillin combined with clavulanic acid has become the preferred medication for these resistant organisms. Sulfisoxazole plus erythromycin is another effective substitute in penicillin-allergic patients. All medications should be administered for at least 10 to 14 days, and a follow-up examination is a must to assure complete resolution.

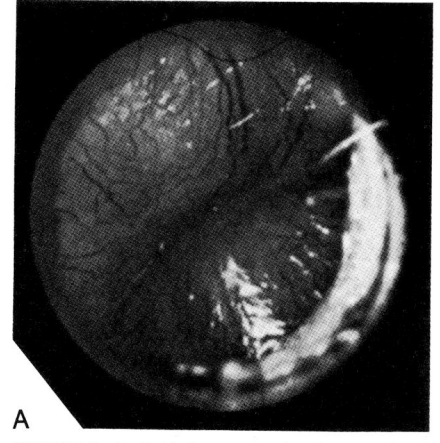

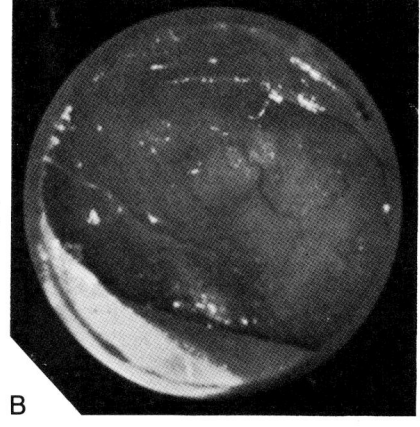

FIGURE 6–3. *A*, Early stage of acute purulent otitis media. *B*, Later stage of acute otitis media. (Courtesy of Dr. Richard A. Buckingham and Dr. George E. Shambaugh, Jr.)

In addition to antibiotic therapy as described above, dry heat application helps provide relief, analgesics may help, and some physicians recommend anesthetic ear drops. The patient is preferably seen two days after initiating treatment. If there is no evidence of resolution, either clinically or by examination, then a myringotomy should be performed to lessen the complications, which will be discussed later.

Otitis-Prone Children

Otitis-prone child:
—male
—under age 2
—Native American, white
—first episode usually under age 6 months
—S. pneumoniae episode

Otitis media is one of the most common infections in children. In some studies it is estimated to occur in 25 per cent of children. It is more common in Native American and Eskimo children than in whites and least common in blacks. The majority of episodes occur in the first two years of life, with a second peak incidence during the first year of school. Those who have had six or more episodes of otitis media before age six have been termed "otitis-prone." A study by Howie showed that an episode of *S. pneumoniae* infection in the first year of life was associated with continuing incidence of repeated episodes of acute otitis media. Boys are affected more than girls. These children did not have an increased incidence of allergic conditions. Eight serotypes of *S. pneumoniae* are responsible for more than 75 per cent of episodes of acute otitis media. Thus, the development of a pneumococcal vaccine could be an important step in controlling these repeated episodes.

Treatment of children with this high propensity to develop otitis media is either medical or surgical. Medical management includes administration of antibiotics in low dosage for periods of up to three months in the winter. Another alternative is placement of ventilation tubes. The decision to perform myringotomy is generally based on failure of medical prophylaxis or the development of allergic reactions to commonly employed antimicrobials, either the sulfa drug group or the penicillins.

Serous Otitis Media

Serous otitis media and mucoid otitis media have similar etiologies. Serous otitis media is caused by a transudation of plasma from the blood vessels into the middle ear space largely due to hydrostatic pressure differences, whereas mucoid otitis media results from active secretion from glands and cysts in the lining of the middle ear cleft. Eustachian tube dysfunction is a major underlying factor. Other causative factors include hypertrophy of the adenoids, chronic adenoiditis, cleft palate, tumors in the nasopharynx, barotrauma, associated inflammation such as sinusitis or rhinitis, radiation therapy, and immunologic or metabolic deficiencies. Allergy can play an adjunctive role in causing middle ear effusions.

Middle ear effusion is the most common cause of hearing loss in school-age children.

Middle ear effusion often has no symptom other than hearing loss. It is often recognized on pre-school screening.

These middle ear fluid problems are most common in children and usually manifest as a conductive loss. This is the most prevalent cause of hearing loss in school-age children. There may be recurrent attacks of acute purulent otitis media between which the ears never return to normal. Language delay may occur when this becomes prolonged. A conductive hearing loss, which seldom exceeds 35 dB, is frequently picked up in a school or screening audiogram. Children seldom volunteer that they have any difficulty. The child may be described by the teacher as inattentive. Adults generally describe their symptoms more dramatically, and the symptoms include a "plugged up" feeling in their ears and decreased hearing acuity. They may note an improvement in hearing with position changes of the head. Tinnitus may result from movement of middle ear fluid; dizziness is rarely a problem.

Physical examination reveals drumhead immobility as assessed with a pneumatic otoscope. Positive and negative pressures (see Fig. 1–2) are applied to the ear canal after obtaining an adequate seal. If there is air in the tympanum, it will be compressed and the drumhead will move inward with the application of positive pressure and outward with negative pressure. Movement is either damped or does not occur in the presence of serous otitis media or mucoid otitis media. In serous otitis media an amber or yellow drumhead may be seen, whereas in mucoid otitis media the drumhead has a duller and more opaque appearance. The malleus appears short, retracted, and chalky white. Occasionally in serous otitis media fluid levels or bubbles are seen through a semitransparent tympanic membrane (Fig. 6–4). The tympanic membrane may appear blue or purplish if blood products are also present in the middle ear.

Pneumatic otoscopy demonstrates decreased drumhead mobility. It may also demonstrate "bubbles" behind the tympanic membrane.

Serous fluid has been collected for study at the time of myringotomy. Cultures have been positive for bacterial organisms in about 40 per cent of cases. The organisms are identical to those obtained by tympanocentesis for acute otitis media. Thus, antimicrobial selection is similar for acute and serous otitis media. The frequency and type of positive cultures are the same for both the mucoid and serous types of otitis media.

Treatment for these conditions is first medical and then, if need be, surgical. Medical treatment includes antibiotics, antihistamines, decongestants, eustachian tube ventilation exercises, and allergic hyposensitization. Allergic hyposensitization is reserved for cases in which definite allergies are demonstrated by skin testing. Dietary limitation is advised when food allergy is demonstrated. Antihistamines are used only in children or adults with associated nasal or sinus congestion. Neither antihistamines nor decongestants are of value when there is no associated nasopharyngeal congestion. The patient is evaluated for other associated problems such as chronic sinusitis, nasal polyps, nasal obstruction, and adenoid hypertrophy. Medical management for mild serous otitis media is continued for a period of three months. By this time, 90 per cent of patients will have resolved the fluid.

Antihistamines are of value only when there is demonstrable nasal or sinus congestion.

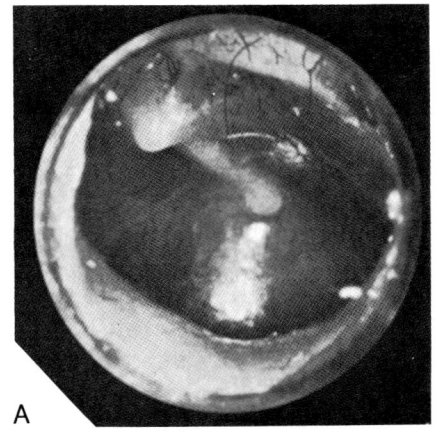

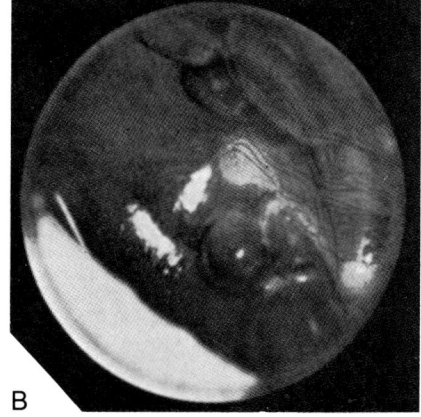

FIGURE 6–4. *A*, Serous otitis media. *B*, Bubbles in the middle ear are seen in serous otitis media after inflammation. (Courtesy of Dr. Richard A. Buckingham and Dr. George E. Shambaugh, Jr.)

Fluid persisting after 3 months of medical management with hearing loss is an indication for myringotomy.

Persistence of fluid is an indication for surgical correction. This consists of a myringotomy incision, removal of the fluid, and often insertion of a pressure equalization tube. The pressure equalization tube acts as a vent to allow air to enter the middle ear. This relieves the vacuum and lets the fluid drain or be absorbed.

The decision to proceed to surgical intervention is not made on duration alone. Severity of the hearing impairment and frequency and severity of preceding problems are considered. The problem is most often bilateral, but a child with a thin fluid, minimal hearing loss, or unilateral problem may be treated for a longer period by a more conservative approach. On the other hand, thinning of the tympanic membrane, deep retraction, significant hearing impairment, and poor school performance may be indications to proceed to myringotomy sooner.

Unilateral serous otitis media in an adult requires investigation of the nasaopharynx for tumor.

The ventilation tubes are left in place until spontaneously extruded—usually within a period of six months to one year (Fig. 6–5). Unfortunately, because of recurrence of the fluid, some children require insertion of special tubes designed to stay in for longer than one year. The disadvantage of these longer-lasting tubes has been the persistence of a perforation after extrusion. Ventilation tube insertions have provided immediate restoration of hearing and correction of severely retracted tympanic membrane, especially when there is persistent negative pressure.

The greatest disadvantage of ventilation tubes has been the need to keep the middle ear dry. Various plugs have been devised for this purpose. Myringotomy incision and tube placement have also been on rare occasion associated with the development of a cholesteatoma. Drainage through the tubes is not unusual and may be associated with upper respiratory infections or allowing water to enter the middle ear, and, in certain cases, can be a persistent, unexplained problem. In these instances, medical management with systemic antibiotics or antibiotic ear drops has to be continued for long periods of time, even while tubes are in place. Failure to respond to this type of management necessitates mastoid radiographs and further evaluation. The value of adenoidectomy for chronic serous otitis media is still controversial. Certainly in individuals with large adenoids causing nasal and nasopharyngeal obstruction, there is a role for this procedure. The majority of children do not fit this category. The value of adenoidectomy in children with moderate adenoid tissue and recurrent problems is still being evaluated. The most recent study (Gates) reports adenoidectomy is beneficial even when the adenoid tissue is not obstructing.

Persistent drainage through a ventilation tube requires culture, systemic antibiotics, and appropriate topical antibiotic drops.

Radiologic Assessment of the Middle Ear and Mastoid

Temporal Bone. After obtaining a thorough history and careful otoscopic evaluation of the external and middle ear, it may be determined that x-ray examination of the temporal bone will be necessary. As with any x-ray examination, the most useful information can be obtained if the physician and radiologist confer with each other and discuss the specific problem being evaluated. In this way the most helpful radiologic studies can be performed, and the information obtained will be of greater value to the clinician.

Conventional radiographs of the temporal bone are specifically useful in studying the mastoid, middle ear, labyrinth, and internal auditory canal. The most common views are the Law, Schüller, Mayer, Owens, Towne, and

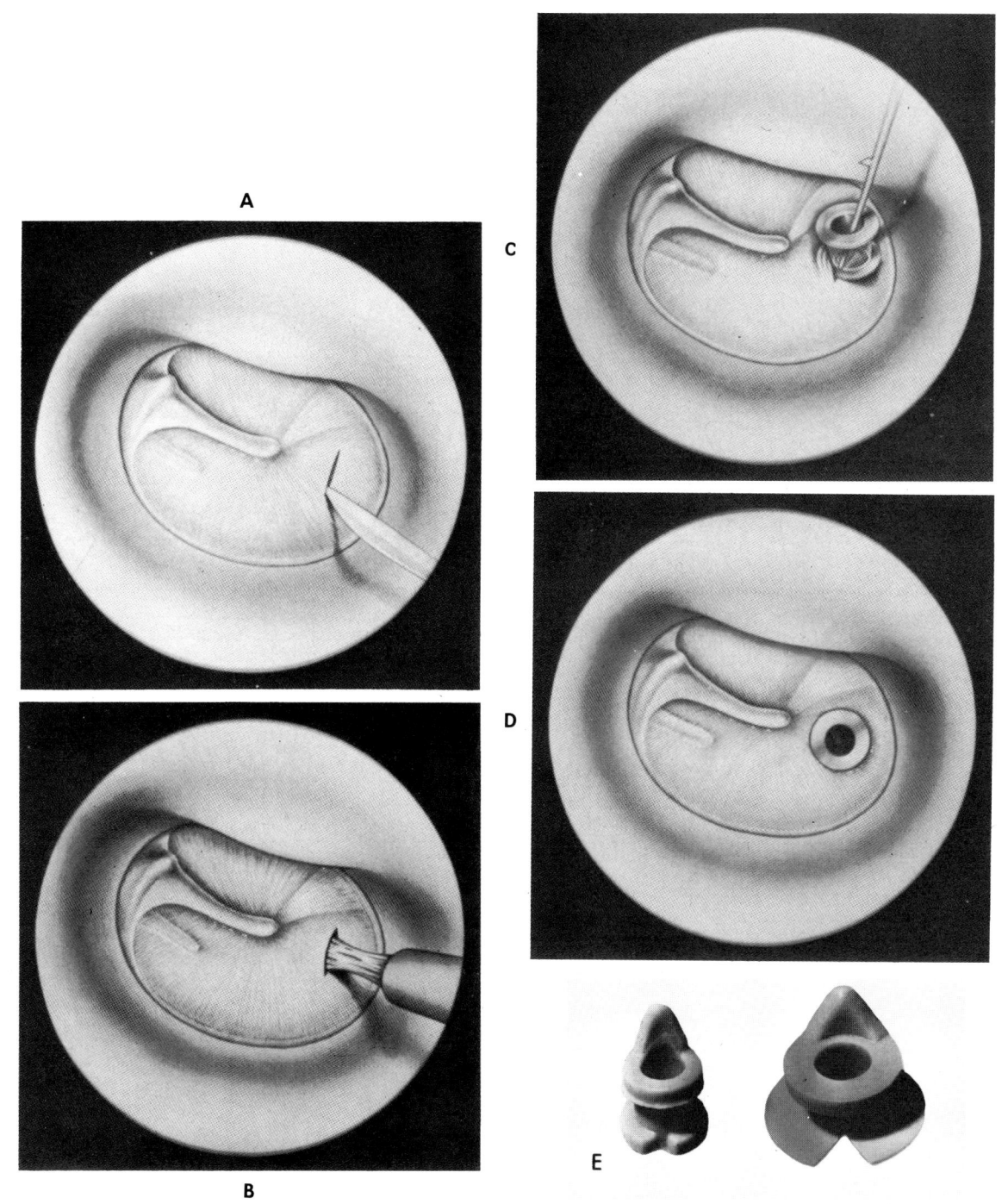

FIGURE 6–5. *A,* Myringotomy incision. *B,* Aspiration of fluid. *C,* Insertion of ventilation tube. *D,* Ventilation tube in place. *E,* Type I, standard ventilation tube (left) and type II, larger ventilation tube with larger inner flange and opening for chronic, obstinate cases (right). Both tubes are made of silicone rubber. (*A* to *D* from Paparella MM, Shumrick DA (eds): Otolaryngology, Vol 2. Philadelphia, WB Saunders Co, 1973, p 90. *E* from Paparella MM, Payne E: Otitis media. *In* Northern J (ed): Hearing Disorders. Boston, Little, Brown and Company, 1976, Fig 10–2.)

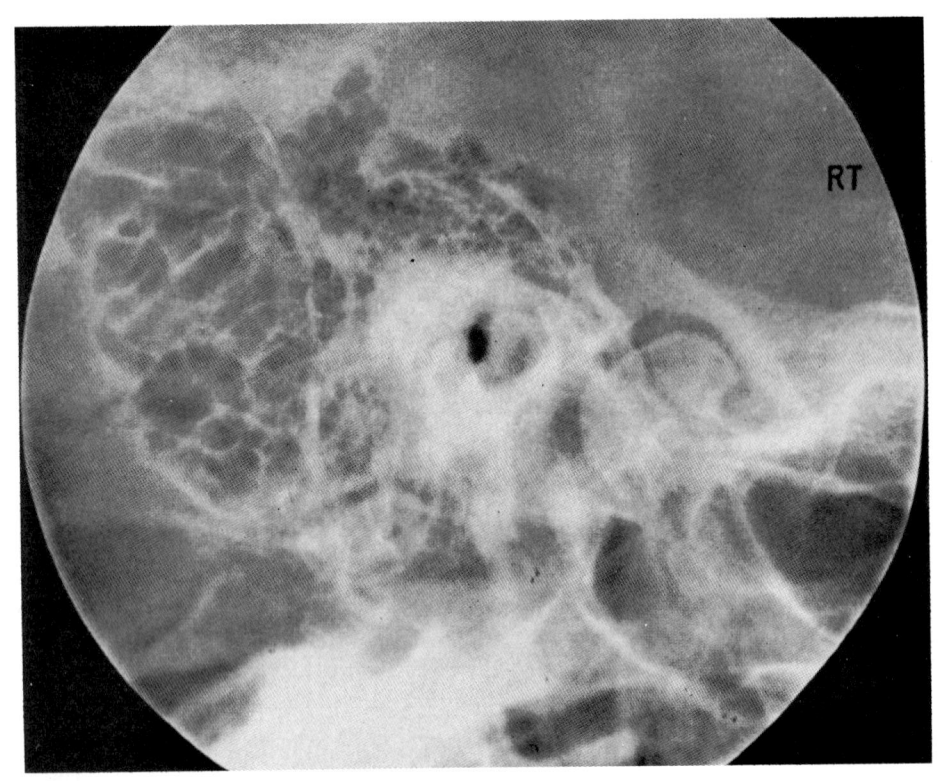

FIGURE 6–6. Law position. The external canal, tympanic cavity, vestibule, and internal canal are shown by an area of diminished density behind the mandibular condyle. The attic-aditus-antral areas are obscured entirely. The pneumatic cells of the mastoid process are well visualized. (From Compere WE Jr: Conventional radiologic examination of the temporal bone. *In* Shambaugh GE Jr (ed): Surgery of the Ear, 2nd ed. Philadelphia, WB Saunders Co, 1967, p 103.)

Stenvers views (Figs. 6–6 to 6–10). Prior to the advent of antibiotics, the *Law* view was of particular value in evaluating acute mastoiditis. This is a nearly direct lateral view. Even today it is usually obtained prior to any mastoid surgery to determine the position of major landmarks such as the mastoid tegmen and sigmoid sinus as well as the general overall size of the mastoid. The additional lateral elevation of the x-ray beam in the *Schüller* view not only shows those structures seen in the Law position, but also permits visualization of the attic or epitympanum. By angulation of the head 45 degrees, the *Mayer* position is obtained. This film demonstrates the region of the antrum and the head of the malleus. By a modification of the direction of the x-ray beam, it is also possible to demonstrate the incus and the area of the epitympanum. The *Owens* view is similar to the modification of the Mayer position, but less angulation of the beam provides a better visualization of the ossicles and epitympanic recess as they are now visualized above the petrous ridge. Another modification of an oblique view is known as the *Chausse III* projection. It provides additional information about the structures in the middle ear.

The *Stenvers* position views the long axis of the petrous pyramid to demonstrate the internal auditory canal, the labyrinth, and the antrum. The *Towne* view shows both petrous pyramids through the orbits, permitting direct comparison of the petrous pyramids and internal auditory canals on the same film. When the physician is most interested in structures of the middle ear, the standard Schüller, modified Mayer, and Chausse III views

FIGURE 6–7. Schüller position. By increasing the elevation of the beam, the labyrinth is depressed and the head of the malleus is visible above the crest of the petrosa. Compare with Figure 6–6. (From Compere WE Jr: Conventional radiologic examination of the temporal bone. *In* Shambaugh GE Jr (ed): Surgery of the Ear, 2nd ed. Philadelphia, WB Saunders Co, 1967, p 104.)

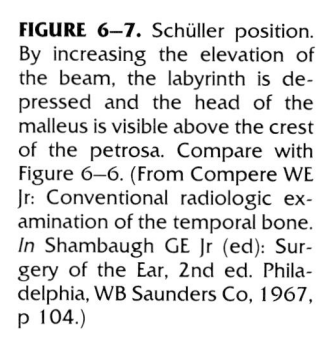

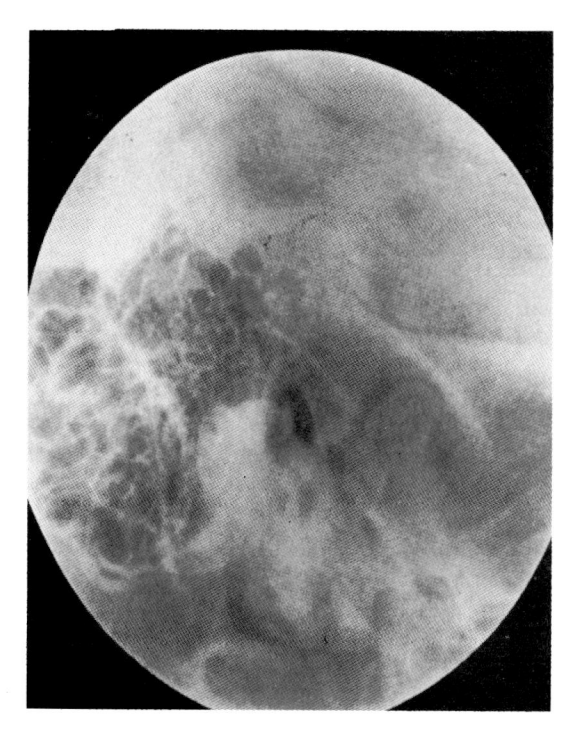

KEY TO THE LINE DRAWING
1. Root of the zygoma
2. Condyle of the mandible
3. Temporomandibular joint
5. Tympanic cavity
6. Epitympanic cavity
7. Malleus
10. Area of the aditus
11. Area of the antrum
12. Mastoid cells
13. Mastoid tip
14. Anterior plate of the lateral sinus
15. Tegmen plate
16. Arcuate eminence
21. Petrosa
22. Anterior crest of the petrosa
25. Auricle

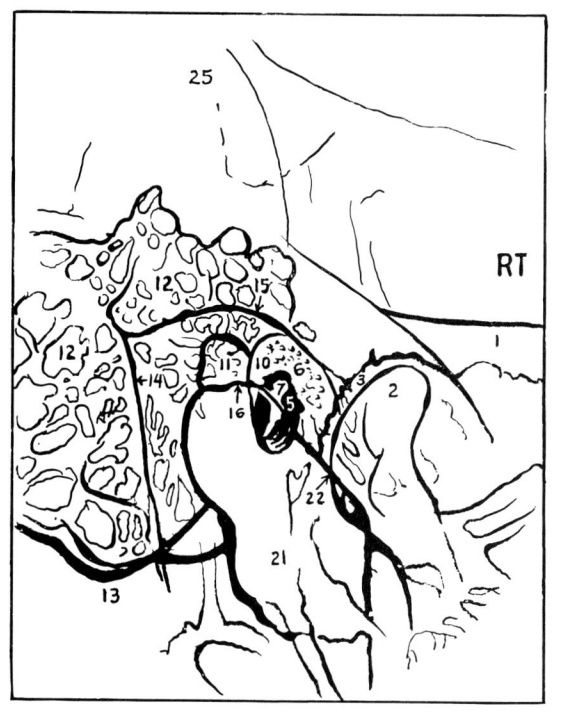

will provide the most information. If, however, there is a possibility of an acoustic neuroma or abnormality in the petrous region or internal auditory canal, the Towne, Stenvers, and transorbital views should be obtained.

The degree of mastoid cell development is described on radiographs by the terms pneumatic, diploic, sclerotic, and undeveloped. The generally accepted view of mastoid development is the following: When normal pneumatization of a mastoid occurs unhindered by recurrent episodes of infection in childhood or other developmental abnormalities, the resultant well-developed mastoid air spaces are referred to as *pneumatic*. When the pneumatization of the mastoid is disturbed by some infectious process there

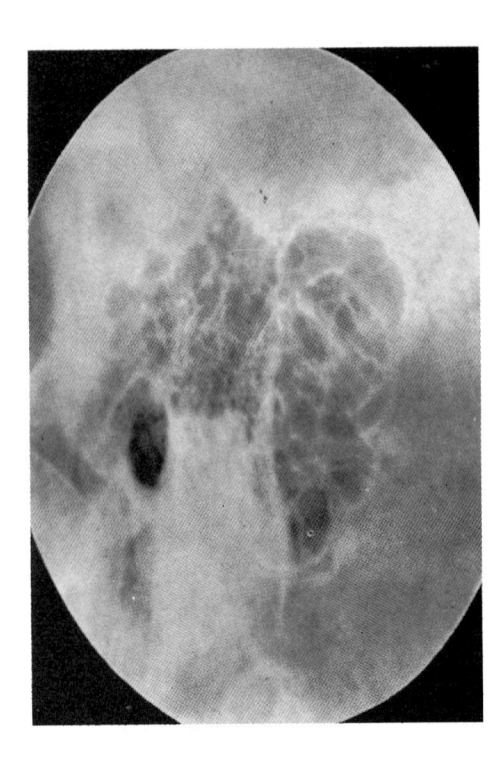

FIGURE 6–8. Mayer position showing malleus and incus in tympanic cavity with cells of attic. The antrum is partially obscured by the arcuate eminence. (From Compere WE Jr: Conventional radiologic examination of the temporal bone. *In* Shambaugh GE Jr (ed): Surgery of the Ear, 2nd ed. Philadelphia, WB Saunders Co, 1967, p 106.)

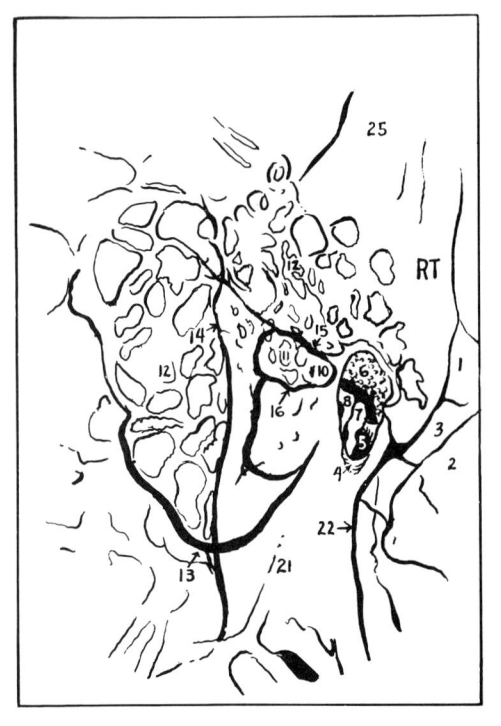

KEY TO THE LINE DRAWING
1. Root of the zygoma
2. Condyle of the mandible
3. Temporomandibular joint
4. External auditory canal
5. Tympanic cavity
6. Epitympanic cavity
7. Malleus
8. Incus
10. Area of the aditus
11. Area of the antrum
12. Mastoid cells
13. Mastoid tip
14. Anterior plate of the lateral sinus
15. Tegmen plate
16. Arcuate eminence
21. Petrosa
22. Anterior crest of the petrosa
25. Auricle

FIGURE 6–9. Owens position. Incus and malleus are clearly seen in the tympanic cavity, with epitympanum and antrum in normal relationship. (From Compere WE Jr: Conventional radiologic examination of the temporal bone. *In* Shambaugh GE Jr (ed): Surgery of the Ear, 2nd ed. Philadelphia, WB Saunders Co, 1967, p 108.)

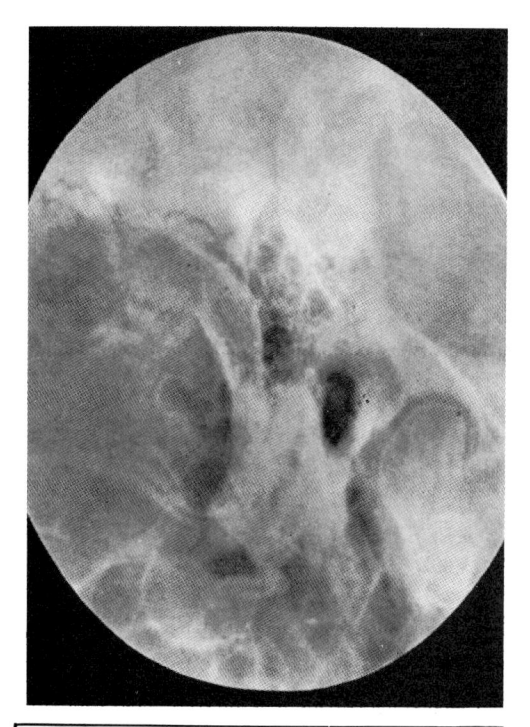

KEY TO THE LINE DRAWING
1. Root of the zygoma
2. Condyle of the mandible
3. Temporomandibular joint
4. External auditory canal
5. Tympanic cavity
6. Epitympanic cavity
7. Malleus
8. Incus
10. Area of the aditus
11. Area of the antrum
12. Mastoid cells
13. Mastoid tip
14. Anterior plate of the lateral sinus
15. Tegmen plate
16. Arcuate eminence
21. Petrosa
22. Anterior crest of the petrosa
25. Auricle

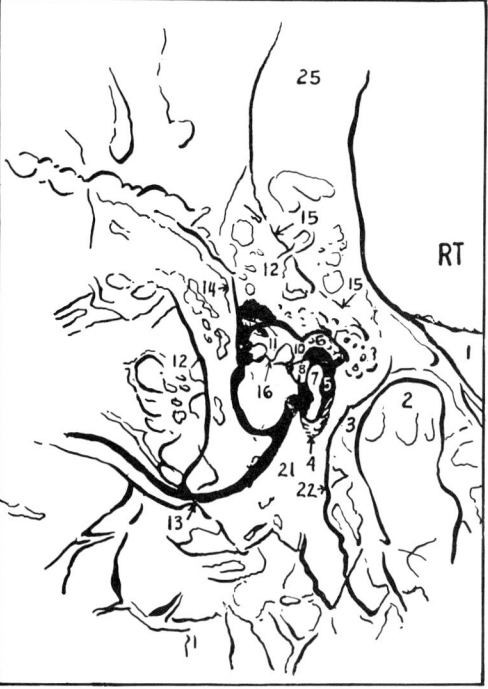

may be only a few groups of large cells present. Such an appearance is referred to as diploic. A small number of patients will have dense bone in the region of the mastoid. This probably results from osteoblastic activity stimulated by the repeated or chronic infection. This pattern is referred to as a *sclerotic* mastoid. It is common to find cholesteatoma development in this type of mastoid.

108 PART TWO—THE EAR

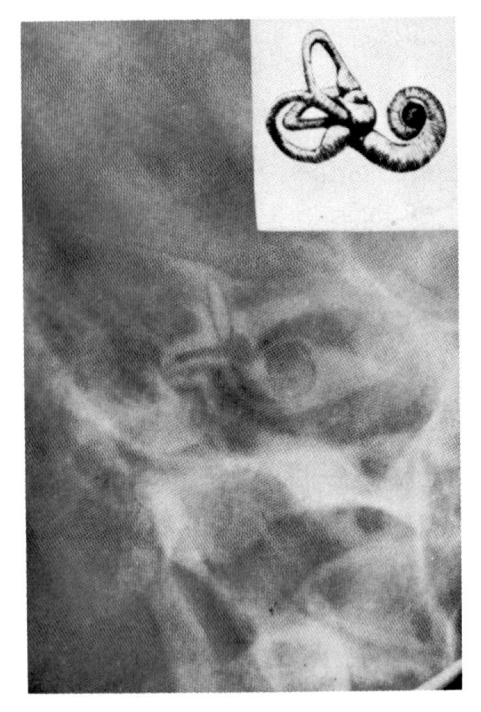

FIGURE 6–10. Stenvers position showing internal auditory canal, labyrinth, and antrum. (From Compere WE Jr: Conventional radiologic examination of the temporal bone. *In* Shambaugh GE Jr (ed): Surgery of the Ear, 2nd ed. Philadelphia, WB Saunders Co, 1967, p 109.)

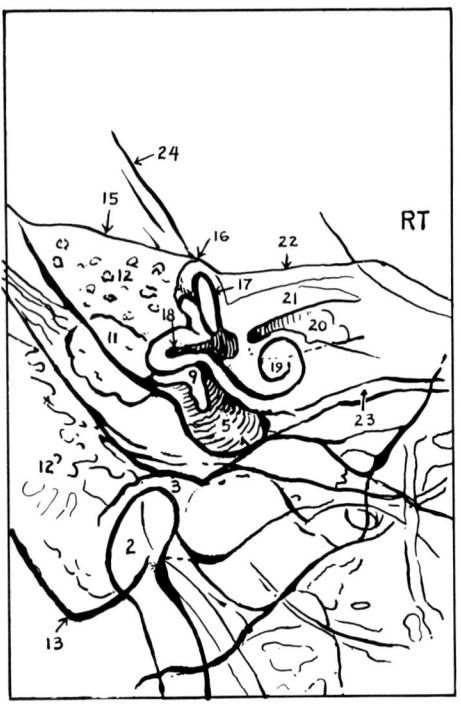

KEY TO THE LINE DRAWING
 2. Condyle of the mandible
 3. Temporomandibular joint
 5. Tympanic cavity
 9. Combined shadow of malleus and incus
11. Area of the antrum
12. Mastoid cells
13. Mastoid tip
15. Tegmen plate
16. Arcuate eminence
17. Superior semicircular canal
18. Horizontal semicircular canal
19. Cochlea
20. Internal auditory canal
21. Petrosa
22. Anterior crest of the petrosa
23. Petro-occipital suture
24. Sagittal crest of the occipital bone

CT Scanning

Computed tomography has in most instances become the preferred method of diagnosing middle ear, mastoid, and inner ear abnormalities (Fig. 6–11). Initially used for determining the presence of acoustic neuromas, the more refined CT scanners are capable of demonstrating ossicular discontinuity,

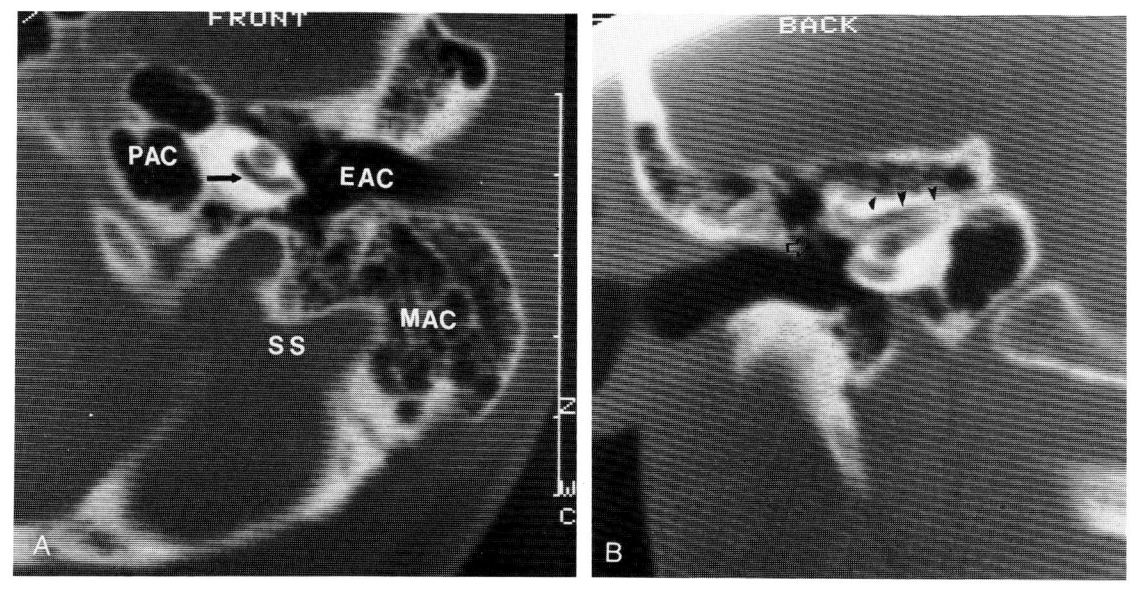

FIGURE 6–11. CT scans of a normal ear and mastoid. *A,* PAC, large petrous air cell; EAC, external auditory canal; SS, sigmoid sinus; MAC, mastoid air cells. Arrow points to the basal turn of the cochlea. *B,* A series of small arrowheads outlines the course of the facial nerve through the fallopian canal. The large arrow points to the malleus, showing how the head of the malleus lies within the attic of the middle ear space.

congenital anomalies, and extent of middle ear diseases such as cholesteatoma. This permits the operating surgeon to know whether the facial nerve is dehiscent by erosion of the cholesteatoma. In certain situations CT scans can even demonstrate fistulization into the horizontal semicircular canal. In congenital disorders CT scans have even been able to demonstrate the absence of a normally patent cochlea. Standard CT scanning is done in the axial plane. When special information is necessary, the sections can be retaken in the coronal plane or computerized reconstruction can be performed in the coronal plane.

Acute Coalescent Mastoiditis

Fortunately, this serious complication in the preantibiotic era is seldom seen today. Yet, for some reason, it is seen once or twice a year in major institutions. The diagnosis may be missed by the fact that the patient has received some antibiotics that were effective in altering the classic physical findings but not in eliminating the infection. In the untreated case, there is fever, pain, and hearing loss occurring in association with acute otitis media. The tympanic membrane bulges outward; there is sagging of the posterior superior canal wall, postauricular swelling displacing the pinna outward and forward, and mastoid tenderness, especially posterior and slightly superior to the level of the external canal (Macewen's triangle).

Radiologic examination in coalescent mastoiditis reveals opacification of the mastoid air cells by fluid and interruption of the normal trabeculations of the cells. The loss of the individual cell outlines distinguishes the findings from those of serous otitis media, in which the cell outlines remain intact.

Mastoiditis can occur in patients who have been immunosuppressed or who have neglected acute otitis media; it is possibly related to the virulence

Acute mastoiditis:
—*fever*
—*pain*
—*hearing loss*
—*bulging tympanic membrane*
—*sagging posterior canal wall*
—*postauricular swelling*
—*mastoid tenderness*
—*radiologic findings*

of the causative organism. The usual responsible organisms are the same as those that cause acute otitis media.

Treatment initially is a wide myringotomy, culture, and appropriate intravenous antibiotics. When the radiologic examination shows loss of the trabecular pattern or there is progression of disease, an urgent, complete mastoidectomy is mandatory to prevent serious complications such as petrositis, labyrinthitis, meningitis, and brain abscess.

CHRONIC INFECTION OF THE MIDDLE EAR AND MASTOID

Since the middle ear is connected to the mastoid, chronic otitis media is accompanied by chronic mastoiditis. These inflammatory problems can be considered active or inactive. Active refers to the presence of infection with drainage from the ear or otorrhea resulting from underlying pathologic changes such as cholesteatoma or granulation tissue. Inactive refers to the sequelae from a previously active infection that has "burnt out"; thus otorrhea is absent.

Patients with inactive chronic otitis media often complain of a hearing loss. There may be other symptoms of vertigo, tinnitus, or a sense of fullness as well. A dry perforation of the tympanic membrane is usually seen. Other changes may indicate tympanosclerosis (white patches in the tympanic membrane), loss of ossicles which is sometimes visible through the tympanic membrane perforation, and fixation or disruption of ossicles from previous infection. If there is sufficient disability and hearing loss, surgical correction or tympanoplasty can be considered.

Signs and Symptoms

Active chronic otitis media means there is an aural discharge. The otorrhea and chronic suppuration of the middle ear may indicate on first examination the nature of the pathologic process. In general, the otorrhea from chronic otitis media may be purulent (thick, white) or mucoid (watery and thin), depending upon the stage of inflammation. A mucous discharge results from activity of secretory glands in the middle ear and mastoid. A very foul-smelling, putrid discharge of dirty grayish yellow color suggests cholesteatoma and its degenerating products. Small, white, shiny flakes may be seen. Bacteriologic examination of the discharge from chronic middle ear suppuration provides little practical information for management. Secondary invaders, such as staphylococci, *Proteus vulgaris,* and *Pseudomonas aeruginosa,* and numerous anaerobic bacteria as part of a mixed flora are invariably found in chronic aural discharge. The most common anaerobes are members of the *Bacteroides* species. A thin, watery discharge and a history of painless onset should suggest the possibility of tuberculosis. If there is a thin, fetid discharge with blood, the possibility of malignancy should be considered.

Another important symptom in chronic otitis media is hearing loss, which is usually conductive but may be mixed. When the hearing loss is slight even though the pathologic involvement is extensive, the diseased area, or cholesteatoma, may be effectively conducting sound to the oval window. Pain is an uncommon symptom in chronic middle ear suppuration, and its presence is a serious sign. It may mean that a complication is impending due

FIGURE 6–12. In cases of chronic suppuration of the middle ear the fistula test is used to determine the presence of an erosion through the horizontal semicircular canal. The Politzer bag fitted with an atomizer tip supplies a convenient means of compressing the air in the external canal. If a fistula is present, the compression of the air will cause vertigo and usually nystagmus. If the test is negative, there is no fistula or the labyrinth is dead.

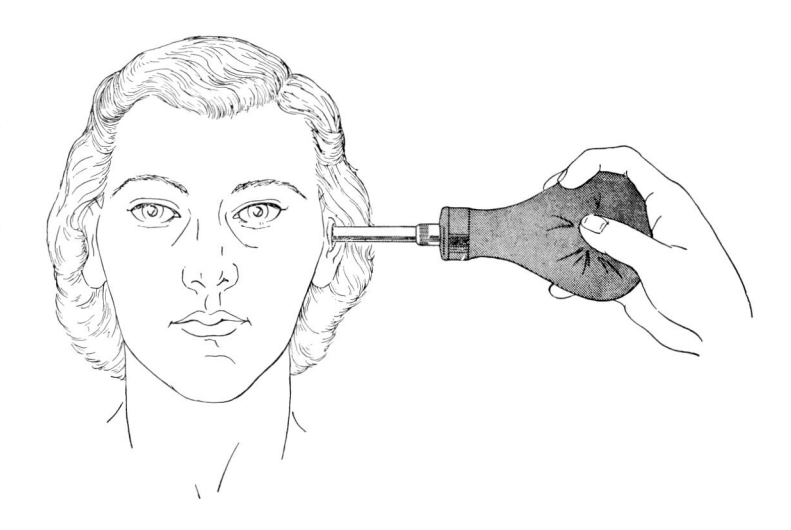

to blockage of secretion, exposure of dura or lateral sinus wall, or imminent brain abscess formation. Vertigo in a patient who has chronic middle ear suppuration is another serious symptom. This suggests the presence of a fistula, which means an erosion of the bony labyrinth, most commonly the horizontal semicircular canal. This is a serious finding, since infection can then pass from the middle ear and mastoid into the inner ear, thereby causing labyrinthitis (complete deafness) and, from there, possibly meningitis. A fistula test should be performed in every case of chronic middle ear suppuration when there is a history of vertigo. A fistula test requires application of both positive and negative pressure to the tympanic membrane and thereby across the middle ear space. The pneumatic otoscope, if an excellent seal can be obtained, may be suitable for this purpose. The test should be routinely done in patients with chronic otitis media, since a fistula may be present in the absence of vertigo (Fig. 6–12). A negative fistula test, however, does not exclude the possibility of a fistula.

Vertigo in a patient with chronic middle ear disease suggests erosion of the horizontal semicircular canal.

Fistula test: positive pressure applied by pneumatic otoscope causes vertigo and nystagmus.

Tympanic membrane perforations may be marginal or central. If the perforation is marginal or in the attic, cholesteatoma should be suspected. Granulation tissue may be seen filling the perforation or, in some instances, will form a sizable polyp extruding into the ear canal. Special care is required when this polyp is removed under the microscope to avoid injury to the ossicular chain. Multiple perforations in the tympanic membrane in adults suggest the possibility of tuberculous infection of the middle ear.

Radiologic examination usually reveals a sclerotic-appearing mastoid, often smaller and less pneumatized than the opposite or normal side. Bone erosion, especially in the area of the attic (scutum missing), suggests cholesteatoma.

Treatment

Conservative treatment for chronic otitis media consists essentially of advising the patient to keep water out of the ear and cleansing in the office with careful spot suctioning. Hydrogen peroxide or alcohol can be used for cleansing with a soft cotton-tipped wire applicator for removal of diseased tissue and inspissated suppuration. Local powders and ear drops, usually containing antibiotics and steroids, can be applied. Attention is directed to regional infections of the upper respiratory system. Antibiotics can be helpful in ameliorating the acute exacerbations of a chronic otitis media. However, antibiotics are not generally useful in treating this condition because, by definition, chronic otitis media means that intractable pathologic changes already exist, and antibiotics will not prove useful in curing this condition. If surgery is planned, systemic antibiotic treatment for several weeks prior to surgery may reduce or eliminate active drainage and enhance the surgical results.

Cholesteatoma is usually first evident through a perforation in the posterior superior quadrant of the tympanic membrane.

One of the pathologic conditions one sees in chronic otitis media and mastoiditis is cholesteatoma, which is keratinizing squamous epithelium ("skin") that becomes entrapped in the middle ear space and mastoid. This usually occurs secondarily to invasion of epithelial cells from the adjacent external auditory canal through the attic into the mastoid. Rarely, this can occur congenitally by entrapment of epithelial cells behind an intact tympanic membrane. Cholesteatoma in the middle ear could be called an epidermal cyst, a lesion sometimes seen in the cerebellopontine angle as well. The epithelium gradually increases in size, as if trapped in a bottle with a narrow neck. Release of enzymes and products of degradation as well as pressure will result in adjacent bone erosion. Until it becomes infected or impairs hearing, a cholesteatoma can reach considerable size with resultant loss of mastoid bone, ossicles, and bony protection of the facial nerve. Another pathologic change seen in chronic otitis media is granulation tissue, which can also cause osseous destruction and severe changes throughout the middle ear and mastoid. Granulation tissue can appear in an immature (soft) or mature (fibrous) form. A specific kind of granulation tissue is cholesterol granuloma, in which cholesterin clefts are seen within a bed of granulation tissue with interspersed giant cells (Fig. 6–13). This disorder is always treated by surgery and requires a mastoidectomy.

A cholesteatoma develops as a blind epithelium-lined sac with a small bottleneck opening. It gradually expands eroding the surrounding bone.

It may remain asymptomatic until it becomes acutely infected or erodes the ossicular chain, horizontal canal, or facial nerve.

Surgery

Surgery is aimed at eradicating infection and obtaining a safe, dry ear through a variety of tympanoplasty and mastoidectomy procedures. The primary purpose of surgery is removal of disease and is achieved if proper

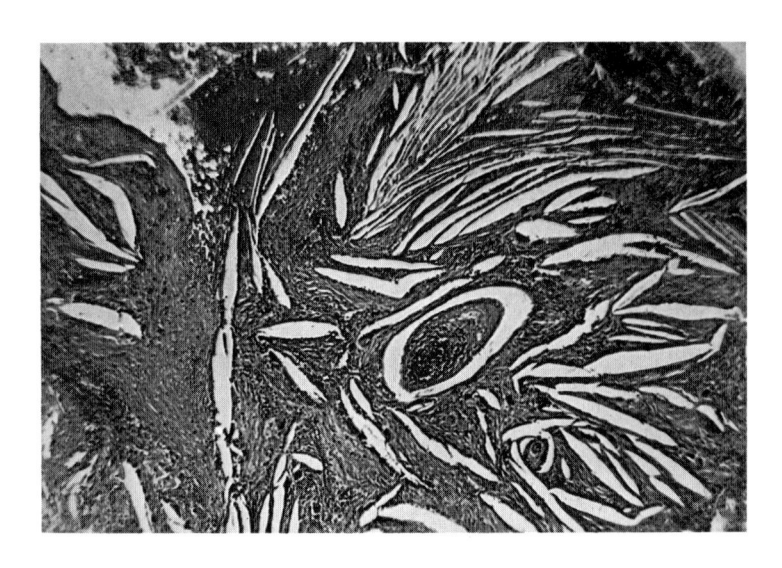

FIGURE 6–13. Cholesterol granuloma. Cholesterin clefts are seen in a bed of dense fibrous granulation tissue with interspersed giant cells. (From Paparella MM, Shumrick DA (eds): Otolaryngology, Vol 2. Philadelphia, WB Saunders Co, 1973, p 109.)

healing results (Fig. 6–14). The purpose of mastoidectomy is to eradicate infected tissue, creating a safe, dry ear; the purpose of tympanoplasty is the preservation and restoration of hearing, using procedures to graft the tympanic membrane and reconstruct the middle ear. The secondary objective is, when possible, to maintain or improve hearing (tympanoplasty). If chronic otitis media and mastoiditis are serious, and especially if a complication exists or is impending, mastoid surgery can be considered at any age. In general, tympanoplasty is performed less commonly in children below the age of five. This is because of the high incidence of ear infections in these children, who have not yet achieved adequate eustachian tube function. Many different tympanoplasty techniques exist, including grafting (skin, fascia, homologous tympanic membranes) and reconstruction (homologous ossicles, cartilage, alloplastic materials). In Figure 6–15, the classic tympanoplasty types are described.

COMPLICATIONS OF ACUTE OTITIS MEDIA AND MASTOIDITIS

The complications of acute or chronic middle ear disease and mastoiditis can involve changes directly occurring within the middle ear and mastoid or secondary infection of the surrounding structures. The structures immediately adjacent to the mastoid are shown in Figure 6–16. There are preformed pathways of extensions of infection into the area as well as extension of disease process by bony destruction with erosion as in the cholesteatoma or middle ear and mastoid with chronic granulation tissue. Erosion of the hard bony covering protecting the labyrinth and the tegmen can occur with chronic infection. The preformed pathways existing along these channels are more likely to be the route of dissemination of infection in the acute processes.

Middle Ear Complications

Conductive hearing loss can result from chronic otitis media. If a tympanic membrane is intact, the middle ear contains air, and there is a disruption of the ossicular chain, a maximum conductive hearing loss of 60 dB will result. The magnitude of the conductive loss may not always correlate with the severity of the disease, since pathologic tissues can also conduct sound to the oval window. Sensorineural deafness can result from acute otitis media as well as chronic otitis media. Any time there is an infection in the middle ear space, especially under pressure, there is a possibility that the products of infection will spread through the round window membrane into the inner ear, causing sensorineural hearing loss. The infection is usually limited to the basal turn of the cochlea, a portion that is not tested routinely when hearing is measured. Over time, however, the hearing loss can spread until it does become a problem later in life. This emphasizes the need for more aggressive treatment to prevent possible permanent sensorineural loss from developing in patients with acute otitis media who do not undergo resolution within 48 hours with appropriate antibiotic therapy (Fig. 6–17).

The maximum conductive loss occurs when there is ossicular discontinuity in the presence of an intact tympanic membrane.

Facial Nerve Paralysis. The facial nerve can be injured by either chronic or acute otitis media. In the case of acute otitis, the nerve is affected by purulent material directly in contact with the nerve. Because there may be

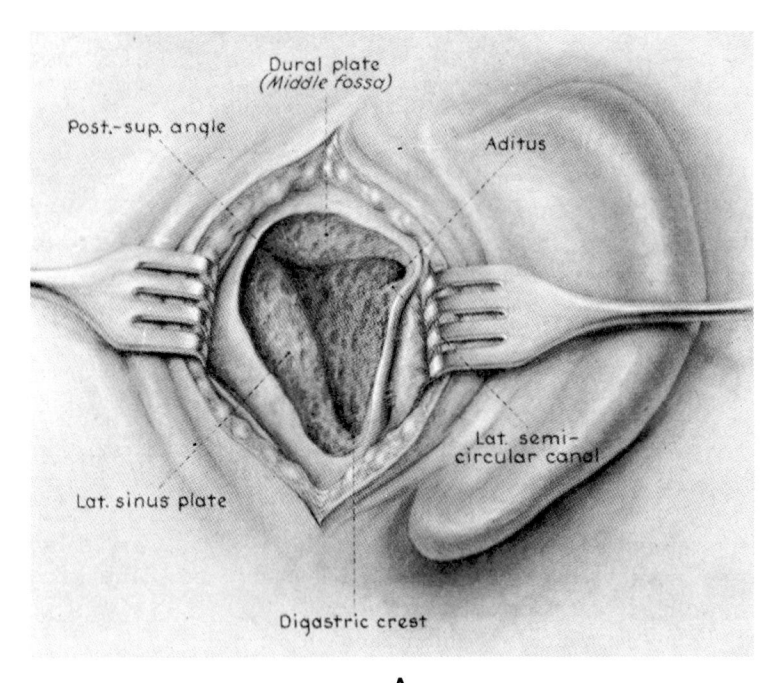

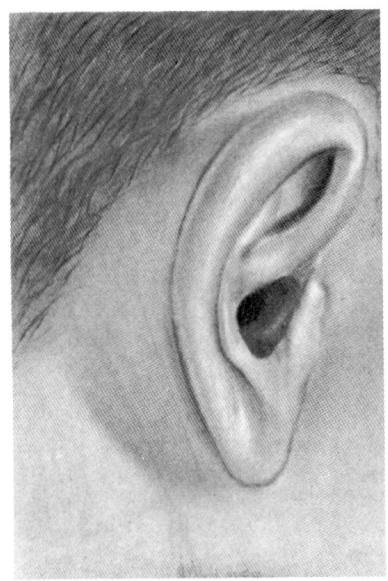

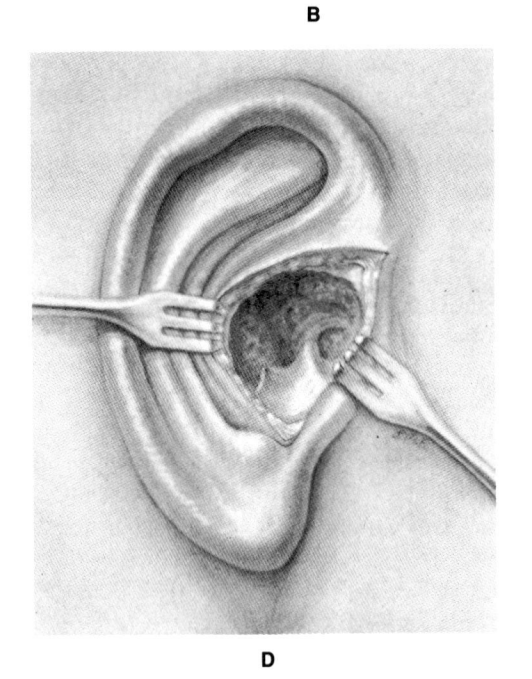

FIGURE 6–14. *A*, Simple mastoidectomy. The external auditory canal and middle ear are left intact while the mastoid is exenterated of disease and cell structures. *B*, Mastoid surgery can also be approached endaurally, as seen here. A larger opening (meatus) into the ear canal remains. *C*, Modified radical mastoidectomy. In this operation the mastoid is exenterated and the posterior canal wall is removed. The middle ear may be normal or nearly normal; however, often, tympanoplasty techniques need to accompany the mastoid procedure. Postoperatively, one sees a mastoid cavity and a relatively normal appearing tympanic membrane. *D*, Classic radical mastoidectomy indicates removal of all diseased tissues in the middle ear and mastoid. The otologist usually attempts to preserve or restore hearing through tympanoplasty as well.

FIGURE 6–14 *Continued* E, Completed radical mastoidectomy from surgeon's point of view demonstrates the important anatomic structures. a, Epitympanum; b, tegmen tympani; c, tegmen mastoideum; d, sinodural angle; e, lateral sinus; f, digastric ridge; g, mastoid tip; h, floor of middle ear (jugular dome); i, eustachian tube (protympanum); j, semicanal of tensor tympani muscle; k, horizontal facial nerve; l, cochleariformis process and tensor tendon; m, lateral semicircular canal; n, vertical facial nerve and ridge; o, round window; p, stapes; q, pyramidal process and stapes tendon; r, promontory. (*E* from Paparella MM, Shumrick DA (eds): Otolaryngology, Vol 2. Philadelphia, WB Saunders Co, 1973, p 290.)

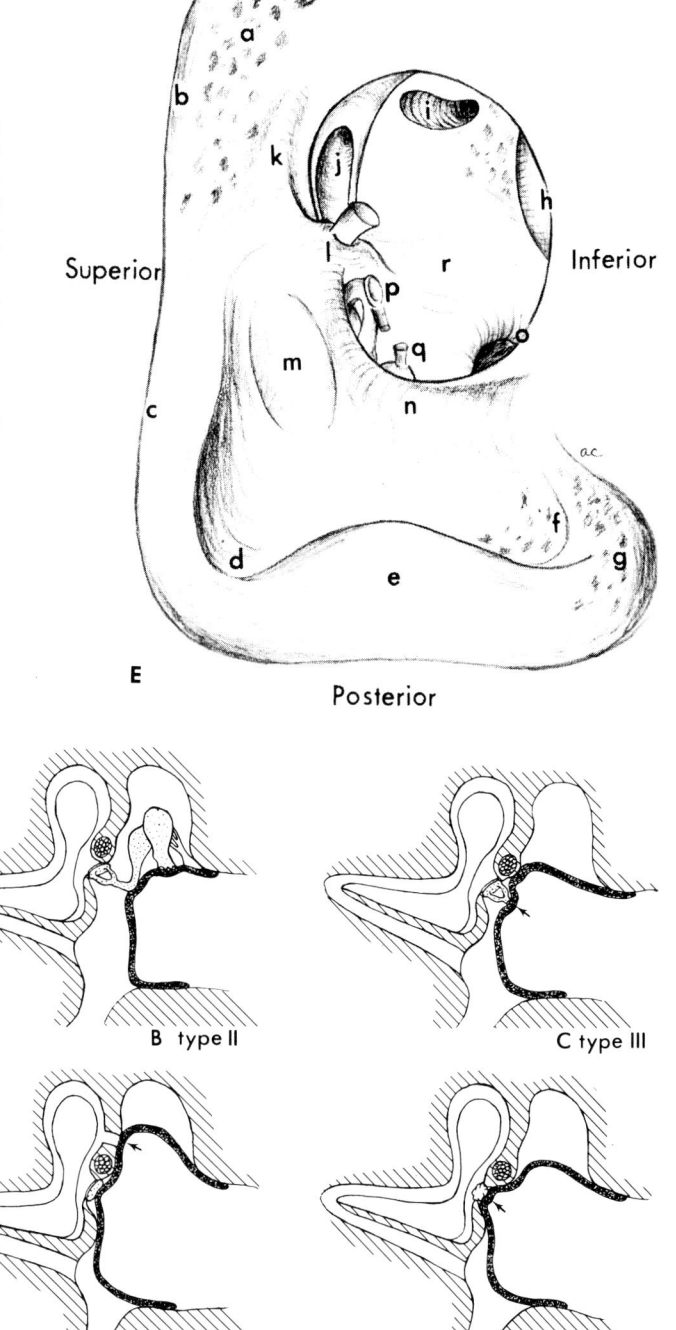

FIGURE 6–15. Tympanoplasty types. Middle ear spaces (mainly mesotympanum) decrease in size from type I to type IV. Assuming many other factors, the most common of which is good eustachian tube function, to be stable and under control, hearing results are decreasingly good as one proceeds from type I through type IV tympanoplasty. Under favorable conditions, type I tympanoplasty should result in normal or nearly normal restoration of conductive hearing, whereas type IV should result in approximately a 30 db air-bone gap. *A,* Type I—graft rests on malleus. *B,* Type II—grafts rests on incus. *C,* Type III—graft attaches to head of stapes. *D,* Type IV—graft attaches to footplate of stapes. *E,* Type Va—fenestration of lateral semicircular canal (arrow). *F,* Type Vb—stapedectomy (arrow). (From Paparella MM, Shumrick DA (eds): Otolaryngology, Vol 2. Philadelphia, WB Saunders Co, 1973, p 292.)

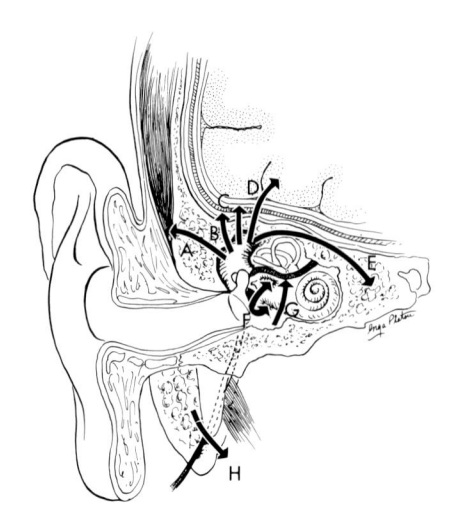

FIGURE 6–16. To understand complications of otitis media, one should consider spread of infection to regional structures. A, Subperiosteal space; B, subdural space; C, meninges; D, brain: E, petrous apex; F, labyrinth; G, facial nerve; H, neck. Another area, not shown here, is the lateral sinus in the back of the mastoid. (From Paparella MM, Payne E: Otitis media. *In* Northern J (ed): Hearing Disorders. Boston, Little, Brown and Company, 1976, Fig 10–8.)

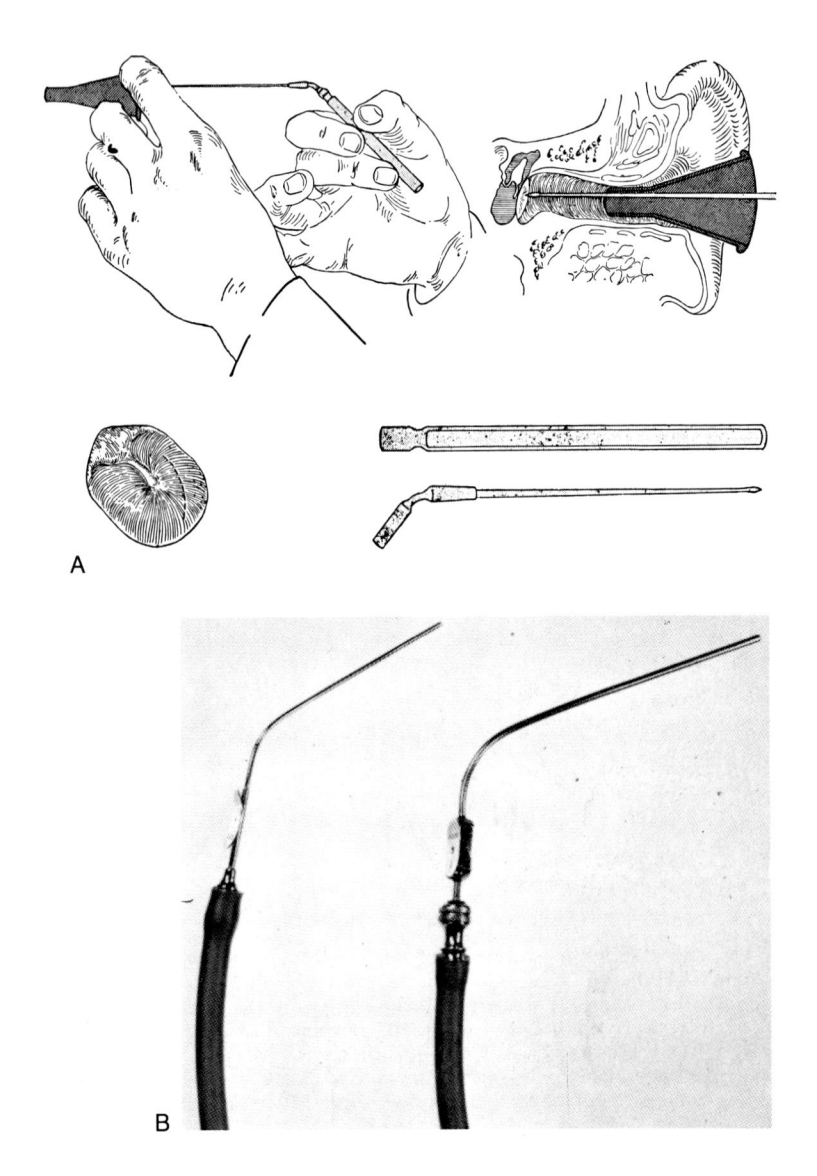

FIGURE 6–17. *A,* Accurate visualization of the drumhead under magnification and complete immobilization of the patient, using general anesthesia for children, are essential. The myringotomy knife should incise only the drumhead. *B,* Two sizes of suction tubes which can be used to aspirate middle ear fluid. When the fluid is thick, use of the larger suction tube is indicated.

natural areas of bony dehiscence exposing the facial nerve in the middle ear, the toxic products of infections can cause a facial palsy. Treatment involves an immediate wide myringotomy, obtaining cultures, and appropriate intravenous antibiotics. If resolution does not occur, surgical exploration is indicated.

Chronic otitis causes facial paralysis by a different mechanism. Granulation tissue or cholesteatoma adjacent to the nerve releases toxic products and causes pressure. Antibiotics will neither eliminate nor ameliorate this process, and surgery is required—the sooner the better.

Inner Ear Complications

Extension by destructive processes such as cholesteatoma or by direct passage of infection to the labyrinth may produce signs of inner ear disease manifested by severe vertigo or sensorineural hearing loss.

Labyrinthine Fistula and Labyrinthitis. Chronic otitis media, especially with cholesteatoma, may result in destruction of the vestibular labyrinth. A fistula into the labyrinth allows infection into the inner ear, causing labyrinthitis, which can lead to deafness. The patient with a fistula usually has vertigo in addition to other symptoms. A fistula test is performed by creating a negative and then a positive pressure against the middle ear and examining the patient for the development of vertigo and associated nystagmus (see Fig. 6–12). While a positive test is highly suggestive of the presence of a fistula, a negative test does not preclude the possibility of a fistula. CT evaluation may assist in the demonstration of the presence of a fistula, usually in the horizontal semicircular canal. It is possible for a fistula to be present in the absence of vertigo. Surgical treatment is necessary to eradicate all infection and to properly seal the fistula, thereby allowing the inner ear to recover, if destruction is not already too extensive.

Suppurative Labyrinthitis. Suppurative labyrinthitis can result from extension into a fistula (as just described), infection that has invaded the round window, or meningitis resulting from otitis media. Generalized labyrinthitis can invade all parts of the inner ear spaces, resulting in severe vertigo and ultimately complete deafness. When localized, it may cause either cochlear or vestibular symptoms and dysfunction alone. Labyrinthitis results from extension of infection into the perilymphatic space. Two forms of labyrinthitis exist: serous, in which chemical toxins cause dysfunction, and suppurative, in which actual pus invades the inner ear, resulting in its destruction. In either case it is extremely important to alleviate infection through appropriate surgery of the middle ear and mastoid.

Extradural Complications

Petrositis. Approximately one third of temporal bones have air cells in the petrous apex. These cells can become infected by direct extension of middle ear and mastoid infection. There are a variety of other routes of spread of infection to the petrous bone. Petrositis becomes evident when a weakness of the sixth cranial nerve occurs in a patient with otitis media. Pain often accompanies this because of irritation of the fifth cranial nerve. This syndrome was described by Gradenigo as a classic feature of petrositis. Petrositis, however, may exist without the classic triad, especially in patients who continue with suppuration or pain after appropriate surgery. Treatment

Gradenigo's syndrome: retro-orbital pain, 6th nerve paralysis, supportive otitis media.

Petrositis occurs in individuals with pneumatized petrous apetic cells.

of chronic petrositis is surgical, and during surgery for chronic ear infection petrous air cells are explored and diseased tissue is evacuated using a variety of techniques.

Lateral Sinus Thrombophlebitis. Infectious invasion of the sigmoid sinus, as it courses through the mastoid, results in thrombophlebitis of the lateral sinus. Small fragments of the thrombus break off, creating a shower of infectious emboli. Fever, unexplained by other findings, is the first sign of this invasion. It tends to fluctuate considerably and, as the disease develops fully, a septic or "picket fence" (spiking) pattern results. Chills often accompany a rise in temperature; pain is isolated to the area of the mastoid emissary vessels, which can become red and tender. This is called Griesinger's sign. The diagnosis is confirmed by magnetic resonance imaging (MRI) or digital subtraction angiography. Blood cultures may be positive, particularly if made at the time of the chill. Treatment is surgical and consists of removing the focus of infection in the infected mastoid cells, necrotic lateral sinus plate, or an infected and often necrotic lateral sinus wall. Drainage of the sinus and evacuation of the infected clot are indicated. Ligation of the internal jugular vein to prevent escape of the infected emboli into the lung and to other parts of the body is performed.

Extradural abscess:
—pulsatile, purulent discharge
—severe earache
—ipsilateral headache
—low grade fever
—develops during episode of acute otitis media.

Extradural Abscess. Extradural abscess represents a collection of pus between the dura and the bone overlying either the mastoid cavity or the middle ear. It is most frequently assciated with chronic suppurative otitis media with granulation tissue or cholesteatoma with erosion of the tegmen in this region. Symptoms include severe earache and headache.

Subdural abscess:
—develops from chronic otitis media
—headache
—fever, restlessness
—focal seizures
—difficulty speaking
—coma
—CSP may be normal, no organisms.

Subdural Abscess. A subdural abscess may develop as direct extension of an extradural abscess or by extension of thrombophlebitis through the venous channels. Symptoms include fever, headache, and the development of coma in a patient with chronic suppurative otitis media. Multiple central nervous system findings include seizures, hemiplegia, and a positive Kernig's sign. While an extradural abscess is frequently drained through the mastoid cavity at the time of radical mastoidectomy, a subdural abscess requires primary neurosurgical drainage.

Central Nervous System Complications

Meningitis. The most common intracranial complication from suppurative otitis media is meningitis. It can result from acute or chronic otitis media and can be localized or generalized. Although these two types are clinically similar, the spinal fluid of patients with generalized meningitis will often reveal bacterial organisms, whereas in localized meningitis, viable microorganisms cannot be recovered from the spinal fluid. Clinical features of meningitis include stiffness of the neck, increased temperature, nausea and vomiting (sometimes projectile), and headache. In advanced cases, there is also coma and delirium. On clinical examination there is resistance to flexion of the neck and a positive Kernig's sign. Usually sugar is low and protein is elevated in the spinal fluid. Treatment of meningitis is chemotherapeutic, and the patient is treated intensively with antibiotics specific for the organisms involved. Meningitis is treated first, and subsequently, if necessary, the ear infection is corrected through surgery. Any case of recurrent otitic meningitis requires that the ear infection be eradicated surgically.

Brain Abscess. As a complication of otitis media and mastoiditis, brain abscess can affect the cerebellum in the posterior cranial fossa or the temporal lobe in the middle cranial fossa. Brain abscess is usually formed as a consequence of direct extension of the otologic infection or thrombophlebitis. An extradural abscess usually forms prior to development of the brain abscess. Symptoms of a cerebellar abscess are generally stormier than those of the temporal lobe abscess. Cerebellar abscess may present with symptoms of ataxia, dysdiadochokinesia, intention tremor, and past pointing. Focal seizures or aphasia may be present with temporal lobe abscesses, and other symptoms include toxicity, headache, fever, vomiting, and a lethargic state suggesting cerebral involvement. A slow pulse and convulsive seizures are significant signs. Papilledema may also be present. Contrast CT scan or MRI allows localization of the lesion. The treatment is primarily surgical, and the abscess must be drained by traditional methods or needle aspiration and the patient placed on an intensive course of antibiotics. Following recovery after neurosurgical treatment of the brain abscess, combined otologic and neurosurgical approaches will be necessary to prevent recurrences.

Otitic Hydrocephalus. This condition consists of an increase in intracranial pressure with normal cerebrospinal fluid findings except for a marked increase in pressure. It may accompany an acute or chronic ear infection. Symptoms of this condition include intense persistent headache, diplopia, blurring of vision, nausea, and vomiting. Papilledema is present. Treatment consists of repeated lumbar punctures and management of persistent ear infection as well. It is believed that involvement of the lateral sinus leads to the inability of arachnoid granulations to absorb cerebrospinal fluid that is formed.

Myringotomy

Myringotomy is the incision of the tympanic membrane, either to provide ventilation to the middle ear, to permit drainage of middle ear fluid, or to obtain cultures. The procedure is performed under the operating microscope using general or local anesthesia. In the office setting, local anesthetic appropriately injected into the external canal or iontophoresis using a 2 per cent xylocaine solution placed in the ear canal provides sufficient anesthesia. Local anesthesia is particularly useful in older children or adults with serous otitis media but is less effective when the tympanic membrane is acutely inflamed. It is not used in the presence of external otitis. A curvilinear incision is made about 2 mm from the margin of the drumhead starting below and continuing upward anteriorly or posteriorly. Incisions are made in the anterior inferior or posterior inferior quadrant to avoid injury to the ossicular chain. It is technically easier to make the incision in the posterior inferior quadrant, and this area is less sensitive. The blade is never inserted more than 2 mm in order to prevent touching the medial wall of the middle ear, which can cause pain and bleeding. Further, there can be a dehiscence or bulge of the jugular vein coming onto the floor of the middle ear. Disruption of the ossicular chain is avoided by placing the incision in the inferior quadrants. Damage to the round window is avoided by making an incision only through the tympanic membrane and by limiting the depth of the incision (Fig. 6–17).

Myringotomy incisions are made in the anterior inferior or posterior inferior quadrants.

Myringotomy is performed for treatment of complications of otitis media such as mastoiditis or facial nerve paralysis developing during a course of otitis media. A wide "smile" type of incision is made. In these situations no tube is inserted. Continuous drainage, supportive care, and intravenous antibiotics are given. The wide myringotomy allows an opportunity to obtain a culture and Gram's stain. Special small collection devices are available to obtain secretions for study. Current indications for myringotomy in acute otitis media are (1) persistent pain after 48 hours of antibiotic treatment; (2) potential development of complications such as acute mastoiditis or facial nerve paralysis; (3) development of acute otitis media while on a systemic antibiotic; (4) development of otitis media in an immunosuppressed patient.

Myringotomy is required to obtain a culture in immunocompromised patients.

One of the most common indications for myringotomy today is persistent chronic serous otitis media that has failed medical management. In this case ventilation tubes are frequently inserted at the time of myringotomy. This prevents closure of the myringotomy site, as the tube may remain in place up to six months. Myringotomy incisions without tube placement often heal within 48 hours. Current indications for ventilation tube placement (PE tubes) at the time of myringotomy are the following:

1. Recurrent episodes of acute otitis media in spite of continuous prophylactic antibiotics
2. Persistent serous otitis media that has not responded to conservative management (usually a period of three months after an episode of acute purulent otitis media)
3. Persistent negative middle ear pressure and resultant atelectasis of the tympanic membrane, especially retraction into the posterior superior quadrant
4. Development of persistent negative middle ear pressure in patients undergoing hyperbaric oxygen treatment
5. In association with certain middle ear reconstructive procedures in which eustachian tube dysfunction is considered marginal

TUMORS OF THE MIDDLE EAR AND MASTOID

A variety of tumors, benign and malignant, can originate in the middle ear, mastoid, and adjacent regions, especially the external auditory canal. These tumors can be considered primary, indicating their origin in the temporal bone, or secondary, indicating that they have metastasized to the temporal bone from a distant site or invaded the middle ear from an adjacent area, usually the parotid gland.

Primary Tumors

Of the primary tumor types, the glomus jugulare or glomus tympanicum tumor is the most important and most common. The tumor originates from glomus bodies that relate to the jugular bulb in the floor of the middle ear, or they can originate from nerve distributions elsewhere in the middle ear. The tumor is histologically similar to carotid body tumors or chemodectomas. A malignant variety has been reported but is extremely rare. Through expansion this tumor can cause adjacent destruction resulting in hearing loss and a sense of fullness, and in some cases it may extend to the base of the skull, causing cranial nerve and intracranial complications. It is a highly vascular tumor and can often be seen as a bulging purplish mass in the floor of the middle ear through a semitransparent tympanic membrane. The blanching that occurs by pressure from a pneumatic otoscope is called Brown's sign. The CT scan with contrast is the most useful diagnostic test. In some instances angiography and retrograde jugular venography are necessary to make the diagnosis and determine the blood supply and extent of the tumor. Certainly a tissue diagnosis requires surgical exploration of the site, and in most instances surgery is the preferred modality of treatment. If the tumor is extensive, combined surgery and radiotherapy often are indicated. Unresectable tumors do show response to radiation therapy. Other benign tumors include neurofibroma of the facial nerve, hemangioma, and osteoma.

Primary malignant tumors that can involve the middle ear space include squamous cell carcinoma, rhabdomyosarcoma, adenoid cystic carcinoma, and adenocarcinoma.

Rhabdomyosarcoma occurs in young children. This disease was once considered universally fatal, whereas in recent years there have been reported cures with combined radiotherapy and chemotherapy.

Many squamous cell carcinomas originate primarily from the ear canal and then invade the middle ear and mastoid secondarily. It is especially important to suspect any lesion in the external canal which does not heal spontaneously or with appropriate medical treatment as representing a possible malignancy. Persistent chronic external otitis is a definite indication for biopsy of the external ear canal. If these tumors are found early, the patient has a much better chance of being cured than if the lesion progresses, necessitating total temporal bone resection and yielding a much lesser chance for survival. Occasionally, tumors, especially with superimposed infection, will present with symptoms of drainage, especially bloody drainage. Other symptoms include pain, a sense of fullness, hearing loss, and if the vestibular labyrinth is involved, vertigo. Facial nerve paralysis develops if the tumor erodes through the posterior canal wall and involves the facial nerve, but this generally occurs late in the course of the disease. The tumor will also extend anteriorly through fissures into the region of the parotid gland and pterygomaxillary fossa.

When external otitis does not resolve with usual treatment, a biopsy is indicated.

Facial nerve paralysis is a late sign of malignancy of the temporal bone.

The most common malignant tumors of the middle ear in adults are adenoid cystic carcinoma and adenocarcinoma. The most common malignancy to extend from the external canal to the middle ear is squamous cell carcinoma. Other less common tumors capable of arising in the external canal and then invading the middle ear are adenoid cystic carcinoma, malignant melanoma, and neglected basal cell carcinoma.

Secondary Tumors

Tumors that arise from distant primary foci and metastasize to the middle ear, mastoid, and temporal bone include adenocarcinoma of the prostate, mammary carcinoma, hypernephroma or renal carcinoma, bronchogenic carcinoma, gastrointestinal carcinoma, and melanoma.

In addition, the middle ear and mastoid can be invaded by tumors from adjacent areas such as meningioma, acoustic neuroma, glioma, neurilemoma, adenoid cystic and mucoepidermoid carcinoma of the parotid gland, and nasopharyngeal cancers extending up the eustachian tubes.

Hematologic malignancies such as malignant lymphoma and leukemia frequently involve the temporal bone, almost always involving the bone marrow of the petrous apex, and can also cause infiltration of the middle ear and eustachian tube, resulting in conductive hearing losses and effusions. In terminal or severe leukemia, actual hemorrhage can take place in the inner ear, causing sudden profound deafness as well as vestibular symptoms.

References

Bluestone CD, Stool SE: Pediatric Otolaryngology. Philadelphia, WB Saunders Co, 1983, p 16.

Draf W, Schulz P: Insertion of ventilation tubes into the middle ear: Results and complications. Ann Otol Rhinol Laryngol 89(Suppl 68):303, 1980.

Gates GA, Avery CA, Cooper JC, Prihoda TJ: Chronic secretory otitis media: Effects of surgical management. Ann Otol Rhinol Laryngol 98(Suppl 138):1, Jan 1989.

Healy GB, Teele DW: The microbiology of chronic middle ear effusions in children. Laryngoscope 87:1472, 1977.

Holm VA, Kunze L: Effects of chronic otitis media in language and speech development. Pediatrics 43:833–839, 1969.

Howie VM, Ploressard JH, Sloyer JL: The "otitis prone" condition. Am J Dis Child 129:678–688, 1975.

Jokipii AMM, Karma P, Ojala K, et al: Anaerobic bacteria in chronic otitis media. Arch Otolaryngol 103:278, 1977.

Klein JO: Microbiology of otitis media. Ann Otol Rhinol Laryngol 89(Suppl 68):98, 1980.

Miglets AW, Saunders WH, Paparella MM: Atlas of Ear Surgery. St Louis, The CV Mosby Co, 1986.

Moller P: Long-term otologic features of cleft palate patients. Arch Otolaryngol 101:605–607, 1975.

Paparella MM, Shumrick DA (eds): Otolaryngology. Vol 1: Basic Sciences and Related Disciplines. Vol 2: Ear. Vol 3: Head and Neck. Philadelphia, WB Saunders Co, 1980.

Paradise JL, Bluestone CC, Taylor FH, et al: Adenoidectomy with or without tonsillectomy for otitis media. Ann Otol Rhinol Laryngol 92(Suppl 107):36, 1983.

Shambaugh GE Jr, Glasscock ME: Surgery of the Ear. 3rd ed. Philadelphia, WB Saunders Co, 1980.

Teele DW, Klein JO, Rosner BA: Epidemiology of otitis media in children. Ann Otol Rhinol Laryngol 89(Suppl 68):5, 1980.

7

DISEASES OF THE INNER EAR

by Samuel C. Levine, M.D.

Patients who experience disease of the inner ear have symptoms of hearing loss, tinnitus, and disequilibrium. The physiology of hearing and balance has been covered in previous chapters. Here we discuss the clinical presentation of these problems and review by disease process the disorders of the inner ear. After discussing the clinical presentation of these problems in a general way, the chapter is divided into two large sections. The first deals with diseases that predominantly affect the cochlea and the later section deals with diseases that primarily affect the vestibular system. Since the two systems are physically interrelated, it is rare that a process involves only one of the structures. For this reason, there is some repetition.

Clinical Issues

History. The history of hearing loss is often one of the most difficult to ascertain. A frequently heard clinical complaint is "My hearing is fine. My wife insisted that I come in and have my hearing tested." Patients will also have significant trouble describing when they first noticed that they had a hearing problem. This is often associated with a time that they first were unable to use a telephone or found that while they were in a car with competing noise they had a problem with their hearing. It is important for diagnostic reasons to ascertain whether the patient has fluctuation in his or her hearing or a distinctly one-sided problem. Some factors in the history may even suggest the type of hearing loss which a patient has experienced. Patients who have high-tone sensorineural hearing loss will describe an inability to hear a female speaker or may have problems with certain words with high-tone consonants such as "f," "s," or "th."

It is important to obtain a work and social history in any case related to hearing loss. Patients who have had military exposure to noise often will have high-frequency sensorineural hearing loss. Similarly, adults who have worked for many years in loud work places will develop hearing problems. Ototoxic drugs may cause similar complaints. Finally, certain families appear to be prone to familial hearing loss. If this is not elicited in the history, it can be easily overlooked.

Tinnitus. Tinnitus is defined as an abnormal ringing noise in the ear. It is extremely common and is associated most frequently with sensorineural hearing loss. Anyone who complains of a pulsatile sound must be examined for an anatomic source. Anatomic sources for the tinnitus include vascular problems such as aberrant vessels or middle ear tumors. Patients who have

Tinnitus is any abnormal noise that the patient hears.

a sensorineural etiology to their tinnitus will describe worsening of tinnitus in quiet environments where competing noise is not covering the problem. They often will complain of bothersome tinnitus surrounding the time of falling asleep and first awakening.

Dizziness. In obtaining a history of dizziness, it is first important to attempt to differentiate dizziness of vestibular origin from that of central origin or from those causes that are unrelated to the balance system. If the patient suggests that he has had a loss of consciousness or has the sensation that he is about to faint during any of his attacks of dizziness, a nonvestibular etiology is likely.

In obtaining the history, it is important to get as accurately as possible the date of onset, the character of the initial phase of dizziness, the activity that the patient was carrying on at the time of onset, the duration of the symptoms, and finally the recovery period. The course of the illness is also clarified by obtaining a history of the frequency of recurrences (Table 7–1).

Dizziness caused by vestibular disorders is characterized by nausea, spinning sensations, and blurry vision.

Classically, vestibular dizziness creates a sensation of whirling or spinning, either of the patient or the environment. In more chronic cases and in bilateral cases of peripheral dizziness, patients may experience only a "drunken" feeling or a feeling of severe unsteadiness.

Vestibular symptoms of dizziness are often associated with somatic symptoms as well. Patients will complain of severe nausea and occasionally vomiting during attacks of vestibular dizziness.

Patients with vestibular symptoms often complain of blurred vision or difficulty focusing on a given object. They rarely complain of symptoms of double vision, scotomata, or blind spots. These unusual visual changes suggest a nonvestibular etiology.

Physical Examination

A thorough examination of the head and neck is absolutely essential to diagnose disorders of the inner ear. A full neurologic examination is also required. It is of importance to examine every cranial nerve, especially those immediately above and below the eighth cranial nerve, including an examination of visual acuity as well as range of eye motion. The eyes need to be examined for evidence of nystagmus. Neurologic tests such as the Romberg, in which a patient is asked to stand and close his eyes, are extremely informative. Sway and unsteadiness seen with the eyes closed which goes

TABLE 7–1. DIFFERENTIAL DIAGNOSIS OF DIZZINESS

	CENTRAL	PERIPHERAL
Onset	Variable	Sudden
Nature/description	Unsteady (swimming), "lightheaded"	Spinning, turning
Duration	Constant, varying	Episodic, motion-related, <2–3 days
Fatigable	Rarely	Yes
Visual effects	Closing eyes does not alter	Closing eyes makes symptoms worse
Visual symptoms	Double vision, blind spot	Blurry vision
Auditory symptoms	No	Yes
Headaches	Yes	No (but aural fullness)
Systemic effects	None	Nausea, vomiting
ENG results	Abnormal saccades; difficulty following a target	Decreased unilateral caloric

away when the patient can see again is suggestive of labyrinthine pathology. Patients should be examined for joint position sense and peripheral sensation. Cerebellar function can be tested by finger-to-nose and rapid alternating movements.

Laboratory Evaluation

Any patient who complains of hearing loss or tinnitus *must* have a thorough audiologic evaluation. This includes hearing threshold evaluation in frequencies from 250 Hz to 8 kHz. When appropriate, bone conduction, tympanograms, and reflexes need to be examined. If the patient's symptoms suggest a vestibular etiology or the etiology of a patient's dizziness cannot be ascertained by history alone, an electronystagmography (ENG) examination is necessary. Thorough ENG testing requires visual tracking, rapid deviation of eye movement, and caloric testing; optionally the patient may have bithermal caloric stimulation or rotational chair testing. ENG test equipment and procedures vary widely. The person performing the test needs to have experience in the operation and standardization of the equipment.

Any patient who complains of hearing loss or tinnitus must have an audiogram.

Laboratory tests may be obtained when it is considered appropriate. A suggested battery might include a CBC, urinalysis, coagulation function, glucose tolerance tests, thyroid and lipid testing, and an FTA-ABS test. Metabolic causes of dizziness or hearing loss are few, but they represent correctable causes for the patient's symptoms.

DISEASES PRIMARILY AFFECTING THE HEARING MECHANISM

More than 16 million Americans are classified as having a significant hearing loss. These hearing loss patients can be classified into two basic categories, one being congenital causes and the second being acquired etiologies. It is estimated that between 2000 and 4000 infants are born deaf every year (Fig. 7–1). Only half of these are of genetic etiology and about one third of the cases have no cause that is ever found. In those cases that have genetic causes, roughly two thirds are recessive, one third are dominant, and only 2 per cent are X-linked. Recent changes in audiology have enabled earlier detection and therapy for the profoundly deaf child. Most institutions

Only half of all congenital hearing loss is of a genetic cause; of these one third are dominant, two thirds are recessive, 2 per cent are X-linked.

FIGURE 7–1. Pie chart. There are 2000 to 4000 deaf infants born each year in the United States; only half have genetic causes. Of those infants with a known genetic cause of hearing loss, most are recessive. Only 2 per cent of the known genetic causes of hearing loss are X-linked.

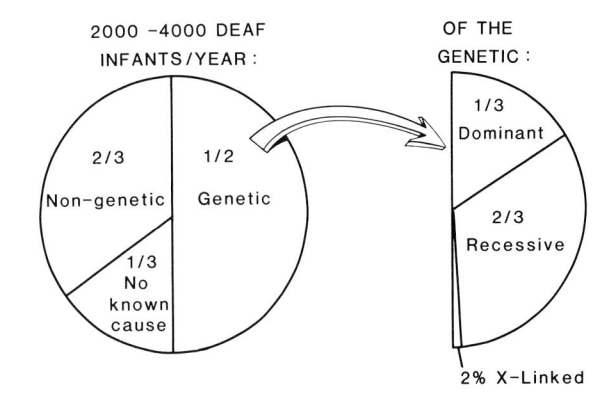

now have screening procedures in their neonatal intensive care units to attempt to detect hearing loss in infants.

The impact of hearing loss on older individuals has been known for a long time. From 1980 until 1985, the average age of the United States population has increased by two years. Government estimates of spending for special education, hearing aids, and compensation for those with hearing problems amounts to $500 million each year and, in the face of an aging population, there is serious concern about the ability of any insurance program to cover the tremendous cost of hearing loss.

Congenital Deafness

The list of genetic causes of hearing loss is extremely long. This is reviewed in Table 7–2. The most common causes of sensorineural hearing loss in children are reviewed in Table 7–3. Proctor reviewed these causes and showed that eight leading causes account for almost half of all hereditary hearing loss. Leading the list is diabetes. Hyperlipidemia is the second leading cause and otosclerosis is third. The remaining five causes represent less than 1 per cent each.

Congenital Deafness of Genetic Origin

Deafness of Genetic Origin Occurring Alone

MICHEL'S DEAFNESS. This entity, described by Michel in 1863, is characterized by total lack of development of the inner ear. Michel's deafness is thought to be autosomal dominant in transmission.

MONDINI'S DEAFNESS. In 1791, Mondini described a partial aplasia of the bony as well as membranous labyrinth. This malformation results in a flattened cochlea with development only of the basal turn so that instead of 2½ turns there are only 1½ turns, while the middle and apical turns occupy a common space. The osseous vestibular labyrinth may also be malformed. Dysgenesis of the organ of Corti causes the hearing loss. This condition is transmitted as an autosomal dominant trait.

TABLE 7–2. GENETIC HEARING LOSS IN CHILDREN

Without associated anomalies	**With integumentary disease**
Inner ear anomalies	Waardenburg's syndrome
Michel's aplasia	Oculocutaneous albinism
Alexander's aplasia	Ectodermal dysplasia
Mondini's dysplasia	
Scheibe's dysplasia	**With renal disease**
	Alport's syndrome
With eye disease	Potter's syndrome
Usher's syndrome	
Refsum's syndrome	**With metabolic disease**
Cockayne's syndrome	Pendred's syndrome
Optic atrophy	Mucopolysaccharidosis
Cataracts	
	With cardiovascular disease
With musculoskeletal disease	Jervell and Lange-Nielson syndrome
Albers-Schönberg disease	Hyperlipidemia
Paget's disease	
Treacher Collins syndrome	**With chromosomal anomalies**
Goldenhar's syndrome	Down's syndrome
Crouzon's syndrome	Other
Apert's syndrome	
Klippel-Feil syndrome	
Osteogenesis imperfecta	

7—DISEASES OF THE INNER EAR

TABLE 7–3. MAJOR CAUSES OF SENSORINEURAL HEARING LOSS IN CHILDREN

Diabetes	Paget's disease
Hyperlipoproteinemias	Rubella
Otosclerosis	Retinitis pigmentosa
Rh incompatibility	Pendred's syndrome

SCHEIBE'S DEAFNESS. Scheibe, in 1892, described this type of aplasia, in which the bony labyrinth is fully developed but the pars inferior (saccule and cochlear duct) is represented by mounds of undifferentiated cells. Scheibe's aplasia is the most common of all inherited congenital deafness disorders and is usually transmitted as an autosomal recessive trait. Pathologic findings are similar to those seen in animals with congenital genetic deafness. There may be some residual hearing in the low frequencies (Fig. 7–2).

which the bony labyrinth is fully developed but the pars inferior (saccule in 1904, described this type of inherited deafness characterized by aplasia of the cochlear duct. The organ of Corti and adjacent ganglion cells of the basal coil of the cochlea are most severely affected, resulting in a high-frequency hearing loss. Bony and membranous labyrinths otherwise appear normal.

Deafness Associated with Other Abnormalities

WAARDENBURG'S DISEASE. This syndrome is transmitted as a dominant trait. The primary features include lateral displacement of the medial canthi and lacrimal points, a flat nasal root, hyperplasia of the eyebrows, partial or total heterochromia of the irides, partial albinism in the form of a white forelock, and congenital deafness in approximately one fourth of these patients. The degree of deafness may be severe or mild.

ALBINISM. Albinism may be autosomal dominant, recessive, or sex-linked. Deafness associated with albinism may be bilateral and severe.

HYPERPIGMENTATION. Severe sensorineural deafness has been found in persons affected by hyperpigmented areas of skin. The pigmentary defects

FIGURE 7–2. Labyrinthine capsule in Albers-Schönberg disease in an infant 13 months of age. A.L., Apposition line. G.O., Globuli ossei. E.C., Endosteal capsule. L.B., Lamellar bone. P.C., Periosteal capsule. S.B., Skeinlike bone. I.L.B., Incompletely lamellar bone. (From Jackson C, Jackson CL: Diseases of the Nose, Throat and Ear (ed 2). Philadelphia, WB Saunders Co, 1959.)

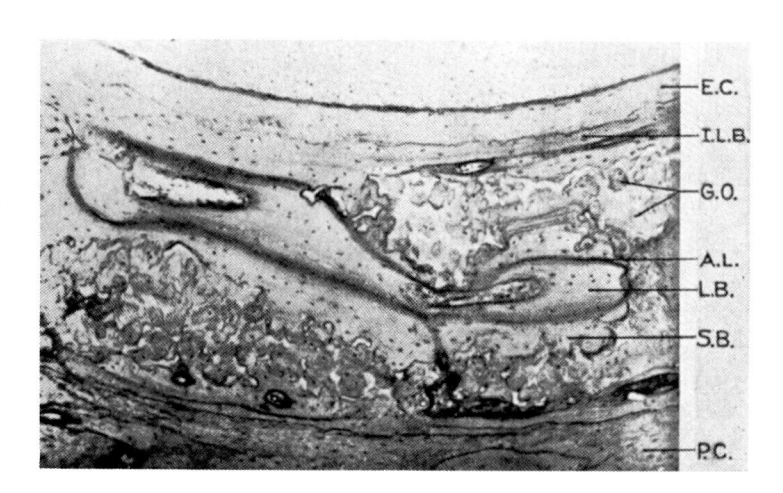

progress from small spots in localized areas in childhood to larger lesions over the entire body in adults.

ONYCHODYSTROPHY. The association of congenital male dystrophy and congenital sensorineural deafness is probably a recessive trait. The affected siblings have small, short fingernails and toenails and severe high-frequency deafness.

PENDRED'S DISEASE (NONENDEMIC GOITER). It has been estimated that this syndrome may account for as many as 10 per cent of the cases of recessive hereditary deafness. It is characterized by abnormal iodine metabolism resulting in thyroid enlargement which usually appears in adolescence, with nodular development in adulthood. The affected persons are usually born with severe hearing loss.

JERVELL'S DISEASE (JERVELL AND LANGE-NIELSEN DISEASE). The main characteristics of this syndrome include a prolongation of the Q-T interval, Stokes-Adams attacks, and congenital bilateral severe hearing loss. It has been estimated that this disease is related to 1 per cent of all recessive hereditary deafness. Syncopal attacks begin to occur in childhood, and affected persons usually die suddenly in childhood.

USHER'S DISEASE. The main features of this syndrome are progressive retinitis pigmentosa and congenital severe to moderate sensorineural hearing loss. Inheritance of this disease is usually through recessive transmission, but it may be sex-linked or dominant. The hearing loss is bilateral and severe.

Chromosomal Abnormalities

Chromosomal anomalies account for some types of congenital deafness. They are not truly hereditary but represent cases in which an extra chromosome has been added to one of the 22 pairs of autosomal chromosomes.

TRISOMY 13-15 (D). This syndrome may include low-set ears, undifferentiated pinnae, absence of the external auditory canals or the middle ear, cleft lip, cleft palate, microphthalmia, coloboma irides, and aplasia of the optic nerve. Infants with this syndrome usually die within a short time.

TRISOMY 18 (E). This syndrome may include low-set ears, malformed pinnae, micrognathia, flexion of the index finger over the third finger, and prominent occiput. Patients with this syndrome fail to thrive and usually die in infancy.

Congenital Deafness of Nongenetic Origin

Deafness Associated with Other Abnormalities

RUBELLA. Still one of the most common causes of nongenetic congenital deafness is rubella (German measles). With the use of the present rubella vaccine, this particular disease should eventually be eliminated. If a woman contracts German measles within the first three months of pregnancy, the probability is high that her child will suffer some degree of sensorineural hearing loss. A child with congenital rubella may also suffer from other defects, such as cardiac defects, mental retardation, and blindness. Pathologic examination shows aplasia of the organ of Corti and of the saccule (pars inferior). The pars superior is generally normal.

Women who contract rubella in the first trimester have children at higher risk for hearing loss.

ERYTHROBLASTOSIS FETALIS. Kernicterus in the newborn may result from Rh blood incompatibility of the parents. This disease is characterized by a deposition of bilirubin in the central nervous system, and jaundice, mental retardation, cerebral palsy, and deafness may be present shortly after birth in these infants. Postpartum exchange transfusion is the treatment for this problem; however, the child may still have some high-tone sensorineural loss. Therefore, the physician should be alert to this possibility.

CRETINISM. Thyroid disease may be associated with deafness, as in this syndrome, which is usually referred to as endemic cretinism. It is generally accepted that iodine deficiency is responsible for the cretinism. This condition is usually found in certain geographic locations, such as the Alps. The hearing loss is of a mixed type, being both sensorineural and conductive.

Nongenetic Deafness Occurring Alone

Causes of congenital deafness which may occur without associated abnormalities include premature birth, hypoxia, and prolonged labor. There is also the possibility that the mother received ototoxic drugs during pregnancy which may impair the hearing of the child. The pathology in these diseases has not been well studied.

Delayed or Acquired Genetic Deafness

It is important for the clinician to recognize deafness as early as possible and to advise the patient accordingly.
abnormalities include premature birth, hypoxia, and prolonged labor. There DEAFNESS). The genetic nature of this type of hearing loss may be overlooked owing to its clinical similarity to other types of sensorineural hearing loss. Correct diagnosis depends primarily upon a careful history of the problem in relation to its occurrence in other members of the family. The diagnosis is often made by excluding all possible extrinsic causes, leaving only an intrinsic cause—namely, genetic hearing loss—as the most likely possibility. The deafness is usually bilateral and is considered to be an autosomal dominant disorder. It can appear in childhood or in early adulthood and will progress in severity during the remainder of the patient's life. Genetic progressive deafness is characterized by a bilateral, generally flat or basin-shaped sensorineural configuration on the audiogram with fairly good discrimination. There may be absence of the organ of Corti and spiral ganglion cells in the basal turn and, most important, irregular degeneration of the stria vascularis (Fig. 7–2).

OTOSCLEROSIS. Otosclerosis is an autosomal dominant disorder and has been described in Chapter 6. It causes primarily a conductive hearing loss, which may be associated with a progressive sensorineural hearing loss.

Deafness Associated with Other Abnormalities

The number of described genetic syndromes involving deafness is so large that a detailed discussion of each is impossible. Therefore, the more common syndromes that may be encountered will be discussed.

ALPORT'S DISEASE. This dominantly transmitted syndrome is a progressive renal disease (glomerulonephritis) that usually begins in childhood. Kidney degeneration is usually accompanied by a progressive sensorineural hearing loss that increases as renal malfunction worsens. Hearing loss associated with Alport's syndrome is bilateral, symmetric, and greater in the high frequencies. Response to caloric tests may be reduced. Males are affected more frequently than females.

Any syndrome with renal disorders, retinitis pigmentosa, facial anomalies or cardiac problems may have hearing loss as part of the clinical picture.

VON RECKLINGHAUSEN'S DISEASE. This syndrome is a localized form of neurofibromatosis which includes bilateral acoustic tumors. Peripheral signs of the disease such as hyperpigmented spots on the skin are often present. The disease is usually transmitted through dominant inheritance.

HURLER'S SYNDROME. This disease begins in early childhood and results in skeletal deformity, dwarfism, mental retardation, enlargement of the spleen and liver, blindness, and profound sensorineural hearing loss. It appears to be transmitted as a recessive trait and may be sex-linked. It is usually fatal.

KLIPPEL-FEIL SYNDROME. This syndrome consists of skeletal defects, which may include fusion of the cervical vertebrae, spina bifida, scoliosis, and torticollis. Vestibular dysfunction and profound sensorineural deafness may also be present. The disease is inherited as an autosomal recessive trait.

REFSUM'S DISEASE. This disease is characterized by retinitis pigmentosa, ichthyosis, polyneuropathy, ataxia, and hearing loss. Approximately half of the patients with Refsum's disease have a progressive sensorineural hearing loss. The disease is transmitted as an autosomal recessive trait.

ALSTROM'S DISEASE. The primary features of this syndrome are retinitis pigmentosa, diabetes mellitus, obesity, and progressive deafness. Hearing loss appears around age 10 and is slowly progressive. The syndrome is inherited through autosomal recessive transmission.

PAGET'S DISEASE. Osteitis deformans, or Paget's disease, is characterized by skeletal deformities of the skull and the long bones of the legs. The disease usually begins in middle age. This disease is inherited as an autosomal dominant trait (Fig. 7–3).

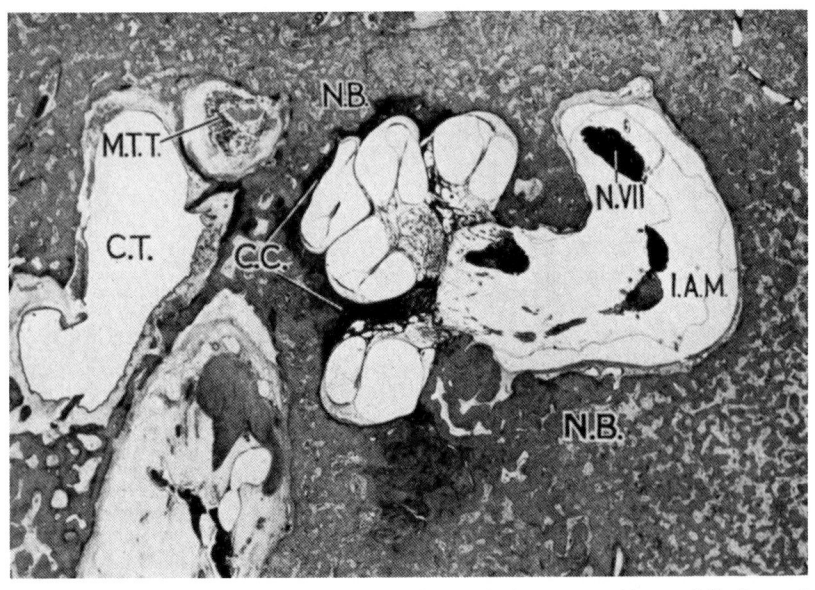

FIGURE 7–3. Paget's disease, vertical section through the temporal bone. C.C., Remants of the old cochlear capsule. C.T., Cavum tympani. I.A.M., Internal auditory meatus. M.T.T., Tensor tympani muscle. N.B., Newly formed bone. N.VII, Facial nerve. (Photomicrograph from Otological Research Laboratory, College of Physicians and Surgeons, Columbia University.) (Reprinted from Jackson C, Jackson CL: Diseases of the Nose, Throat and Ear (ed 2). Philadelphia, WB Saunders Co, 1959.)

RICHARDS-RUNDLE SYNDROME. The main features of the syndrome include mental deficiency, ataxia, hypogonadism, and severe deafness. All these symptoms appear in childhood. Hearing loss is total by five or six years of age. Transmission is through autosomal recessive inheritance.

CROUZON'S DISEASE. Craniofacial dysostosis is characterized by premature synostosis of the cranial suture, exophthalmos, parrot or hook nose, short upper lip and protruding lower lip, atresia of the auditory meatus, and a mixed hearing loss. The syndrome is inherited as an autosomal dominant trait.

Infectious Causes of Hearing Loss

MIDDLE EAR INFECTIONS. An infectious process in the middle ear can obtain access to the inner ear. Metabolic products pass from the middle ear into the cochlea or vestibule through the round or oval window. The frequency and severity of this process are not well documented. It can occur in acute otitis but is seen more often in chronic cases. If a cholesteatoma forms and invades the inner ear, deafness is the usual result.

Middle ear infections can lead to sensorineural hearing loss by passing toxic byproducts through the round or oval window.

VIRUSES. Viral infections that cause hearing loss include mumps, chickenpox, measles, influenza, herpes zoster, and adenoviruses. Mumps is the leading cause of unilateral acquired hearing loss in children. Measles remains the leading cause of bilateral hearing loss. Viral etiologies are usually seen in children. Their role in adults is less well defined.

MENINGITIS. Meningitis is a major cause of hearing loss in children. The loss is usually bilateral but may on occasion be unilateral. The hearing loss usually occurs in patients who are comatose for some period of time. The hearing loss appears to occur early in the process, which may not be aborted even with appropriate antibiotic therapy (Fig. 7–4).

SYPHILIS. Congenital syphilis should always be considered as a cause for acquired sensorineural hearing loss. A fluctuating unilateral or bilateral hearing loss with changes in balance may appear at any time during a

FIGURE 7–4. Microphotograph showing invasion of the meninges of the internal meatus from labyrinthitis. Soft tissue parts of the cochlea are destroyed. A collection of pus (P) has formed in the base of the modiolus. Note thickened dura mater and granulation tissue (D). (From Jackson C, Jackson CL: Diseases of the Nose, Throat and Ear (ed 2). Philadelphia, WB Saunders Co, 1959.)

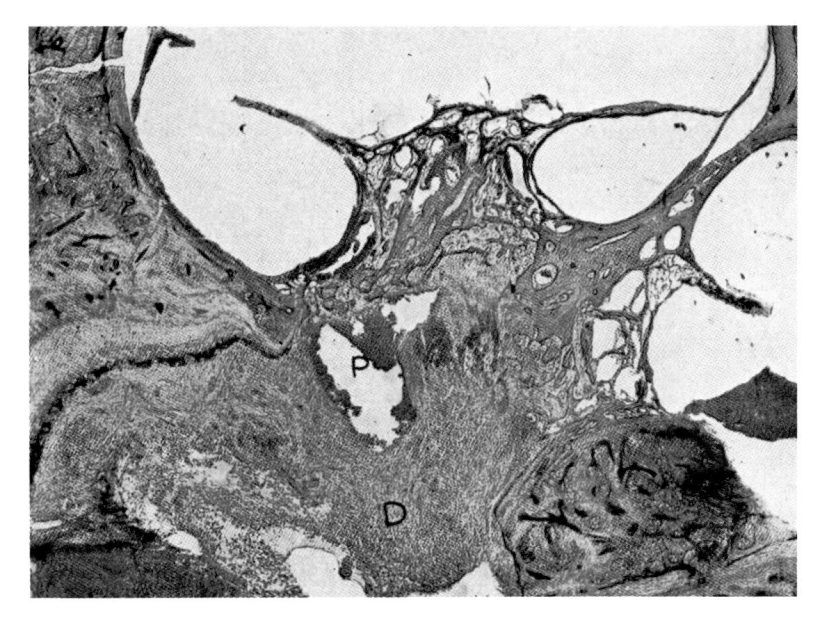

patient's life. Only FTA-ABS tests are reliable in the diagnosis of later phases of syphilis.

BULLOUS MYRINGITIS. This is an infectious process involving the middle layer of the tympanic membrane. It is a painful process that has been associated with high-tone sensorineural hearing loss.

Ototoxic Drugs

Table 7–4 presents an extensive list of drugs and chemicals that affect the inner ear and hearing mechanism. As a general rule, any drug or chemical that causes a renal toxic effect can and usually does cause some ototoxicity. Each of the listed drugs can cause both vestibular and hearing symptoms. Most of the medications listed are irreversible in their effects, although if the effect is detected early enough and the drug discontinued some hearing loss can be reversed. Drugs with otoxic effects that are particularly reversible include salicylates. Salicylate poisoning results in a 30- to 40-dB flat hearing loss that is reversible when the drug is discontinued. Similarly, erythromycin causes hearing loss only when given intravenously and in relatively high doses. When this drug is withdrawn, the hearing loss is also reversed. Medications such as dihydrostreptomycin have been banned in the United States because of their long-term effects on the auditory system. Even after dihydrostreptomycin is discontinued, effects on the hearing system can occur as late as a month following discontinuation of the drug.

When using any ototoxic agent: (1) get baseline hearing levels, (2) test for balance, (3) warn the patient of the potential toxicity.

In handling patients who are on potentially ototoxic drugs, the first rule is that the patient must be warned about the potential side effects. If possible, baseline studies including balance and hearing tests should be performed before the drug is prescribed. At the first warning sign, a repeat

TABLE 7–4. OTOTOXIC AGENTS

Antibiotics	**Antineoplastics**
Aminoglycosides	Bleomycin
Streptomycin	Nitrogen mustard
Dihydrostreptomycin	*cis*-Platinum
Neomycin	
Gentamicin	**Miscellaneous**
Tobramycin	Pentobarbital
Amikacin	Hexadine
Other Antibiotics	Mandelamine
Vancomycin	Practolol
Erythromycin	
Chloramphenicol	**Chemicals**
Ristocetin	Carbon monoxide
Polymyxin B	Oil of chenopodium
Viomycin	Nicotine
Pharmacetin	Aniline dyes
Colistin	Alcohol
	Potassium bromate
Diuretics	**Heavy Metals**
Furosemide	Mercury
Ethacrynic acid	Gold
Bumetanide	Lead
Acetazolamide	Arsenic
Mannitol	
Analgesics and Antipyretics	
Salicylates	
Quinine	
Chloroquine	

Acoustic Tumors

The most common inner ear tumor causing hearing loss is an acoustic neuroma. Acoustic neuromas are benign tumors of the Schwann cells covering the eighth nerve. These schwannomas occur most often on the balance portion of the eighth nerve. Other causes of hearing loss by tumors in the internal auditory canal include seventh nerve neuromas, meningiomas, hemangiomas, and aberrant vessels. Tumors in younger individuals or a family history of acoustic neuromas may represent an early manifestation of von Recklinghausen's syndrome. Von Recklinghausen's disease causes all cases of bilateral acoustic neuromas. The usual course of an acoustic neuroma is that the patient develops a unilateral sensorineural hearing loss. This is at first mild, but as the tumor continues to grow, it slowly crushes the nerves of the internal auditory canal. Rarely, patients complain of vestibular symptoms. The hearing loss progresses slowly in most cases. Acoustic neuromas can, however, cause sudden hearing loss or Meniere-like syndromes as well. **Any unilateral or asymmetric hearing loss is an acoustic neuroma until proved otherwise.** Discovery of small acoustic neuromas is made by having a high degree of suspicion leading to ABR (auditory brainstem response) testing and radiologic confirmation. Acoustic tumors are seen only on enhanced CT scans with high-resolution thin slices. MRI also provides an excellent view of these tumors and is probably more sensitive than CT scanning (Fig. 7–5).

Any asymmetric hearing loss requires further work-up with ABR, CT, or MRI.

Acoustic tumors may be removed surgically by three major routes. They can be resected from the middle fossa, from the posterior fossa, or across

FIGURE 7–5. A right cerebellopontine angle tumor is seen on MRI. The signal is more intense than nearby brain. The black line behind it is a large blood vessel. Acoustic neuromas are usually seen extending into the internal acoustic canal.

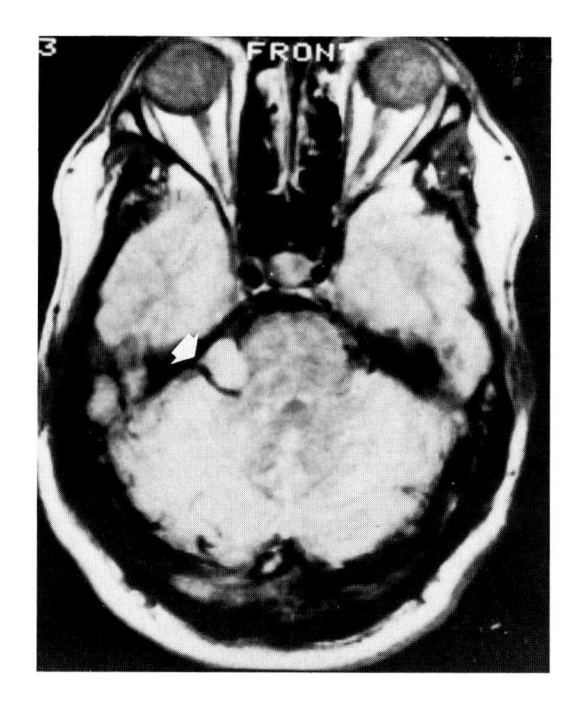

the labyrinth. The selection of a given procedure or combination of procedures is based on tumor size, potential for hearing preservation, and surgical experience.

Trauma

Trauma to the inner ear can be divided into two primary forms. One is acoustic energy and the second is mechanical energy. In injuries causing mechanical trauma to the temporal bone, temporal bone fractures are possible. Structurally, the temporal bone is made of some of the densest bone in the human body. It is protected by its central location. When the temporal bone fractures, it rarely does so without associated problems. These can and usually do include loss of consciousness, subdural or epidural hematoma, or concussion. Ultimately, this means that the patient's hearing is not a critical problem given (or requiring) acute treatment. These patients often will need neurosurgical procedures.

Temporal bone fractures are 80 per cent longitudinal, 20 per cent transverse.

Temporal bone fractures are divided into two general groups (Fig. 7–6). One is longitudinal fractures; the second is transverse fractures. Statistically, 80 per cent of the fractures are longitudinal and 20 per cent are transverse. Longitudinal fractures begin at the foramen magnum and travel out to the external auditory canal. The ear usually bleeds and there is a conductive hearing loss. Transverse fractures account for a high proportion of injuries to the labyrinth and facial nerve because the fracture line travels through the petrous apex or the labyrinth. Labyrinthine injuries can be less severe, causing a concussion phenomenon with recovery of balance and hearing, or more severe, with total loss of hearing.

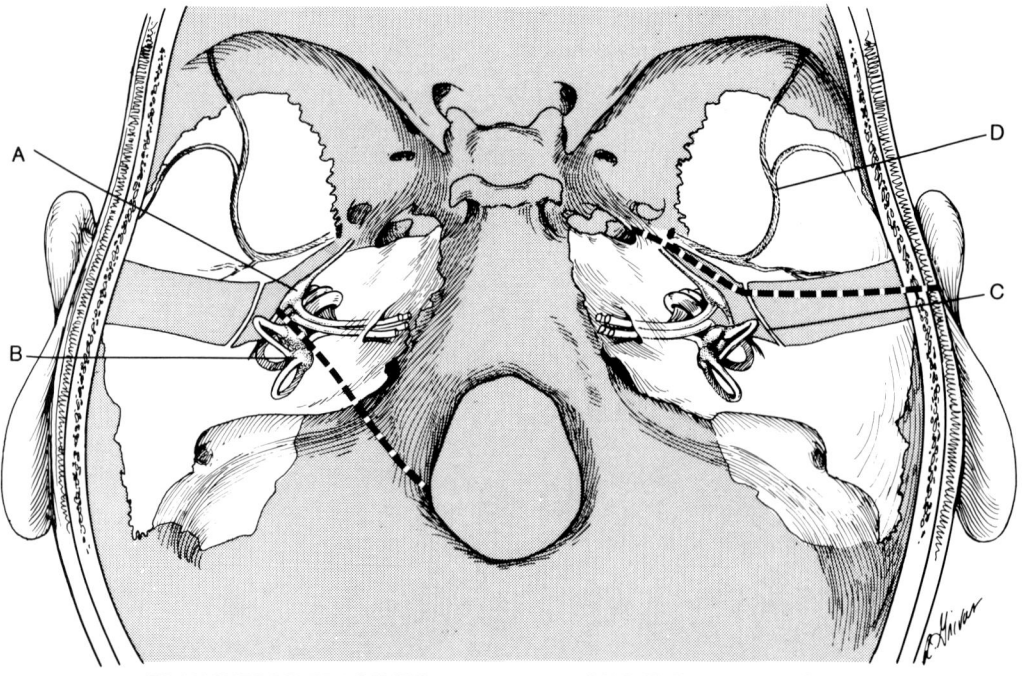

FIGURE 7–6. A temporal bone fracture. Temporal bone fractures are divided into longitudinal and transverse types. Transverse fractures usually involve the geniculate ganglion (A) and the inner ear (B). Longitudinal fractures go through the tympanic membrane (C). Either type can injure the middle meningeal artery (D).

Blast injuries cause a concussion wave that does more damage to the middle ear than to the inner ear, but high-tone sensorineural hearing loss can result from this type of injury. Acoustic trauma is perhaps the most common cause of sensorineural hearing loss. Sensorineural hearing loss is caused by both loudness and length of exposure. The Occupational Safety and Health Administration (OSHA) has established standards that are believed to relate hearing loss to the exposure of workers to loud noises over time in the work place. While levels of 80 dB for 8 hours are thought to be safe, exposure to 110 dB noise over a relatively brief period of time is considered dangerous to the long-term safety of the hearing mechanism. Experience has shown that high-tone hearing loss occurs first, and this is believed to be related to the acoustic energy and the natural frequency of the inner ear hearing mechanism. Early on, noise exposure results in a temporary threshold shift. These generally improve in less than two weeks. Repeated trauma results in permanent threshold changes.

Presbycusis

Presbycusis is the loss of hearing over time due to the aging mechanism in the inner ear. There are four pathologic types that have been classified by Schuknecht. The first phenomenon is sensory presbycusis. In this form of pathology hair cells are lost first. Later, this leads to a loss in cochlear neurons. Usually this involves hair cell loss on the basal turn of the cochlea and high-tone hearing loss. Neuropresbycusis, on the other hand, involves a primary loss of cochlear neurons with relative preservation of the hair cells. There is relatively greater loss of word discrimination in this case and only a gradual loss of hair cells over time. Strial presbycusis leaves excellent word discrimination scores after a degenerative process causes moderate to severe hearing loss that is relatively flat in nature. Pathologically, the stria vascularis appears to degenerate and shrink. Finally, cochlear-conductive hearing loss leaves a normal neuronal and hair cell population without damage to the stria vascularis but shows a hearing loss that is thought to be related to a limitation of movement in the basilar membrane. The exact nature of the pathologic process is not clear.

Idiopathic Causes of Hearing Loss

Meniere's disease is believed to be a disorder caused by swelling of the endolymphatic space. Patients with Meniere's disease of a cochlear nature describe fluctuation in hearing loss with a low-tone tinnitus. Attacks can last several minutes to hours. Losses are usually temporary but can become permanent over longer periods of time. Usually Meniere's disease involves vestibular changes and for that reason it is discussed in the next section.
Multiple sclerosis is also a cause of varying degrees of hearing loss. The structural location of the hearing loss is not clearly explained. It is relatively rare that multiple sclerosis patients develop total sensorineural hearing loss and deafness. It is of value to note that next to visual symptoms, the most common manifestation of MS can be in the eighth cranial nerve.

Issues of Sudden Hearing Loss

Sudden hearing loss can be a very frightening experience for a patient. It warrants the immediate attention of the physician. The problem can be related to a known cause or may be idiopathic. The loss may be minimal or severe, temporary or permanent. The disorder is only a symptom complex and it is not exceedingly common. Few good studies have been done to document the pathophysiology or relative success of different treatment regimens.

In approaching a patient with sudden hearing loss, every effort should be made to try to discover the cause of the hearing loss and measure its severity. Attention should be devoted to ruling out cardiovascular, diabetic, or other systemic causes. An otologic and audiologic exam as well as a CT scan may be required.

More often than not, no cause is found. Patients should be informed of their prognosis and treatment options. Prognosis is best if treatment was sought within 24 hours of onset and if hearing is still at a relatively good level. Prognosis deteriorates rapidly with longer time periods of severe hearing loss in older patients who develop dizziness.

Idiopathic sudden hearing loss is thought to be caused by thromboembolic or immune events.

Treatment is directed at several potential causes of idiopathic sudden hearing loss. One thesis suggests the cause to be thromboembolic in small vessels of the ears. Proponents of this theory treat patients with vasodilators, plasma expanders, or anticoagulants. An alternate thesis suggests that an unknown virus or immunologic event leads to the sudden hearing loss. The proponents of this thesis suggest the use of high-dose steroids to reduce inflammatory products. These drugs are used for short periods of time. Overall, patients who are put at bed rest and treated seem to have a higher recovery rate than those who are not treated.

Treatment Concepts

Any patient suffering from a known etiology of hearing loss should first have that etiology controlled. Any patient on ototoxic drugs should have the drugs stopped if at all possible. Patients who are in noisy work places should wear protection and should limit their exposure to loud noise. Once trauma to the acoustic mechanism has occurred by whatever method, hearing loss is usually permanent. Currently, treatment of hearing loss involves amplification using an external hearing aid. While implantable devices are considered, the common application of such devices is not yet available. In severe cases, cochlear implantation with an electrode array is possible at this time. Only the totally deaf patient is currently considered for implantation in this manner.

Tinnitus poses one of the most complex problems to treatment. It is purely a psychoacoustic phenomenon and, therefore, cannot be measured. It has been estimated that 13 million people suffer with this problem. Perhaps one million patients suffer severe or debilitating tinnitus. Often masking of the tinnitus is the most practical alternative. Recommendations to patients involve the use of masking with a fan or "pink" noise such as an FM radio tuned off of the station. If these simple measures do not help and the patient has a hearing loss, then treatment with an amplification method is recommended. In severe cases that have failed these methods, a tinnitus device or instrument is prescribed. In these cases, producing the pitch or frequency of the tinnitus can sometimes create a masking inhibition that persists even after the device is turned off. A small number of patients respond to this form of therapy. Other methods such as DC stimulation have been tried and occasionally are of value. More often, patients respond well to biofeedback or other psychologic methods to help them deal with their symptoms in a better manner.

DISEASES THAT PRESENT WITH VERTIGO AS A PRIMARY SYMPTOM

Balance depends upon four separate and interdependent systems. First, the vestibular system senses accelerating movement and perceives gravity. Proprioceptive cues from joint position senses and muscle tone provides information concerning the relationship of the head to the remainder of the body. Third, vision gives perceptions of position sense, speed, and orientation. Finally, all of these senses are integrated through the brain stem and cerebellum.

Balance comes from vestibular, ocular, proprioceptive, and central (neural) sources.

Nonvestibular Causes of Dizziness

HYPERVENTILATION. Hyperventilation is one of the more common causes of nonvestibular dizziness. Symptoms of lightheadedness and paresthesia in the distal extremities occur with rapid ventilation. The circumoral area is particularly prone to sensations of paresthesias. This is often associated with hysterical types of personalities.

HYPOGLYCEMIA. Hypoglycemia is a transient reduction in blood glucose which occurs in chemical diabetics. It is often accompanied by symptoms of nausea and vomiting, but true spinning vertigo is rare. Patients complain of symptoms of unsteadiness and lightheadedness associated with severe sweating and pallor.

VASCULAR CAUSES. Any vascular phenomenon that compromises the blood supply to the brain stem and cerebellum can lead to symptoms of dizziness or unsteadiness. The most common form of this is a migraine variant. Patients who complain of classic symptoms of migraine headache also can occasionally complain of dizziness. This phenomenon is caused by vertebrobasilar spasm. Longer-term disequilibrium and unsteadiness of similar etiologies are caused by vertebrobasilar artery insufficiency. Often this is associated with atherosclerotic heart disease and embolic phenomena. Rarely is the vertebrobasilar system involved in an isolated manner; more commonly, the carotid arteries are also involved. In order to cause symptoms of dizziness, vertebrobasilar blood flow must be significantly compromised to flows below 50 per cent of normal.

CERVICAL VERTIGO. The exact role of cervical vertigo is uncertain. Initially, this was thought to be a variant of vertebrobasilar insufficiency. Recently the definition has changed in that cervical joint position sense is thought to be lost in some patients, and this produces symptoms of dizziness. The only form of therapy is physical therapy to restore strength in the neck.

Vertigo on a Vestibular Basis (Table 7–5)

BENIGN POSITIONAL VERTIGO. Benign positional vertigo is usually seen in patients who note that, with a certain position of the head, they have

TABLE 7–5. COMMON DISORDERS OF THE VESTIBULAR SYSTEM

	PROCESS	TYPE AND LOCATION
Infections	Labyrinthitis	Bacterial, viral, syphilitic, cholesteatoma, herpes zoster
	Petrositis	Bacterial
	Meningitis	Bacterial, viral
	Encephalitis	Viral
Vascular	Occlusion	Vertebral, basilar, internal auditory artery, PICA, AICA
	Aneurysm	
	Infarction	
	Arteriovenous malformation	
	Migraine	
Trauma	Bone fracture	Longitudinal and transverse
	Barotrauma	Round or oval window fistula
	Concussion	Labyrinth, brain stem, cerebellum
	Avulsion	Eighth nerve
Neoplasm	Cancer	Metastases and primary malignancy of temporal bone involving labyrinth
	Glomus	
	Schwannoma	Eighth nerve
	Meningioma	Internal auditory canal
	Epidermoid	Labyrinth
	Primary brain tumor	
Metabolic	Diabetes mellitus	
	Otosclerosis	
	Paget's disease	
	Thiamine deficiency	
	Familial ataxia	
	Osteopetrosis	
Toxins	See Table 7–4	
Unknown causes	Meniere's disease	Autoimmune, idiopathic
	Vestibular neuronitis	Viral?
	Cupulolithiasis	Cupular
	Multiple sclerosis	

acute attacks of transient dizziness. This is accompanied by nystagmus that fatigues on repeated testing. Typically, there is a brief delay from the onset of the change in position to the onset of vertigo. The first attack is usually the most severe, and repeated attacks become less severe in nature. Pathologically the calcified cupula is thought to fracture, leading to this syndrome. For this reason, the disease is sometimes referred to as cupulolithiasis. Treatment is usually directed toward symptomatic relief and reassurance that the process usually resolves spontaneously.

VESTIBULAR NEURONITIS. Vestibular neuronitis is caused by an unknown source. It is essentially a clinical disorder in which the patient complains of severe dizziness with intractable vomiting, nausea, and inability to stand or walk. These symptoms can go on for three to four days. Some patients need to be hospitalized for symptoms of dehydration. Attacks leave the patient with unsteadiness and imbalance for several months. Repeated episodic attacks can occur. There is usually no change in hearing with this phenomenon.

LABYRINTHITIS (Fig. 7–7). Labyrinthitis is an inflammatory process involving the inner ear mechanism. There are different clinical and pathologic classifications. The process can be either acute or chronic and can be either toxic or suppurative. Acute toxic labyrinthitis is caused by an infection of nearby structures; whether it be the middle ear or the meninges makes little

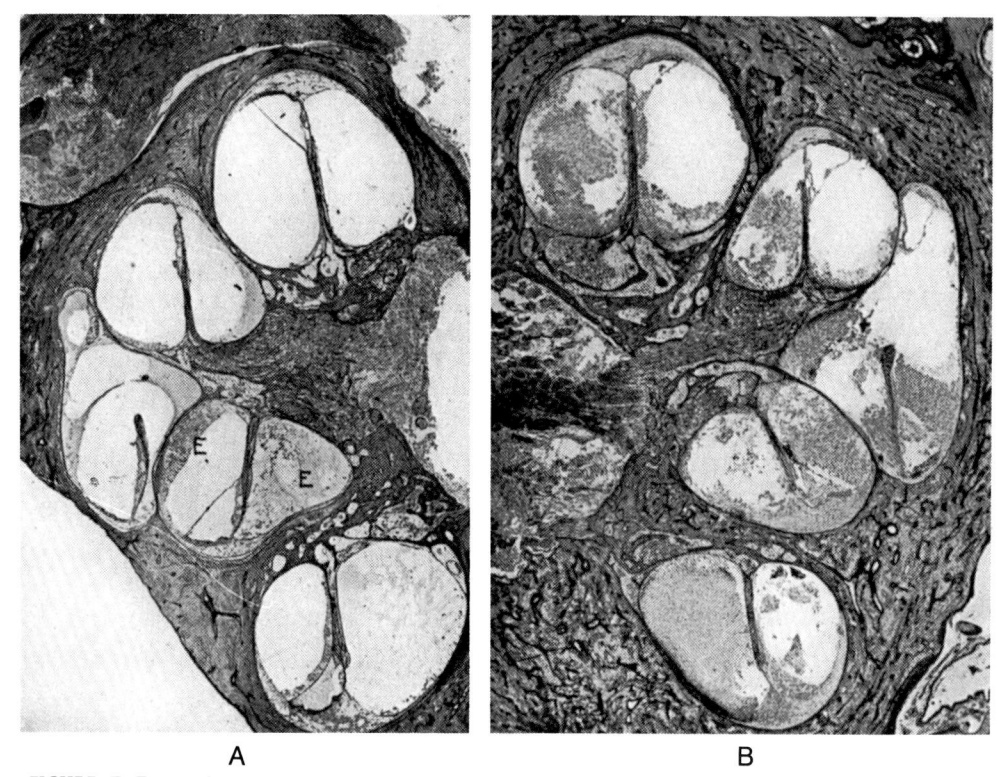

FIGURE 7–7. *A,* Microphotograph showing the early serofibrinous stage of meningitic labyrinthitis. Serofibrinous exudate (E) has collected mainly in the middle coil. Pus cells have invaded the modiolus but not the labyrinthine fluids. *B,* Microphotograph showing the diffuse purulent stage of meningitic labyrinthitis. Pus cells are diffusely distributed throughout the cochlear spaces and the modiolus. Destruction of the cochlear duct has already occurred in the basal coil. (From Jackson C, Jackson CL: Diseases of the Nose, Throat and Ear (ed 2). Philadelphia, WB Saunders Co, 1959.)

difference. Toxic labyrinthitis usually resolves with some loss of hearing and vestibular function. This is thought to be caused by toxic products from an infection and not by viable organisms. Acute suppurative labyrinthitis occurs with an acute bacterial infection that extends into the structures of the inner ear. The chances of complete loss of hearing and vestibular function are quite high. Finally, chronic changes can exist from any source and may lead to endolymphatic hydrops or pathologic changes ultimately sclerosing the labyrinth.

MENIERE'S DISEASE (Fig. 7–8). Meniere's disease is a disorder of swelling in the endolymphatic space. This pathologic process is referred to as hydrops. Pathologically, Meniere's disease is caused by a swelling of the endolymphatic compartment. When this process reaches a pinnacle, a Reissner's membrane ruptures, mixing endolymph and perilymph. This causes a temporary hearing loss that resolves when the membrane reseals and the chemical composition of the endolymph and perilymph returns to normal. Classically, the patient develops a low-tone sensorineural hearing loss followed by a symptom of low-pitched tinnitus. Patients describe aural fullness and then become acutely vertiginous. Attacks last between 15 minutes and several hours in duration. This classic picture can be modified to involve only the vestibular portion of the labyrinth when symptoms involve only changes in balance and aural

Meniere's disease is characterized by hearing loss, tinnitus, dizziness, and pressure or fullness in one ear.

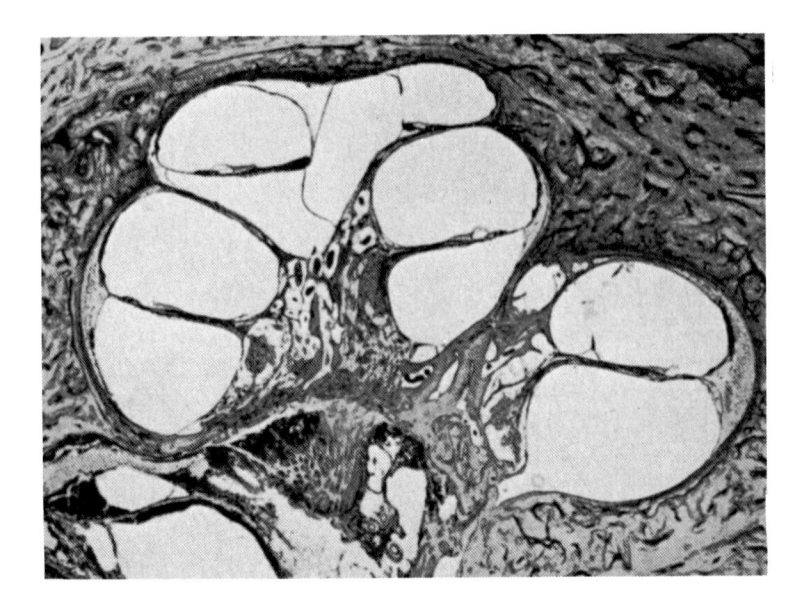

FIGURE 7–8. Meniere's disease. This shows the enlargement of the scala media. The Reissner's membrane is stretched to the point that it is plastered on the superior wall of the cochlea.

fullness. Meniere's disease is an unpredictable disorder that can occur at any time, although primarily it affects middle-aged women. The disease fluctuates over long periods of time without significant variation, but in certain cases the disease can progress rapidly, leading to total hearing loss and lack of reliable vestibular function in the ear. Unfortunately, fluctuation over a long period of time is the norm. Meniere's syndrome is a similar clinical picture that is caused by a known etiology. These causes include hypothyroidism and syphilis. Treatment of the idiopathic process involves limitation of salt in the diet and the prescription of a mild diuretic to prevent the formation of endolymphatic hydrops. Symptomatic treatment with vestibular suppressants is recommended. In cases of medical failure, surgical therapy is directed either at improving the flow of endolymph through the endolymphatic duct and sac or at sectioning the vestibular nerve through a number of surgical routes.

Recent literature suggests that some cases of bilateral Meniere's disease may be caused by an immune phenomenon. This has not been well documented, although treatment with steroids has resulted in dramatic improvement in both hearing and function in selected patients.

Perilymph Fistula

Patients who have sudden barotrauma in the area of the ear can experience sensorineural hearing loss and dizziness. This is seen in divers, flyers, and anyone who has a sudden change in pressure in the middle ear space. These sudden changes can cause a disruption of the round or oval window membrane, allowing perilymph to leak into the middle ear space. The role of minor pressure changes such as sneezing has not been determined. Some cases of perilymph fistula have developed without apparent pressure change. The fistula can be repaired by sealing a leak with fat grafts. Resolution of the symptoms of dizziness occurs in only a few cases. The rates of occurrence and cure are still debatable.

Treatment

A majority of the diseases listed here cause a change in the vestibular function. This means that neural firing from the nerves is still present, but the data transmitted to the brain are unreliable. Treatment is directed toward reducing the level of function of the vestibular nerve in the brain stem. Vestibular suppressants include antihistamines and benzodiazepines. The two primary drugs used for this are Antivert and Valium. Both drugs give symptomatic relief but do not generally make symptoms completely disappear.

Severe and persistent cases of vestibular vertigo can be treated with vestibular nerve sections through one of at least three routes. First, the nerve can be sectioned through the middle fossa. This procedure is primarily limited to patients under 60 years of age in good health and those willing to accept a half-head shave. A second route involves the posterior fossa, where a suboccipital craniectomy is performed and the nerve is identified in the internal auditory canal. The procedure carries some risk to the facial nerve as well as the cochlear nerve but can usually be accomplished without significant difficulty. The degree of completeness of the section has been under question in recent literature. The final route is a translabyrinthine approach with removal or destruction of the entire vestibular system. In this case, there is a high degree of success, but all patients will lose hearing in the affected ear.

References

Hughes G: Clinical Otology. New York, Thieme, Inc., 1986.
Konigsmark BW, Gorlin RJ: Genetic and Metabolic Deafness. Philadelphia, WB Saunders, 1976.
Schuknecht HF, Gulya AJ: Anatomy of the Temporal Bone. Philadelphia, Lea & Febiger, 1986.

8
DISORDERS OF THE FACIAL NERVE

by Robert H. Maisel, M.D., and Samuel C. Levine, M.D.

Paralysis of the facial musculature produces abnormalities of facial expression, difficulty eating, and problems maintaining clear vision. Patients who suffer this disorder immediately notice the severe cosmetic and functional deformities. Often, they relate no apparent reason for the onset of this disorder. Bell's palsy is a peripheral seventh nerve paralysis for which no apparent explanation can be found. The term assumes that a thorough evaluation for some of the known causes of facial paralysis has been completed. The first examining physician should evaluate the patient, assess facial nerve function, and obtain appropriate laboratory studies. This chapter includes the anatomy and pathophysiology of the facial nerve. The diagnostic tests necessary for evaluation of facial nerve function are discussed and the differential diagnosis is reviewed.

GROSS ANATOMY OF THE FACIAL NERVE

In order to evaluate the causes of facial paralysis, it is necessary to understand the anatomy and function of the nerve. The seventh cranial nerve begins at the brain stem and follows a course through the temporal bone, ending in the muscles of the face. There are at least five major branches. While the seventh cranial nerve carries innervation to facial motion, it also provides lacrimation, salivation, impedance regulation of the middle ear, and the senses of pain, touch, temperature, and taste (Fig. 8–1).

The seventh nerve nucleus is in the region of the pons. Here, it receives information from the precentral gyrus of the motor cortex, which innervates the ipsilateral and contralateral forehead. The cerebral cortical tracts also innervate the contralateral portion of the remainder of the face. The motor nucleus innervates only the ipsilateral facial nerve. As the nerve leaves the brain stem, a branch of the eighth nerve referred to as the nervus intermedius separates and joins the seventh nerve as it enters the internal auditory canal. The nerve turns anteriorly and enters the geniculate ganglion. The ganglion contains the cell bodies for taste to the anterior tongue and those for touch, pain, and temperature to the external auditory canal. A number of nerve fibers pass through the ganglion and form the greater superficial petrosal nerve (parasympathetic). This runs along the floor of the middle fossa and enters the pterygoid canal. It then passes into the sphenopalatine ganglion

The facial nerve makes two sharp turns (first and second genua) as it passes through the temporal bone.

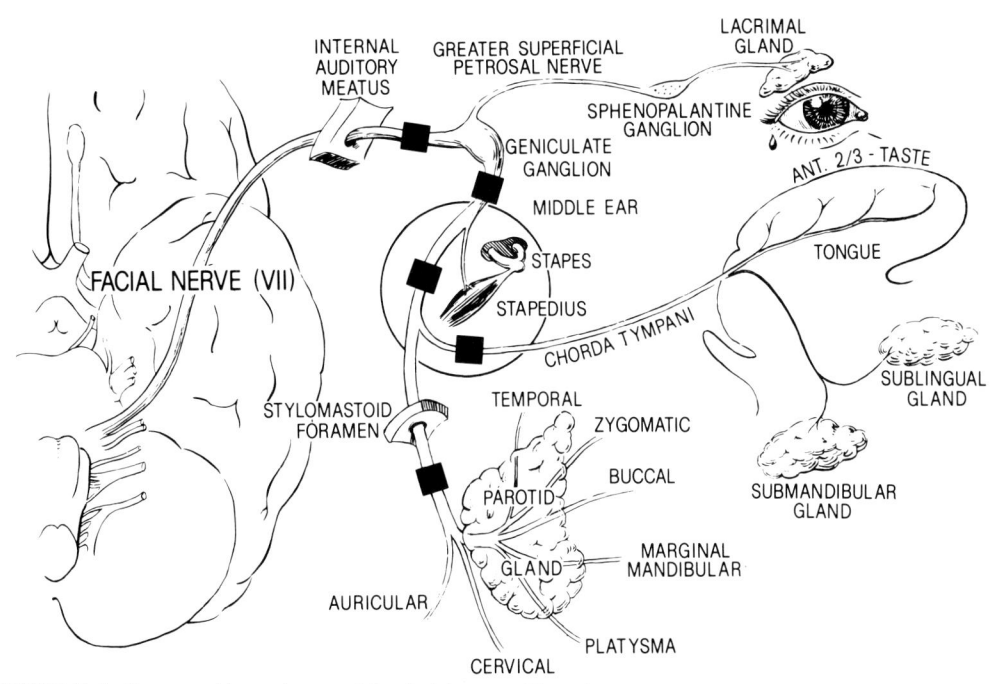

FIGURE 8–1. Topographic anatomy of the facial nerve. Physiologic testing permits determination of the site of the injury. Lesions medial to the geniculate ganglion will cause diminished tearing. A lesion within the middle ear may cause absence of the stapedial reflex. Injury to the chorda tympani will diminish taste and salivation.

and anastomoses with fibers that innervate the lacrimal apparatus. The facial fibers make a sharp turn posteriorly at the geniculate ganglion and descend through the labyrinthine segment to the tympanic segment of the nerve. The nerve enters the tympanic segment and makes a second genu (or turn). It is here, near the oval window, that the nerve can become exposed and may be palpable in the middle ear. The nerve descends from the genu vertically and gives a branch to the stapedius muscle. Below this level, a second branch emerges and backtracks through the ear as the chorda tympani nerve. The chorda carries fibers of touch, pain, temperature, and taste to the anterior two thirds of the tongue. It also controls salivation from the submandibular glands. It passes between the malleus and incus (Fig. 8–2) and exits the temporal bone through the iter anterior. The major portion of the facial nerve carries motor fibers that exit from the stylomastoid foramen just medial to the mastoid process. Seventy per cent of the fibers at this point represent motor fibers to the face. The nerve subsequently turns anteriorly and divides into five major branches—the temporal, zygomatic, buccal, mandibular, and cervical. The branches may anastomose with one another as the nerve passes through the parotid gland (Fig. 8–3).

The bony covering over the facial nerve in the middle ear can be dehiscent.

PHYSIOLOGY AND PATHOPHYSIOLOGY

Facial movement is a result of up to 7000 motor fibers moving in synchrony to initiate muscular contraction. Each axon connects synaptically to several muscle fibers. Neurotransmitter chemicals (acetylcholine) and enzymes (cho-

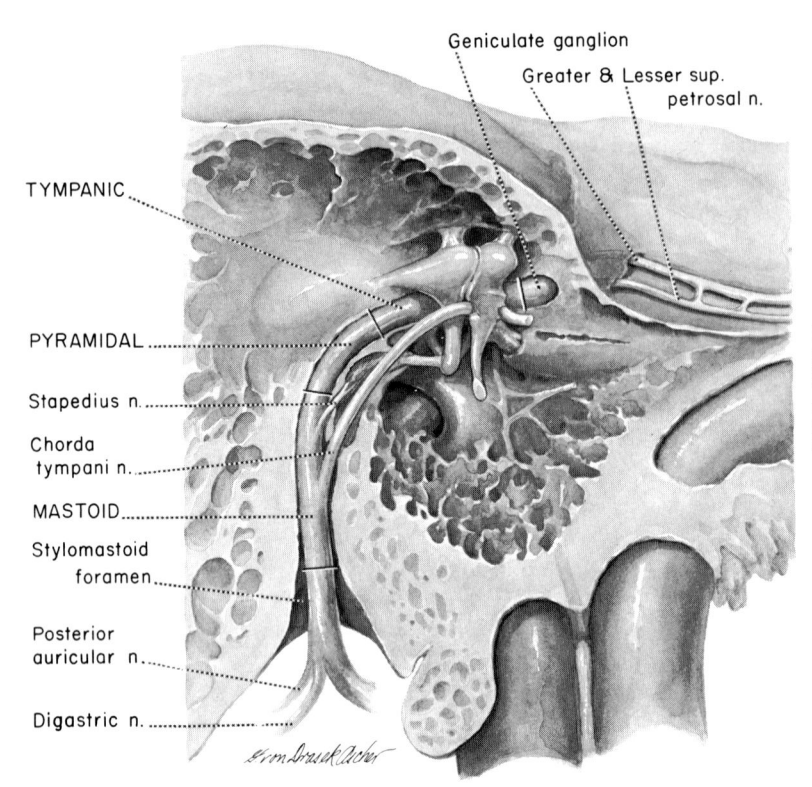

FIGURE 8–2. Course of the facial nerve in the temporal bone. (From Shambaugh GE, Clemis JD: Facial nerve paralysis. *In* Paparella MM, Shumrick DA (eds): Otolaryngology. Vol 2. Philadelphia, WB Saunders Co, 1973, p 265.

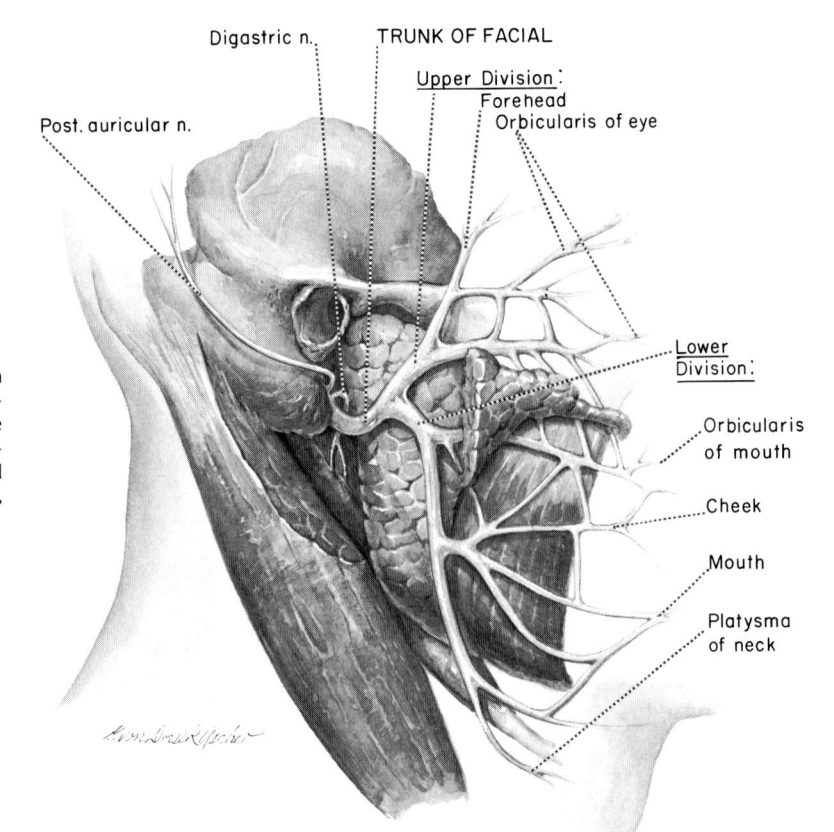

FIGURE 8–3. Peripheral distribution of the facial nerve. (From Shambaugh GE, Clemis JD: Facial nerve paralysis. *In* Paparella MM, Shumrick DA (eds): Otolaryngology. Vol 2, Philadelphia, WB Saunders Co, 1973, p 266.)

line transferase) are manufactured by the nerve cell body in the pons and are transported along the nerve to the motor end plate through the microtubular systems. It is believed the neurometabolites are carried proximally by similar transport mechanisms from each axon. The facial nerve has a single motor neuron that is located within the central nervous system (CNS). The sensory cell bipolar neurons have their nuclei outside of the central nervous system, with one axon from the periphery to the cell body and another from there to the central nervous system. The motor cell axon is covered by Schwann cells, which form the neural tubule for nonmyelinated nerves and which themselves lay down the insulating myelin for myelinated nerves. A node of Ranvier, which represents the junction between Schwann cells, is seen every millimeter. The basement membrane on the outside of the Schwann cell is continuous so that the axon is never in contact with extracellular spaces (even at the nodes of Ranvier). The axon receives its oxygen from the Schwann cells and rejuvenates its axoplasm from the parent neuron. The rate of axoplasmic metabolism as well as its rate of movement appears to be about 1 mm a day. It progresses from the central nervous system cell distally; this is the rate of regeneration of an axon where the nerve is completely transected.

NEUROPHYSIOLOGY-NEUROPATHOLOGY OF INJURY

When an axon is injured either by direct trauma or due to metabolic events, marked histologic and measurable biochemical changes may occur all the way back to the cell body. Pressure on a nerve may result in a damming of the flow of axoplasm. Nerve injuries have been classified in a system of five degrees of increasing complexity and decreasing likelihood of uncomplicated recovery. A first-degree injury, or conduction block, is also called neurapraxia. This occurs when the conduction of impulses is blocked, damming axoplasm transport (in both directions) with some axoplasm transport continuing (Fig. 8–4A).

The first-degree conduction block is called neurapraxia.

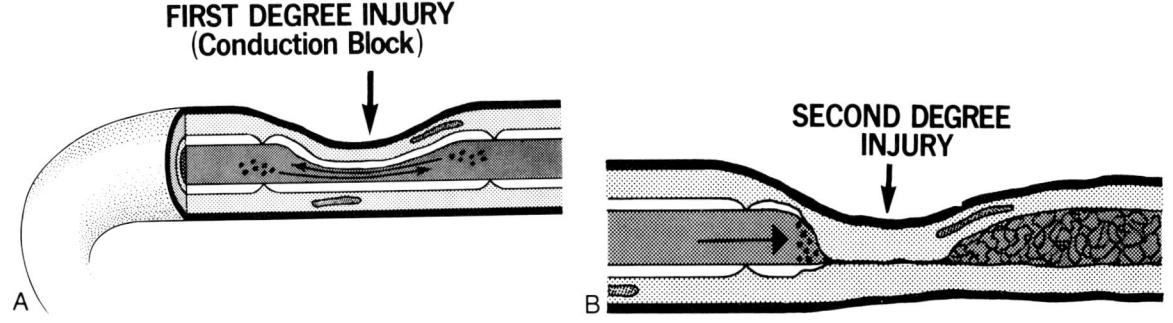

FIGURE 8–4. *A,* First-degree injury. Nerve fiber is twisted or compressed in such a way as to distort intraneural anatomy yet allow axoplasmic flow in both directions. Note that the myelin layer is also maintained in these injuries. *B,* Second-degree injury. With continued pressure, torsion, or both, axoplasmic continuity is disrupted. The distal axon's trophic influence on myelin layer is lost, resulting in distal degeneration of the myelin layer. Schwann cell and endoneurium, which together constitute the endoneurial tube, remain intact. (From Johns ME, Crumley RL: Facial nerve injury, repair, and rehabilitation [a self-instructional package]. Washington, DC, American Academy of Otolaryngology, 1979, pp 19–20.)

The distance from the site of injury to the cell body in the pons determines to some degree the amount of injury to the entire nerve. If the injury occurs in the internal auditory canal with axon disruption, long distances of axoplasm are lost and the permanent damage is greater than when such an injury occurs distally near the motor end plates. Younger people make a more complete recovery from the same nerve injury (if repaired) than do older people and people with chronic diseases (e.g., diabetes) or metabolic disorders. If the amount of pressure on the nerve is sufficient to completely block the movement of axoplasm past the site of injury over several days, axonotmesis (second-degree injury) occurs with loss of axonal continuity (Fig. 8–4B). This results in wallerian degeneration distally. The axons may continue for several days being electrically responsive to external stimulation (distally) but with no voluntary motor movement or electrical conductivity across the site of injury. Histologically, the proximal nerve remains normal but biochemical changes occur. Axonotmesis and neurotmesis have several histologic correlates. The Schwann cells become swollen and phagocytic. They then multiply until they fill the connective tissue tubule surrounding each nerve fiber. The neuron deprived of nutrients normally brought back through the axons loses Nissl substance with swelling of cytoplasm (chromatolysis). The distant nerve continues to undergo changes, which are usually not evident until three or four days after injury. The formation of Büngner's bands occurs. These are thought to provide a biochemical mode of attraction for new nerves. When the nerve fiber is cut, repairing nerve produces in its healing phase a growth cone at the proximal end of the axon. It begins to grow toward the original distal end where the new motor end plates are. There are multiple protoplasmic processes of the growth cone, and a single regenerating axon will branch and enter Schwann cells of many tubules, while similarly a single Schwann cell may be shared by many small axons. Similarly, growth to another nerve may occur. Histochemical analysis of a regenerating neuron shows increasing levels of RNA synthetase and glucose-6-phosphate dehydrogenase, maximizing at about 21 days. Some theorists have suggested, on the basis of this information, that cut nerves heal best if repaired at this time, but immediate repair is still the treatment of choice. Delay is unwarranted owing to scarring and physical changes in the wound.

There is theoretical evidence to suggest that the repair of a cut facial nerve is more likely to be effective if done 21 days after the injury.

Facial muscles are branchiomeric muscles, and greater muscle wasting is seen in somatic muscle than in branchiomeric muscle after loss of motor nerves. In humans it has been noted that there is a progressive but mild decrease in facial muscle fiber size over the two weeks after complete denervation. Observation has not shown complete degeneration of facial muscle fibers following denervation. For these reasons, it is believed that rehabilitation of the facial muscles by nerve transfer or reanastomosis of the original injured nerve is reasonable for periods of at least 24 months after injury. The facial nerve really goes through three stages after injury. Stage 1, which occurs up to 21 days, involves the physiologic events described above, in which the cell body undergoes metabolic transformation and begins to regenerate to create axoplasm that will inhabit the now empty neurotubules.

Stage 2, which lasts up to two years, is a period when the cell body and the proximal segment can regenerate using the Büngner's bands or reserved endoneural tubes through which the regenerating axons can reach the facial muscles. Therefore, certainly up to two years after an injury, it should be considered plausible to reanastomose the severed nerve, interpose a cable graft between the two points of loss of continuity, or transfer another functioning motor nerve to the distal nerve segments. Stage 3, which is usually characterized by distal neural scarring and muscle degeneration, obviously precludes consideration of restoring neuromuscular continuity.

It is possible to repair the facial nerve up to two years after the injury.

DIAGNOSTIC TESTING

A number of diagnostic tests are used to evaluate facial nerve function. Since a major portion of the facial nerve is in the temporal bone, tests directed toward hearing are frequently used to evaluate the nearby structures. The goal of testing is to locate the lesion and to project the ultimate outcome of the paralysis.

AUDIOLOGIC TESTING

Any patient who suffers a facial nerve palsy needs to have a complete audiogram. Testing must include air conduction and bone conduction thresholds, as well as tympanometry and stapes reflexes. The function of the eighth cranial nerve can be evaluated using auditory brain stem evoked response (ABR) tests. This test is most helpful in detecting pathology in the internal auditory canal. A conductive hearing loss suggests an abnormality in the middle ear space, and in view of the exposure of the facial nerve in this area infectious sources need to be considered. Reflex testing is much more complex. A loud tone is presented, either to the ipsilateral or contralateral ear, which evokes a reflex movement of the stapedius muscle. This changes the tension on the tympanic membrane and results in a change in the impedance of the ossicular chain. If the tone is presented to the opposite, normal-hearing ear and the reflex is elicited, the seventh nerve is thought to be intact at this point. Absence of this reflex when either ear is stimulated suggests an abnormality of the afferent seventh cranial nerve.

If facial nerve paralysis develops during acute otitis media, the nerve may be dehiscent in the middle ear.

TEAR TESTS

By using a Schirmer test, the tearing function of the eye can be evaluated. These strips are commercially available and are placed over the lower lid into the conjunctival sac on both sides (Fig. 8–5). After three minutes, the length of the strip that is moist is compared to the opposite side. A difference of greater than 25 per cent suggests potential involvement of the seventh cranial nerve. The side of less tearing is interpreted to represent greater superficial petrosal nerve activity due to loss of action in the parasympathetic nerve of Wrisberg (Table 8–1).

The Schirmer test compares tearing on both sides.

Decreased tearing on the Schirmer test means injury to the greater superficial petrosal nerve or to the facial nerve proximal to the geniculate ganglion.

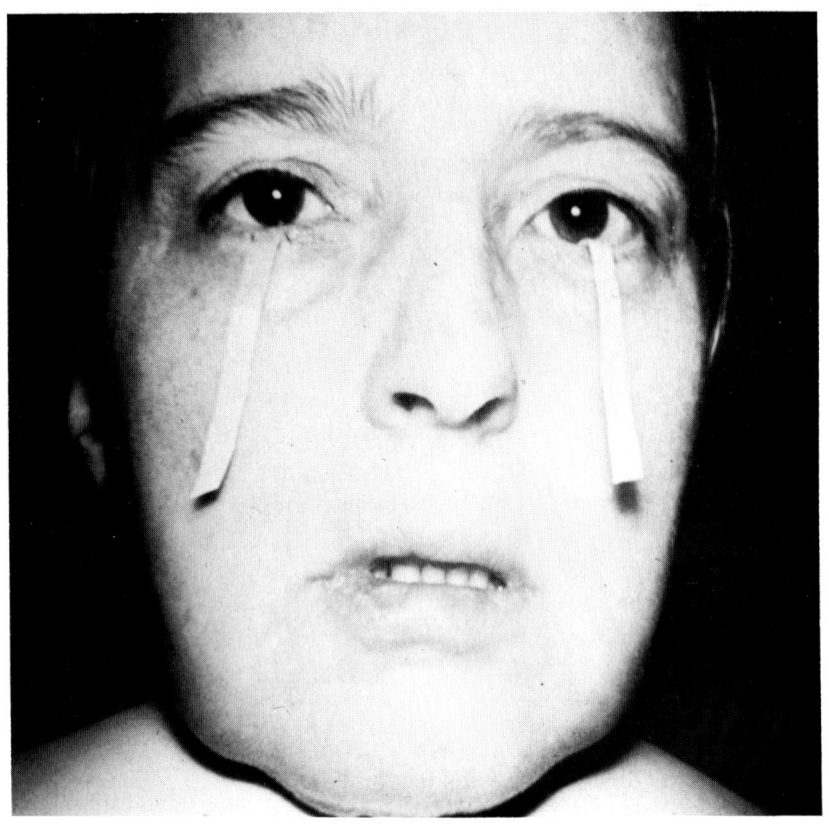

FIGURE 8–5. A Schirmer's test demonstrating decreased lacrimation of the right eye in comparison to the left eye.

TASTE

Measurement of taste is a reliable indicator of the interruption of the function of the chorda tympani nerve. Salt and lemon juice are two easy taste tests to obtain. Saccharine or sugar can also be used. Loss of taste due to injury is limited to the anterior two thirds of the tongue and stops at the midline.

TABLE 8–1. FACIAL NERVE TEST RESULTS

SITE OF LESION	SCHIRMER'S LACRIMATION TEST	SALIVARY FLOW TEST	STAPEDIUS REFLEX IMPEDANCE TEST	TASTE TESTING
Cerebral hemisphere	−	−	−	−
Brain stem	±	±	±	±
Cerebellopontine angle to geniculate ganglion	+	+	+	+
Geniculate ganglion to stapedius muscle	−	+	−	+
Stapedius muscle to stylomastoid foramen	−	+	−	+
Face	−	−	−	−

Key: − usually normal
± possibly abnormal
+ often abnormal

SALIVATION

Salivation tests can be performed by cannulating the submandibular glands. A small section of No. 50 polyethylene tubing is inserted into Wharton's duct. A piece of cotton saturated with lemon juice is placed in the mouth, and one must see the flow of saliva in both tubes. The volume can be compared at one minute. A reduction in salivary flow of 25 per cent is considered abnormal. The same problems exist with this pathway as with taste, since both are transmitted by the chorda tympani nerve.

Tests such as the Schirmer test, acoustic reflex, taste, and salivary flow were once thought to have localizing value. That is to say, they could point to the specific site of a lesion. This is not a reliable phenomenon but may be of topognostic value.

NERVE FUNCTION TESTS

A number of nerve function tests are available. They include electromyography (EMG), electroneuronography (ENOG), and maximal stimulation tests. EMG's are frequently performed by neurology services. They have value later in determining the patient's course in reinnervation responses. EMG's can be classified as showing a normal response, a denervation, a fibrillation, or a bizarre pattern suggestive of a myopathy or a neuropathy (Fig. 8–6). Unfortunately, before 21 days following an acute paralysis, the value of an EMG is limited. Prior to 21 days, if the face does not move, the EMG will show denervation potentials. Fibrillation potentials are a positive sign showing recovery of some fibers. These potentials are not seen before 21 days.

ENOG obtains more information at an earlier time. ENOG carries out a stimulation at one point and measurement of the EMG at a more distal point on the nerve. Nerve conduction velocity can be calculated. If there is a 90 per cent reduction in ENOG versus the other side at ten days, the chances of recovery are significantly reduced. Fisch and Eselin reported that a 25 per cent drop resulted in incomplete recovery in 88 per cent of their patients, whereas 77 per cent who maintained a response greater than that had normal recovery of their facial nerve.

Finally, the maximal stimulation test is easy and convenient. In this test,

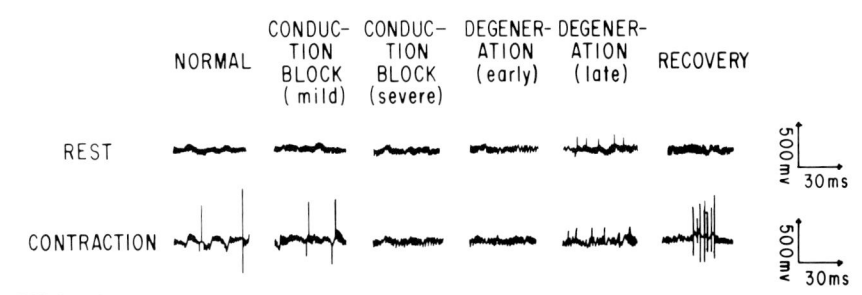

FIGURE 8–6. Schematic representation of electromyographic recordings of facial paralysis. (From Mathog RH, Hudson WR: Electrodiagnosis in facial paralysis. South Med J 63:37–40, 1970.)

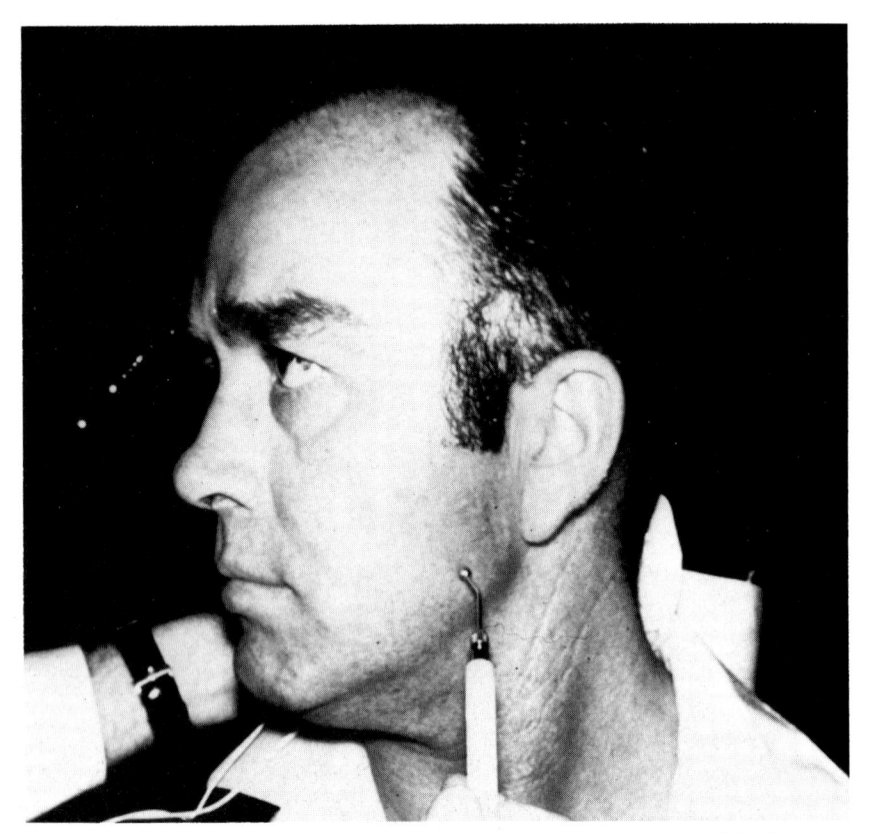

FIGURE 8–7. The facial nerve excitability test demonstrating stimulation of the lower division of the facial nerve just anterior to the stylomastoid foramen.

the probe is pressed against the face in the area of the facial nerve. The current is slowly increased to 5 ma, or until the patient has discomfort (Fig. 8–7). The forehead, eyebrow, periorbital area, cheek, nasal ala, and lower lip are tested by gently sweeping the electrode. Any movement in the area indicates a normal response. A small difference in response between the paralyzed side and the normal side is considered to be a sign of recovery. Marked decrease means that twitch on the paralyzed side occurs at 25 per cent of the current used on the normal side. When compared at ten days, 92 per cent of the Bell's palsy patients had some return of function. When the electrical response was lost, 100 per cent had incomplete return of function. In those patients in whom there was a marked decrease, 73 per cent had incomplete return of facial function. The statistics suggest that the most reliable form of testing is direct nerve function tests.

DIFFERENTIAL DIAGNOSIS

The differential diagnosis of facial nerve paralysis is lengthy. It involves congenital, infectious, traumatic, neoplastic, vascular, and finally idiopathic causes. The following list covers major causes but is not meant to be complete.

CONGENITAL LESIONS

Congenital causes of facial nerve paralysis are uncommon. One of the more common causes in this category is Möbius' syndrome. In this case, the facial nerve forms but it is a fibrotic tract. And while muscle development may be present in some cases, it usually rapidly degenerates to fibrosis. Unfortunately, these children have no response to any electrical testing at birth and will not develop any form of facial movement because of the abnormality.

More often, facial nerve paralysis is a result of childbirth trauma. During the process of childbirth, fractures of the temporal bone can occur. The use of forceps has been indicated as a potential cause of many of these lesions. Any neonate identified with a seventh nerve paralysis should have tests as soon as possible. Stimulation of the face after birth will differentiate congenital causes from birth trauma. If the injury occurs in the birth process, electrical stimulation will be possible for several days. This is an important finding in both the diagnosis and prognosis of the facial palsy.

Möbius' syndrome: (1) external and middle ear anomalies, (2) involvement of cranial nerves III, V, VI, VII, and XII.

INFECTIONS

Infections occurring anywhere along the path of the facial nerve can lead to paralysis. Rarely, meningitis will present with facial nerve palsy. Abscesses in the parietal cortex region can create a central paralysis. This is diagnosed by the ability to move the forehead on the affected side but the inability to move the remainder of the face on that side. Ramsay Hunt syndrome, or herpes zoster oticus, involves the nerve and creates a rash in the external auditory canal and pinna. Small pustules form in the external auditory canal and are extremely tender (Fig. 8–8).

Bacterial infections of the middle ear can paralyze the face. Infections can be acute or chronic. They can involve only inflammatory materials, or cholesteatomas may also be present. An uncommon tick-borne illness called Lyme disease can also cause paralysis of the facial nerve among other cranial nerve palsies.

FIGURE 8–8. Ramsay Hunt syndrome demonstrating a vesicular rash of the pinna. (From Becker W, et al: Atlas of Otorhinolaryngology. Philadelphia, WB Saunders Co, 1969, p 11.)

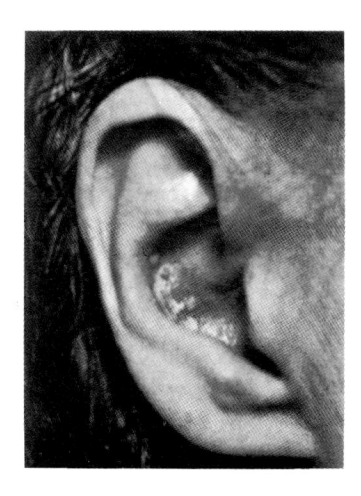

TRAUMA

Facial nerve evaluation should be performed immediately on any patient with a basilar skull fracture. The prognosis is better if the nerve functions partially, even if it is later found to be paretic.

Trauma to the temporal bone is a common cause of facial palsy. Fractures can be both longitudinal and transverse (see Chapter 2). While longitudinal fractures are much more common, transverse fractures injure the nerve many times more frequently. The energy needed to cause a temporal bone fracture is substantial, and many of these palsies are not noticed until the patient awakens from coma following a motor vehicle accident.

VASCULAR LESIONS

The role of vascular lesions in facial nerve function is an area of dispute. While the presence of aneurysms or thrombosis of major vessels is an uncommon cause of facial palsy, it is indisputable. Recently, there has been discussion of abnormal loops of normal vessels being located near the internal auditory canal. These loops have been blamed for facial spasm and tics but not overt paralysis. The importance of these vascular loops is not yet clear.

NEOPLASMS

The development of facial nerve paralysis in a patient with external otitis suggests malignancy.

Tumors of the cerebellopontine angle, particularly acoustic neuromas and meningiomas, are the most common neoplasms causing facial nerve paralysis. Facial nerve neuromas are distinctly uncommon. Other neoplasms of the middle ear can result in facial paralysis. These include benign causes such as glomus jugulares or more malignant causes such as histiocytosis, rhabdomyosarcomas, and squamous cell carcinomas.

IDIOPATHIC CAUSES

Some causes of facial paralysis are more difficult to determine. Some metabolic causes include diabetes mellitus and a genetic disorder known as Melkersson-Rosenthal syndrome. A large number of patients with facial nerve palsies never have a cause discovered. While a viral source has been suggested and vascular causes have been sought, no real etiology has ever been determined for many facial nerve palsies. Although Sir Charles Bell first described facial nerve palsies that were of traumatic origin, we now associate his name with idiopathic facial palsies.

Bell's palsy means unilateral, idiopathic, peripheral facial nerve paralysis. Before diagnosing as Bell's palsy, other etiologies of facial nerve paralysis must be ruled out.

The most common cause of unilateral facial paralysis remains Bell's palsy. The pathogenesis of this disorder is still unclear, probably because it represents many inciting agents. Some cases result from viral inflammation, while others may represent a polyneuropathy due to systemic or central nervous system disorder. Bell's palsy is a unilateral weakness or paralysis of the face with no readily identifiable cause and virtually always has some recovery of function within six months. It has been hypothesized that ischemic and immunologic factors may be related directly to the pathogenesis of this disorder. There is always a peripheral facial nerve dysfunction with involvement affecting all five major branches. The onset is acute, with a progressive course reaching the stage of greatest muscle weakness within three weeks. Upper respiratory inflammation symptoms may precede the onset of paralysis. Severe ear pain may occur early; dysacusis and other signs such as dysgeusia relating to parasympathetic nerve paresis accompanying the facial motor hypofunction are consistent with the diagnosis.

Careful history-taking and physical examination including otoneurologic work-up are necessary to exclude disorders that may, at first glance, mimic a Bell's palsy and, therefore, deserve their own diagnosis. Once the diagnosis is secured by the absence of historic events such as a slowly progressive or recurring facial paralysis and the absence of either active middle ear disease or palpable masses in the parotid gland, a treatment plan should be derived and explained to the patient.

TREATMENT

The value of topognostic-prognostic testing and treatment remains a matter of frequent debate. Some physicians do nothing except observe the patient periodically. Often, however, an audiogram is obtained which suggests a retrocochlear mass lesion (acoustic neuroma). If a facial weakness occurs with an ipsilateral sensorineural hearing loss, careful neuroradiographic evaluation of the posterior fossa and skull base is firmly indicated to completely rule out a small acoustic neuroma. Improvement of the facial paralysis is insufficient with associated findings to ignore the need for radiographs.

Sensorineural hearing loss + facial nerve paralysis = internal auditory canal tumor.

Topognostic testing has been used for the past 20 years to help locate the site of lesion. It was particularly valuable for the surgeon contemplating surgical decompression of the facial nerve. Intact tearing indicates that decompression to the level proximal to the cochlear air form process may be sufficient. Similarly, an intact stapedial reflex suggests that the vertical segment of the facial nerve is involved while the horizontal segment in the middle ear has been spared.

Surgeons who consider surgical decompression on the theory that the nerve is compressed either by fiber sheath or by edema of the nerve within the bony canal have used facial nerve stimulation tests. In this test, the normal side of the face is compared to the paralyzed side; using either the minimal test or the maximal stimulation test, as described above, a decision is reached about the likelihood of axonotmesis which, if present, would suggest the value of surgical decompression. If electrical tests remain equal between the two sides, neurapraxia is the diagnosis and excellent spontaneous recovery is to be expected. Many clinicians use the ENOG prognostic test following the proposed guidelines of Esslen and Fisch (Fig. 8–9). Patients who have 90 per cent or greater reduction of amplitude within ten days of onset have a 50 per cent chance for a poor prognosis. For these patients, surgery can be considered.

When electrical tests show identical responses on both sides, the prognosis for recovery of nerve function is excellent.

Patients with facial nerve paralysis have complications during the early phase due to the paralysis itself. There are problems with control of oral secretions which create drooling, inability to whistle, trouble with speaking clearly, biting the buccal mucosa because of loss of motor tone, and popping of food in the paralyzed buccal pouch. This requires manipulation with finger

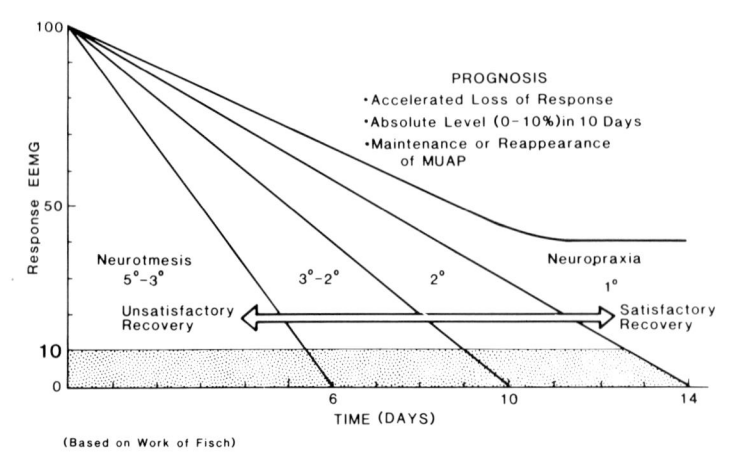

FIGURE 8-9. The prognosis for recovery follows the response to evoked electromyography noted within the first 10 days. Prognosis is poor if the response to evoked electromyography is lost within the first 5 days and is favorable if the response is maintained beyond 10 days, and especially 14 days. Early return of voluntary motor unit action potentials noted by EMG within the first 14 days indicates that the nerve is recovering and portends a favorable prognosis. (Reprinted by permission from May M: Office medical management of acute facial palsies. In May M (ed): The Facial Nerve. New York, Thieme Medical Publishers, Inc, 1986, p 334.)

Grafts from cranial nerves XI or XII are used for ipsilateral nerve VII.

or tongue to easily swallow the food. There have been recommendations by physical therapists that stimulation of the muscles to preserve tone is important during the paralyzed phase in anticipation of spontaneous or surgical recovery. This is under strong debate and currently we do not recommend this to our patients, although if they have decided upon it themselves we do not condemn such treatment.

When facial nerve grafting is not possible, other cranial nerves in the area can be used. The spinal accessory nerve can be used to innervate the facial nerve and has occasionally been used in circumstances in which radical neck dissection was necessary but the proximal eleventh nerve was free of tumor. However, because of the morbidity to the shoulder, this graft is rarely used. A much more common nerve graft is the hypoglossal nerve to facial nerve. This nerve, even when split and shared between the tongue muscles and the facial muscles, may cause paralysis of the tongue muscles; until facial reanimation occurs, the combined missing function of both nerves makes speech as well as chewing and swallowing difficult. In patients with multiple cranial neuropathy of nerves such as 10 and 12, the 12 and 7 anastomosis is less certain.

Medical therapy for Bell's palsy requires attention to the paralyzed eyelid. Most patients will have some drying of the eye, and corneal protection using either eye drops or ointments is necessary. A moisture chamber or glasses should be worn when the patient is exposed to wind or dust.

When a relatively long period of paralysis is expected or when the paralysis will be permanent, surgical treatment of the eye is necessary. A tarsorrhaphy has been used in the past, but it is a complicated procedure that produces significant patient morbidity and can be difficult to reverse should the patient request it or should facial nerve function return. A reasonable alternative is to place gold springs in the eyelids. Similarly, fascial slings to create a symmetric resting facial tone are useful, and in the course of surgical

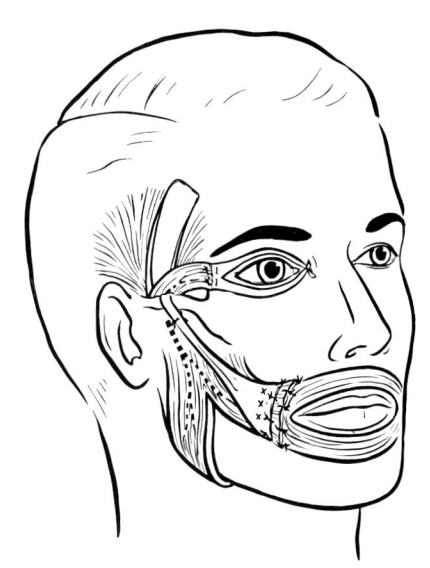

FIGURE 8–10. Masseter and temporalis muscle transfer to facial muscles. (From Freeman BS: Facial palsy. In Converse JM (ed): Reconstructive Plastic Surgery. Vol III. Philadelphia, WB Saunders Co, 1964, p 1151.)

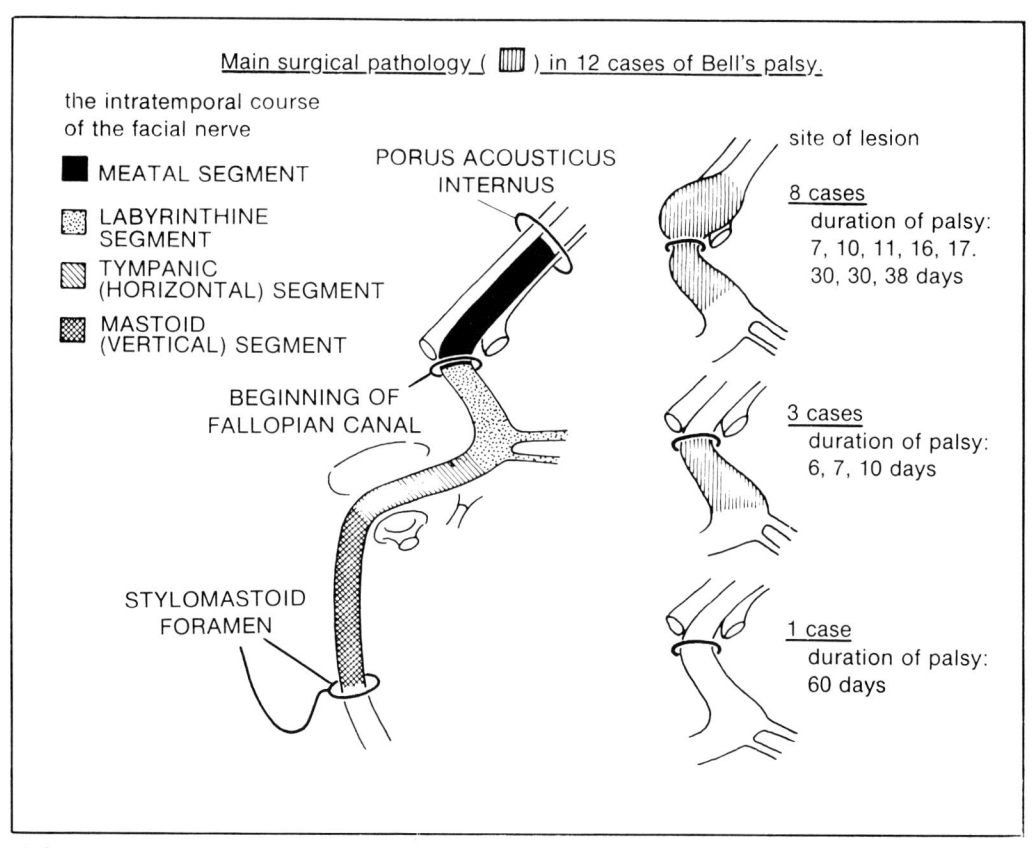

FIGURE 8–11. Localization of the pathologic changes observed in the meatal and labyrinthine segments of the facial nerve following total intratemporal exposure for Bell's palsy. Note that, in 8 of 11 cases, the observed pathologic alteration of the facial nerve fibers was particularly evident in the distal part of the internal auditory canal. (From Fisch U, Esslen E: Total intratemporal exposure of the facial nerve: Pathological findings in Bell's palsy. Arch Otolaryngol 95:337. Copyright 1972, American Medical Association.)

treatment a unilateral face lift to tense the skin on the paralyzed side similarly makes a more pleasant presentation of the patient with paralysis (Fig. 8–10).

Some clinicians recommend prednisone at a dose of 1 mg/kg/day for up to 14 days as medical therapy for Bell's palsy. There is little agreement in the literature on the effect of steroids in preventing denervation, synkinesis, autonomic mass movement, and crocodile tearing, and little evidence that they alter the course of the paralysis or palsy. Steroids do stop the otalgia, and for patients with severe otalgia this is a good medical treatment. All other medications are unproven in this disease. From 1970 to 1985 the best surgical treatment was either a transmastoid facial nerve decompression from the geniculate ganglion distally to the level of the stylomastoid foramen or a middle fossa decompression as advocated by Fisch. Figure 8–11 shows the location of the surgical pathology in 12 cases of Bell's palsy.

More otologists are at present reluctant to recommend transmastoid surgery; when electrical tests and clinical evaluation suggest surgery, a neuro-otologic approach through the middle cranial fossa is often the treatment undertaken.

References

Adour KK, Bell DM, Wingord J: Bell's palsy: Dilemma of diabetes mellitus. Arch Otolaryngol 99:114–117, 1974.
Alford BR, Jerger JF, Coats AC, et al: Neurophysiology of facial nerve testing. Arch Otolaryngol 97:214–219, 1973.
Cannon CR, Jahrsdoerfer RA: Temporal bone fractures, review of 90 cases. Arch Otolaryngol 109:285–288, 1983.
Fisch U: Surgery for Bell's palsy. Arch Otolaryngol 107:1–11, 1981.
Harner SG, Daube JR, Ebersold MJ, Beatty CW: Improved preservation of facial nerve function with use of electric monitoring during removal of acoustic neuromas. Laryngoscope 96:65–69, 1986.
Kettel K: Peripheral facial paralysis in fractures of the temporal bone. Arch Otolaryngol 51:25–41, 1960.
Malone B, Maisel RH: Anatomy of the facial nerve. Am J Otolaryngol 9(6):497–504, 1988.
May M, Hughes GB: Facial nerve disorders, update 1987. Am J Otolaryngol 8:167–180, 1987.

9

FACIAL PAIN, HEADACHE, AND OTALGIA

by Lawrence R. Boies, Jr., M.D.

The otolaryngologist is routinely called upon to diagnose and treat head pain; he or she may also be consulted by another physician in an attempt to diagnose headache resulting from a less than obvious cause. Probably the most overdiagnosed condition, particularly on the part of the laity, is "sinus headache," possibly due in part to the continual barrage of television ads promoting over-the-counter drugs for the relief of "sinus headache." Furthermore, there has been a tendency on the part of the physician to indict the sinuses when the cause of a headache cannot be easily explained, an indictment that is not difficult to understand owing to the frequency of nasal obstruction and hypersecretion from the nasal mucosa, as well as the anatomic position of the nasal fossae and the accessory sinuses in the general area in which headaches are often centered.

"Sinus headache" is overdiagnosed by the laity.

The intention here will not be to encompass the entire subject of facial pain and headache, but rather to outline a diagnostic approach to these problems while emphasizing the elements of the otolaryngologic physical examination related to them. Therefore, only those diagnostic entities of particular interest to the otolaryngologist will be discussed here; appropriate chapters in a standard textbook of neurology are recommended for concurrent study.

CLASSIFICATION OF HEADACHE

In the early 1960's a committee was formed to classify the causes of head pain according to etiology so that the student and practicing physician might approach the problem in a more organized manner.* The report distinguished between migraine headaches, considering them vascular in nature, and tension headaches, relegating them to the musculature. This classification has been widely applied since that time; however, in the interim, there have been significant questions raised concerning this dichotomy and the consequent treatment of these disorders. Rather than separate entities, the view is currently being postulated that migraine, tension, and cluster headaches are differing manifestations of central nervous system disturbances involving the upper brain stem, limbic system, and/or hypothalamus. These distur-

---

*The Committee was composed of Drs. Arnold P. Friedman (chairman), Knox H. Finley, John R. Graham, E. Charles Kunkle, Adrian M. Ostfeld, and Harold G. Wolf.

bances are thought to biochemically affect perception of and sensitivity to pain as well as cause the observed vascular and/or muscular changes. These new data will greatly broaden the understanding and treatment of headaches; however, a new, replacement classification system encompassing these various findings has not yet been formulated. Until that time, for ease of discussion, we will continue to rely on the original classification system, which is herein included in its entirety.

The term headache commonly denotes head pain from brow level up. This outline defines headaches somewhat broadly: It covers both painful and nonpainful discomforts of the entire head, including the face and upper nucha. Since so much that a man describes as headache may be any abnormal head sensation, it is essential for proper treatment to determine whether the complaint is actually one of pain. A useful scheme for the classification of the varieties of headache is one based on pain mechanisms. The divisions rest on experimental and clinical data, together with reasonable inference; the story is far from complete. Yet the arrangement can serve as a framework for diagnostic criteria for the major clinical types of headache, and by emphasis on basic mechanisms it offers a logical approach to the planning of therapeutic trials. For convenience, short and simple names are suggested for certain major entities and are indicated in boldface type.

Essential in the study of headache in most instances is an appraisal of its close link to the patient's situation, activities, and attitudes. Sometimes in obvious ways, more often in subtle ones, headache may be the principal manifestation of temporary or sustained difficulties in life adjustment. These relationships are notably evident in groups I through V.

Major Categories

- I. Vascular headache of migraine type
    - A. "Classic" migraine
    - B. "Common" migraine
    - C. "Cluster" headache
    - D. "Hemiplegic" and "ophthalmoplegic" migraine
    - E. "Lower-half" headache
- II. Muscle-contraction headache
- III. Combined headache: vascular and muscle-contraction
- IV. Headache of nasal vasomotor reaction
- V. Headache of delusional, conversion, or hypochondriacal states
- VI. Nonmigrainous vascular headaches
- VII. Traction headache
- VIII. Headache due to overt cranial inflammation
- IX–XIII. Headache due to disease of ocular, aural, nasal and sinus, dental, or other cranial or neck structures
- XIV. Cranial neuritides
- XV. Cranial neuralgias

Descriptions

I. Vascular Headaches of the Migraine Type. Recurrent attacks of headache, widely varied in intensity, frequency, and duration. The attacks are commonly unilateral in onset and are usually associated with anorexia and sometimes with nausea and vomiting; some are preceded by, or associated with, conspicuous sensory, motor, and mood disturbances; they are often familial.

Evidence supports the view that cranial arterial distention and dilatation are importantly implicated in the pain phase but cause no permanent changes in the involved vessel. Listed below are particular varieties of headache, each sharing some, but not necessarily all of the mentioned features:

A. "Classic" Migraine. Vascular headache with sharply defined, transient visual and other sensory or motor prodromes or both.

B. "Common" Migraine. Vascular headache without striking prodromes and less often unilateral than *A* and *C*. Synonyms are "atypical migraine" or "sick headache." Calling attention to certain relationships of this type of headache to environmental, occupational, menstrual, or other variables are such terms as "summer," "Monday," "week-end," "relaxation," "premenstrual," and "menstrual" headache.

C. "Cluster" Headache. Vascular headache, predominantly unilateral on the same side, usually associated with flushing, sweating, rhinorrhea, and increased lacrimation, brief in duration and usually occurring in closely packed groups separated by long remissions. Identical or closely allied are erythroprosopalgia (Bing), ciliary or migrainous neuralgia (Harris), erythromelalgia of the head or histaminic cephalgia (Horton), and petrosal neuralgia (Gardner et al.).

D. "Hemiplegic" Migraine and "Ophthalmoplegic" Migraine. Vascular headache characterized by sensory and motor phenomena that persist during and after the headache.

E. "Lower-Half" Headache. Headache of possible vascular mechanism centered primarily in the lower face. In this group there may be some instances of "atypical facial" neuralgia, sphenopalatine ganglion neuralgia (Sluder), and vidian neuralgia (Vail).

II. Muscle-Contraction Headache. Ache or sensations of tightness, pressure, or constriction, widely varied in intensity, frequency, and duration, sometimes long-lasting, and commonly suboccipital. It is associated with sustained contraction of skeletal muscles in the absence of permanent structural change, usually as part of the individual's reaction during life stress. The ambiguous and unsatisfactory terms "tension," "psychogenic," and "nervous" headache refer largely to this group.

III. Combined Headache: Vascular and Muscle-Contraction. Combinations of vascular headache of the migraine type and muscle-contraction headache, prominently coexisting in an attack.

IV. Headache of Nasal Vasomotor Reaction. Headaches and nasal discomfort (nasal obstruction, rhinorrhea, tightness, or burning), recurrent and resulting from congestion and edema of nasal and paranasal mucous membranes, and not proven to be due to allergens, infectious agents, or local gross anatomic defects. The headache is predominantly anterior in location and mild or moderate in intensity. The illness is usually part of the individual's reaction during life stress. This is often called "vasomotor rhinitis."

V. Headache of Delusional, Conversion, or Hypochondriacal States. Headaches of illnesses in which the prevailing clinical disorder is a delusional or conversion reaction and a peripheral pain mechanism are nonexistent. Closely allied are the hypochondriacal reactions in which the peripheral disturbances relevant to headache are minimal. These also have been called "psychogenic" headaches.

N.B.: The foregoing represent the major clinical disorders dominated by headache—those which are particularly common and in which headache is frequently recurrent and disabling.

VI. Nonmigrainous Vascular Headaches. Associated with generally nonrecurrent dilatation of cranial arteries.

A. Systemic infections, usually with fever.

B. Miscellaneous disorders, including hypoxic states, carbon monoxide poisoning, effects of nitrates and other chemical agents with vasodilator properties, caffeine-withdrawal reactions, circulatory insufficiency in the brain (in certain circumstances), postconcussion reactions, postconvulsive states, "hangover" reactions, foreign protein reactions, hypoglycemia, hypercapnia, acute pressor reactions (abrupt elevation of blood pressure, as with paraplegia or pheochromocytoma), and certain instances of essential arterial hypertension (e.g., those with early-morning headache).

VII. Traction Headache. Headache resulting from traction on intracranial structures, mainly vascular, by masses.

A. Primary or metastatic tumors of meninges, vessels, or brain.

B. Hematomas (epidural, subdural, or parenchymal).

C. Abscesses (epidural, subdural, or parenchymal).

D. *Postlumbar puncture headache* ("leakage" headache).

E. Pseudotumor cerebri and various causes of brain swelling.

VIII. Headache Due to Overt Cranial Inflammation. Headaches due to readily recognized inflammation of cranial structures—resulting from usually nonrecurrent inflammation, sterile or infectious.

A. *Intracranial disorders*—infectious, chemical, or allergic meningitis, subarachnoid hemorrhage, postpneumoencephalographic reaction, arteritis, and phlebitis.

B. *Extracranial disorders*—arteritis and cellulitis.

IX-XIII. Headache Due to Disease of Ocular, Aural, Nasal, and Sinus, Dental, or Other Cranial or Neck Structures.

IX. Headaches due to spread of effects of noxious stimulation of *ocular structures* (as by increased intraocular pressure, excessive contraction of ocular muscles, trauma, new growth, or inflammation).

X. Headaches due to spread of effects of noxious stimulation of *aural* structure (as by trauma, new growth, or inflammation).

XI. Headaches due to spread of effects of noxious stimulation of *nasal* and *sinus* structures (as by trauma, new growth, inflammation, or allergens).

XII. Headaches due to spread of effects of noxious stimulation of *dental* structures (as by trauma, new growth, or inflammation).

XIII. Headaches due to spread of pain from noxious stimulation of other structures of the cranium and neck (periosteum, joint ligaments, muscles, or cervical roots).

XIV. Cranial Neuritides. Caused by trauma, new growth, or inflammation.

XV. Cranial Neuralgias. Trigeminal (tic douloureux) and glossopharyngeal. The pains are lancinating ("jabbing"), usually in rapid succession for several minutes or longer, are limited to a portion or all of the domain of the affected nerve, and are often triggered by end-organ stimulation. Trigeminal neuralgia must be distinguished in particular from "cluster headache" (**I**, *C*), with which it is often confused.

N.B.: So-called chronic post-traumatic headache may arise from any one of several mechanisms. Such headache may represent sustained muscle contraction (**II**), recurrent vascular dilatation (**I**, *B*), or rarely, local scalp or nuchal injury (**XIII**). In some patients, the post-traumatic pain is part of a clinical disorder characterized by delusional conversion or hypochondriacal reactions (**V**).

EVALUATION OF HEADACHE

History

The patient with a headache problem invariably deserves a complete medical history review. First, the given head pain profile should be established with emphasis on the following aspects:

1. Time relationships
    a. Age of patient at onset
    b. Duration of problem
    c. Duration of single attacks
    d. Frequency of attacks
    e. More frequent occurrence at a certain time of day
    f. Onset following trauma or development of another medical problem
2. Prodromal or associated symptoms (if any)
3. Location
4. Quality
5. Precipitating factors

6. Factors intensifying pain
7. Response to medication (type)
8. Recent or previous dental work
9. Psychosocial history

A family history of headache, emotional disturbance, or organic disease states should not be overlooked; 75 per cent of migraine sufferers have a relative also afflicted. Occupational as well as sociologic factors may be of interest; stress and environmental pollutants have been implicated. Items of significance in the past medical history include allergy, cardiovascular disease, hypertension, head or neck trauma, neurologic disorders, glaucoma, and emotional problems in addition to ear, dental, and sinus disease. Drug use should be documented. Occasionally a precise diary of all dietary intake and headache attacks must be kept by the patient.

Clinical Examination

Manifestations of systemic conditions mentioned in the headache classification should be searched for. A complete neurologic examination may be indicated in certain cases. Specific points relating to the examination of the head and neck might include the following:

Auscultation for bruit (e.g., neck, parietotemporal areas)
Eye examination (visual acuity, visual fields, abnormal eye movements, funduscopic examination, ocular tension)
Evaluation of cranial nerve function
Palpation for arterial tenderness
Palpation for muscle spasm and tenderness (including muscles of mastication)
Evaluation for nuchal rigidity
Complete otolaryngologic examination, including evaluation of occlusion
Palpation of temporomandibular joints

Certain physical findings noted on the general otolaryngologic examination and relating to head pain may seem obvious. The preceding classification suggests areas and types of pathologic changes to be aware of. However, some areas that are frequently overlooked by the physician include the temporomandibular joints, portions of the pharynx requiring indirect examination, and the teeth. Mirror (or fiberoptic) examination of the pharynx is especially important in evaluating otalgia in patients with no apparent signs of ear disease; occult neoplasms in the pharynx may present in this manner. Physicians should become acquainted with the more common forms of dental disease. The nasal spaces should be examined carefully in all patients with headache possibly related to the nose or sinuses. The rhinoscopic examination should include a fiberoptic exam of nasal and posterior nasal spaces. After initial rhinoscopy the physician should decongest the nasal mucosa with ephedrine, phenylephrine, or cocaine solution. Reexamination is then performed. Noteworthy findings might include septal irregularities, contact points between septum and turbinates, suppurative drainage, polyps, or other neoplasms. The response of the patient to nasal shrinkage is an important diagnostic point if head pain is present at the time of examination. Likewise, relief of pain following specific cocainization of the sphenopalatine ganglion, which is located lateral to the posterior tip of the middle turbinate, is helpful in establishing a diagnosis.

Mirror or fiberoptic examination of the pharynx is important in evaluation of unexplained otalgia.

Rhinoscopy following decongestion is emphasized.

In certain patients laboratory and radiographic examinations are indicated. Some of the studies to consider include the following:

1. Paranasal sinus, skull, dental, cervical spine, temporomandibular joint radiographs
2. CT scan of head
3. MRI scan of head
4. Lumbar puncture (cerebrospinal fluid examination)
5. Personality profile (e.g., Minnesota Multiphasic Personality Inventory)
6. Electroencephalogram
7. Thermography

Differential Diagnosis

Dorland's Illustrated Medical Dictionary (27th Ed) defines headache or cephalgia (cephalalgia) simply as pain in the head. Neuralgia, on the other hand, is a paroxysmal pain that extends along the course of one or more nerves. It is usually of a severe, stabbing character. Both primary and secondary causes of neuralgia should be considered.

Head pain may be divided into acute and chronic (or chronic recurring) types. Obviously, acute types may become chronic. Generally, one would associate the term acute with head pain related to acute febrile states; acute infections involving the ears, sinuses, or teeth; intracranial hemorrhage; meningitis, cerebritis, and brain abscess; and with primary attacks of migraine, cluster headache, the cranial neuralgias, and glaucoma. The remainder would be termed chronic.

Friedman has stated that most patients with headache as a major complaint

TABLE 9–1. FEATURES OF CERTAIN HEAD PAIN CONDITIONS

CONDITION	LOCATION	ASSOCIATED SYMPTOMS
Cluster headache	Behind or above one eye with extension to temple or maxilla	Nasal congestion, lacrimation, conjunctival injection; may occur at night
Muscle-contraction headache	"Hatband," bitemporal, occipital, suboccipital	Chronic anxiety; in some cases may be related to occupational muscle fatigue
Nasal vasomotor reaction	In and around nose, ethmoid, and maxillary areas; may radiate into frontal area	Nasal obstruction and rhinorrhea often occur
Temporal arteritis	In area of temporal (often bilateral) or other involved branches of extracranial arteries	Ischemic optic neuritis
Acute sinusitis	Pain in area of involved sinus; sphenoid sinusitis may cause retro-orbital, occipital, or vertex pain	Fever, malaise, tenderness over involved sinus, nasal discharge and congestion, associated upper respiratory tract infection
Chronic sinusitis	Infrequently causes chronic head pain; may be confused with vasomotor reaction, since symptoms are in same general area	Nasal polyposis, chronic suppurative nasal discharge
Temporomandibular joint dysfunction	In and around ear with radiation into neck or temporal area	Aural fullness; clicking in joint
Trigeminal neuralgia	Face; any of the three divisions of the trigeminal nerve may be involved, alone or in combination	Usually associated trigger zones that respond to light contact
Glossopharyngeal neuralgia	Pharynx with radiation into ear	Salivation; trigger zones in tonsillar region

do not have a serious organic disease. Roughly 90 per cent of chronic headaches, in his experience, are either migraine vascular headaches, muscle-contraction headaches, or a combination of the two. Nevertheless, one should carefully rule out organic disease or serious psychologic problems in all patients with chronic recurring head pain. Some puzzling patients require close observation and symptomatic or trial therapy to establish a diagnosis. Van Allen and Friedman point out that time, patience, and careful re-examination can solve many difficult problems.

There are several components that make up a head pain profile. Table 9–1 has been constructed as a guide to differential diagnosis using location and associated symptoms in outlining certain clinical entities of particular interest to the otolaryngologist. The remainder of this chapter will be devoted to an expanded discussion of these entities.

CLINICAL ENTITIES OF PARTICULAR INTEREST TO THE OTOLARYNGOLOGIST

Cluster Headache

According to the classification presented earlier, cluster headache is now considered a vascular headache of the migraine type. Previously used terms for this condition are mentioned in the outline (**I, C**). The predominantly unilateral facial and head pain occurs primarily in men, with sudden onset and abrupt cessation. It is said to be the most excruciating of the vascular headaches. There is no prodrome. Frequent attacks, one to three per day, of short duration, typically 45 minutes to one hour, tend to occur in clusters or clumps during a period of up to three months. Periods of remission may last from months to even years, averaging two years. The focus of pain is usually centered behind one eye, with radiation to involve the entire side of the face and neck. The pain is often associated with flushing, sweating, increased lacrimation, and rhinorrhea on the involved side. It is not unusual for an attack to occur at night, awakening the patient from his sleep. An attack may be precipitated by alcohol, histamine, and other vasodilators. The mechanism involving dilatation of the extracranial and dural arteries is generally accepted; however, the interrelationships and specific nature of neurologic, humoral, and psychologic factors are not understood completely.

Cluster headaches are said to be the most excruciating of the vascular headaches.

The focus of pain is usually behind one eye.

The main entities to consider in the differential diagnosis include trigeminal neuralgia, acute glaucoma, intracranial aneurysm, and acute sinusitis, particularly with sphenoid involvement. Features such as lack of trigger points, unilateral lacrimation, lack of other eye findings, and the general pattern of attacks help distinguish cluster headache in the differential diagnosis.

The following modes of treatment are available:

1. The inhalation of 100 per cent oxygen may abort an acute attack. Some patients keep an oxygen tank at their bedside.
2. Ergotamine has been the most dependable drug. However, because of gastroparesis, oral ergotomine is not always appropriate. Ergotomine inhalation has been found to be suitably fast and effective. Also available are sublingual, parenteral, and rectal forms.
3. Local application of anesthetic (lidocaine) nose drops has been reported to be an effective abortive agent.
4. Methysergide has been used successfully as prophylactic treatment.

Propranolol (Inderal) has been advocated in preventive therapy by some neurologists.

5. The most effective approach to managing cluster headaches is the prophylactic daily administration of various drugs during the cluster period. These include ergotamine, methysergide maleate, corticosteroids, lithium carbonate, calcium channel blockers (especially verapamil), and indomethacin.
6. Psychotherapy may be helpful in this and other forms of vascular head pain.

Histamine desensitization has been shown to be of little value.

Muscle-Contraction Headache

Otolaryngologists frequently encounter headache originating in the muscles and fibrous structures about the head. The pain is often of a chronic nature and is located in the frontal, temporal, occipital, and suboccipital regions (Fig. 9–1). Tension is a common cause, although fatigue and inflammatory disturbances may be factors. Fortunately, many tension headaches are of a mild character. The patient complains of the sensation of a tight band ("hat band") around the head, but it is not severe enough to be painful. This sensation is produced by a mild, involuntary increase in

"Hat band" headaches are commonly caused by tension.

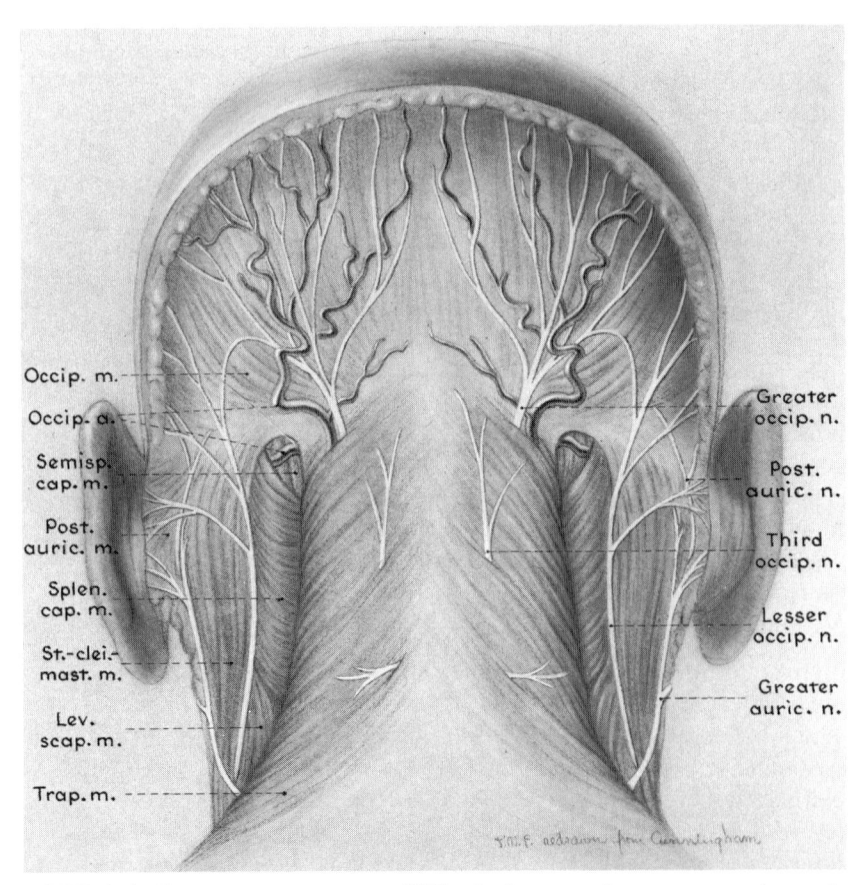

FIGURE 9–1. There are numerous possibilities in the muscular, nervous, and vascular structures in the posterior neck and occiput for the production of headache or neuralgia.

temporal muscle tension. Treatment consists of sympathetic listening and practical advice such as heat and massage.

A more severe form occurs with a chronic state of tension of the postural muscles of the head and neck, often bilateral. In particular, the muscles of the shoulder girdle and back of the neck are affected, becoming hypertonic with resultant occipital pain referred to the vertex. A frequent cause is simple anxiety; muscular fatigue seen with certain occupations or athletic sports may also be a cause. Biofeedback and relaxation have both been used successfully by many practitioners to treat this type of headache, with training aimed at relaxing the specific muscles involved as well as general relaxation involving the entire body.

Muscle-contraction headaches that are secondary to structural abnormalities in the neck are often included in the tension group but should not be considered as such. These include cervical spondylosis, a condition often observed in the elderly. In cervical spondylosis, the headache pain tends to be dull and is moderated by massage and/or heat. Other therapies include nonsteroidal anti-inflammatory drugs, other forms of physical therapy, antidepressants, and muscle relaxants.

Structural abnormalities of the neck should be considered in evaluating occipital headaches.

Irritation of one or more of the cervical roots (cervical radiculopathy) may lead to headaches, often present upon waking. Treatment of these headaches focuses upon the involved roots, e.g., use of a cervical collar, particularly at night, intermittent cervical traction, or injection of sensitive areas.

Rooke and Rushton state that there is a tendency to label as tension any chronic cervico-occipital headache that occurs in the absence of demonstrable organic disease, especially when other anxieties or tensions exist in the patient. Suspicion that the diagnosis of tension headache is *incorrect* should be aroused by the following features:

1. It is unilateral.
2. It responds favorably to simple analgesia.
3. It is modified by position or activity.
4. It is described in simple, accurate terms.
5. Despite chronicity, there are periods of clear-cut relief.
6. There is an element of progression.

Other terms may be brought up in discussions involving muscle-related pain. Myalgia is defined as simple muscle pain that has been linked with physical allergy and autonomic instability. Myofascitis refers to a localized inflammatory condition involving muscle and overlying and adjacent fasciae with resultant fibrosis. Other inflammatory processes from a variety of causes may specifically involve muscle (myositis) or fibrous structures (fibrositis, fasciitis, tendinitis). These conditions, alone or in combination, do involve appropriate structures around the head and neck. Many do result in muscle spasm but would more likely be classified under group **XIII** of the outline presented earlier in this chapter.

Fibrositis, or fibromyalgia, is a common condition that has long been the subject of controversy. Many physicians have not recognized it as a discrete entity but rather have viewed the reported pain as psychogenic in origin, representing a manifestation of a reactive disorder. This conclusion was supported by the lack of significant histopathology or laboratory and radiographic changes. However, as criteria evolve to standardize the diagnosis of this condition, its existence has gained a greater degree of credibility.

Fibromyalgia continues to be a controversial subject.

Goldenberg cites the primary standard to be a minimum number of tender points (ranging from 4 to 12) at characteristic locations. Other important symptoms include disturbed sleep, fatigue, and morning stiffness.

Therapy for fibrositis is nonspecific, with many patients benefiting from a multifaceted approach, including reassurance that this condition is not life-threatening or progressive, simple analgesics or nonsteroidal anti-inflammatory medications, tricyclic agents, psychotherapy, and physical therapy.

Nasal Vasomotor Reaction

This condition is discussed further in Chapter 12 under the heading of vasomotor rhinitis. The majority of patients who suffer from the nasal congestion and engorgement caused by it complain mainly of nasal obstruction with or without rhinorrhea. Headache associated with vasomotor rhinitis is the exception rather than the rule. Pain originating in the nose or sinuses may be caused by the following:

1. Contacts within the nasal fossae
2. Environmental or other changes resulting in a temporary negative pressure in one or more of the paranasal sinuses (e.g., barosinusitis)
3. Disease within a sinus, causing pressure or tension

McAuliffe et al. have demonstrated pain-sensitive areas in the nasal space and the regions to which pain originating therein is referred. These pain-sensitive areas are the following:

1. Nasofrontal area
2. Middle meatus, especially around the ostia
3. Generally, the septum and lateral nasal wall

Stimulation of the anteroinferior portion of the septum, middle and inferior turbinates, and ostia of the maxillary sinus refers pain to the malar and zygomatic regions of the ipsilateral side. Stimulation of the superior portion of the nasal fossa refers pain to the eye, intraorbital area, and lower portion of the frontal bone.

Pain produced by these contacts is more often acute and somewhat temporary but may become recurrent. Emotional factors may play a role in chronicity. Holmes pointed out that anxiety, conflict, frustration, and resentment may result in nasal hyperemia, swelling, hypersecretion, and, ultimately, pain.

A "vacuum" type pain mechanism is frequently mentioned as a cause of recurring nasofrontal headaches.

The concept of a "vacuum" type pain mechanism has enjoyed intermittent attention among rhinologists, beginning with the writings of Sluder, in which he described an acute frontal headache that was frequently present upon arising and characterized by tenderness in the area of the floor of the frontal sinus on the involved side. He believed that this entity arose from temporary closure of the nasofrontal duct and resultant negative pressure within the sinus cavity. As Shapiro pointed out, this would be analogous to the middle ear condition occurring with a blocked eustachian tube. Obviously, such a mechanism could be invoked by several other pathologic processes besides vasomotor rhinitis. Also, individual local anatomic variants undoubtedly play a role in the production of symptoms. The clear-cut entity of aerosinusitis or sinus barotrauma makes Sluder's proposed mechanism more plausible.

Treatment for headache related to vasomotor rhinitis is relatively limited, provided that one has ruled out allergic conditions, infections, and anatomic deformities. Nasal sprays such as Afrin may be efficacious on a short-term basis. Systemic decongestants have been used with good results in some patients. In unyielding cases partial turbinectomy or electrocautery of the turbinates may be performed. Vidian nerve section may be considered in extreme cases.

"Lower-half" Headache

This term has been used in reference to lower facial pain. Included in this grouping are atypical facial neuralgia, sphenopalatine ganglion neuralgia (Sluder), and vidian neuralgia (Vail). Current thought is that, in general, most pain syndromes involving this area are vasodilating in origin and are not due to neuropathic processes, unless one might implicate the autonomic nervous system in specific cases. True neuralgias involving only the sensory fibers of the maxillary division of the trigeminal nerve which pass through the sphenopalatine ganglion may exist but probably are rare. Greater involvement of the maxillary trunk should give a picture indistinguishable from a second-division trigeminal neuralgia. However, these atypical lower face pain syndromes have generally been more diffuse, deep-seated, and poorly localized. They have occurred in a younger age group and have been void of trigger zones. Few have been relieved by nerve section. Certainly a careful intranasal examination (including sphenopalatine ganglion cocainization) is recommended in such cases. Contacts between the nasal septum and lateral wall should be considered as causes of this type of head pain; however, treatment generally is directed toward a vasodilating etiology.

Atypical "lower-half" headaches are currently thought to be of vascular origin.

A careful intranasal examination is recommended.

Temporal Arteritis

Temporal arteritis is a condition of unknown cause. Although originally described as involving the temporal arteries, it is now referred to generally as extracranial arteritis, since it may involve other branches of the external carotid system. Moreover, arteries elsewhere in the body may be affected. Classically, the arteritis is of the giant cell type.

The condition often causes constant, moderately severe head pain that tends to be bilateral and is associated with tenderness in the area of the involved arteries; it may mimic migraine, muscle-contraction, or cluster headache. The pain is not influenced by cough or head movements. Most commonly, temporal arteritis occurs in older individuals and may be accompanied by generalized weakness and anemia. Diagnosis is made by biopsy and microscopic examination of a suspected vessel. The sedimentation rate is often markedly increased. Blindness may occur owing to ischemic optic neuritis; therefore, prompt treatment with high-dose, prolonged prednisone is recommended to minimize or prevent this complication.

Diagnosis is made by biopsy and microscopic examination of a suspected vessel.

Sinusitis

Acute rhinosinusitis certainly can result in contacts within the nasal fossae in addition to pressure or tension within a given sinus. Contact pain patterns have been discussed. Individual sinus involvement will tend to produce the following general pain locations:

1. Maxillary: anterior facial (cheek) with radiation into teeth, orbital, and malar regions
2. Ethmoids: interocular with spread into frontal location
3. Frontal: forehead, interocular, and temporal areas
4. Sphenoid: retro-orbital, radiation toward vertex and occasionally the mastoid areas

One must remember that several or all sinuses (pansinusitis) may be involved on one or both sides.

When headache with chronic sinusitis is encountered, it is usually due to pathologic conditions such as a mucocele or osteoma or is related to an intercurrent acute flare-up. Certainly any chronic inflammatory process in the nasal region can result in contact pain, as previously noted. Tumors, although rare in this area, must be considered.

Diagnosis and treatment of sinusitis are discussed in Chapter 13.

Inflammation involving dental structures may mimic sinus pain and may also actually cause maxillary sinusitis.

Otalgia

Otalgia, or ear pain, may be due to primary or secondary causes. In some cases the term reflex or referred otalgia has been used for the secondary type. Primary causes of otalgia are usually apparent on careful otologic examination. Such conditions are outlined in the first portion of Table 9–2.

Often when a patient has ear pain, particularly when it is of a mild degree, he or she is not able to identify the location of the pain more specifically

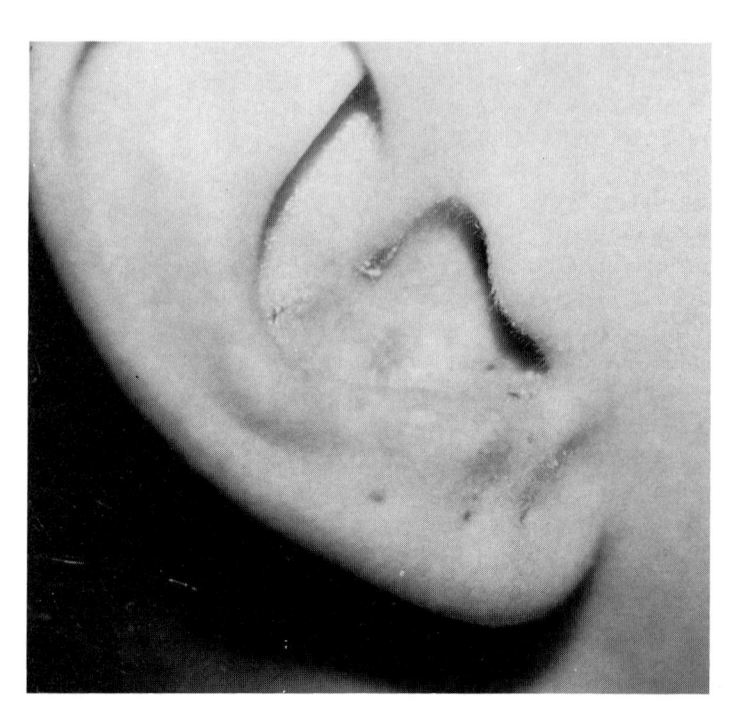

FIGURE 9–2. Right ear showing vesicular lesions of herpes zoster oticus. The patient presented with facial paralysis and severe pain in the region of the right ear.

TABLE 9–2. CAUSES OF EAR PAIN

I. **Primary Pain (Originating in Ear)**
  A. External ear
   1. Furunculosis
   2. Foreign body in external ear canal
   3. External otitis
   4. Abscess of auricle
   5. Perichondritis of auricle
   6. Eczema of meatus
   7. Impacted cerumen
   8. Frostbite of auricle
   9. Herpes simplex and herpes zoster oticus (see Fig. 9–2)
   10. Malignant and benign growth of external ear
   11. Fungal infections (otomycosis)
   12. Acute myringitis and myringitis bullosa
   13. Trauma of tympanic membrane and external canal
  B. Middle ear or mastoid
   1. Acute otitis media
   2. Acute mastoiditis
   3. Acute aerotitis media (barotrauma)
   4. Acute eustachian tube obstruction
   5. Complications of otitis media and mastoiditis
     a. Petrositis
     b. Facial paralysis
     c. Labyrinthitis
     d. Inner ear deafness
     e. Subperiosteal abscess
     f. Extradural abscess
     g. Subdural abscess
     h. Brain abscess
     i. Venous sinus thrombophlebitis
     j. Meningitis
   6. Malignant and benign growth of middle ear and mastoid process
  C. Idiopathic (tic-like pain confined to the ear) causes
   1. Geniculate complex of the seventh cranial nerve
   2. Tympanic branch of the ninth cranial nerve
II. **Secondary (Referred) Pain**
  A. Larynx
   1. Cancer
   2. Ulceration
   3. Perichondritis and chondritis
   4. Arthritis of cricoarytenoid joint
  B. Pharynx (naso-, oro-, and hypopharynx)
   1. Pharyngitis
   2. Acute tonsillitis (palatine, lingual, pharyngeal)

II. **Secondary (Referred) Pain** *Continued*
   3. Peritonsillar abscess
   4. Retropharyngeal abscess
   5. Ulceration
   6. Postadenoidectomy or posttonsillectomy
   7. Nasopharyngeal fibroma
   8. Malignant growth
  C. Oral cavity
   1. Dental neuralgias
     a. Dentine exposed, pulp inflamed, or nerves dying
     b. Unerupted or impacted wisdom or molar teeth
     c. Traumatic occlusion of teeth, faulty closure of jaw, and improper fit of dentures
   2. Acute diffuse glossitis or stomatitis
   3. Carcinoma of tongue
  D. Esophagus
   1. Foreign body
   2. Hiatus hernia
   3. Inflammation
   4. Malignant and benign growths
  E. Miscellaneous causes
   1. Mumps
   2. Acute thyroiditis
   3. Trigeminal neuralgia
   4. Sinuses
     a. Inflammation
     b. Malignant and benign growth
   5. Temporomandibular arthritis
   6. Erysipelas
   7. Raynaud's disease
   8. Chilblains
   9. Postauricular lymphadenitis
   10. Glossopharyngeal neuralgia
   11. Sphenopalatine ganglion cephalgia
   12. Elongation of the styloid process
   13. Involvement of upper three cervical nerves
     a. Whiplash injury and other cervical spine lesions
     b. Inflammation such as tabes dorsalis or herpes
   14. Angina pectoris
   15. Thoracic aneurysm
   16. Innominate artery aneurysm
   17. Affections of nasal passageway
   18. Affections of lung and bronchus

Source: Nelms CR, Paparella MM: Otalgia. Minn Med 52:955, June 1969.

than in the general area of the external ear and deeper. Therefore, when there is no evidence of acute middle ear inflammation or disease in the external ear, it is important to determine which lesions might be present in the distribution of the sensory fibers of the several cranial nerves that supply these structures but have ramifications in more distant areas.

The fifth, seventh, ninth, and tenth cranial nerves have sensory fibers in some areas of the auricle, the external canal, and the tympanum, with considerable overlap in the areas supplied. Also, the second and third cervical nerves supply sensation to the postaural area, while the auriculotemporal branch of the fifth nerve innervates some of the external ear and a considerable area in front of the auricle and around the temporomandibular

Pharyngeal and laryngeal malignancies must be ruled out in cases of unexplained otalgia.

joint. For the most part, in cases of secondary or referred otalgia, one cannot determine the nerve through which pain is being referred until a lesion is found. The most important lesions that demand early detection are, of course, malignancies. The patient with a lesion on the rim of the larynx, in the piriform sinus, or on the epiglottis may complain of earache on the involved side. The reference is through the superior laryngeal branch of the vagus nerve. Any lesion, including early carcinoma, in the area of the palatine tonsils, the adjacent tongue, and lingual tonsils may cause earache via the glossopharyngeal nerve. Otalgia that occurs following tonsillectomy may be explained in the same manner (Fig. 9–3).

Dental disease may cause earache referred through a branch of the trigeminal nerve. Molar impaction and dental infection are common causes.

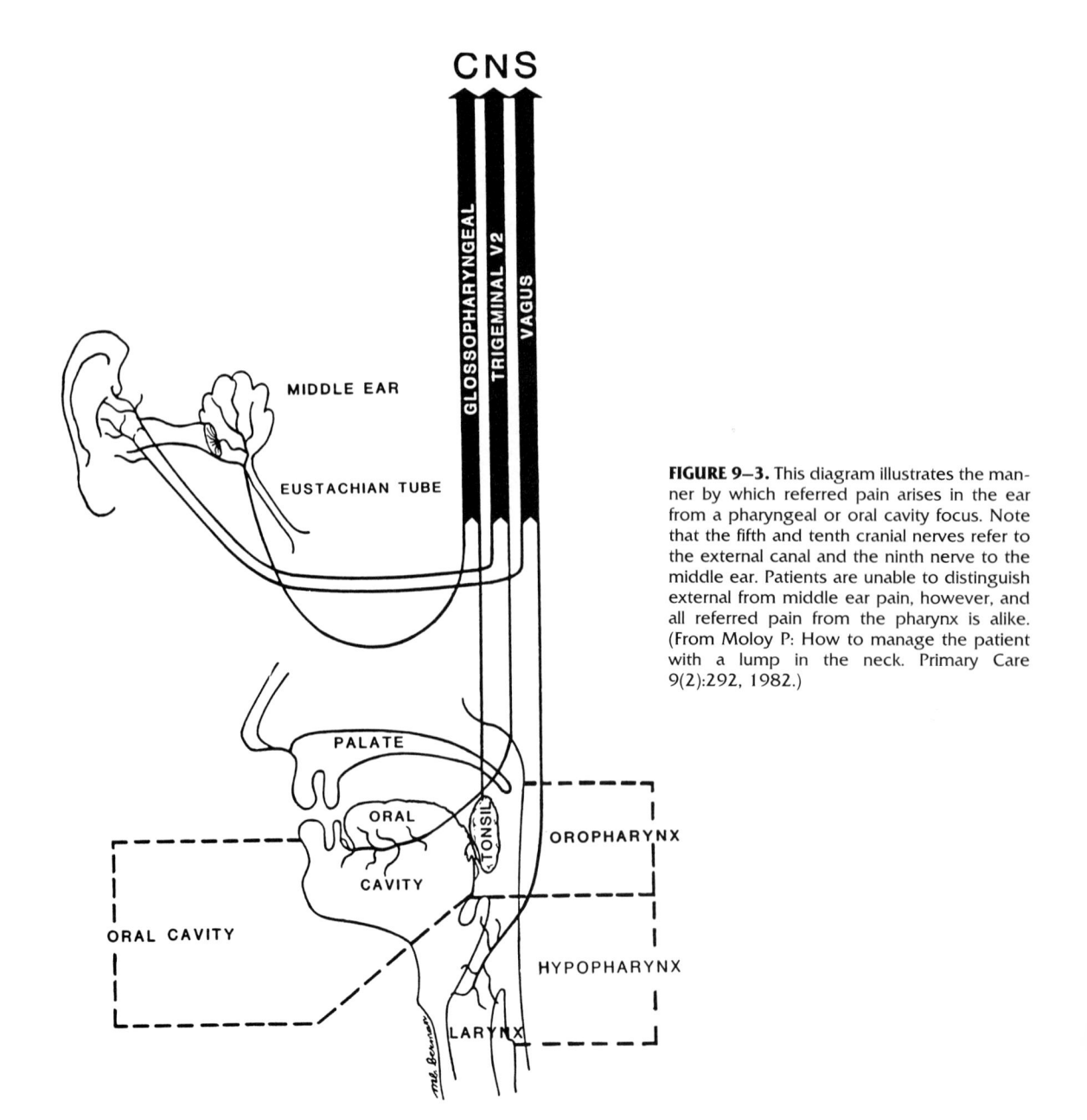

FIGURE 9–3. This diagram illustrates the manner by which referred pain arises in the ear from a pharyngeal or oral cavity focus. Note that the fifth and tenth cranial nerves refer to the external canal and the ninth nerve to the middle ear. Patients are unable to distinguish external from middle ear pain, however, and all referred pain from the pharynx is alike. (From Moloy P: How to manage the patient with a lump in the neck. Primary Care 9(2):292, 1982.)

Temporomandibular Joint Dysfunction

Temporomandibular joint (TMJ) dysfunction is a common cause of secondary otalgia, with the patient frequently complaining of ear infection. The pain may be perceived as a deep, boring pain in the ear mimicking acute otitis media; however, the classic hearing loss associated with infection is not present in these patients. Muscle spasm may accompany temporomandibular joint dysfunction. The temporalis, masseter, and medial and lateral pterygoid muscles are primarily involved, with the trapezius, suboccipital, frontal, and occipital muscles involved occasionally on a secondary basis. Many times the patient exhibits malocclusion and, on occasion, malposition of the maxilla and/or mandible. It is important to know whether the patient has had any recent dental work or has a past history of orthodontic treatment. A past history of gout, rheumatoid arthritis, trauma, Paget's disease, hyperparathyroidism, or arteritis is important in the differential diagnosis of temporomandibular joint dysfunction. Bruxism, or grinding of the teeth, may cause joint dysfunction or muscle spasm, with nocturnal grinding being manifested as morning headache and unconscious stress-induced daytime grinding producing evening headache.

TMJ dysfunction is a common cause of secondary otalgia.

Muscle spasm may accompany TMJ dysfunction.

A history of bruxism is of interest.

A complete otolaryngologic examination should be performed, with special attention to the dentition and function of the masticatory muscles. The teeth should be examined for dental caries and for malocclusion as well as for missing or extracted teeth and crown or bridge work. If the patient is edentulous, the degree of stability of the dentures, particularly the lower, should be evaluated, as ill-fitting dentures may cause symptoms of temporomandibular joint dysfunction. The temporomandibular joint should be palpated for evidence of opening or closing click, crepitus, or restricted anterior motion on opening, also referred to as translation. The muscles of mastication should be palpated, including the temporalis muscle, the masseter muscle, and the pterygoids, which are palpated intraorally. Jaw opening and closing should be observed, with any changes or deviation of the jaw to the right or left noted. Measurements should be made on maximal mouth opening between the edges of the upper and lower incisors; this measurement in the average adult is greater than 40 mm. Measurement of less than 40 mm may indicate decrease in joint function and in translation. A complete cranial nerve examination should also be performed; on rare occasions parapharyngeal tumors or tumors at the base of the skull can cause restricted mouth opening and temporomandibular joint symptoms; however, these tumors frequently cause sensory and/or motor changes, particularly involving cranial nerves V, VII, IX, X, and XI. Radiographic evaluation should include a panoramic dental radiograph to visualize the joints and, if indicated, further joint imaging techniques such as contrast arthrotomography or magnetic resonance imaging.

Dental examination including palpation of the TMJ and muscles of mastication is important.

Initial symptomatic treatment includes a soft to liquid diet, heat applied over the affected muscles, and anti-inflammatory drugs such as aspirin or other nonsteroidal anti-inflammatory agents. Many times oral splints are the initial treatment for these patients to disocclude the teeth and allow the mandible to assume the normal position, thereby allowing the muscles of mastication to relax and assume a more normal function. If the cause of the joint dysfunction is related to the occlusion, then correction of the malocclusion is extremely important. This may range from very minimal grinding of the occlusal surface of the teeth, known as occlusal equilibration, to ortho-

Conservation treatment is often sufficient.

Correction of malocclusion may be necessary in some cases.

dontic treatment for more severe malocclusions; in some cases, orthognathic surgery, that is, elective osteotomies with repositioning of the maxilla, mandible, or both, is required. In frank degenerative joint disease or with disk dislocation, joint surgery may be indicated as the treatment of choice. This may include a tightening of the joint capsule with removal of the meniscus of the joint, or, in more extensive cases, joint replacement with either alloplastic materials or autogenous grafts.

Trigeminal Neuralgia

The sharp, lancinating pain with trigger zones is characteristic of trigeminal neuralgia.

The diagnosis of primary trigeminal neuralgia (tic douloureux) is usually not difficult because of the character of the pain. In this type of headache the pain is of sudden onset, sharp and lancinating, and initiated at trigger zones about the face which react to light physical contact or drafts of air. It usually occurs in persons beyond middle age and may involve one or more of the divisions of the trigeminal nerve. The ophthalmic division is least frequently affected. Attacks may occur every few seconds, with intervals of freedom. Periods of recurrent attacks may last from a few days to a few weeks. Remissions of months to years are seen. The disease is usually unilateral and the cause is unknown.

Specific causes must be ruled out before making the diagnosis of a primary neuralgia.

In the secondary type of trigeminal neuralgia, the pain as a rule is of a chronic nature, with longer episodes and less severe attacks. Trigger zones are uncommon. The cause is found to be some lesion involving one of the nerve roots. Tumors, both intra- and extracranial, must be ruled out. While occasionally multiple sclerosis is found to be the cause, dental, nasal, and sinus diseases are the more common causes. In actuality, the neurologic disturbance associated with the aforementioned temporomandibular joint dysfunction may involve a branch of the trigeminal nerve and, therefore, technically would be considered a secondary form.

Drug treatment consists of use of phenytoin (Dilantin), baclofen, clonazepam, valproic acid, or carbamazepine (Tegretol) alone or in combination. When prescribing Tegretol in particular, the physician must be aware that severe, sometimes irreversible, adverse reactions involving the hematopoietic system can result. Early detection of hematologic change is important, since in some patients the resultant aplastic anemia is reversible.

Patients unresponsive to the medical treatment described are managed by alcohol injection or rhizotomy of the involved nerve or nerve root. Currently, percutaneous radiofrequency rhizotomy seems to be the method of choice. Other treatment possibilities include surgical ablation of the gasserian ganglion or nerve decompression.

Glossopharyngeal Neuralgia

A common secondary form may be seen briefly after tonsillectomy.

Primary glossopharyngeal neuralgia, a tic douloureaux of this nerve, is relatively rare. The paroxysms of stabbing pain in the ear, with trigger zones in the tonsillar area of the involved side, accompanied by salivation, provide a picture in which the diagnosis is not difficult. A secondary form that is common is seen in the earache following tonsillectomy or with any inflammatory or neoplastic process involving the tonsillar area and adjacent areas in the absence of middle ear disease. As previously discussed, one must consider the many causes of referred otalgia when entertaining the diagnosis of glossopharyngeal neuralgia.

Medical treatment of the primary form is identical to that discussed for trigeminal neuralgia, i.e., Dilantin and Tegretol. Patients unresponsive to drug therapy are handled surgically by suboccipital craniectomy and rhizotomy.

Carotidynia

Carotidynia, pain upon palpation of the common carotid arteries, is a condition that appears to have two forms. The first is acute, lasting one to two weeks, with no recurrence, and the other form shows a chronic pattern, possibly related to migraines. Corticosteroids have proved effective in both forms of this condition.

References

Baker AB, Baker LH: Clinical Neurology. Philadelphia, JB Lippincott Co, 1987.
Biber MP, Warfield CA: Headache, Otolaryn Clin North Am 19:55–63, 1986.
Boies LR: The modern role of the rhinologist in the diagnosis and therapy of the etiology of head pain. Ann Otol 59:507, 1950.
Classification of headache. Arch Neurol 6:173, 1962; JAMA 179:717, 1962; Neurology 12:378, 1962.
Costen JB: A syndrome of ear and sinus symptoms dependent on disturbed function of the temporomandibular joint. Ann Otol 43:1, 1943.
Dalessio DJ: Wolff's Headache and Other Head Pain. New York, Oxford University Press, 1972.
Friedman AP: When your patient complains of headaches. Med Times 103:67–77, 1975.
Friedman AP: Symposium on headache and related pain problems. Med Clin North Am, Vol 62:3, 1978.
Gelb H: Symposium on temporomandibular joint dysfunction and treatment. Den Clin North Am, 27:3, 1983.
Goldenberg DL: Fibromyalgia syndrome: An emerging but controversial condition. JAMA 257:2782–2787, 1987.
Hilger JA, et al: Symposium on headache: Mechanisms, management, nasal function and headache. Trans Am Acad Ophthalmol Otolaryngol 66:757, 1963.
Holmes TH, et al: The Nose. Springfield, IL, Charles C Thomas, Publisher, 1950.
Indihar F, Alter M: Trigeminal neuralgia. Minn Med 53:655, 1970.
McAuliffe GW, Goodel H, Wolff HG: Experimental studies on headache; pain from nasal and paranasal structures. Assoc Res Nerv Ment Dis Proc 23:185, 1943.
Nelms CR, Paparella MM: Otalgia. Minn Med 52:955, 1969.
Paparella MM, Shumrick DA (eds): Otolaryngology. Vol 2: Ear. Philadelphia, WB Saunders Co, 1973.
Raskin NH, Appenzeller O: Headache, Philadelphia. WB Saunders Co, 1980.
Rooke ED, Rushton JG: Headache: A discussion of its office management. Med Clin North Am 44:925, 1960.
Rushton T: Cranial nerve neuralgia. Med Clin North Am 44:969, 1960.
Sandoz Pharmaceuticals: Headache and Commonest Symptom. East Hanover, NJ, 1975 (monograph).
Shapiro SL: Vacuum headache. Eye Ear Nose Throat Mon 49:46, 1970.
Sluder G: Headaches and Eye Disorders of Nasal Origin. St Louis, The CV Mosby Co, 1920.
Vail HH: Vidian neuralgia. Ann Otol 41:837, 1932.
Van Allen MW, Friedman AP: Headaches which merit neurologic investigation. CMD:1069–1078, 1968.

PART THREE

THE NOSE AND PARANASAL SINUSES

10

APPLIED ANATOMY AND PHYSIOLOGY OF THE NOSE

by Peter A. Hilger, M.D.

The nose is an important organ that deserves more consideration than it normally receives; it is one of the body's most important protectors against an unfavorable environment and has been for millenia.

In an era in which an ever-increasing number of scientific studies and publications have been devoted to airborne occupational hazards and airborne pollutants, a basic understanding of the anatomy and physiology of the nose is important.

The nose performs a number of functions: it subserves the sense of smell, prepares inhaled air for use in the lungs, furnishes the air resistance necessary for normal functioning of the lungs, exerts certain reflex effects upon the lungs, and modifies speech.

ANATOMY

External Nose

The midline structure projecting outward from the plane of the cheeks and upper lip, the external nose may be divided structurally into three divisions: the bony vault, the most superior, is immobile; below it comes the slightly movable cartilaginous vault; and lowest is the movable nasal lobule. Considering the bony skeleton only, the lower half of the pyriform aperture divides the internal from the external nose. Superiorly, the external nasal skeletal structures include the ascending processes of the maxillae and the two nasal bones, all supported by the nasal process of the frontal bone and a portion of the perpendicular plate of the ethmoid bone. The anterior nasal spine, representing the portions of the embryologic medial maxillary process that engulfs the anterior premaxilla, may also be considered a part of the external nose. The next division, the slightly movable cartilaginous vault, is made up of the upper lateral cartilages, fused with each other in the midline and also fused with the upper margin of the quadrangular septal cartilage. The lowest third of the external nose, the nasal lobule, has its shape maintained by the lower lateral cartilages. The lobule encloses the nasal vestibule and is delineated medially by the columella, laterally by the alae of the nose, and anterosuperiorly by the nasal tip (Fig. 10–1). Mobility of the nasal lobule is necessary for facial expression, sniffing, and sneezing. The subcutaneous muscles of expression over the nasal bones, anterior cheeks, and upper lip assure this mobility. Subcutaneous connective tissue

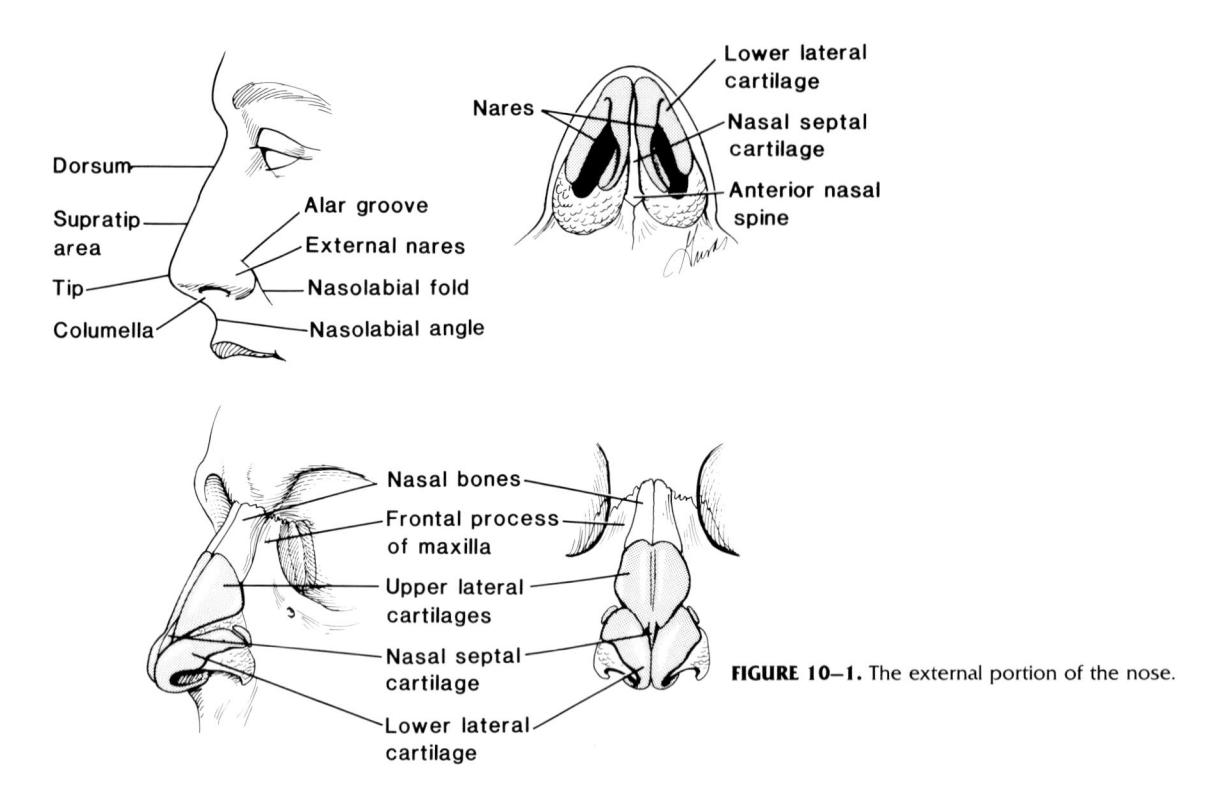

FIGURE 10–1. The external portion of the nose.

and skin complete the needed tissues of the external nose. The soft tissue division between the internal and external nose has as its inferior margin the pyriform crest with its skin cover, the nasal septum medially, and, as its superior and lateral delineation, the lower margin of the upper lateral cartilage. This narrowest structure of the entire upper respiratory tract is referred to by the anatomist as the limen nasi or the os internum, and by the physiologist as the nasal valve of Mink. The designation "valve" is appropriate because it moves with, and helps regulate, respiration.

The nasal valve is the narrowest structure in the upper respiratory tract.

Internal Nose

This structure extends from the os internum anteriorly to the posterior choana, which divides the nasal cavity from the nasopharynx. The nasal septum, a bony midline structure, anatomically divides the organ into two noses. The internal lateral nasal walls are further structured by the turbinates and the irregular air spaces between them—the inferior, middle, and superior meati (Fig. 10–2). While the skeletal outlines appear to assure rigid diameters of the air spaces, the soft tissue coverings of the internal nose tend to vary greatly in thickness, altering the resistance, and, consequently, the pressures and flow volumes of the inspiratory and expiratory air currents. The varying diameters come about from strictly mucosal congestion and decongestion, from changes in the vascular swell bodies of the turbinates and upper septum, and from crusts and deposits or drainage of mucosal secretions.

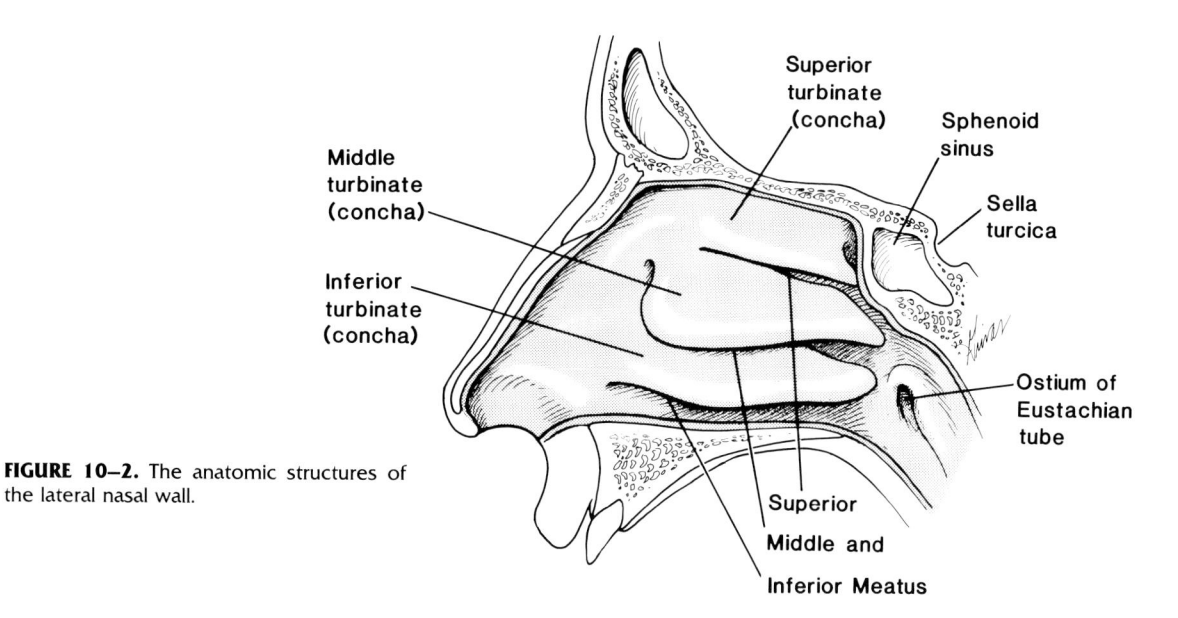

10—APPLIED ANATOMY AND PHYSIOLOGY OF THE NOSE

FIGURE 10–2. The anatomic structures of the lateral nasal wall.

The nasolacrimal duct empties into the inferior meatus anteriorly. The hiatus semilunaris of the middle meatus provides sinus ostia for the frontal, anterior ethmoid, and maxillary sinuses. The posterior ethmoid sinus cells drain into the superior meatus, and the sphenoid sinus drains into the sphenoethmoid recess (Fig. 10–3).

The frontal, maxillary, and anterior ethmoid sinuses open into the middle meatus.

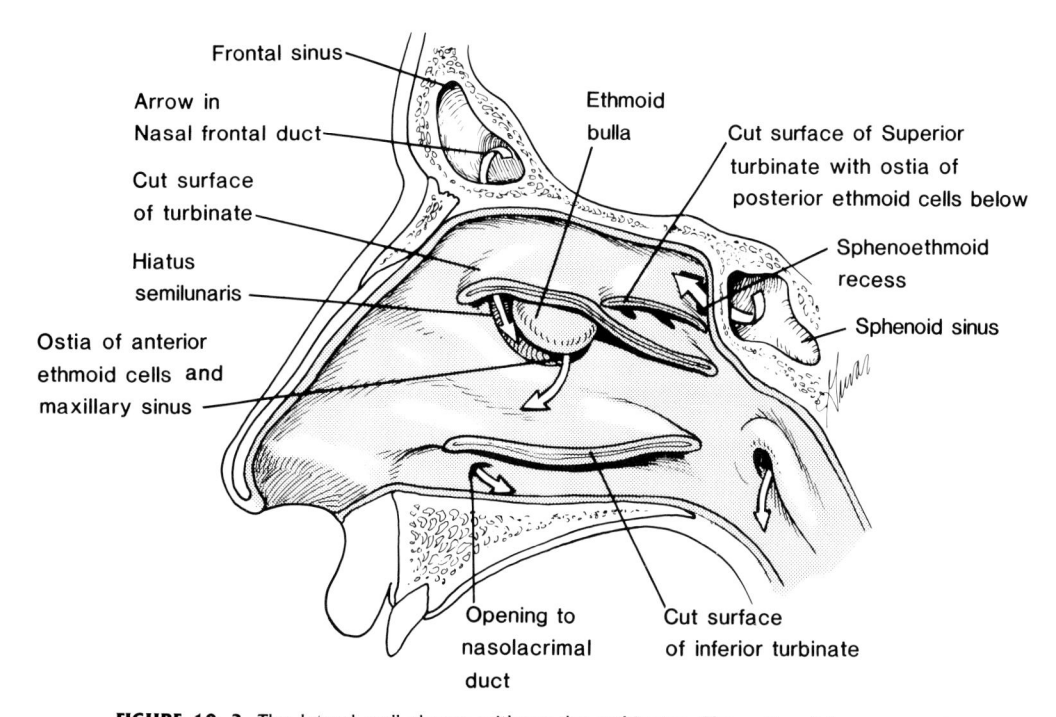

FIGURE 10–3. The lateral wall shown without the turbinates. The ostia of the paranasal sinuses as well as the nasolacrimal duct can be seen opening into the appropriate meatus.

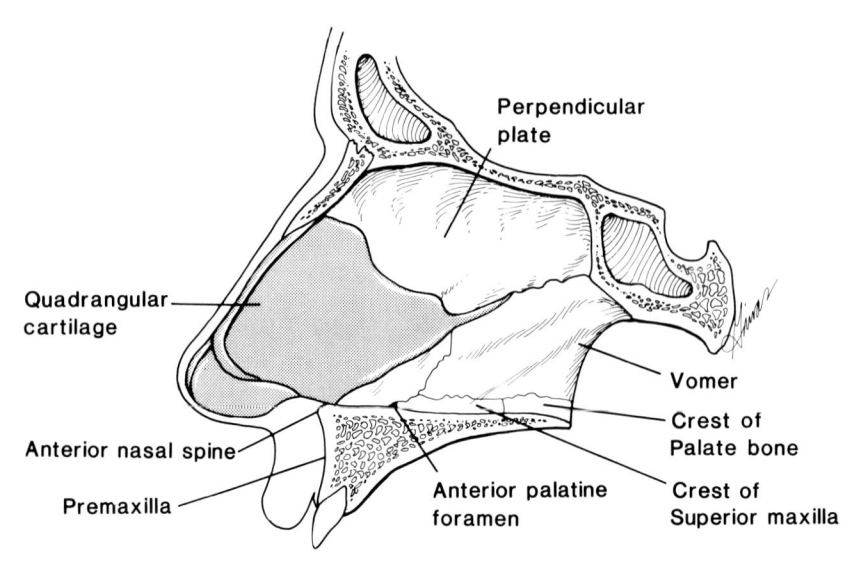

FIGURE 10–4. The nasal septum and adjacent structures.

The olfactory nerve endings occupy fairly small areas on the medial and lateral internal nasal wall, high up in the nasal vault. Structural deformities, as well as excessive mucosal thickening or edema, can prevent the inspired air streams from reaching the olfactory area and, thus, severely interfere with olfaction.

The skeletal portion of the septum is composed of the septal cartilage (quadrangular) anteriorly, the perpendicular plate of the ethmoid above, the vomer and rostrum of the sphenoid posteriorly, and a ridge below comprising the crest of the maxillas and the crest of the palatines (Fig. 10–4). Ridges and spurs, which sometimes require removal, occur not infrequently. Warping of the septum, which may be due to growth factors or trauma, may be so great that it interferes with the air flow and must be corrected surgically. The adjacent turbinates commonly compensate for irregularities in the septum (if they are not too great) by increasing in size on the concave side and decreasing on the other side in such a way as to maintain the optimum width of the air spaces. Thus, even though the septum is warped, air flow may be even and normal. Areas of erectile tissue on both sides of the septum serve to adjust its thickness under varying atmospheric conditions.

Minor septal deformities rarely alter nasal air flow because of turbinate compensation.

Paranasal Sinuses

Human beings have about 12 cavities along the roof and lateral aspects of the nasal air space, varying in number, shape, size, and symmetry. These sinuses are hollows within the several facial bones and are accordingly named maxillary, sphenoid, frontal, and ethmoid sinuses (Figs. 10–3 and 10–5). The latter usually consist of interconnected small groups of anterior and posterior ethmoid cells, each group having an ostium draining into the nose. All of the sinuses are lined with a modified respiratory epithelium capable of producing mucus and, having cilia, of emptying secretions into the nasal cavities. In health, the sinuses are essentially air-filled.

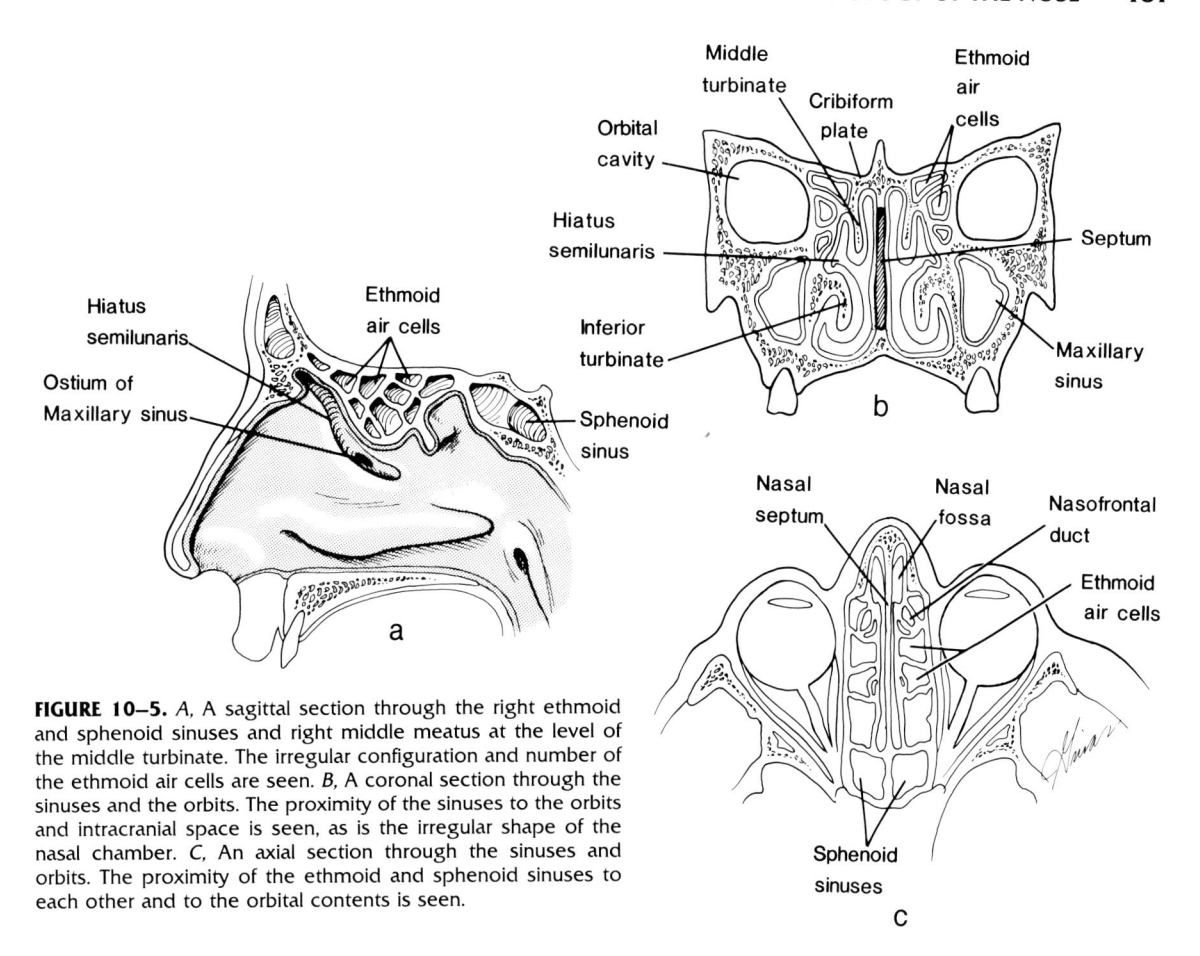

FIGURE 10–5. *A*, A sagittal section through the right ethmoid and sphenoid sinuses and right middle meatus at the level of the middle turbinate. The irregular configuration and number of the ethmoid air cells are seen. *B*, A coronal section through the sinuses and the orbits. The proximity of the sinuses to the orbits and intracranial space is seen, as is the irregular shape of the nasal chamber. *C*, An axial section through the sinuses and orbits. The proximity of the ethmoid and sphenoid sinuses to each other and to the orbital contents is seen.

A rudimentary maxillary sinus, or antrum, is most consistently present at birth. The other paranasal sinuses appear in early childhood within the facial bones. These bones outgrow the cranium while supporting it. As their firm centers are resorbed, nasal mucous membranes are drawn into the newly forming cavities.

The maxillary sinus is the only sinus routinely present at birth.

HISTOLOGY

The Respiratory Mucosa of the Nose

The usually ciliated, pseudostratified columnar epithelium of the respiratory apparatus varies considerably in different portions of the nose, depending on pressure and velocity of the air streams, their temperatures, and their predominant moisture content (Fig. 10–6). Thus, the anterior ends of the turbinates and the septal mucosa for a short way past the os internum are still lined by a stratified squamous epithelium without cilia—an extension of the skin of the nasal vestibule. Along the main path of the inspiratory currents the cells become columnar; the cilia are short and slightly irregular. Cells of the middle and inferior meatuses, handling most of the expiratory flow path, grow long and evenly spaced cilia. The sinuses contain cuboidal

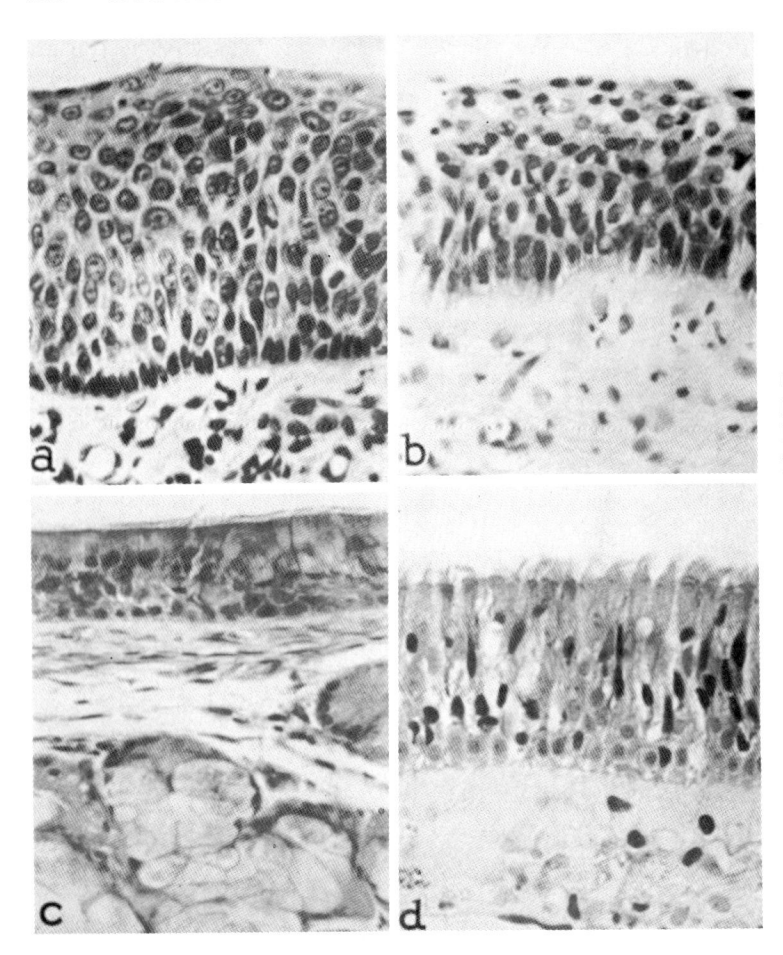

FIGURE 10–6. Photomicrographs of respiratory epithelium as related to the impact of respired air. *a*, Preturbinal area; *b*, anterior end of inferior turbinate; *c*, inferior meatus showing glands containing serous and mucous cells; *d*, middle third of inferior turbinate. Within the sinuses, the epithelium is of the cuboidal type.

epithelium and cilia uniform in length and spacing. The force of the air currents passing through the various localities also influences the thickness of the lamina propria and the number of glands in this mucosa. It is thin where there is a low or gentle air flow and thick where the air streams are strong. Secretion-producing glands and goblet cells, the sources of the mucous blanket, are found in proportion to the thickness of the lamina propria. The very viscous and sticky mucous blanket catches dust, inspirated foreign bodies, and bacteria and, through the action of the cilia, carries these substances to the pharynx, to be swallowed and destroyed in the stomach. Lysozyme and immunoglobulin A (IgA) are found in the mucous blanket and give further protection against pathogens. The mucous blanket in the nose is renewed about three to four times an hour. The cilia—tiny, hairlike structures—move in unison rapidly in the direction of the blanket's flow, then bend and recover much more slowly. Their stroke rate is 700 to 1000 cycles per minute.

Cilia

The cilia, about 5 to 7 microns in length, are located on the end plates of the surface cells in the epithelium and number about 100 per square micron, with about 250 per cell in the upper respiratory tract. The cilia seem to work almost automatically. For example, it is possible to tear a cell into small bits without stopping ciliary movement; a single cilium will continue to stroke as long as a tiny bit of cytoplasm containing its basal body remains attached to it. All of the cilia in an area of epithelium are coordinated in a marvelous manner. Each, as it strokes, moves metachronously with the surrounding cilia. As one observes them stroking, the ranks bow in unison and the files in sequence. Not only are the strokes of adjacent cilia coordinated as to time, but the directions of untold millions in a sinus are so coordinated as to be an important factor in carrying the mucus to the nasopharynx.

The structure of the cilia has been revealed by the transmission electron microscope (Fig. 10–7). They are built up of two single central microtubules surrounded by nine pairs of microtubules, all enclosed within the thin, fragile, trilaminar cell membrane. Each cilium consists of a shaft, a tapered tip, and a basal body. Not all microtubules extend completely to the tip. The two central single microtubules do not extend below the level of the cell surface. However, just below the level of the cell surface, each pair of peripheral microtubules is joined by a third microtubule in the basal body, a structure found in the apical cytoplasm. These triplets then continue to descend further in the apical cytoplasm as rootlets, gradually tapering off.

In stroking, the individual cilia do not merely move back and forth like wheat stalks in a grain field. Each stroke has a powerful, rapid phase in the direction of flow with the cilium straight and stiff, followed by a slower phase of recovery during which the cilium bends. The time relationship between the effective phase and the phase of recovery has been worked out experimentally on the rat. The ratio is 1:3; i.e., the effective phase takes one third the time of the phase of recovery. The stroke is not unlike the arm stroke of a swimmer.

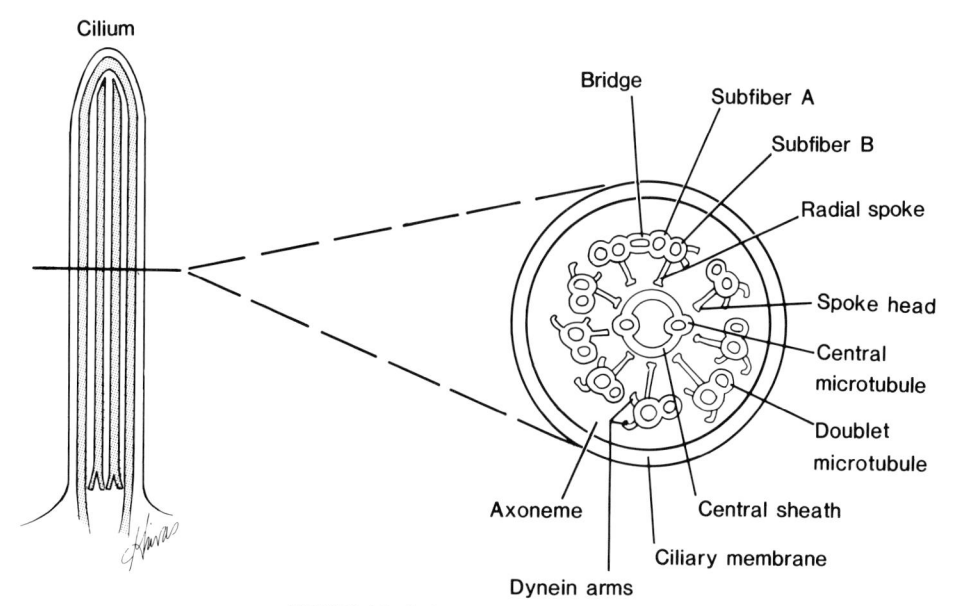

FIGURE 10–7. Anatomic detail of a cilium.

Olfactory Area

Great interpersonal variations characterize the structure of the olfactory region; these differences may be in the thickness of the mucosa (it is usually about 60 microns thick), in the size of the cells, and in the olfactory vesicles. The border between the respiratory and olfactory regions is generally very sharply defined but irregular. In man the olfactory pseudostratified columnar epithelium is composed of three cell types: (1) olfactory bipolar nerve cells; (2) sustentacular, supporting cells, which are the most numerous; and (3) a few, small basal cells, which are probably stem cells for the sustentacular cells (Fig. 10-8).

Each olfactory cell is a bipolar neuron. In the epithelium they are evenly distributed among the supporting cells. These olfactory sense cells constitute the only portion of the central nervous system that reaches the surface of the body. The distal end of such a cell is a modified dendrite that protrudes above the surface of the epithelium, forming the so-called olfactory vesicle. On the surface of this vesicle are 10 to 15 nonmotile cilia. The proximal end of each cell tapers to a thin process about 0.1 micron in diameter, which is the axon. This axon joins with other similar axons to form the olfactory nerves, which pass through the cribriform plate into the olfactory bulb, where they form synapses with the dendrites of a second set of neurons. The axons of this second set of neurons form the olfactory tract, which passes to the brain to connect with numerous nuclei, fasciculi, and other tracts. The central olfactory apparatus is highly complex.

The supporting sustentacular cells probably do more than just support; it is postulated that the sustentacular cells provide lateral support and also represent a means of intraepithelial ionic communication via their junctional complexes with the olfactory bipolar neurons. They are supplied at the

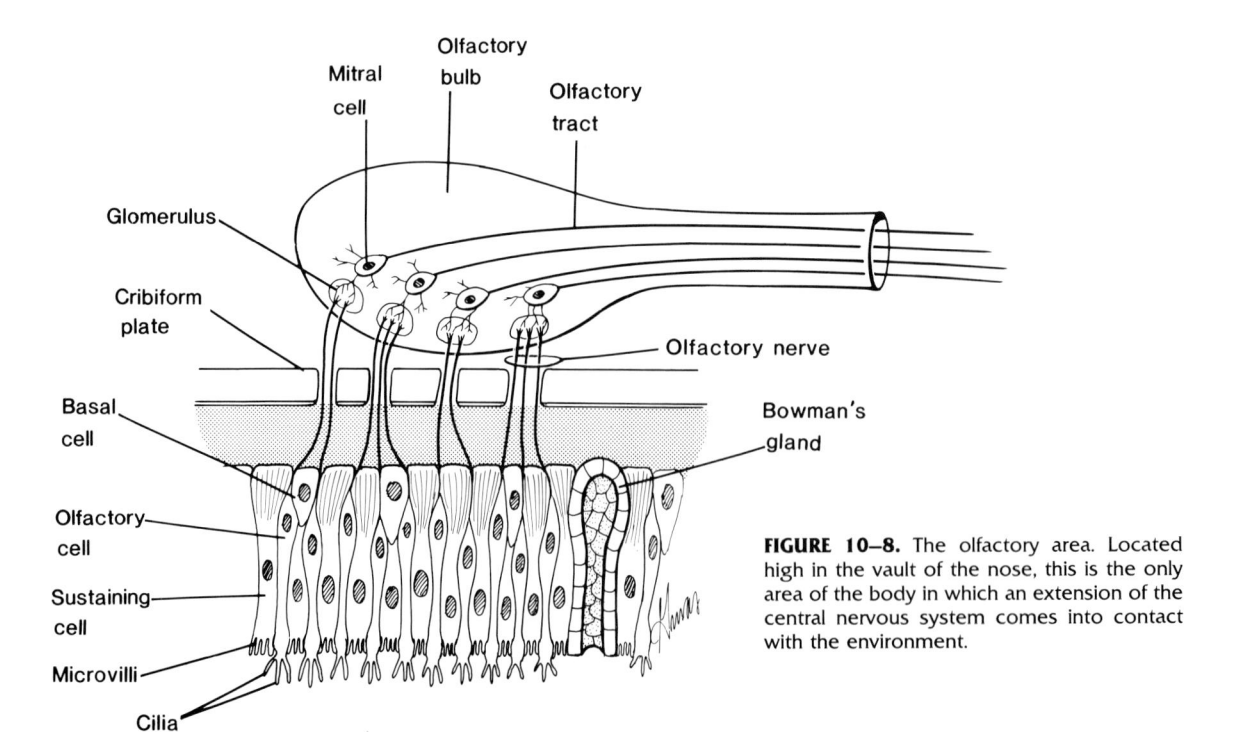

> The olfactory bipolar neurons represent the only portion of the central nervous system that reaches the body's surface.

FIGURE 10-8. The olfactory area. Located high in the vault of the nose, this is the only area of the body in which an extension of the central nervous system comes into contact with the environment.

surface with numerous microvilli—up to a thousand on a cell—which form a thick brush border. These cells have no motile cilia. The microvilli are tiny outpouchings of the cell membrane, like the fingers on a rubber glove, and are not at all like the usual respiratory cilia (see Fig. 10–7). These microvilli increase the surface area enormously, but their function is not yet well understood.

A great number of glands (glands of Bowman) lie in the lamina propria in the olfactory region. Opening onto the surface through rather wide ducts, their cells are cuboidal or low cylindrical.

Blood Supply

The sphenopalatine branch of the internal maxillary artery supplies the conchae, meatus, and septum. The anterior and posterior ethmoidal branches of the ophthalmic artery supply the ethmoidal and frontal sinuses and the roof of the nose (Figs. 10–9 and 10–10). A branch of the superior labial artery and the infraorbital and alveolar branches of the internal maxillary artery supply the maxillary sinus, and the pharyngeal branch of the same artery is distributed to the sphenoid. The veins form a close cavernous plexus under the mucous membrane. This plexus is especially well marked over the middle and inferior conchae and the lower portion of the septum, where it forms the erectile tissue. Venous drainage is accomplished principally through the ophthalmic, anterior facial, and sphenopalatine veins.

The superior portions of the nasal cavity are nourished by the ethmoid arteries, while the posterior and inferior portions are supplied by the maxillary artery.

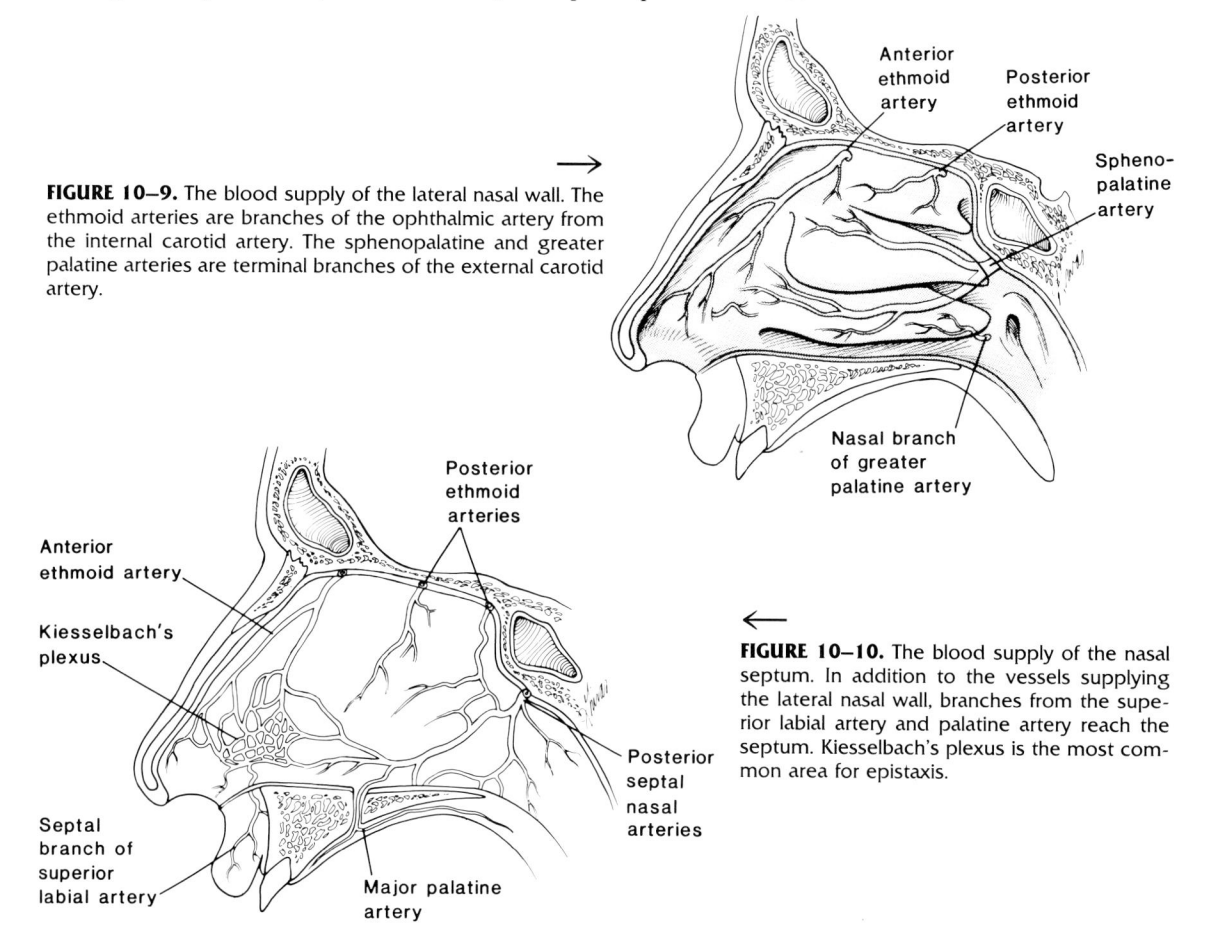

FIGURE 10–9. The blood supply of the lateral nasal wall. The ethmoid arteries are branches of the ophthalmic artery from the internal carotid artery. The sphenopalatine and greater palatine arteries are terminal branches of the external carotid artery.

FIGURE 10–10. The blood supply of the nasal septum. In addition to the vessels supplying the lateral nasal wall, branches from the superior labial artery and palatine artery reach the septum. Kiesselbach's plexus is the most common area for epistaxis.

Lymphatic System

The nose has a rich supply of lymphatics occurring in an anterior and a posterior network. The anterior network of lymphatics is small and drains along the facial vessels to the neck. They serve the most anterior portion of the nose—the vestibule and the preturbinal area.

The posterior network serves the majority of the nasal anatomy, joining three main channels in the posterior area of the nose—the superior, middle, and inferior channels. The superior group, from the middle and superior turbinates and that portion of the nasal wall, pass above the eustachian tube and empty into the retropharyngeal lymph nodes. The middle group, passing below the eustachian tube, drain the inferior turbinate, inferior meatus, and a portion of the floor and go to the jugular chain of lymph nodes. The inferior group, from the septum and part of the floor of the nose, pass through the lymph nodes along the internal jugular vessels (Fig. 10–11).

Nerve Supply

Directly involved are the first cranial nerve for olfaction, the ophthalmic and maxillary divisions of the trigeminal nerve for all other sensory afferent impulses, the facial nerve for movement of the respiratory muscles of the external nose, and the autonomic nervous system. This last is mainly by way of the sphenopalatine ganglion, to control the diameters of veins and arteries in the nose as well as mucous production, thus modifying air flow conductance, temperature, and moisture regulation of the air streams (Fig. 10–12).

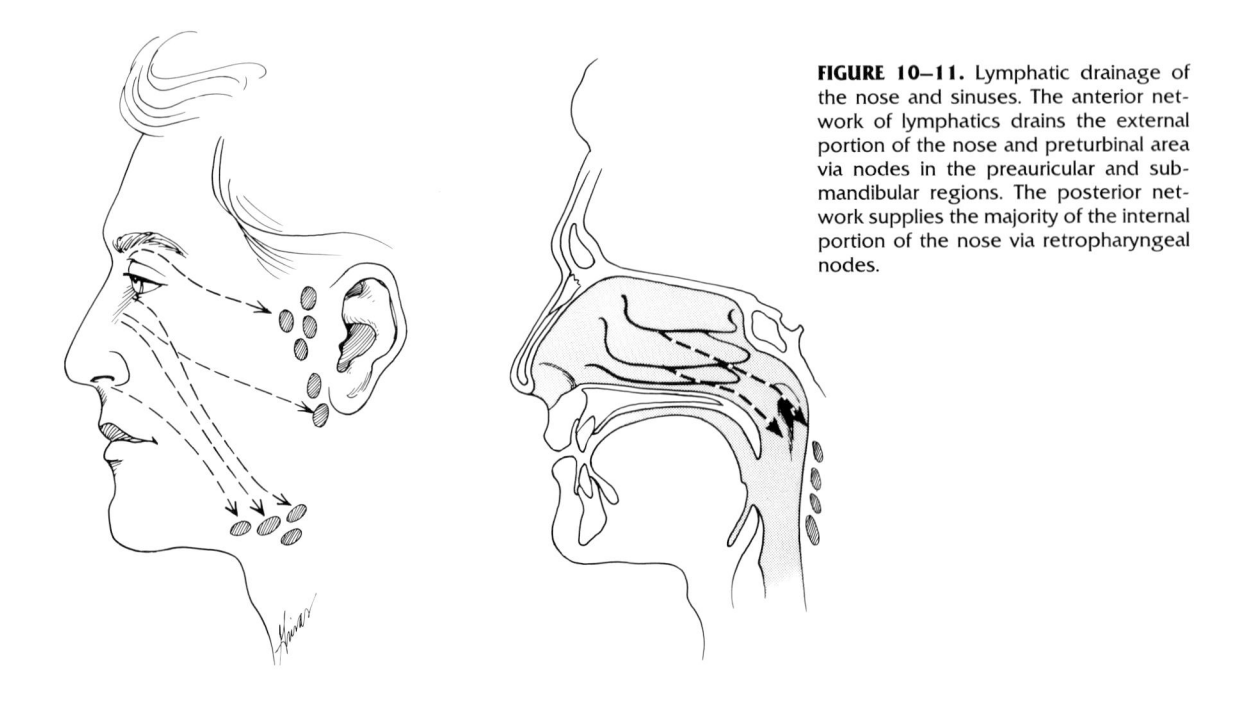

FIGURE 10–11. Lymphatic drainage of the nose and sinuses. The anterior network of lymphatics drains the external portion of the nose and preturbinal area via nodes in the preauricular and submandibular regions. The posterior network supplies the majority of the internal portion of the nose via retropharyngeal nodes.

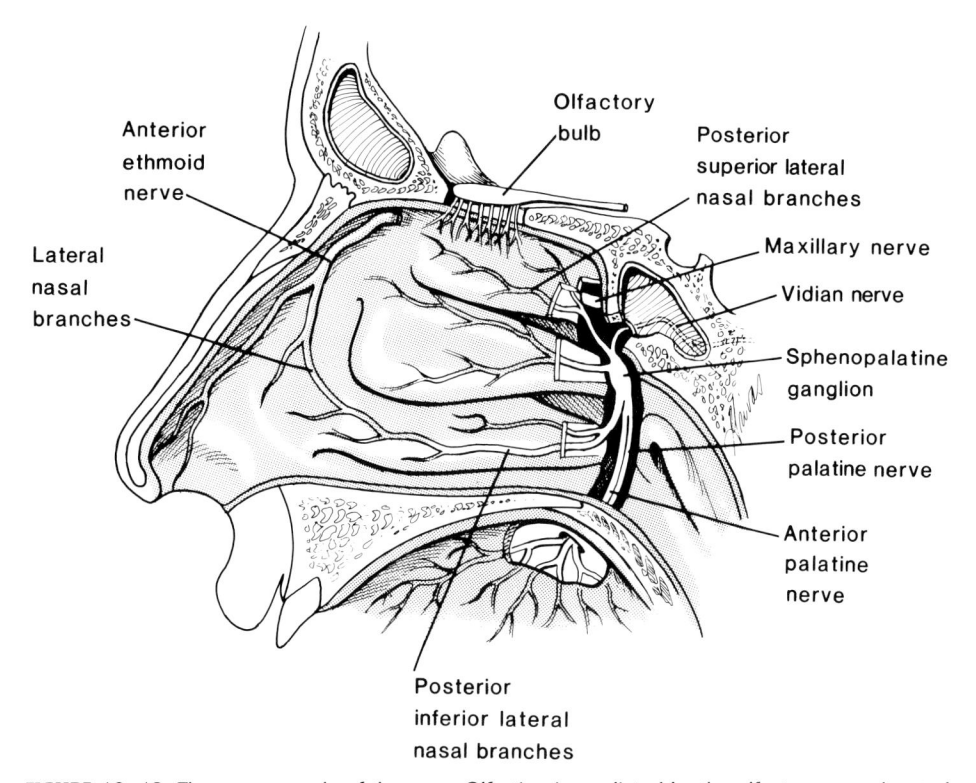

FIGURE 10–12. The nerve supply of the nose. Olfaction is mediated by the olfactory nerve located high in the nasal vault. Autonomic control of nasal physiology is mediated primarily by sympathetic and parasympathetic fibers that reach the nose by way of the sphenopalatine ganglion. Sensation is from the ethmoid branches of the ophthalmic division of the fifth cranial nerve and the maxillary division of the fifth nerve.

PHYSIOLOGY

Olfaction

Just as nasal anatomy makes inspection of the olfactory cleft with a nasal speculum usually not possible, for the same reason inspiratory air flow curves normally do not reach high enough into the cleft to allow us to detect an odor, unless it is very strong. If we are to be successful at identifying a given odor, we usually have to sniff, that is, create additional negative pressure to pull the entering air currents up into the olfactory area. With pathologic nasal airway obstruction a patient will often complain of anosmia before mentioning that he has become a mouth breather. Moreover, since we characterize different foods by a combination of taste and smell, the patient's presenting complaint may be that food does not "taste right" anymore.

A decrease in the sense of smell is often perceived as a decrease in taste.

Man's sense of smell is rudimentary compared to other members of the animal kingdom, yet the sensitivity of this organ is truly startling. McKenzie states that vanillin is perceptible by us as a smell when it is present in concentrations as low as 5×10^{-10} gm/L of air. The process by which odors are perceived has not been determined with certainty, but there are two theories that suggest chemical or undulation mechanisms. According to the chemical theory, particles of odorous substances are distributed by diffusion throughout the air and cause a chemical reaction when they reach the olfactory epithelium. According to the undulation theory, waves of energy similar to light impinge upon the olfactory nerve endings. Regardless of mechanism, the olfactory sense is quickly exhausted.

It is still very difficult to standardize in a laboratory test descriptions of different characteristics of various odors or measurements of comparative odor concentrations. Amoore identified seven main categories of odors, adequate to encompass and describe all the varieties perceived. Although many investigators agree with his theory, his system is still not accepted in routine clinical practice or as the basis for determining disability ratings. Instead, for the most part, investigators try to distinguish between anosmia, hyposmia, normal olfaction, and parosmia (perverted olfaction) by offering an odoriferous substance, such as oil of clove, in various air dilutions to the test subject.

The sinuses have no obvious physiologic function. Negus is of the opinion that they serve the sense of smell by accommodating extension from the ethmoturbinals, especially in the frontal and sphenoid sinuses. Ethmoturbinals covered with olfactory epithelium occur in some of the lower animals. In man, the sinuses are empty and our sense of smell is far inferior to that of, for instance, the dog or cat; man's ethmoturbinals have apparently disappeared during the process of evolution.

Airway Resistance

The human breath begins at the rim of the nostril. The act of breathing conveys air through the upper and lower respiratory tract to the alveoli of the lung in sufficient volume, with sufficient pressure, moisture, warmth, and cleanliness, to assure optimal conditions for oxygen uptake, and in the reverse process optimal elimination of carbon dioxide brought to the alveoli by the blood stream (Fig. 10–13). The nose, with its many inspiratory and

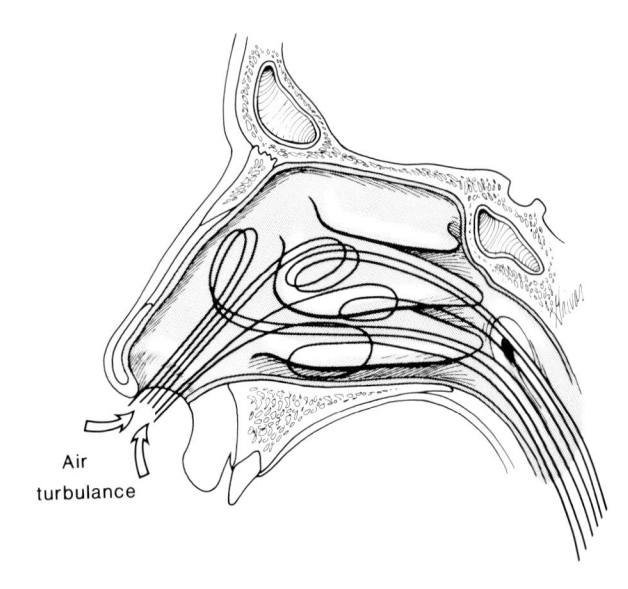

FIGURE 10–13. The pattern of airflow through the nose. The majority of the air stream arcs through the nose near the middle turbinate rather than along the floor of the nose. Turbulent flow enhances the physiologic functions of filtration, humidification, and warming of air as well as regulation of airway resistance.

expiratory baffles and the valvelike action of the erectile tissues in the turbinates and septum, smoothes and shapes the air streams, regulates volumes of passing air and pressure, and conducts most of the air-conditioning activities (air filtration, control of temperature and humidity).

Variations in nasal resistance are due primarily to changes in the erectile tissues of the turbinates.

Changes in air pressure which take place inside the nose during the respiratory cycle have been measured using rhinomanometry. During quiet respiration air pressure changes inside the nose are minimal and normally are not greater than 10 to 15 mm H_2O, with an air flow rate varying between 0 and 140 ml/min. At inspiration a drop in pressure occurs; air flows out of the sinuses. During expiration there is a small increase in pressure; air flows into the sinuses. Sinus air exchange is very minor on the whole, except during the act of sniffing, the mechanism whereby air delivery to the olfactory membranes lining the sinuses is increased.

A wide range in nasal airway resistance has been noted in normal individuals. More than 50 per cent of the total respiratory resistance during normal respiration is due to the total nasal resistance. In striking contrast, only 20 per cent of total respiratory resistance is accounted for by the oral passage during mouth breathing. In the majority of individuals there is a change from nasal to oronasal breathing during exercise with its increased air requirements. A wide variation normally exists, however, as to when this transition occurs. Although oral breathing is demonstrably easier, individuals will usually resort to it as their normal style of breathing only in the case of uncompensated nasal stenosis or when poor pulmonary function cannot overcome normal nasal resistance. With complete nasal obstruction and its resultant necessary transoral respiration, an increase in PCO_2 has been noted by some investigators. This preference for nasal breathing is requisite during the first six months of human life and continues to provide protection against airborne hazards throughout life.

The nose provides more than 50 per cent of normal respiratory resistance.

Several areas of the nose where the air passage narrows can be likened to "valves." In the vestibular segment of the nose there are two such narrowings. The more anterior narrowing is found between the posterior aspect of the upper lateral cartilage and the nasal septum. Any deviations of the nasal septum in this area often cause an increased narrowing with its resultant symptomatic airway obstruction. Such deviations can result from trauma or growth irregularities. The second narrowing is found at the bony piriform aperture. These two areas can be considered highly significant clinically in the greater preponderance of intranasal surgical corrections.

A normally occurring alternation in nasal resistance between the right and left nasal passages has been demonstrated through the use of rhinomanometry. Respiration volumes in the two passages are altered through alternating congestion and decongestion of the erectile tissue covering the nasal turbinates on opposite sides of the septum. Cycles in normal individuals have been found to vary from 1 hour to 6 hours in length, with an average cycle length of 2½ hours. These fluctuations are not normally noted by most individuals, since total nasal resistance tends to remain at a constant level.

An alternating cyclic variation in airway resistance exists between the right and left nasal passages.

Air Conditioning

During the brief time that air traverses the horizontal portion of the nasal passage, 16 to 20 times a minute in normal respiration, the inspired air is warmed (or cooled) to near body temperature and its relative humidity is brought to near 100 per cent.

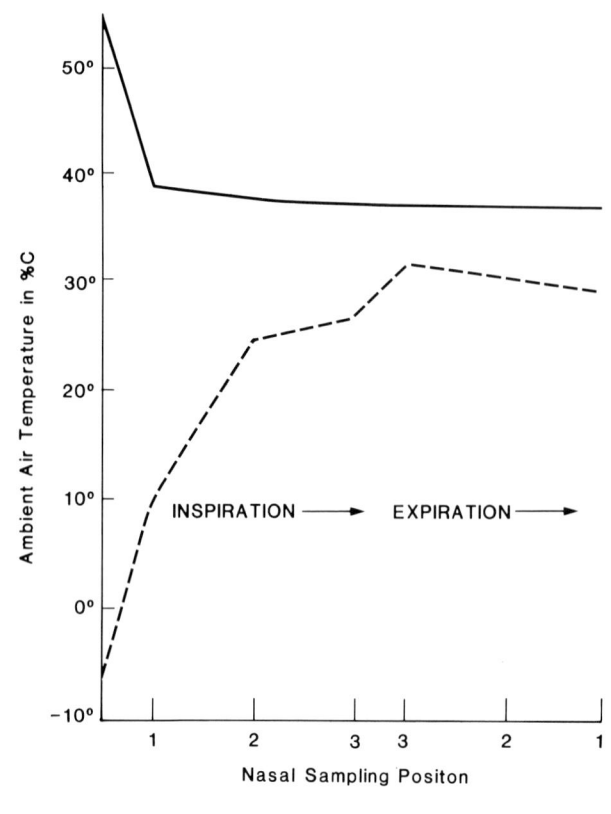

FIGURE 10–14. Nasal temperature regulation. Despite extremes of environmental temperature, as air passes deeper into the nose (from sampling position 1 to position 3) the temperature is adjusted to near body temperature.

Extremes of temperature and dryness of inspired air are compensated for by modification of the air flow (Fig. 10–14). This is carried out by physical changes in the erectile tissues of the nose.

Air Purification

The hairs, or vibrissae, of the skin-lined nasal vestibule play a role in air filtration. More prominent in males, it is not understood what role this sex differentiation plays in air filtration needs.

The irregular internal anatomy of the nasal passages causes eddies in the

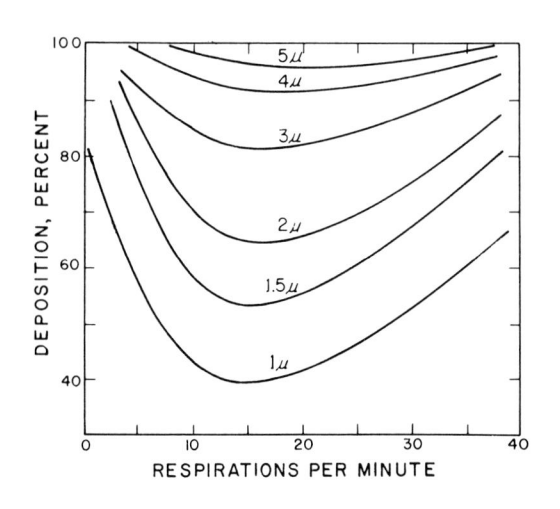

FIGURE 10–15. Variations of total respiratory deposition in relation to breathing frequency for different size particles. (Redrawn from Dennis, 1961; reproduced, with permission, from Scientific Foundations of Otolaryngology editors, London. Hilding A.C.: Nasal filtration. In Harrison, Donald, and Hinchcliffe, Ronald, (Eds.): Scientific Foundations of Otolaryngology. London, Heinemann, 1976.)

FIGURE 10–16. Percentage of inhaled particles passing through (penetrating) the nasal chamber in relation to particle size (mean size), taken from a variety of particles. Airflow, 18 liters per minute. Experimental findings (solid line) are compared with theory (calculated findings). (Redrawn from Landahl, 1950; reproduced, with permission, from Scientific Foundations of Otolaryngology editors, London.)

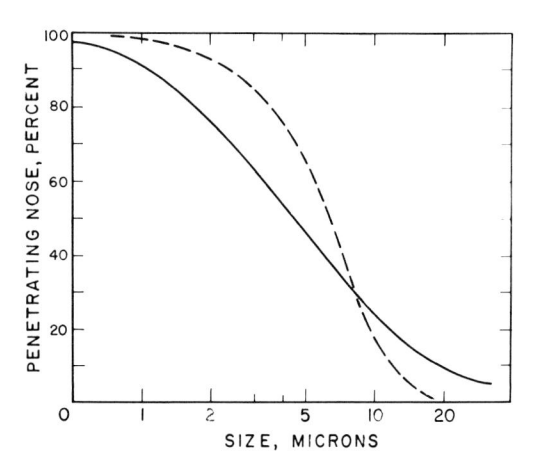

inspired air, resulting in a deposition of particulate matter in the nose and nasopharynx. This foreign material, including bacteria and viruses (which frequently coalesce into large particles), is either expectorated or carried by mucociliary transport to the stomach for sterilization by gastric secretions (Figs. 10–15 and 10–16).

Soluble gases are also removed from the air as it passes through the nose. The greater the water solubility of the gas, the more completely it is removed by the nasal mucosa. Pollutants such as hydrogen chloride, sulfur dioxide, and ammonia are all highly soluble and therefore well-cleansed from the inspired air. Conversely, carbon monoxide and hydrocarbons have a very low solubility and thus pass straight through to the lungs.

Mucociliary Function

The transport of foreign particles deposited from inspired air posteriorly to the pharynx, where they are either swallowed or expectorated, is carried out through action of cilia moving the mucous blanket with its entrapped particles (Fig. 10–17). Nasal airflow turbulence provides extensive exposure

FIGURE 10–17. Direction and relative rate of flow of nasal mucus.

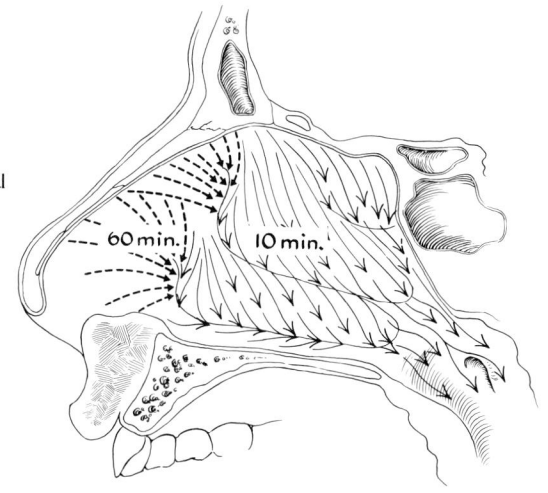

of inspired air to the nasal epithelium with its mucous blanket, a highly viscid, continuous sheet of secretion which extends into all of the spaces and angles of the nose, sinuses, eustachian tubes, pharynx, and the entire bronchial tree.

The upper layer of this exceedingly thin mucous blanket, which is rich in glycoproteins, is the more viscid, with a tensile strength that allows the cilia's stiff forward motion to keep the blanket moving posteriorly in a continuous stream. The lower, periciliary layer is more serous, providing little hindrance to the bending, ciliary recovery stroke. The mucous blanket is renewed by the submucosal glands two to three times an hour.

Just as the ciliary movement of the bronchopulmonary lining propels the mucous blanket toward the pharynx, so, too, do the cilia of the nose and ears. A considerable negative pressure is created by the pulling action of the cilia on the mucous blanket when any of these chambers is blocked by a mucous plug. This may result in intense sinus pain as the plug clears the ostium and, as the mucous plug moves down the auditory canal, may cause atelectasis of the tympanic membrane.

Effective ciliary action has been shown to be compromised by extreme drying of the air, as often occurs in many homes during the winter heating months. It is also important to maintain the normally occurring neutral pH of 7. Air pollution interferes with ciliary effectiveness in various ways. Nitrogen dioxide and sulfur dioxide, frequent components of smog, compromise nasal health. Positively charged particulate matter can neutralize the negative atmospheric ion count normally produced by solar irradiation. Ciliary movement has been shown to be reduced and even to stop as the ion count becomes more positive. As a result, although the patient may present with a complaint of "sinusitis," the real cause is impaired ciliary physiology.

Nasal mucus, in addition to its role in transporting particulate matter deposited from inspired air, also transfers heat, normally warms inspired and cools expired air, and humidifies the inspired air with more than a liter of moisture each day. However, even this amount of moisture is often not sufficient to humidify the highly desiccated air frequently encountered in heated homes during northern winters. This may result in mucosal drying with its many accompanying nasal problems. The degree of moisture in the mucous blanket is determined by neural stimulation of the seromucous submucosal glands in the nasal lining.

The anterior third of the nasal chamber changes in response to changes in the physical properties of the inspired air. With a great deviation from the norm the respiratory epithelium lining the anterior portion of the turbinates, particularly the inferior turbinate, becomes transitional or squamous and no cilia are observed. The mucous blanket in this region becomes more viscid and movement is achieved only through the pulling transmitted along the mucous blanket from still-ciliated areas located posteriorly. If there is a high content of particles in the inspired air, as occurs in certain occupations, crusting is observed around the vibrissae and the anterior turbinal ends.

The direction of mucous streaming in the nose is generally backward. Since the cilia are more active in the protected inferior and middle meatus, they tend to drag the mucous blanket from the common meatus into these recesses. The direction of flow on the septum is back and somewhat downward toward the floor. On the floor, the direction is back, with a tendency to flow under the inferior turbinate into the inferior meatus. On the medial aspect of the turbinates, the flow is back and downward, passing under the inferior margin into the corresponding meatus. The drainage from the nonciliated areas in the anterior third of the nose is practically all through the meatus. This is the area that collects most of the airborne contaminants.

The direction of the flow in the sinuses is spiral, beginning, in humans, at a point remote from the ostium. The rate increases progressively as the ostium is approached, and in the ostium the mucous blanket passes out in the form of a whirling tube at a rate of 15 to 20 mm/min.

The rate of mucous flow determined by ciliary action varies in different portions of the nose; that of the anterior nasal segment may be only one sixth that of the posterior, which is 1 to 20 mm/min. Mucociliary deficiencies, either inherent or acquired, have been demonstrated to relate to significant disease states.

The mucous blanket, in addition to trapping and removing inert particulate matter, also presents a barrier to allergens, viruses, and bacteria. Although viable organisms are readily cultured from the anterior nasal segment, it is difficult to obtain a positive postnasal culture. Lysozyme, present in the mucous blanket, is destructive to the walls of some bacteria. Active phagocytosis in the nasal membrane provides subsurface protection. The respiratory cell membrane also provides cellular-induced immunity.

Quantities of immunoglobulins are produced in the nasal mucosa, perhaps in part by plasma cells normally found in the tissue. According to physiologic need, IgG, IgA, and IgE have been observed. Allergic rhinitis occurs when an inhaled allergen comes into contact with the IgE antibodies to that antigen which are fixed to nasal mucosal and submucosal mast cells, generating and releasing inflammatory mediators that produce characteristic nasal mucosal changes.

Pulmonary Correlations

Normal pulmonary physiology is dependent upon nasal breathing. Bronchial tone is dependent upon nasopulmonary reflexes that also cause changes in total pulmonary resistance and perfusion. Studies have reported instances in which serious cardiorespiratory problems, ranging from moderate cardiomegaly and right ventricular hypertrophy to severe right cardiac failure and pulmonary edema, were caused by partial obstruction of the upper respiratory tract. These changes were reversed after the airway was cleared. However, these observations were made mainly in black children with enlarged adenoids and were attributed to hypoxia and hypercapnia causing a pulmonary vasoconstriction and elevated pulmonary arterial pressure. It is therefore assumed that an individual susceptibility must be prerequisite for these pathologies, since observation of these changes is very rare when compared with the frequency of nasopharyngeal obstruction in children in general.

Pulmonary physiology is influenced by the health of the nose.

Research has demonstrated a reflex transmitted from the nasal mucosa to the homolateral lung. A decreased cardiac output and increased peripheral vascular resistance have also been related to nasal membrane stimulation. The peripheral vascular resistance, however, has not altered carotid flow. This is a similar finding to that described in the "diving reflex," which selectively preserves cerebral blood flow.

SPEECH MODIFICATION

As discussed elsewhere, speech production is a complex process involving the lungs acting as a power source, the larynx acting as a sound generator, and structures in the head and neck, such as lips, tongue, teeth, etc., acting as articulators to change the basic laryngeal sounds into understandable speech. The nose and sinuses as well as the nasopharynx have a role in articulation. In certain sounds such as "m," "n," and "ing," nasal resonation is important.

In general, speech that is abnormal due to alteration in the nasal spaces can be considered hypernasal or hyponasal. Hypernasality results when velopharyngeal insufficiency allows too many sounds to resonate in the nasal spaces. Patients with unrepaired soft palate clefts typically demonstrate this abnormal speech. Hyponasality results when sounds that normally resonate in the nasal spaces are prevented from doing so. Nasal obstruction causing this abnormality may be due to such diverse causes as an upper respiratory infection, adenoid hypertrophy, or nasal tumors.

References

Abramson M, Harker LA: Physiology of the nose. Otolaryngol Clin North Am 6:623–635, 1973.

Acheson ED, Cowdell RH, Hadfield, E, Macbeth RD: Nasal cancer in woodworkers in the furniture industry. Br Med J 2:587–596, 1968.

Aschan G, Drettner B, Ronge H: A new technique for measuring nasal resistance to breathing. Illustrated by the effects of histamine and physical effort. Ann Acad Reg Sci Upsal 2:111, 1958.

Bates JH, Potts WE, Lewis M: Epidemiology of primary tuberculosis in an industrial school. N Engl J Med 272:714–717, 1965.

Bawden H: A bibliography of the literature on the organ and sense of smell. J Comp Neurol 11:1, 1901.

Dalhamn T: Studies on the effect of sulfur dioxide on ciliary activity in rabbit trachea in vivo and in vitro and on the resorptional capacity of the nasal cavity. Am Rev Respir Dis 83:566–567, 1961.

Dalhamn T, Sjoholm J: Studies on SO_2, NO_2, and NH_3. Effect on ciliary activity in rabbit trachea of single in vitro exposure and resorption in rabbit nasal cavity. Acta Physiol Scand 58P:287–291, 1963.

Drettner B: Vascular reactions of the human nasal mucosa on exposure to cold. Acta Otolaryngol, Suppl 166, 1961, 105 pp (Rhinometry, pp 26–35).

Frank NR, Yoder RE, Brain JD, Yokoyama E: SO_2 (^{35}S-labeled) absorption by the nose and mouth under conditions of varying concentration and flow. Arch Environ Health 18:315–322, 1969.

Fry FA, Black A: Regional deposition and clearance of particles in the human nose. J Aerosol Sci 4:113, 1973.

Hatch TF, Gross P: Pulmonary Deposition and Retention of Inhaled Aerosols. New York, Academic Press, 1964.

Hilding AC: The common cold. Arch Otolaryngol 12:133, 1930.

Hilding AC: Summary of some known facts concerning the common cold. Ann Otol Rhinol Laryngol 53:444, 1944.

Hilding AC: Nasal filtration. *In* Harrison D, Hinchcliffe R (eds): Scientific Foundations of Otolaryngology. London, Heinemann, 1976.

Hilding AC, Filipi AN, Elstrom JH: Filtration of cigarette smoke by the nose in rabbits: Effect of depth of anesthesia and death. Arch Environ Health 15:584–588, 1967.

Hoepke H, Maurer H: Z Anat Entwicklungsgesch 108:768, 1938.

Hughes EC, Johnson RL: Circadian and interpersonal variability of IgA in nasal secretions. Ann Otol Rhinol Laryngol 82:216–222, 1973.

Ironside F, Matthews J: Adenocarcinoma of the nose and paranasal sinuses in woodworkers in the state of Victoria, Australia. Cancer 36:1115–1121, 1975.

Landahl HD: On the removal of airborne droplets by the human respiratory tract. II. The nasal passages. Bull Math Biophys 12:161–169, 1950.

Landahl HD, Herrmann RG: Retention of vapours and gases in the human nose and lung. Arch Indust Hyg 1:36–45, 1950.
Lehmann G: The dust filtering efficiency of the human nose and its significance in the causation of silicosis. J Indust Hyg 17:37–40, 1935.
Maurer H: Z Anat Entwicklungsgesch 105:359, 1936.
Maurer H: Z Anat Entwicklungsgesch 107:203, 1937.
McKenzie D: Aromatics and the Soul. New York, Hoeber, 1923, p 39.
Morrow PE: Some physical and physiological factors controlling the fate of inhaled substances. I. Deposition. Health Phys 2:366–378, 1960.
Negus VE: The function of the paranasal sinuses. Acta Otolaryngoal 44:408–426, 1954.
Negus VE: Biology of Respiration. London, E & S Livingston, Ltd, 1965.
Ogura JH, Nelson JR, Dammkoehler R, et al: Experimental observations of the relationships between upper airway obstruction and pulmonary function. Ann Otol Rhinol Laryngol 73:381–403, 1964.
Palm PE, McNerney JM, Hatch T: Respiratory dust retention in small animals: A comparison with man. Arch Indust Health 13:355–365, 1956.
Proctor DF, Wagner HN Jr: Clearance of particles from the human nose. Arch Environ Health 11:366–371, 1965.
Proctor DF: Physiology of the air passages. Clin Anesthesiol 1:13–27, 1965.
Proetz AW: Applied Physiology of the Nose. 2nd ed. St Louis, Annals Publishing Co, 1953.
Rasmussen AT: The Principal Nervous Pathways. New York, Macmillan Co, 1932, pp 48–50.
Ratcliffe HL, Palladino VS: Tuberculosis induced by droplet nuclei infection; initial homogeneous response of small mammals (rats, mice, guinea pigs, and hamsters) to human and to bovine bacilli, and rate and pattern of tubercle development. J Exp Med 97:61–68, 1953.
Speizer FE, Frank NR: The uptake and release of SO_2 by the human nose. Arch Environ Health 12:725–728, 1966.
Taylor M: The nasal vasomotor reaction. Otolaryngol Clin North Am 6:645–654, 1973.
Williams HL: The nose as form and function. Ann Otol Rhinol Laryngol 78:725–740, 1969.
Williams HL: The clinical physiology and pathology of the nasal airways and their adjoining air-filled cavities. Ann Otol Rhinol Laryngol 79:513–518, 1970.

11
ALLERGIC CONDITIONS IN OTOLARYNGOLOGY PATIENTS

by Malcolm N. Blumenthal, M.D.

Allergies are common conditions involving the nose and sinuses. They are defined as adverse immune reactions. Atopy is a type of allergy which is mediated by reagin-type antibodies. They include diseases such as seasonal rhinitis, allergic asthma, and eczema. Although the IgE system is the main immunoglobulin involved in the production of atopic conditions, other immune mechanisms may play a role in the allergic reactions.

CLASSIFICATION OF ALLERGIC REACTIONS

Allergic reactions have been classified into those involving immunoglobulin and those involving the cellular system (Coombs and Gell). This is an arbitrary classification, and these systems may act intra- and interdependently. The final clinical picture may involve nonimmunologic and immunologic mechanisms. In addition, several immune mechanisms may be involved in the final clinical picture.

Immunoglobulin-Mediated Reactions

Antibody Cell–Associated Reactions (Reagin, Cytophilic, Anaphylactic Antibodies). These reactions involve an antibody, usually IgE, attached by the Fc portion to a cell containing mediators, or their precursors (mast cell, basophil, eosinophil, macrophage). The Fab portion of these antibodies interacts with the specific allergen (ragweed, mite, egg). Consequently there is activation of several membrane-associated enzymes. Products of these enzymatic cleavages lead to the release of mediators (Table 11–1). These mediators cause immediate-type reactions, occurring within seconds to minutes, such as edema, as well as late-phase reactions, occurring several hours after the interaction. Late inflammatory reactions most likely result from the release of mediators from the mast cells as well as from eosinophils, macrophages, and platelets. Clinical examples are some cases of asthma, anaphylaxis, and urticaria as well as seasonal rhinitis (Atkins and Zweiman; Matthews; Plaut and Lichtenstein; Schwartz; Wasserman).

This process causes immediate-type reactions like allergic rhinitis.

Antigen Cell–Associated Reactions (Cytotoxic, Blocking and Stimulating Antibodies). These reactions involve an antibody, usually of the IgG and IgM variety, interacting with an antigen that is part of or associated with the cell wall. As a result these reactions, which are usually complement-dependent, can cause damage, stimulation, or blockade. Those involving damage to the cell are conditions such as Rh-positive and penicillin hemolytic anemia and autoimmune thrombocytopenia. Stimulation from this type of

TABLE 11–1. MEDIATORS OF ATOPIC REACTIONS (PARTIAL LIST)

Preformed
   Histamine
   Proteoglycans
     Heparin
     Chondroitin sulfate
   Proteases
    Tryptase
    Chymase
    Hageman factor "activator"
    Prekallikrein-activating elastase
   Neutrophil chemotactic factor (high molecular weight)
   Eosinophil chemotactic factor of anaphylaxis
   Arylsulfatase A and B
   Lymphocyte chemotactic factor
   Eosinophil chemotactic factor oligopeptide
   Inflammatory factor of anaphylaxis
   Superoxide dismutase
   Myeloperoxidase
Newly generated or secondary agents
   Arachidonic acid derivatives
    Leukotrienes C4, D4, and E4 (slow-reacting substance of anaphylaxis)
    Hydroperoxyeicosatetraenoic acid
    Hydroxyeicosatetraenoic acid
    Prostaglandins
    Thromboxanes
   Platelet-activating factor
   Adenosine
   Prostaglandin-generating factor of anaphylaxis

reaction may explain thyrotoxicosis. The blocking activity may be involved in myasthenia gravis, insulin-resistant diabetes, and bronchial asthma and rhinitis. The latter may be due to blocking antibodies directed against the beta receptor site, causing an imbalance between the beta and alpha receptors and resulting in a hyperreactive respiratory tract.

Antigen-Antibody Reactions and Cell-Independent Reactions (Arthus Reaction, Immune Complex). These involve interaction of the antigen and antibody independent of the cell, activating the complement and other amplifying systems, resulting in an adverse reaction. The antibody usually is of the IgG or IgM variety. Clinical examples of these reactions are serum sickness, post-streptococcal glomerulonephritis, and some types of hypersensitivity pneumonitis.

Cell-Mediated Reactions

Antigen interacting with T lymphocytes leads to the release of various mediators, resulting in the clinical picture. Antibodies may assist in the selection of the lymphocyte to interact. Clinical examples are contact dermatitis and some transplantation reactions.

CLINICAL APPROACH TO THE DIAGNOSIS OF ALLERGIC PROBLEMS OF THE NOSE AND SINUSES

The clinical evaluation of immunologically related diseases involves understanding the immune system as well as its interaction with the external environment. The clinical evaluation of allergies is complicated because of the many variables influencing the clinical picture. Both immunologic and nonimmunologic factors are involved. The following criteria should be satisfied before a diagnosis of allergy is made.

Clinical Picture Compatible with an Immunologic Reaction

The history and physical examination help to determine whether the clinical picture is compatible with known allergic reactions. Typical occurrences of hay fever, hives, angioedema, and asthma are easily recognized as allergic reactions. For the less common manifestations such as fever, fatigue, headaches, or dizziness, the diagnosis must be made with great care. In the latter cases, nonimmunologic factors possibly contributing to the symptoms must be carefully excluded.

Routine laboratory studies such as determination of the number of eosinophils and serum IgE levels may be useful adjuvants to suggest the diagnosis of an allergic problem. Eosinophils are associated with several types of immune as well as nonimmune reactions (Cohen and Ottesen; Weller). Interpreting eosinophils is difficult because of problems of definition and because eosinophils are influenced by exertion, certain drugs such as steroids and beta-adrenergic agents, time of day, and techniques of assay, as well as by their kinetics.

Eosinophil interpretation is difficult.

Immunologic and nonimmunologic reactions can result in eosinophilia in the blood, tissues, and secretions (Table 11–2). Therefore eosinophils are compatible with but not diagnostic of allergy.

Studies of the immunoglobulin levels in the blood will provide information about the presence or absence of immunologically mediated diseases. In general, increased levels are of little diagnostic value because they represent a nonspecific manifestation of a variety of chronic diseases. Elevations of IgE have been observed with many conditions, including some immunolog-

TABLE 11–2. CLINICAL EOSINOPHILIA (PARTIAL LIST)

Atopic conditions
  Allergic rhinitis (hay fever)
  Allergic asthma
  Eczema
Parasitic infections (helminthic disease)
Immunodeficiency diseases (Wiskott-Aldrich syndrome,
  hyper-IgE syndrome, graft-versus-host disease)
Bronchopulmonary aspergillosis
Drug reactions
Tropical pulmonary eosinophilia
Aspirin-sensitive asthma
Vasculitis (hypersensitivity angiitis, Churg-Strauss syndrome,
  hypersensitivity vasculitis)
Löffler fibroplastic endocarditis
Connective tissue diseases (dermatomyositis, rheumatoid arthritis,
  polyarteritis nodosa)
Eosinophilic gastroenteritis
Hypereosinophilic syndrome
Adrenal insufficiency
Neoplastic diseases (Hodgkin's disease, immunoblastic
  lymphadenopathy, eosinophilic leukemia)

TABLE 11–3. ELEVATED SERUM IGE LEVELS (PARTIAL LIST)

Atopic conditions
    Allergic asthma
    Allergic rhinitis
    Eczema
Infections
    Viruses (infectious mononucleosis)
    Parasitic infections (helminths)
Allergic bronchopulmonary aspergillosis
Immunodeficiency states
    Wiskott-Aldrich syndrome
    Nezelof syndrome
    Hyperimmunoglobulin syndrome (Hill Quie syndrome)
Neoplastic conditions
    Multiple myeloma
    Hodgkin's disease
Acute graft-versus-host disease

ically mediated conditions (Geha; Welliver). IgE levels are more often elevated than not with such atopic diseases as asthma, rhinitis, eczema, and allergic bronchopulmonary aspergillosis. In addition, elevated levels are also found with many other diseases (Table 11–3). There are a large number of commercial immunoassays for total serum IgE levels that use a variety of assay techniques. Elevated IgE levels, like eosinophils, are compatible with but not diagnostic of allergic reactions.

IgE elevation is compatible with but not diagnostic of allergy.

Many other laboratory procedures such as complement studies and radiography are available to provide information that the disease process is compatible with an immunologically mediated disease. None of these tests are sufficient for the diagnosis. Therefore, the next step is to identify the allergen and determine how it is related to the symptom.

Identification of the Allergen and Its Relationship to the Clinical Picture

Historical information and provocative and elimination testing are the main methods used to satisfy this criterion. At the present time there are no in vitro studies available.

The patient's history is of the utmost importance in determining which factor or factors may precipitate or aggravate the allergic clinical picture. For respiratory allergies the time of year should be noted. Typically the trees pollinate earliest in the spring, followed by the grasses. Weeds pollinate in the fall. Molds such as *Cladosporium* may occur all through the year depending upon the climate. They are usually highest during the late summer. Mites, one of the major components of house dust, may be present all through the year but occur in greater numbers in the warmer, more humid months (Platts-Mills et al; Solomon and Mathews).

In addition to the history, provocation tests and elimination procedures may be helpful to demonstrate relationships between allergens and the clinical picture. The clinical significance of allergenic inhalants, contactants, and ingestants may be determined by placing them in direct contact with the involved organ. Inhalation or oral challenges are the common provocative tests performed. Elimination diets as well as avoidance of suspected aeroallergens or contactants are also useful to establish the triggering factor.

The patient's history, provocation tests, and elimination methods are valuable.

Demonstration of an Immune Mechanism Involving the Suspected Allergen

The third criterion to be satisfied is the demonstration of an immune mechanism that can interact with the suspected allergen. Proving a direct cause and effect is difficult. Demonstration that an antibody interacts with an allergen does not verify the cause of the disease. Despite this limitation, methods are available to provide evidence that an immune mechanism is involved and what the mechanism may be. These tests are done to confirm the presence of an immune mechanism, not to identify the causative agent.

In Vivo Methods. Many in vivo methods are used to study the immunoglobulin as well as the cellular system. Skin testing is the main in vivo method to identify IgE or reaginic antibody (Belin and Norman; Gleich et al). This reaction occurs within minutes after introduction of the allergen. It interacts with the reaginic antibodies attached to cells which release mediating substances. As a result, an immediate wheal/flare as well as a late-phase reaction may develop. Testing can be performed using a prick or scratch and an intradermal injection. Their exact relationship is not well defined. Intradermal testing is more sensitive but more likely to produce systemic reactions in highly sensitive individuals, is less clinically significant, is more time consuming to perform, and is more uncomfortable for the patient. Intradermal testing is used if prick or scratch tests are negative or questionable.

Skin testing is the most common way to demonstrate reaginic antibodies.

It should be realized that skin tests need to be interpreted in view of the clinical picture. There are no absolute cut-offs defining a positive or negative reaction.

In Vitro Methods

QUANTIFICATION OF SPECIFIC IgE. After the IgE was characterized in 1968 it was possible to raise antisera against this immunoglobulin class. This opened up the area of performing immunoassays (Emanuel; Gleich et al). The most widely used version is the radioallergosorbent test (RAST), which employs allergen insolubilized on a cellulose paper disc (allergosorbent) that binds specific IgE (and other antibody classes) from serum during a first incubation. The immunoglobulin-bound solid phase is then washed, and I-125 isotope–labeled anti-IgE (fc) or enzyme-labeled anti-IgE (Fc) is incubated with the washed disc in a second incubation. After further washing the radioactivity bound to the IgE on the disc is counted, or, in the case of enzyme-labeled antibody, a substrate is incubated to produce a colored or fluorescent product. The radioactivity bound to the disc or the quantity of product generated by enzyme activity is related to the disc-bound IgE by a reference serum source from which unknown specimens are interpolated. It should be stressed that the scoring systems for all of these procedures have not been well related to the clinical picture. In general, a high value will include fewer nonallergic patients but will also exclude allergic subjects. A low score will include more allergic subjects as well as nonallergic individuals. All the results must be interpreted in relationship to the history. The advantages and disadvantages of this assay are summarized in Table 11–4.

The RAST method is the most popular way to quantify IgE.

The RAST results do not always correlate with clinical allergy.

During the past several years modifications of the original RAST have been marketed for the measurement of specific IgE in the human serum. The relative performance of these newer systems is still largely unevaluated.

TABLE 11–4. COMPARISON OF SKIN TESTS, HISTAMINE RELEASE, AND RAST

	SKIN	HISTAMINE	RAST
Least patient risk	3	1	1
Most quantitative	3	2	1
Least affected by drugs	3	2	1
Can be performed on most patients	3	1	1
Most sensitive	1	2	3
Rapid results	1	3	2
Largest number of allergens	1	3	2
Least expensive	1	3	2
Not influenced by IgG	1	2	3

Scale: 1 = high; 3 = low.

In principle, most of the assays are of similar design to the RAST. They differ mainly in the solid phase used to fix the allergen, the type of tracer attached to the anti-IgE detection protein, and the instrument required to read the final signal (Emanuel).

MEASUREMENT OF THE RELEASE OF MEDIATORS. IgE can be measured using assay systems of the release of mediating substances (Gleich et al). The most common is the histamine release assay. This method involves using peripheral leukocytes that contain basophils assumed to have attached IgE. Increasing amounts of test allergen are added to the cells, and the release of histamine is measured using a biologic, fluorometric, or immunoassay system. The amount of histamine released is expressed as a percentage of total histamine in the cells. These methods have been expensive and time-consuming. New methodology may allow this procedure to be more economical and easier to perform. The histamine release systems measure not only IgE antibody but possibly other reaginic antibodies as well as their ability to attach to cells and release mediating substances. Their other advantages and disadvantages are summarized in Table 11–4.

COMPARISON OF IN VIVO AND IN VITRO TESTING FOR REAGINIC ANTIBODIES. The clinical evaluation of immunologically mediated disease can be performed using in vivo and in vitro methods. One of the major problems with all these tests has been the variability of allergens from lot to lot and from supplier to supplier. Another has been the lack of reliable information on the relevant biologic potency of extracts. Better standardization procedures are resolving these problems (Blumenthal et al).

Generally a significant positive correlation is found between RAST tests, skin tests, histamine release assays, and histories. The skin test is the most sensitive assay at the present time for IgE-mediated reactions.

The skin test is the most sensitive method.

Indications for performing the RAST and the histamine release assay are (1) situations in which the patient cannot be skin tested such as the presence of dermatographism, dependence on medication that interferes with skin testing, extreme youth and age when skin testing is difficult to perform and interpret, and previous extreme sensitivity to the test allergen, (2) the need to confirm the significance of a positive skin test, and (3) a strong history of allergen sensitivity but a negative skin test.

At the present time, skin testing is the initial method used to confirm the presence of an IgE mechanism involving the suspected allergen. This is due to the lower cost and greater sensitivity of this method. If RAST or the histamine release assay is to be performed first, it is with the knowledge that these methods are less sensitive and more expensive and skin testing still may have to be done if the in vitro tests are negative.

ALLERGIC RHINITIS, NASAL POLYPS, AND SINUSITIS

Rhinitis, nasal polyps, and sinusitis have been noted to be associated with allergic mechanisms (Smith).

Allergic rhinitis occurs in 10 per cent of the population.

Incidence. Although the exact incidence of allergic rhinitis is not definitely known, approximately 10 per cent of the general population appears affected (Norman, 1985). Nasal polyps and sinusitis appear to be increased in subjects with allergic rhinitis. A triad of aspirin sensitivity, nasal polyps, and bronchial asthma has been described in 2 to 28 per cent of individuals with bronchial asthma (Giraldo et al; McDonald et al). These individuals will frequently have problems with other nonsteroidal anti-inflammatory agents such as indomethacin and ibuprofen.

Pathogenesis. Allergic rhinitis is thought to involve reaginic antibodies, basophils, mast cells, and the release of such mediating substances as histamine, prostaglandin, and leukotrienes, which, in turn, act on the nasal passages to produce the clinical manifestations. Other immunologic mechanisms may be involved in producing an inflammatory reaction in the nose. The role of allergic mechanisms in the development of nasal polyps and sinusitis is not well defined.

Clinical Picture and Diagnosis. Allergic rhinitis typically begins at an early age with symptoms of nasal congestion or obstruction, sneezing, watering and itching of the eyes, and postnasal drip. The most common complaints associated with nasal polyps are nasal obstruction and rhinorrhea. The symptoms and signs from the development of sinusitis will depend upon the sinuses involved. Typically there may be headaches, tenderness or pain in the area of the involved sinuses, nasal occlusion, nasal discharge, and sore throat. It has been suggested by some that active sinusitis can aggravate bronchial asthma.

Physical examination in subjects with allergic rhinitis will reveal excessive lacrimation and reddening of the sclera and conjunctiva, periorbital darkness (allergic shiners), moderate to marked swelling of nasal turbinates, which will be pale to purplish in color, clear thin nasal secretions, and a lateral crease of the ridge of the nose. Nasal polyps are most commonly seen in the upper part of the lateral nasal wall around the middle turbinate. Typical allergic nasal polyps are smooth, soft, glistening, and bluish in color. Pain and tenderness over the involved sinuses may be seen in sinusitis.

Laboratory findings compatible with immunologic reactions include increased eosinophils in the nasal secretion and peripheral blood and an elevated serum IgE level. Sinus films may help diagnose sinus polyps and sinusitis. Bilateral involvement is more compatible with an allergic mechanism than is unilateral disease.

Inhalant allergies usually cause allergic rhinitis.

The antigen usually can be identified on the basis of the history, such as seasonal variation or symptoms after exposure. If the antigen is not identified by these means, provocative testing may be undertaken. Although usually an inhalant, the allergen may be of another classification, such as an ingestant or injectant.

Evidence should be found that the suspected antigen is interacting with the immunologic system. Because the main immune mechanism producing allergic rhinitis involves the reaginic antibody (IgE), skin testing for immediate wheal/flare reactions and/or radioallergosorbent test (RAST) is recommended.

Skin testing and/or RAST evaluation is recommended.

Treatment. Therapy for allergic rhinitis, nasal polyps, and sinusitis falls into five major areas.

AVOIDANCE OF THE CAUSATIVE ALLERGEN. This may be accomplished by isolating the patient from the allergen, placing a barrier between the patient and the allergen, or removing the allergen from the patient.

SYMPTOMATIC TREATMENT WITH DRUGS. Oral antihistamines are chemical compounds that antagonize the action of histamine through the competitive inhibition of histamine at the histamine-receptor sites. They should be given in a rational way. Since patients exhibit marked variability in response to various antihistamines, individualization of doses and frequency of administration is important. Commonly used H_1 antihistamines are ethanolamines, ethylenediamine, alkylamines, phenothiazines, and miscellaneous agents such as cyproheptadine, hydroxyzine, and piperazine. Common side effects seen with these antihistamines are sleepiness, loss of appetite, constipation, anticholinergic effects such as drying of the mucous membranes, and difficulty in urination. A new generation of H_1 antihistamine is under development. As a group they lack any direct chemical relationship to histamine but have a common structure of an aromatic nitrogen in the form of a piperidine, piperazine, or pyridine. Furthermore, these structures are more polar and so their access into the central nervous system is limited, thereby reducing or eliminating related side effects. These include antihistamines such as terfenadine, loratidine, and astemizole. They also promise to be longer acting (Dockhorn and Shellenberger).

Oral medications include a wide variety of antihistamines and decongestants.

It has been suggested by some investigators that H_2 antihistamines such as cimetidine and ranitidine may be useful when given along with the H_1 antihistamines if there is significant nasal obstruction. Symptomatic use of H_1 and H_2 antihistamines has given disappointing results in the treatment of nasal polyps (Havas et al).

A decongestant may be given either alone or in combination with an H_1 antihistamine orally or locally for the treatment of allergic rhinitis. The oral route is usually preferred. Chronic use of local antihistamines and decongestants is not routinely recommended. Some information suggests that local antihistamines may be sensitizing. In addition, use of local decongestants over a long period of time may cause irritation and a "rebound phenomenon" such as rhinitis medicamentosum (Blue). Their use for nasal polyps has been disappointing.

Cromolyn sodium may be given intranasally. This drug will decrease the release of mediating substances. It is considered a preventive medication that is given before the onset of symptoms. Side effects are minimal and have been mainly those of local irritation. Its use for nasal polyps has not been well demonstrated (Norman, 1983).

Topical therapy includes cromolyn and corticosteroids.

Corticosteroids may be used for the treatment of allergic rhinitis. They may be given systemically as well as intranasally with a poorly absorbed corticosteroid such as beclomethasone or flunisolide. The local medications are preferred because of their more direct action and lower risk of side effects. They usually take several days to weeks to become effective. These agents also have been reported to decrease the size of nasal polyps (Norman, 1983).

Hyposensitization can be used if conservative care fails.

ALLERGEN INJECTION, IMMUNOTHERAPY, OR HYPOSENSITIZATION. When more conservative measures are not successful, allergen injection may be indicated. The procedure involves injecting gradually increasing doses of the causative allergen to induce a tolerance to them in the allergic subjects. Although effective for the treatment of allergic rhinitis, their effectiveness for the treatment of nasal polyps has not been well established (Van Metre and Adkinson).

MANAGEMENT OF COMPLICATIONS OR AGGRAVATING FACTORS. Fatigue, emotional stress, sudden temperature change, intercurrent infections, septal deviation, and exposure to other air pollutants may precipitate, aggravate, and perpetuate symptoms associated with allergic rhinitis, nasal polyps, and sinusitis. Their treatment may be just as important as that directed to the particular allergen.

SURGICAL TREATMENT. Surgery is usually done for nasal polyps and sinusitis associated with an infectious factor if medical therapy fails. This may provide the nose and sinuses with adequate ventilation and drainage and also relieve any obstruction. Surgery may be used to eradicate chronic mucosal disease of the sinuses and complications of sinusitis.

Prognosis. The prognosis and natural course of allergic rhinitis, nasal polyps, and sinusitis have been very difficult to ascertain. Although early reports have noted a high incidence of associated bronchial asthma, this has not been well documented. There is the clinical impression that symptoms of allergic rhinitis lessen with age. Individuals with nasal polyps appear to have recurrences despite medical and/or surgical treatment (Smith).

Differential Diagnosis. Allergic rhinitis needs to be differentiated from idiopathic or vasomotor rhinitis, infectious rhinitis, rhinitis secondary to medications—both local (Neo-Synephrine, cocaine) and systemic (beta-blocking agents, aspirin, reserpine, morphine), rhinitis secondary to mechanical factors, nasal tumors, nasal polyps, cerebrospinal rhinorrhea, chemical irritants, psychological factors, and nasal mastocytosis. In addition to allergies, individuals with nasal polyps should be evaluated for infectious sinusitis and, in children, for cystic fibrosis. Sinusitis of nonallergic etiologies such as trauma, chemicals, immunodeficiency, cystic fibrosis, Kartagener's syndrome, chronic granulomatous disease, and infections should be considered in the differential diagnosis.

SUMMARY

Three criteria should be satisfied before diagnosis and treatment.

Before a physician can confidently diagnose and treat an allergy, the following criteria should be satisfied: (1) The clinical picture is compatible with an allergic reaction. (2) The causative agent has been identified. (3) The immune mechanism has been established. After these criteria have been satisfied, treatment can be given to interfere with the various ongoing processes that result in the final allergic clinical picture.

References

Atkins P, Zweiman B: The IgE-mediated late phase skin response—unraveling the enigma. J Allergy Clin Immunol 79:12, 1987.

Belin H, Norman PS: Diagnostic tests in the skin and serum of workers sensitized to *B. subtilis* enzymes. Clin Allergy 7:55, 1977.

Blue JA: Rhinitis medicamentosa. Ann Allergy 26:425, 1968.

Blumenthal MN, Fish L, Morris R, et al: Adverse health effects from allergens. Minn Med 70:278, 1987.
Cohen S, Ottesen E: The eosinophil, eosinophilia, and eosinophil related disorders. *In* Middleton E, Reed C, Ellis E (eds): Allergy: Principles and Practice. St Louis, CV Mosby Co, 1983, p 701.
Coombs RRC, Gell PGH: Classification of allergic reactions. *In* Gell RRA, Coombs PGH (eds): Clinical Aspects of Immunology, 2nd ed. Oxford, Blackwell Scientific Publications, Ltd, 1968.
Dockhorn R, Shellenberger MK: Antihistamines: The new generation. Immunol Allergy Pract 9:124, 1987.
Emanuel I: Comparison of in vivo allergy diagnostic methods. Immunol Allergy Pract 7:483, 1983.
Geha R: Human IgE. J Allergy Clin Immunol 74:109, 1984.
Giraldo B, Blumenthal M, Spink W: Aspirin intolerance and asthma: A clinical and immunological study. Ann Intern Med 71:479, 1969.
Gleich G, Yunnginger J, Stobo J: Laboratory methods for studies of allergy. *In* Middleton E, Reed C, Ellis E (eds): Allergy: Principles and Practice. St Louis, CV Mosby Co, 1983, p 271.
Havas T, Cole P, Parker L, et al: The effect of combined H_1 and H_2 histamine antagonists on alteration in nasal airflow resistance induced by topical histamine provocation. J Allergy Clin Immunol 78:856, 1986.
Mathews K: Mediators of anaphylaxis, anaphylactoid reactions and rhinitis. Am J Rhinol 1:17, 1987.
McDonald J, Mathison D, Stevenson D: Aspirin intolerance in asthma: Detection by oral challenge. J Allergy Clin Immunol 50:198, 1972.
Norman PS: Review of nasal therapy: Update. J Allergy Clin Immunol 72:421, 1983.
Norman PS: Allergic rhinitis. J Allergy Clin Immunol 75:531, 1985.
Platts-Mills TAE, Heymann PW, et al: Cross-reacting and species-specific determinants on a major allergen from *Dermatophagoides pteronyssinus* and *D. farinae*; development of a radioimmunoassay for antigen P1 equivalent in house dust and dust mite extracts. J Allergy Clin Immunol 78:398, 1986.
Plaut M, Lichtenstein L: Cellular and chemical basis of the allergic inflammatory response. *In* Middleton E, Reed C, Ellis E (eds): Allergy: Principles and Practice. St Louis, CV Mosby Co, 1983, p 119.
Schwartz L: Mediators of human mast cells and human mast cell subsets. Ann Allergy 58:226, 1987.
Smith JM: Epidemiology and natural history of asthma, allergic rhinitis and atopic dermatitis (eczema). *In* Middleton E, Reed C, Ellis E (eds): Allergy: Principles and Practice. St Louis, CV Mosby Co, 1983, p 771.
Solomon W, Mathews K: Aerobiology and inhalant allergens. *In* Middleton E, Reed C, Ellis E (eds): Allergy: Principles and Practice. St Louis, CV Mosby Co, 1983, p 1143.
Van Metre TE, Adkinson NF: Immunotherapy for aeroallergen disease. *In* Middleton E, Reed C, Ellis E, et al (eds): Allergy: Principles and Practice. St Louis, CV Mosby Co, 1988, p 1327.
Wasserman S: Mediators of immediate hypersensitivity. J Allergy Clin Immunol 72:101, 1983.
Weller PF: Eosinophilia. J Allergy Clin Immunol 73:1, 1984.
Welliver R: Allergy and the syndrome of chronic Epstein-Barr virus infection. J Allergy Clin Immunol 78:278, 1986.

12

DISEASES OF THE NOSE

by Peter A. Hilger, M.D.

Although the nose sits in the center of the middle third of the face, it is a structure often overlooked when human disease is discussed. Alterations of nasal physiology create disturbances that run the gamut from temporary inconvenience and mild illness, such as an upper respiratory infection, to life-threatening disorders such as choanal atresia in the neonate. The effects of altered nasal physiology can be seen locally, as in nasal allergy; regionally, as in dental deformities and mouth breathing secondary to chronic nasal obstruction; and systemically, such as cardiopulmonary failure secondary to chronic nasal obstruction.

SYMPTOMS AND PHYSICAL FINDINGS

Symptoms of nasal disease include local as well as distant manifestations. Local symptoms include nasal congestion or obstruction, rhinorrhea, bleeding, pain, anosmia or other alterations in the sence of smell, and postnasal discharge. Similarly, systemic disease may present with nasal symptoms and observable tissue changes. Examination of the nose may reveal mucosal edema as a source of headache or a contributing factor to chronic otologic disease.

Inspection and palpation are the most commonly employed and important techniques of physical examination; however, we must not overlook other methods, including listening to the patient's respirations and speech, which can point to abnormalities in the nose (Fig. 12–1). A satisfactory examination is, of course, expedited by the judicious use of various instruments, such as nasal specula, forceps, applicators, aspirators, mirrors, and optical instruments, which make it possible to visualize the dark recesses of the nasal spaces and even photograph or televise the illuminated images (Fig. 12–2). Tests to quantify alterations in olfaction and to provide objective measure of nasal breathing are also available but less frequently used. Radiographic evaluation of the nose and paranasal sinuses can range from simple sinus films to more sophisticated CT scans and NMR images. Application of these more sophisticated tests will be discussed when appropriate.

Thorough evaluation of the nose requires evaluation before and after decongestion.

A systematic approach to physical examination of the nose is valuable in that it ensures that a comprehensive examination is performed and that gross abnormalities do not distract the examiner from more subtle, but nonetheless significant, alterations. Examination usually starts with inspection of the external nose. Observation and palpation may disclose such abnormalities as previous scars and underlying malunited fractures, which can create nasal

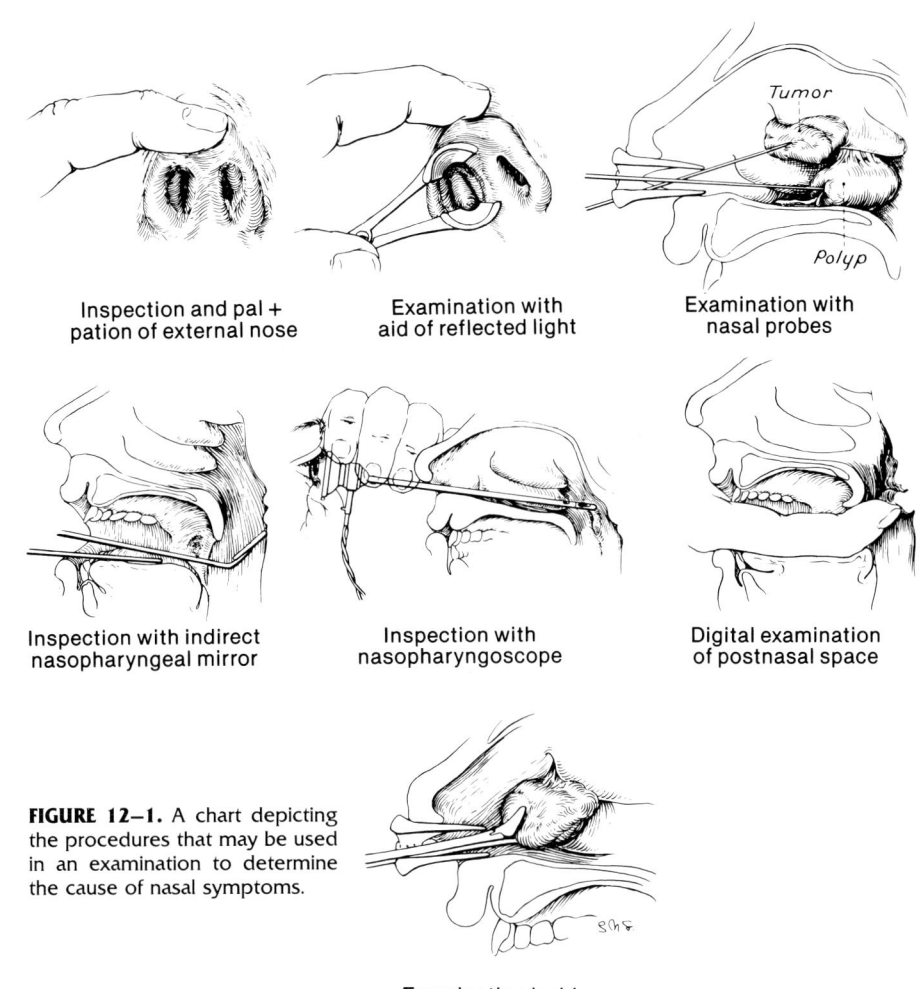

FIGURE 12–1. A chart depicting the procedures that may be used in an examination to determine the cause of nasal symptoms.

- Inspection and palpation of external nose
- Examination with aid of reflected light
- Examination with nasal probes
- Inspection with indirect nasopharyngeal mirror
- Inspection with nasopharyngoscope
- Digital examination of postnasal space
- Examination by biopsy

obstruction. Examination of the internal portions of the nose can then be carried out before introducing a nasal speculum. It is worthwhile to note the position and configuration of the nasal vestibule. Local problems such as friable, superficial blood vessels in the anterior portion of the septum which have created recurrent epistaxis may be overlooked if one hurries to look into the recesses of the nose. Similarly, the introduction of the nasal speculum can distort the nasal ala and artificially support a collapsed cartilaginous vault which was creating nasal obstruction. Evaluation of structures deeper within the nasal spaces than the nasal vestibule will require a nasal speculum and a coaxial light source. A head mirror is a simple and inexpensive tool that can provide adequate illumination. A number of electric headlights are available which are simpler to use but are considerably more expensive. Whatever the source of illumination, it is important that it be coaxial so that the deepest portion of the nose can be examined. Inspection of the nasal chambers should include evaluation of the nasal septum or deformities that can obstruct the airway. The status of the turbinates should be evaluated to determine the presence or absence of edema or alterations in the normal

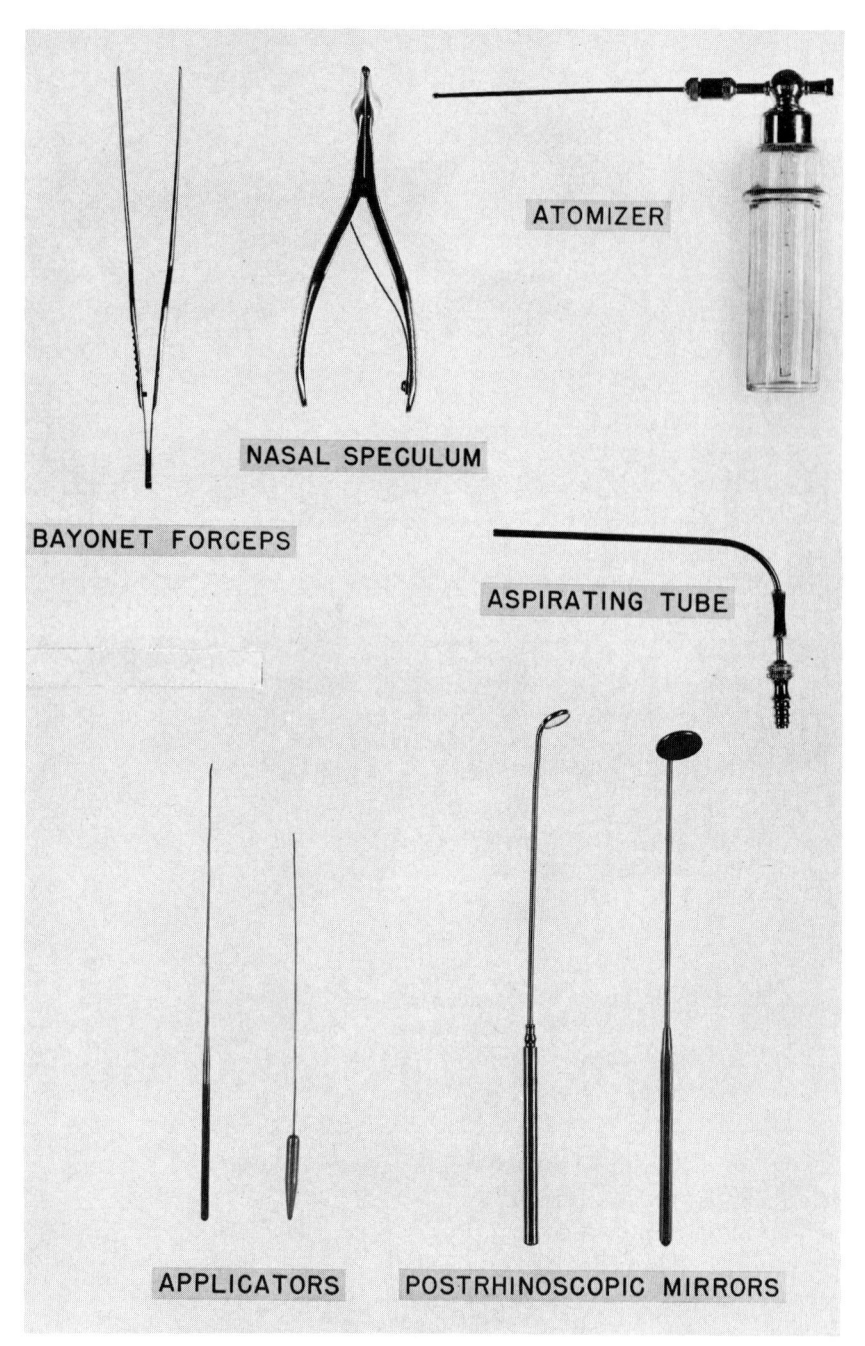

FIGURE 12–2. Instruments necessary for the study of the nasal space.

mucosal color as exemplified by the pale, boggy mucosa of the turbinates in allergic rhinitis. Nasal polyps that typically originate in the middle meatus can also be based directly on the turbinates, the septum, or the superior meatus. Purulent discharge in the middle meatus may be indicative of suppurative disease in the maxillary antrum, anterior ethmoid cells, or frontal sinus. Similarly, discharge present in the superior meatus may indicate an infection in the posterior ethmoid cells. In order to evaluate adequately the intranasal structures, a topical vasoconstrictor such as Neo-Synephrine should be applied without hesitation through an atomizer. Because of the close relationship of the nose and paranasal sinuses, disease processes affecting the nose may also involve the sinuses, and radiographic evaluation may be indicated (see also Chapter 13).

If significant instrumentation within the nose, such as that required for biopsy or control of bleeding, is necessary, application of a topical anesthetic is advised. Cocaine, usually a 4 per cent solution, provides excellent anesthesia as well as vasoconstriction. The solution may be applied through an atomizer or on cotton pledgets. Because of potential toxicity, the total dosage of cocaine in adults should not exceed 3 mg/kg. If the use of cocaine is not advisable or if it is unavailable, lidocaine may be used in conjunction with topical vasoconstriction. Before undertaking nasal biopsy, the physician should be prepared to deal with the adverse affects of the anesthetics as well as possible hemorrhage.

Posterior rhinoscopy is accomplished by placing a small mirror in the oral pharynx with its surface facing directly into the nasopharynx (see Fig. 12–1). A coaxial light source is again essential for adequate visualization and illumination. This technique is valuable to visualize abnormalities such as choanal polyps, hypertrophic turbinates, and purulent discharge from the nose and paranasal sinuses which has been swept posteriorly through the action of the cilia. Flexible fiberoptic nasopharyngoscopes can also be used to examine the nose and nasopharynx. These instruments can be connected to a television camera. The expense of these instruments often precludes their use by most physicians. Rigid endoscopes are also available for similar inspection of the nasal spaces (see Fig. 12–1). These endoscopes can be coupled to delicate surgical instruments. This equipment can then be used to perform procedures within the nose and paranasal sinuses with excellent illumination and magnification under local anesthesia with minimal patient morbidity.

CONGENITAL DISORDERS

Congenital disorders of the nose can range from isolated deformities to abnormalities associated with multiple organ system defects. Furthermore, these disorders can be inherited or acquired. The following discussion will include some of the more common or significant diseases. Congenital nasal deformities that are part of multiple organ system syndromes are discussed in Chapter 15.

Whatever the etiology, it is important to remember that neonates are obligate nose-breathers; therefore, diseases such as choanal atresia can be life-threatening, and intervention to establish an airway, such as a Montgomery nipple or intubation at the time of birth, can be life-saving.

Neonates are obligate nose-breathers and may need an alternate airway established at birth.

Nasal Manifestations of Cleft Lip and Palate

The anatomic proximity of the nose and lip and the shared embryologic precursors of the lip, premaxilla, maxilla, and nose dictate that the child born with a cleft lip and/or palate will also have associated nasal deformities, even if the cleft is incomplete. Although these nasal deformities may be less obvious than the oral abnormalities, the functional and aesthetic changes

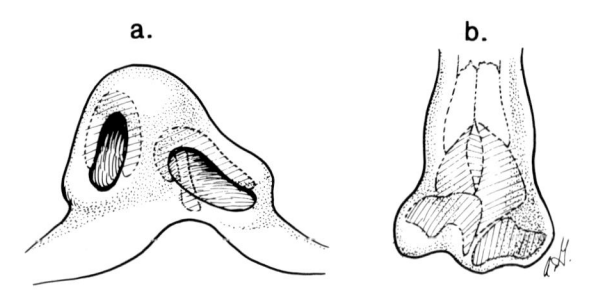

FIGURE 12–3. Base of frontal views demonstrating the typical nasal deformities associated with cleft lip and palate. See text for details.

are always present, change with nasofacial growth, and may become more troublesome as the child matures.

The nasal deformities include septal deflections that are often severe enough to cause significant nasal obstruction. In addition, the lower lateral cartilage and soft tissues of the nasal alae are asymmetric. This often results in a nose with inadequate tip projection, an acute nasolabial angle, sagging of the nasal ala on the cleft side, and irregularities in the position of the nostril sills (Fig. 12–3). The tip deformities may also compromise the nasal airway and compound the nasal obstruction due to septal deflection. Fistulas may also persist through the palate or gingivobuccal sulcus, which will allow the contents of the oral cavity to contaminate the nose, leading to mucosal edema and further nasal obstruction. Reconstructive procedures can provide major improvement of both the functional and aesthetic deformities.

Since it is inappropriate to discuss the oral problems in this section on nasal disease, the interested student is referred to those chapters on oral disease, embryology, and congenital syndromes.

Nasal Dermoid Cysts

Although usually present at birth, congenital nasal dermoid cysts or sinuses may remain unrecognized until later childhood or adult life. They contain all elements of skin: hair follicles, hair, sweat glands, sebaceous glands, and connective tissue. The sinus opening, when present, is usually at the osteocartilaginous junction of the nasal dorsum (Fig. 12–4A and B). It has been theorized that nasal dermoid cysts arise out of ectodermal elements of the fetal trilaminar septum which fail to degenerate. They are noncompressible and nonpulsatile and are evidenced by a pit on the nasal dorsum, associated with which is a group of hairs and an occasional discharge of purulent matter. A CT scan, especially for infants, is the diagnostic tool of choice. The differential diagnosis includes gliomas, encephaloceles, mucoceles, osteomyelitis, hemangiomas, and neurofibromas. Complete excision is the only effective therapy. Optimum age for surgery is between 5 and 6 years, although the risk of infection with its concomitant risk of deformity must be weighed against the inhibition of normal growth that may result from extensive dissection.

Nasal Glioma and Encephalocele

Nasal gliomas and encephaloceles are rare lesions that are quite similar in their embryogenesis and on a histological level, both being composed of extradural glial tissue. However, encephaloceles are connected to the central

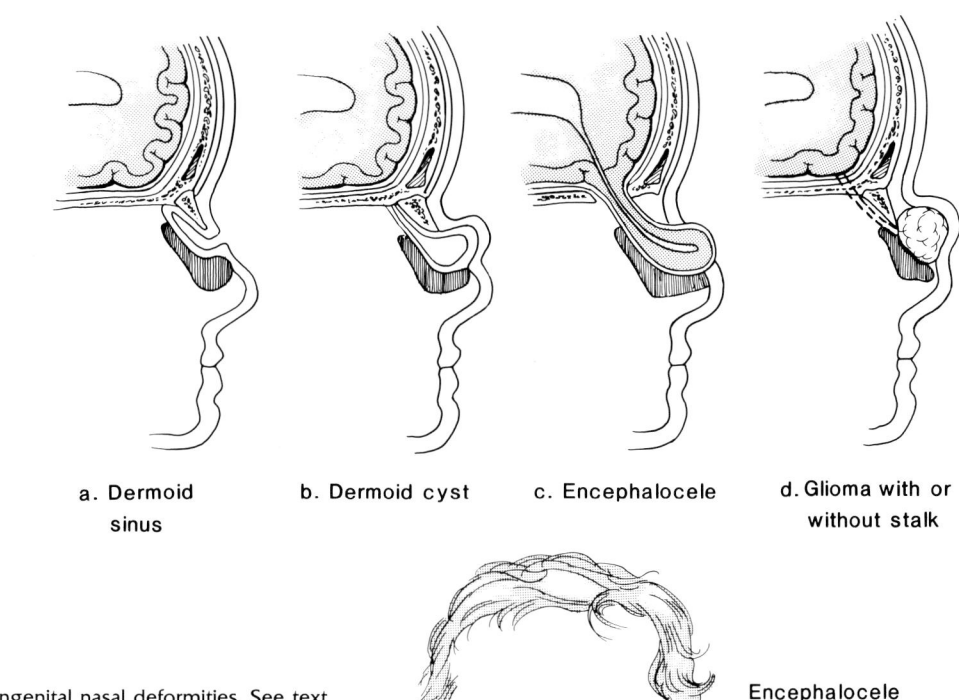

FIGURE 12–4. Congenital nasal deformities. See text for details.

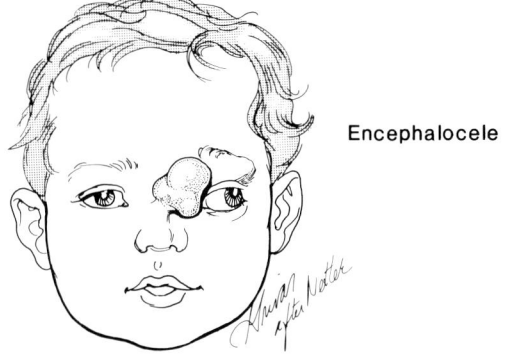

a. Dermoid sinus b. Dermoid cyst c. Encephalocele d. Glioma with or without stalk

Encephalocele

nervous system, whereas gliomas are not (Fig. 12–4C and D). Treatment is always excision; depending upon its location, a neurosurgical approach may be necessary.

A glioma is usually a solid, noncompressible, nonpulsatile gray or purple mass that does not transilluminate and does not produce a positive Furstenberg sign, i.e., no enlargement on compression of the jugular. Gliomas are usually noticed at, or shortly after, birth. Approximately 60 per cent are extranasal, usually occurring along the nasomaxillary suture or near the midline, infrequently in the midline; 30 per cent are intranasal; and 10 per cent have both components. The differential diagnosis most commonly includes dermoid cysts and encephaloceles. CT scanning, NMR, and plain film in three planes are recommended for diagnosis.

Encephaloceles are frequently associated with other midline fusion defects such as cleft lip or palate as well as a high incidence of other central nervous system anomalies. Because an encephalocele is by definition the extracranial herniation of meninges and brain, a cranial defect is always present. Encephaloceles are usually bluish, compressible, pulsatile, may be transilluminated, and produce a positive Furstenberg sign. The differential diagnosis should include dermoid cysts, neurofibromas, and hemangiomas. They are best delineated by CT, NMR scanning, and plain film in three planes. Neurosurgical intervention is necessary.

Choanal Atresia

Choanal atresia will be discussed in the chapter dealing with diseases of the nasopharynx (Chapter 17).

Uncommon Nasal Anomalies

Uncommon nasal anomalies may be associated with genetic syndromes or may result from teratogenic influences. They all share a developmental failure or delay. These conditions include median and lateral nasal clefts. The appearance of median clefts may range from a mild furrow on the nasal dorsum to one approximating polyrhinia. The incidence of associated defects such as coloboma of the lower lid, iris or retina, encephalocele, facial cleft, choanal atresia, and hypertelorism increases with the severity of the median cleft. A CT scan is recommended to rule out any associated dermoid cyst or encephalocele. Surgery is necessary when the deformity is severe.

The appearance of a lateral nasal cleft can range from a simple notch of the lateral nasal ala to a cleft reaching to the eye. Flaps and grafts are used to treat the simple defect. Severe defects frequently are associated with other problems, usually craniofacial and cardiac. Treatment is through a craniofacial approach.

INFLAMMATORY DISEASES—RHINITIS

The Common Cold

Clinical Features. The term "common cold" describes a symptom complex rather than a specific disease. To both physicians and laymen, it has the clearly understood meaning of a short, mild illness in which the main local symptoms are found in the upper respiratory tract and in which nasal symptoms predominate. As long as the illness remains uncomplicated, the diagnosis of a "common cold" is made by the layman and most often does not come to the attention of the physician. To make the differential diagnosis and elucidate a specific etiology of this great variety of acute respiratory disorders with similar initial manifestations may prove to be very difficult or impractical at times. Synonyms for the common cold used by the physician are URI or acute coryza; patients may even call it "sinus."

Nearly 200 viruses are responsible for the common cold.

The student of infectious diseases may think of the common cold as being caused by a "cold" virus, or a specific group of filterable viruses, only to discover that so far nearly 200 different viruses, both of the RNA and DNA types, have been associated with this illness. Moreover, there are many inciting factors other than virus infections that cause symptoms interpreted by the patient as a "cold." The symptoms themselves vary greatly in onset, severity, and associated groups of symptoms, so as to have a variety of disease processes which confuses the etiology.

Most people expect a "cold" to start with nasal airway obstruction, excessive nasal discharge, sneezing, some coughing, and general malaise with or without headache. The body temperature may be normal or slightly elevated. This first stage is usually limited to three to five days. The nasal secretions are at first watery and profuse, then become mucoid, more viscid, and scantier. The illness may terminate at this point. In many patients, however, the illness progresses to a stage of secondary bacterial invasion, characterized by a purulent rhinorrhea, fever, and often a sore throat. The red and swollen secretion-coated mucosa may easily be observed intranasally. The senses of taste and smell are diminished. Sniffling and repeated nose blowing cause reddening of the nostrils and upper lip. This stage may last as long as two weeks, after which the patient recovers without having seen a doctor. The physician is usually consulted only when there are further complications such as pneumonia, laryngitis, middle ear infections, or purulent sinusitis. By that time the inciting illness is clinically unrecognizable as a cold. Interpretation of culture results must take into consideration the fact that the normal flora of the nasopharynx and anterior nose often include *Staphylococcus, Streptococcus pneumoniae, Haemophilus influenzae*, and beta-streptococci.

Etiology. When we limit the definition of the "common cold" to only those cases caused by the well over 100 different rhinoviruses, the "common cold" becomes much less common than the literature leads us to believe. The same complex of symptoms of rhinorrhea, nasal obstruction, sneezing, and coughing may characterize the onset of inhalant or ingestant allergy episodes, the so-called physical allergies, various vasomotor disturbances of the nose brought on by physical or emotional stress, or hormonal or drug-induced body changes, in addition to direct chemical, mechanical, or thermal irritation of the mucous membranes, and last, but not least, a host of other viral and bacterial disorders.

The classifications of respiratory viruses keep changing. Earlier classifications, based on host and tissue affinity and the clinical symptoms of disease, have been gradually replaced by those based on the biochemical composition of the viruses. Thus, we recognize viruses made up primarily of ribonucleic acid (RNA) and those composed mainly of deoxyribonucleic acid (DNA). The RNA viruses include such groups as the rhinoviruses, echoviruses, and influenza, parainfluenza, mumps, measles, and respiratory syncytial viruses. The DNA viruses include the adenovirus group and the herpesviruses that elicit respiratory diseases in animals.

Measles, mumps, and influenza at their onset cause catarrhal upper respiratory symptoms and may be confused with the common cold. The more severe symptoms usually appear later.

Incidence. Frequently occurring illnesses can have a tremendous impact on the world economy. Insurance companies and governmental health agencies the world over provide us with impressive figures. The statistics of several hundred million attacks of the common cold each year in the United States and similar reports in other countries are arrived at by extrapolating absentee figures from schools, the armed forces, and huge industrial firms. In the large majority of instances leading to these statistics, the diagnoses of "common cold" were made by the patients themselves and not by physicians.

Control. The spread of colds caused by various viruses most likely occurs by droplet infection and not by ingestion. Thus, respiratory infections can theoretically be controlled by isolation. Quarantine measures, practiced since the Middle Ages, can be very effective. The general public, however, is not impressed by a "cold," and it is impossible to keep cold sufferers from going to school, going to work, or generally mixing in crowds of people. The conflicting reports throughout the literature on the periods of immunity following an attack are probably best explained on the basis of the great variety of etiologic agents. Susceptibility to colds varies greatly among individuals. There is some indication that children up to age five are more susceptible. The commonly cited experience that chilling, exposure to moisture and cold winds, and fatigue enhance the development of cold symptoms has not been corroborated in well-controlled laboratory studies on known virus-infected volunteers. Exposure to the outdoor elements alone may increase the chances of allergic episodes. It has been postulated that vasomotor changes brought about by hormonal influences similarly enhance the incidence of colds. Conclusions that colds may be aborted by the administration of vasodilators have not been shown to be justified.

Prophylaxis and Therapy. Many useful virus vaccines have been developed since Jenner's fight against smallpox in 1798. Because of the very large number of different viruses involved, it has so far been impossible to develop vaccines to cover even most possibilities of infection. Antibiotics have value only in treating secondary bacterial infections. Chemotherapeutic agents have, to this date, played a very minor role because none has a broad-spectrum effect.

Antihistamines, desensitization, and general antiallergic measures are useful in treating the allergic disorders. Antihistamines used to treat colds, coughs, and allergies are H_1-blocking agents. Little evidence exists that patients with colds experience clinical benefit from their administration. While topical vasoconstrictors such as phenylephrine or oxymetazoline may provide relief of watery rhinitic discharge, they must be used with caution in infants and young children. Oral decongestants decrease some of the profuse nasal discharge, making the patient more comfortable, but they will not effect a cure.

Although cough suppressants are widely used, the Committee of Drugs of the American Academy of Pediatrics has voiced this warning: "Symptomatic treatment may mask serious underlying disease and may be hazardous, particularly in infants whose small airways can be easily plugged with tenacious mucus. . . . When a valid indication exists for antitussive therapy, such as a nonproductive cough that seriously disturbs sleep or school attendance, either codeine or dextromethorphan, which appear to be equiactive, should be recommended." Because of the danger of Reye's syndrome, aspirin should be avoided. Analgesic-antipyretic preparations may provide symptomatic relief, with acetaminophen being the antipyretic of choice.

The best treatment of the uncomplicated viral cold is probably still bed rest and isolation for approximately two days. Adequate hydration can be ensured through the use of a cool mist humidifier, increased fluid intake, and administration of saline nose drops. During the phase of secondary bacterial infection, specific antibiotics may be administered.

In spite of all the advances in virology and tremendous efforts by clinicians everywhere to prevent, control, and treat the common cold, little has been accomplished and much needs to be done in the future.

In addition to the common cold, other viral illnesses encountered, some of which may result in permanent anosmia, include:

Influenzal Rhinitis. Influenzal rhinitis is caused by viruses A, B, and C of the orthomyxoviruses. The sneezing, watery nasal discharge, and stuffy nose are comparable in severity to the common cold; however, secondary bacterial infections and necrosis of the ciliated epithelium occur more frequently with influenza. Vaccination is recommended for high-risk groups. Antibiotics are effective only for secondary bacterial infections.

Rhinitis of Viral Exanthemas. Rhinitis is frequently a prodromal symptom of measles, rubella, and chickenpox, often preceding the exanthema by two to three days. Secondary bacterial infections and complications are more common than with a cold. Although chickenpox will be most frequently encountered, measles and rubella are still a consideration for the clinician, particularly in areas with a high noncompliance with MMR vaccinations.

Rhinitis is a frequent prodromal syndrome of measles, rubella, and chickenpox.

Acute Bacterial Infections

Suppurative Rhinitis. Suppurative rhinitis usually follows a viral rhinitis as a secondary bacterial infection in adults, frequently in association with bacterial sinusitis, and is often associated with adenoiditis in children. Young children, however, will occasionally develop a primary bacterial rhinitis, presenting identically to the common cold. A gray membrane may adhere to the submucosa, with bleeding resulting from attempted removal. *Pneumococcus, Staphylococcus,* and *Streptococcus* are frequently involved in these infections, which, if not treated, can become chronic.

Viral rhinitis is a frequent precursor to suppurative rhinitis.

Furunculosis and Vestibulitis. An extensive and invasive infection of sebaceous glands or hair follicles with some involvement of subcutaneous tissues, a furuncle, or boil, is usually caused by *Staphylococcus aureus* (Fig. 12–5). Analgesics and warm compresses may provide relief from the discomfort. Systemic and topical antibiotics directed against this organism are necessary, as are incision and drainage if an abscess is present.

Staphylococcus aureus is also the causative organism for nasal vestibulitis, a mild inflammation with recurrent crusting and pain. Topical antibiotic ointments two to three times per day will usually suffice.

Septal Abscess. This bacterial infection is usually secondary to a traumatic or surgical hematoma. Treatment is incision and drainage with appropriate systemic antibiotic therapy. Saddling of the nasal dorsum and columellar retraction may result from delayed therapy or a severe infection (Fig. 12–6).

Aggressive early intervention is necessary to avoid disfiguring sequelae.

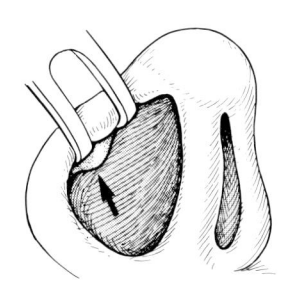

Toxic Shock Syndrome. Although primarily associated with the use of vaginal tampons during menstruation, toxic shock syndrome has also been reported after nasal packing. Caused by *Staphylococcus aureus*, the patient presents with headache, lethargy, myalgia, nausea and vomiting associated with fever, hypotension, tachycardia, generalized erythema of the skin and mucous membranes, and a delayed desquamation of the epithelium of the hands. Packing must be removed immediately and appropriate systemic antibiotics administered.

FIGURE 12–5. Nasal furuncle. This infectious process typically involves that portion of the lateral nasal vestibule containing vibrissae.

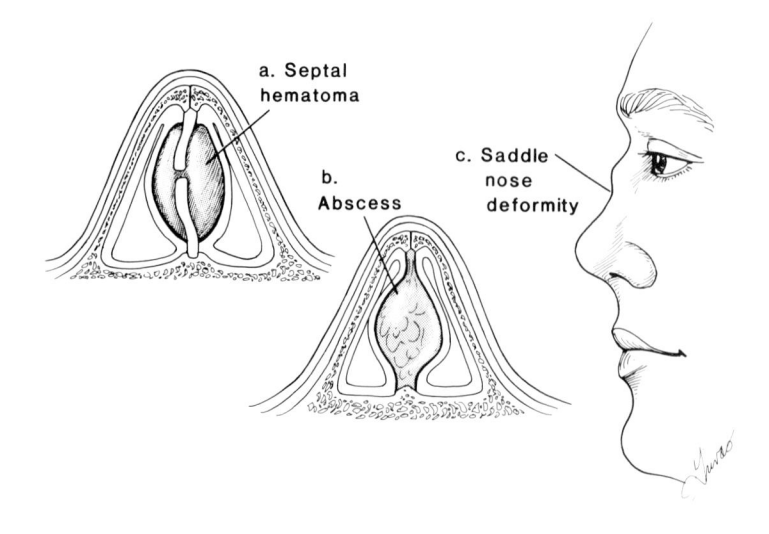

FIGURE 12–6. Septal hematoma and septal abscess. A septal hematoma most frequently develops following nasal trauma with or without associated fracture of the nasal bones. The hematoma dissects the mucoperichondrium from the cartilage. The devascularized cartilage and adjacent hematoma often become contaminated through tears in the mucosa, and an abscess may develop. Cartilage resorption may occur, with loss of nasal support and the development of a saddle deformity.

Chronic Nasal Infections

The differential diagnosis for chronic rhinitis includes both bacterial and fungal diseases.

Fungal

Aggressive nasal fungal infections are usually seen in immunocompromised patients.

Aspergillosis. An infection caused by any of six *Aspergillus* species, aspergillosis most commonly occurs as a chronic pulmonary disease. It may, however, also occur as a chronic granulomatous infection of the paranasal sinuses, nose, middle ear, and external auditory canal. In patients who are debilitated or immunosuppressed, an acute nasal or sinus infection may result. The mucopurulent discharge is characteristically green-brown. Because this organism may be part of the normal oropharyngeal flora, tissues must be sampled under strictly sterile precautions for the culture to have any diagnostic value. Chronic, noninvasive aspergillosis is treated with debridement and topical antifungal drugs. For the acute, life-threatening form, debridement and systemic antifungal drugs, including amphotericin B, are the therapy of choice.

Mucormycosis. Mucormycosis is a malignant, opportunistic infection caused by members of the order Mucorales, principally *Rhizopus oryzae*, found in soil, manure, fruits, and starchy food. The rare occasions when these organisms become pathogenic for man occur in patients with diabetic acidosis or, even more rarely, other debilitated or immunosuppressed conditions. Inhalation of the microorganism inoculates the nasal turbinates and/or ethmoid sinuses, where it spreads along the blood vessels to the retro-orbital areas and cerebrum. The patient presents with headache, fever, internal and external ophthalmoplegia, paranasal sinusitis, and a thick, dark, bloody nasal discharge. This syndrome is identified by a characteristic black or brick-red nasal turbinate. Nonseptate hyphae can be demonstrated microscopically. Treatment consists of immediate intravenous or even intrathecal administration of amphotericin B, debridement of necrotic tissue, and management of the underlying condition.

Candida. *Candida*, along with histoplasmosis, coccidioidomycosis, sporotrichosis, cerocosporamycosis, and blastomycosis, is rarely associated with the nose.

Bacterial

Nasal involvement in the following diseases is often just part of the systemic disease.

Tuberculosis. While primary tuberculosis of the nose is rare in the United States, involvement of the nose is occasionally seen among patients with active pulmonary tuberculosis. Diagnosis begins with a chest radiograph. If this is negative, smears and cultures of sputum and nasal discharge followed by biopsy may be carried out. If these are positive for *Mycobacterium tuberculosis*, an appropriate course of antituberculosis medication must be carried out.

Leprosy. More common in tropical countries, leprosy is also found in the United States, chiefly in Texas, Hawaii, California, Louisiana, Florida, and New York. With a progression very similar to rhinoscleroma, the nose may be the site of the primary infection or it may be part of the systemic disease. Early symptoms include obstruction, crust formation, and bleeding. The upper respiratory tract is more frequently involved in the lepromatous form of leprosy than in the tuberculoid or dimorphous form of leprosy. *Mycobacterium leprae* always involves the nose before spreading to the pharynx and larynx.

Rhinoscleroma. Rhinoscleroma is a granulomatous disease of the nose endemic to Central and Southern Europe and some areas of Asia. Previously rarely seen in the United States, the incidence has been rising in the West and Southwest. Caused by *Klebsiella rhinoscleromatis*, this disorder involves the nose primarily but may later extend to involve any area of the upper respiratory regions, including the larynx. A slowly progressing disease, it begins with an early acute inflammatory reaction with a purulent, foul-smelling rhinorrhea. This is followed by nasal crusting and slow-growing, hard, insensitive nodules that may eventually obstruct the nose. The lower nose and upper lip become prominent if left untreated, causing extensive disfigurement.

Diagnosis is based on the clinical course and pathological examination of the specimen showing characteristic Mikulicz cells and rod-shaped bacteria within the cytoplasm. Granuloma and fibrosis are present. Antibiotic therapy is required. Surgical treatment may be indicated to correct the severe scarring that results.

ALLERGIC RHINOSINUSITIS

Allergic disorders involving the nose occur much more frequently than the lay person or the average physician suspects, affecting approximately 10 per cent of the general population. The nose, as one of the prominent shock organs of allergic disease, is plagued by primary allergic manifestations, chronic rhinitis and sinusitis superimposed on allergic changes, complications of relatively mild anatomic obstructions by edema, and, finally, the late after-effects of chronic allergenic insults, such as mucosal hypertrophy and polyposis. Nasal air flow may be compromised by the nasal congestion and rhinorrhea that occur in allergic rhinitis, directly or indirectly. When confronted by nasal disease, the clinician needs a high index of suspicion and the ability to diagnose and treat allergic disorders.

Allergic rhinitis affects 10 per cent of the population.

Nasal allergy may be seasonal, such as hay fever, or perennial if caused by house dust, animal dander, commonly worn fabrics, or ingestants in the daily diet. Almost all airborne and innumerable ingested substances have been shown to have allergenic properties. Frequently, a patient will be allergic to a number of agents rather than just one inhalant. A cigarette smoker may be allergic to tobacco as well as being chemically irritated by the fumes.

Most allergic patients are sensitive to multiple antigens rather than to a single inhalant.

Allergic rhinitis has been demonstrated to be associated with the occurrence of asthma and atopic eczema. A study of college students with allergic rhinitis demonstrated that 17 to 19 per cent were also asthmatic; however, 56 to 74 per cent of the asthmatic patients had allergic rhinitis. There appears to be an inherited predisposition to these conditions.

Allergy is the altered tissue response to a specific antigen or allergen. Hypersensitivity of the host depends upon antigen dose, frequency of exposure, genetic make-up of the individual, and the relative sensitivity of the host's body.

Allergic reactions are basically considered to be immunoglobulin-mediated, such as rhinitis, asthma, anaphylaxis, and urticaria, or cell-mediated, such as contact dermatitis. These mechanisms are discussed more fully in Chapter 11.

Allergic rhinitis occurs when an antigen to which the patient has been sensitized stimulates one of six nasal neurochemical receptors: the H_1 histamine receptor, the alpha-adrenoceptor, the $beta_2$-adrenoceptor, the cholinoceptor, the H_2 histamine receptor, and the irritant receptor. Of these, the most important is the H_1 histamine receptor, which, when stimulated by histamine, leads to increased nasal airway resistance, causing sneezing, itching, and rhinorrhea.

Diagnosis

This section is concerned specifically with allergy in relation to the tissues of the nose and paranasal sinuses. The differential diagnosis of nasal allergy includes nonallergic rhinitis, infectious rhinitis, and the common cold.

The symptoms of nasal allergy differ from those of infectious rhinitis. The allergic response is usually characterized by sneezing, nasal congestion, and profuse, watery rhinorrhea. No fever is present and the secretion does not progress from thin to thick and purulent, as it does in infectious rhinitis. There is a rapid onset of symptoms after allergen exposure, including watery, itchy eyes or palate. A seasonal pattern or association with animal dander, dust, smoke, or other inhalants can usually be elicited. Associated symptoms such as nausea, belching, bloating, diarrhea, somnolence, or insomnia may also suggest an ingested allergen and differentiate these patients from those with viral rhinitis. Another important difference is that the duration of allergic rhinitis is generally considerably longer than that of viral rhinitis. In patients with allergic diatheses, a positive family history of allergy or asthma is frequently present. As with viral rhinitis, acute bacterial sinusitis may occur secondary to ostial compromise and pooling of the secretions.

The diagnosis of nasal allergy should be established by a systematic investigation that will include a careful history and some or all of the following: nasal examination, skin tests, and elimination regimens. An elimination regimen may also be used as a treatment.

History

Inquiries begin with a history of any allergic diseases in the family. The patient should also be questioned about allergic disorders other than those of nasal origin, such as asthma, eczema, urticaria, or drug sensitivities. The time of year in which the symptoms are prevalent is helpful in determining seasonal allergies. Correlating onset of symptoms with environmental changes at work or about the home is important. Are the living quarters in a dusty or damp area? Do symptoms start with outdoor activities? Pets in the household often are the cause of difficulties. It is important to obtain a history of previous treatment, especially if hyposensitization was utilized. What medications have been used in the past? Which drugs have been helpful without causing side effects?

Symptoms of food allergy are less obvious and require a very detailed history. The time of day of the onset of the symptoms is important, e.g., relationship to meals. Because the patient may be allergic to some of his favorite foods, it may be difficult for him to associate the fact that symptoms could be related to a frequently ingested substance. Cravings for food can represent allergic symptoms. Specific food idiosyncrasies, on the other hand, may point to allergy-producing ingestants.

Nasal Examination

The nasal mucosa in patients with allergy is generally moist, pale, and grayish pink in color. The turbinates appear swollen (Fig. 12–7). If there is an associated infection, the secretions range from thin and mucoid to thick and purulent; at the same time the mucosa may become red and inflamed, congested, or even dry. Polyps may develop in the maxillary antral and ethmoid region and extend into the middle and superior meatus. In addition, polypoid degenerative changes can occur throughout the nasal mucosa, covering the lateral nasal walls; this classic appearance of the nasal mucosa is not always seen, however. Radiography of the paranasal sinuses is nonspecific but may show a thickened mucosal lining and occasional pooling of secretions (Fig. 12–8). When the natural ostia become obstructed from excessive swelling, an air-fluid level within the sinus cavities or even total opacification may become apparent (Fig. 12–9).

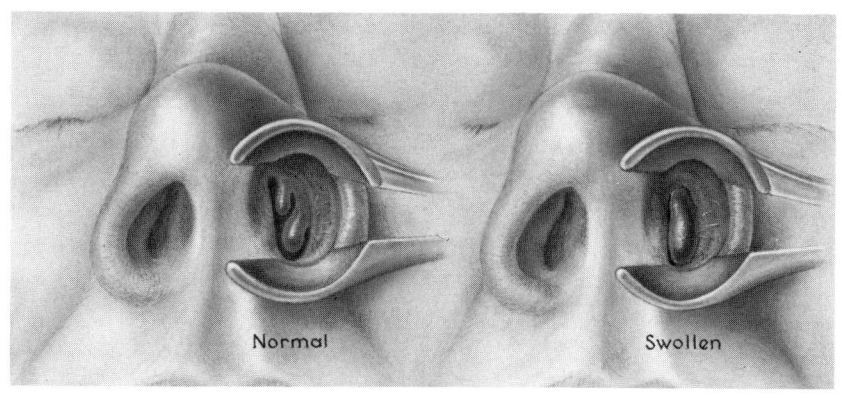

FIGURE 12–7. A comparison of the anterior rhinoscopic views in the normal nose with one in which the turbinates are swollen as in acute allergic rhinitis.

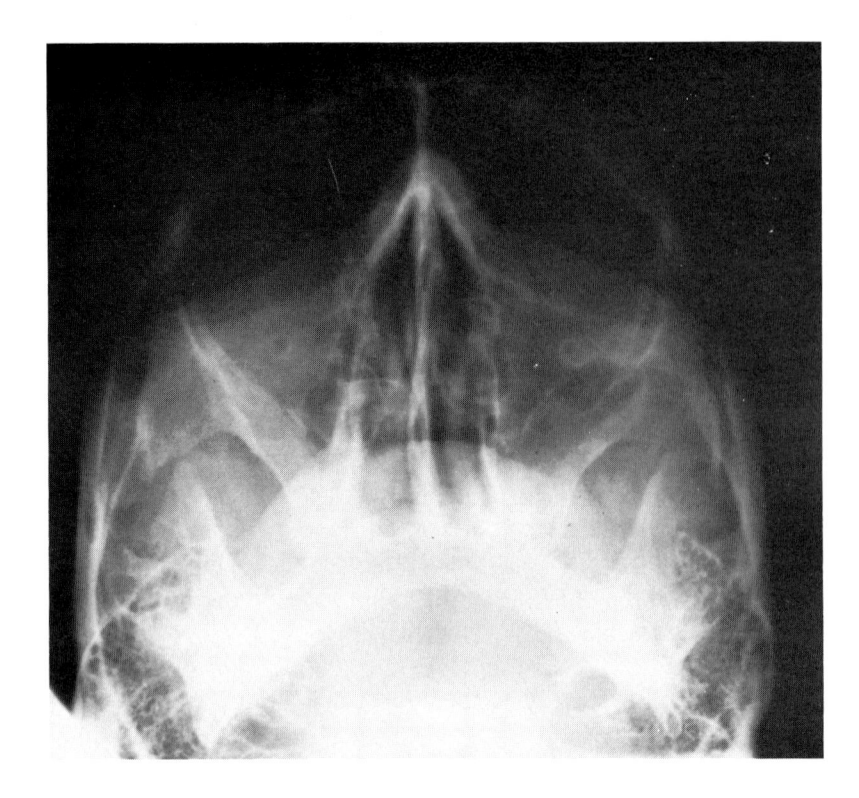

FIGURE 12–8. Waters' view x-ray. Mucosal thickening in maxillary sinuses is often seen in allergic rhinitis.

Nasal Smear

Although some researchers have demonstrated specific diagnoses by cytologic evaluation of a nasal smear, other physicians question their value and feel that smears offer limited additional information. Several smears from beneath the inferior turbinate are obtained at the same time and carefully fixed.

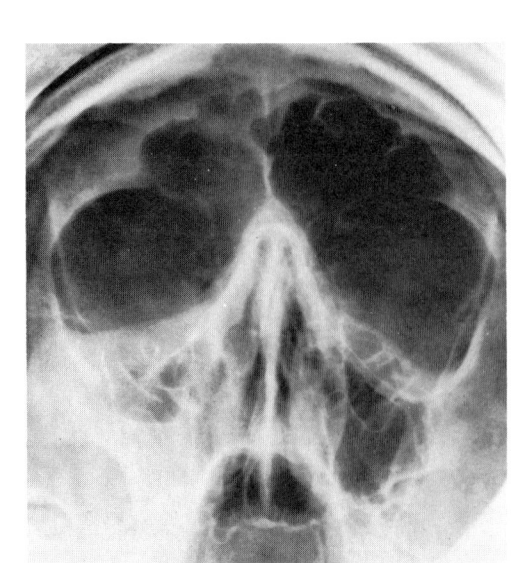

FIGURE 12–9. A Waters' x-ray view. There is a fluid level visible in the involved maxillary sinus.

Clinical Tests for Allergy

Dietary Tests. There are two main categories: the provocative food tests and the various elimination diets. The former essentially consists of abstinence from the suspected food for four to ten days, after which large quantities of the food are ingested. The patient reports subjective changes and is observed for objective data. Elimination diets have been developed for cereals, milk, eggs, and fruit, with the examiner arbitrarily selecting a diet for the patient. It is difficult for the patient to be involved with more than one of these diets at a time.

In Vitro Tests. The cytotoxic food test is used as a screening test. When leukocytes from the buffy coat of the patient's plasma are destroyed in the presence of the food antigen, sensitivity is suspected.

Radioallergosorbency Test. This test requires incubation of the patient's antibodies with specific concentrations of antigen coupled to radioactive paper. It measures the concentration of IgE antibodies and has been found to be a valuable test for the immediate type hypersensitivity.

A more detailed discussion of allergy testing is presented in Chapter 11.

Treatment

Elimination of Allergens

Treatment of nasal allergy is dependent upon several factors. First, if possible, the offending allergenic agent should be eliminated. In the case of pollen allergy, the patient should make proper alterations in his/her environment, such as preventing unnecessary exposure to ragweed pollen. Air-conditioning of the car and home as well as utilization of electronic air filters may be helpful. The patient sensitive to dust should live in as clean an environment as possible, with every effort made to keep the rooms free of dust-collecting items such as shag carpeting and draperies. A patient sensitive to mold should avoid sleeping in damp areas, such as basement bedrooms. Windows should be kept closed at night, as the cold night air frequently contains molds. Patients sensitive to smoke should avoid smoke-filled rooms and association with persons smoking in an enclosed area, such as an automobile. Patients who are known to be sensitive to specific foods will have to make every effort to eliminate those foods from their diet. This may not be easy because processed foods frequently contain substances, information about which may not be immediately available to the consumer.

Medical Management

Local nasal treatment is directed at reducing swelling and formation of secretions and increasing the airway. Temporary relief can be obtained from local application of 0.5 per cent ephedrine sulfate, but this becomes less effective with repeated use. Although 0.25 per cent Neo-Synephrine is an effective topical vasoconstrictor, it may affect the nasal pH and reduce ciliary activity. Another effective medication is 0.05 per cent oxymetazoline. Topical application to the nasal mucosa generally provides progressively shorter periods of temporary relief, becoming less and less effective with use, and may lead to rhinitis medicamentosa.

Local injection of steroids, usually in the form of triamcinolone, into the inferior turbinate has been utilized. Topical steroid therapy with beclomethasone or flunisolide can be very effective without causing adrenal suppression or the dangers of intranasal injections. Topical application of cromolyn has also been shown to relieve many nasal complaints by blocking mast cell degranulation.

Surgical Treatment

Benign mucoid polyps of the nose are commonly associated with nasal allergy. They can occur in children but are seen much more often in adults. Because of nasal airway obstruction, polyps become annoying to the patient. After an obstructing lesion is properly identified as a benign polyp, it may be removed. The patient must be warned that, in the presence of allergies, polyps recur, resulting in repeated polyp removal throughout life. However, proper attention to the underlying allergic disorder tends to delay the rate of recurrence. Most polyps originate as an outpouching of the mucosa covering the maxillary or ethmoid sinuses. The ever-growing mucosal enlargement forms a rounded, soft, moist, often gelatinous, sometimes fleshy mass or at times a serum-filled sac, fixed onto a gradually elongating narrow pedicle that reaches from the sinus, through the ostium, into the nasal cavity. Most polyps are amber or grayish blue but may at times become reddened from local irritation or secondary infection. But what looks like a polyp is not always a polyp! When all the polyps are on one side and none is on the other, one should consider a unilateral, localized infection of the nose or sinuses or even a foreign body in the nose. In the toddler and grade schooler, mucoviscidosis and its nasal changes enter the differential diagnosis. The nasal polyp, a pseudotumor, must be differentiated from a host of true benign and malignant neoplasms; these are indeed rare but must not be missed. The unsuspecting surgeon who uses a nasal snare to remove a juvenile angiofibroma of the nasopharynx which looks like a polyp may set off an exsanguinating hemorrhage. The most difficult lesions to distinguish from the true benign nasal polyps are areas of mucosal polypoid degeneration, most frequently encountered in the anterior portion of the swollen inferior and middle turbinates. Differentiation and identification are made easier by using a decongestant spray in the nose, such as 1 per cent ephedrine or a 0.25 per cent Neo-Synephrine solution. Even better is a 4 per cent cocaine solution, which provides some anesthesia in addition to decongestant action. A nasal suction tip may then be utilized, not only to aspirate secretions for easier inspection but to palpate the soft tissue lesion. Although somewhat movable, the polypoid mucosa has a sessile attachment to the turbinate with the relatively firm bone in its center, while the true polyp moves freely on its pedicle.

Prior to nasal polypectomy, adequate premedication and topical anesthesia are applied. The snare wire is then looped around the stalk of the polyp without complete tightening of the wire, and the polyp, its stalk, and the base of the pedicle are avulsed all in one piece (Fig. 12–10). Sinus infections, caused by the obstructive presence of the polyp stalk in the ostium, usually clear up more readily after the polypectomy. If polyps recur and are related to recurrent sinusitis, surgical correction of the sinus disease may be indicated.

Hypertrophic turbinates may require cauterization, cryosurgery, or partial resection to create an adequate airway. Such surgery should be conservative to prevent atrophic rhinitis (Fig. 12–11).

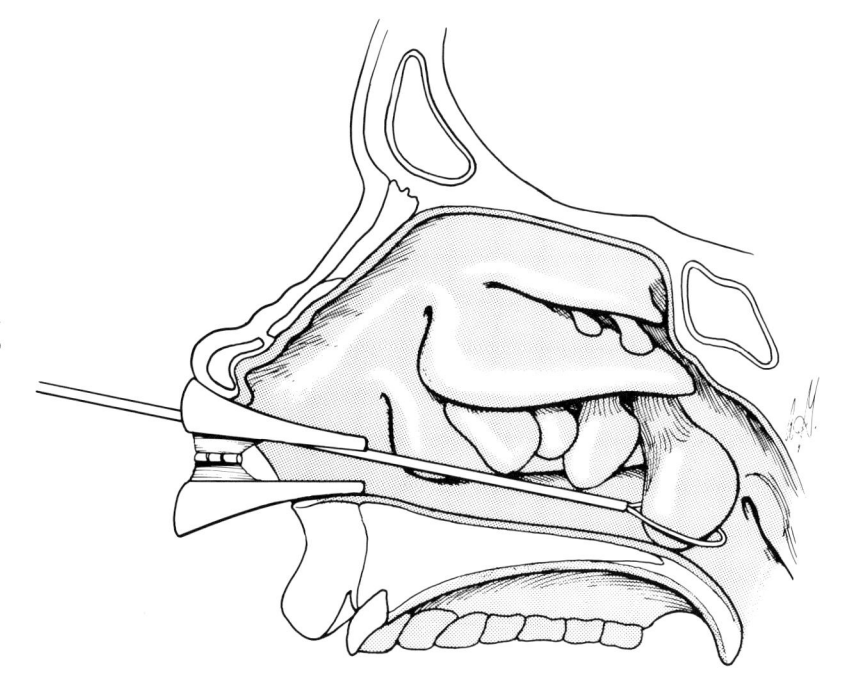

FIGURE 12–10. Nasal polypectomy. A snare is used to grasp and avulse the polyp.

Systemic Treatment

Methods of systemic treatment include medication and allergic desensitization. Allergic rhinitis, whether perennial or seasonal, is most frequently treated with combinations of decongestants and antihistamines. Many such combination drugs are available. Patients with hypertension and those who are taking monoamine oxidase inhibitors should not be given any drug containing an ephedrine-like substance. Such patients can be treated with antihistamine alone.

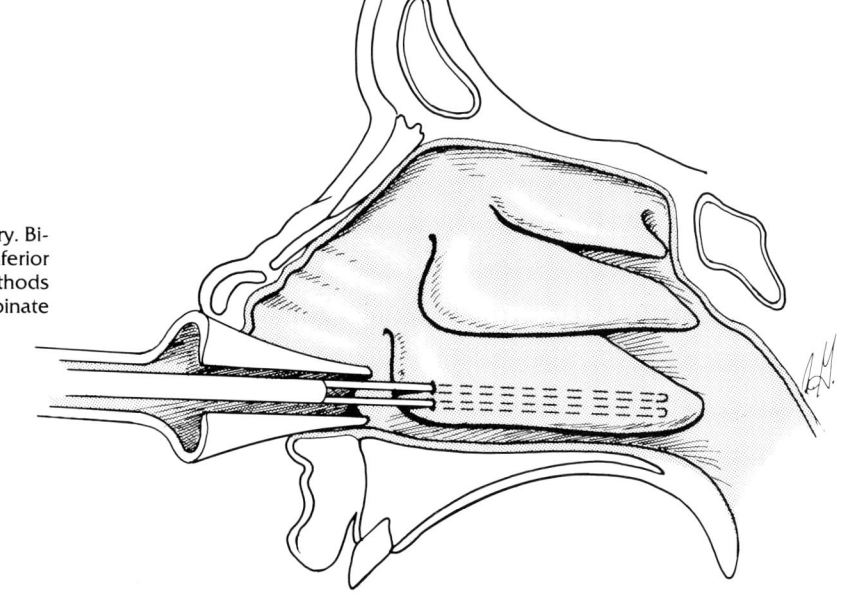

FIGURE 12–11. Turbinate cautery. Bipolar cautery applied to the inferior turbinate is one of several methods to reduce a hypertrophic turbinate and improve the nasal airway.

TABLE 12–1. CLASSIFICATION OF ANTIHISTAMINES

Class 1	**Ethanolamines** are very potent and effective H_1 antagonists. The major side effect is sedation. Gastrointestinal side effects are infrequent.
Class 2	**Ethlenediamines** are highly effective H_1 antagonists. The main side effect is gastrointestinal upset.
Class 3	**Alkylamines** are among the most active H_1 antagonists. Sedation is less frequent. Three out of every four prescription and OTC products contain a Class 3 antihistamine.
Class 4	**Piperazines** are H_1 antagonists with prolonged action.
Class 5	**Phenothiazines** are H_1 antagonists with heavy sedative effects.

Miscellaneous compounds that are not members of one of these categories are also available but are limited in number.

Five classes of antihistamines exist, and it may be necessary to use a trial and error approach to determine the most effective drug with the fewest side effects. Antihistamines of the H_1 class are the drugs of choice in the management of allergic rhinitis. They interfere with histamine action by blocking H_1 histamine receptor sites; although nasal airway resistance remains increased, other allergic effects are reduced. Premedication, therefore, is the preferred mode of administration, since this effectively "ties up" the H_1 receptor sites, thus blocking histamine's effects. Over time a change of drug may be required as tolerance develops to an antihistamine (Table 12–1).

Oral pseudoephedrine and phenylpropanolamine can be used when the primary symptom of allergic rhinitis is congestion. Because of the side effects of excessive stimulation and insomnia, however, they are most effective when paired with an antihistaminic. In certain circumstances, a short course of systemic steroids may be utilized. Prolonged use of cortisone-type drugs for allergic rhinitis generally is not indicated. In seasonal allergic rhinitis prednisone may be administered for five days, after which the dosage is rapidly tapered. A combination of drugs, topical and systemic, may be necessary to achieve the greatest control.

A second method of systemic treatment involves hyposensitization. This topic is discussed in Chapter 11.

Aggravation of asthma has been linked to both chronic and acute sinusitis; treatment of sinusitis and rhinitis is an important step in reducing asthmatic episodes.

Associated Allergic Conditions

There has been an effort to establish a relationship between persistent serous otitis media and chronic allergic rhinitis. Although hyposensitization and medication are frequently effective in treating the allergic rhinitis, the serous otitis media may not resolve. It has been stated that approximately 35 per cent of children with chronic serous otitis media have an underlying allergy problem.

Hyperplastic sinusitis is frequently associated with an underlying allergic rhinitis. In such patients, treatment directed at the rhinitis frequently will relieve the symptoms of headache and sinusitis. However, in certain patients, the changes in the sinuses become so great and are so frequently associated with secondary infection that sinus surgery becomes necessary. Generally, conservative procedures, such as a Caldwell-Luc operation or the creation of a nasal antral window, are performed. Normal mucosa is not removed and generally a drainage procedure is performed. In more severe cases, it may be necessary to perform an ethmoidectomy for removal of irreversibly damaged sinus mucosa and polypoid tissue.

Aspirin Intolerance and Nasal Polyposis

The existence of the triad of aspirin sensitivity, nasal polyposis, and asthma has been well documented. One of the first manifestations of this problem may be a chronic allergic rhinitis. The patient may develop polyps; their removal may precipitate the symptoms of asthma or may worsen the rhinitis. Frequently the patient is middle-aged at the onset of asthma, often becoming steroid dependent. Approximately 2 to 4 per cent of asthmatic patients have aspirin intolerance. The complex is related not to aspirin alone but to other compounds, including aminopyrine, analgesics, and certain dyes. The mechanism is believed to be an alteration in the arachidonic pathway. Surgery should be undertaken only after thorough medical evaluation and perioperative steroid therapy. Administration of a perioperative bronchodilator may also be necessary. Total abstinence from aspirin-containing drugs will not influence the development of polyps, but ingestion of aspirin has been shown to precipitate a definite asthmatic attack. The hallmark of management of such patients is conservative therapy. Proper pre- and postoperative medical care allows the necessary surgery to be performed safely. Treatment revolves around the use of systemic steroids and antihistamines and the avoidance of topical decongestants. Topical corticosteroids may be required. Nasal polyps are removed when they begin to cause complete nasal obstruction. Chronic sinusitis may become part of the clinical picture of required medical and/or surgical care.

2 to 4 per cent of patients with asthma have aspirin intolerance.

NONALLERGIC, NONINFECTIOUS RHINOSINUSITIS

Rather than a single disorder of the nose, this term refers to a group of conditions. Even though the presenting symptoms may be similar, careful history and proper examination are necessary to fully define the given condition so that proper treatment can be instituted. Beginning students in this area of rhinology may be confused by the variety of terms with which they are confronted by both patients and other physicians. Table 12–2 thus outlines some of these terms and their recommended usage.

Vasomotor Rhinitis

This condition of the nasal mucosa results from two opposing forces: Activity of the parasympathetic nerves causes engorgement of the vascular bed with resultant congestion and increased mucous production, while activity of the sympathetic nerves causes vasoconstriction with its resultant nasal patency and decreased mucous production. Factors affecting this balance will be the main subject of the following discussion.

The term vasomotor rhinitis has been applied rather widely; however, it may be considered a misnomer. Vasomotor rhinitis, as it is currently understood, is neither an allergic nor an inflammatory disorder, although, in the strictest sense of the word, the latter implies an inflammatory state of

TABLE 12–2. FORMS OF CHRONIC NONALLERGIC RHINITIS

TERM	COMMENT
Chronic hypertrophic rhinitis	This type of rhinitis is characterized by soft-tissue swelling, excessive secretion, and, in long-standing cases, actual hypertrophy of the mucosa, thickening of the periosteum, and new bone formation. It results from repeated acute nasal infections, from recurrent attacks of suppurative sinusitis, or from vasomotor states independent of local disease.
Vasomotor rhinitis	A form of hypertrophic rhinitis. The etiology is unknown, although psychosomatic factors have been suggested. It may be confused with allergic rhinitis.
Rhinitis medicamentosa	Also generally considered a form of hypertrophic rhinitis related to overuse of topical nasal medication.
Chronic hyperplastic rhinitis	This condition may include elements of hypertrophic rhinitis but generally is associated with nasal polyposis.
Rhinitis sicca	Most commonly considered to be a disorder of altered nasal physiology related to environmental changes, particularly dry inspired air.
Atrophic rhinitis (ozena)	This condition is characterized by a true atrophy of intranasal structures with secondary crusting. Generally idiopathic.
Nasal "catarrh"	An old term referring to chronic nasal symptoms from a variety of causes.

the involved anatomic structures. Factors responsible for the rhinopathia are classified broadly as drug-induced, endocrine, vegetative, and psychoemotional.

Drug-Induced Rhinitis

Antihypertensive drugs, sympathetic blocking agents, may cause nasal congestion.

Rebound vasodilation and congestion are frequent consequences of prolonged use of topical decongestants.

Rebound vasodilation, called rhinitis medicamentosa, can result from the abuse of sympathomimetic decongestant nose drops and nasal spray. The average individual suffering from nasal congestion can obtain immediate initial relief for a period of several hours by utilizing these topical nasal preparations. However, prolonged use results in a chronic congestive state wherein the nasal membrane is sensitive to any irritant, especially when intermittently applied (Fig. 12–12). After an initial vasoconstriction, a secondary vasodilatation occurs which can make the nasal obstruction even worse than before. Moreover, the mucous cells may be unduly stimulated and may increase nasal blockage by excess secretion. The application of these topical drugs may also alter the ciliary action and interrupt the protective mucous blanket present in the nasal cavity. Prolonged use of such medication may result in a hypertrophic rhinitis, treatment of which requires immediate discontinuation of topical nasal medication and a long discussion with the patient about the cause of the problem, careful history-taking, and physical examination to determine and treat the underlying problems that led the patient to initiate the use of topical nasal medications. If the underlying problem is allergy, topical steroids such as flunisolide, beclomethasone, or, rarely, an intraturbinal injection of a corticosteroid may be used. Also recommended is the use of systemic sympathomimetics, e.g., pseudoephedrine.

Other drugs that have been implicated in vasomotor rhinitis include rauwolfia serpentina, alcohol, tobacco, and hashish.

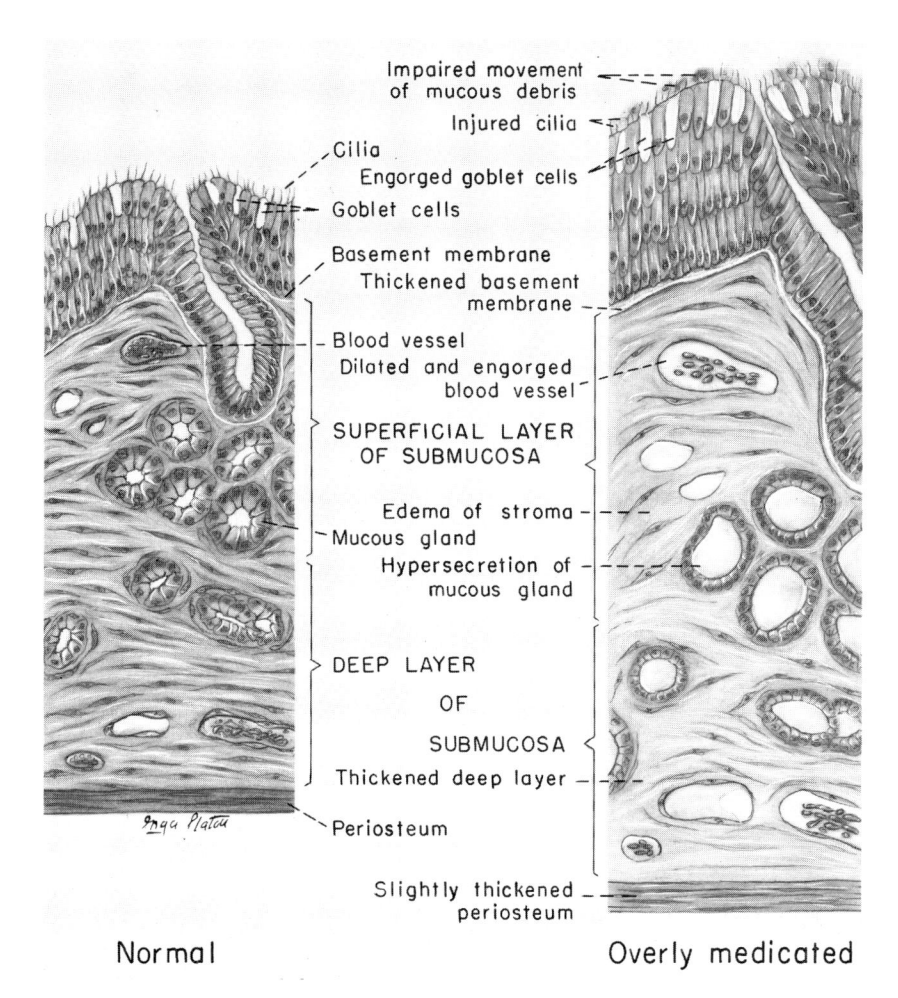

FIGURE 12–12. Pathologic changes in the nasal mucous membrane due to misused medication.

Hormonal

Estrogens stimulate vascular congestion of the nasal membranes as well as engorgement in the uterus, generally peaking in the immediate premenstrual phase when pelvic congestion is at its maximum, causing some women to note nasal congestion at this time. During pregnancy, as the levels of estrogen rise, symptoms of nasal congestion usually begin during the fourth to fifth month and progress to term, paralleling the increased production of estrogen. Symptoms disappear spontaneously at delivery in most patients. In a similar manner, birth control medication may produce nasal engorgement.

Another endocrine cause of nasal engorgement is hypothyroidism, or myxedema. Relief is obtained only with the use of thyroid extract. Conversely, antithyroid drugs may produce congestion.

Temperature

In general, cold air causes vasoconstriction and warm air causes engorgement due to vasodilation. Sudden environmental temperature changes may stimulate nasal congestion and/or rhinorrhea.

Emotional Causes

Studies have shown that the recollection of humiliating and frustrating experiences results in nasal responses identical to those that occurred in response to noxious stimuli. Generally speaking, fear and dejection result in shrinkage and pallor of the nasal mucosa, while anxiety, conflict, frustration, and resentment result in hyperemia, swelling, and hypersecretion.

Nonairflow Rhinitis

If, because of a laryngectomy or tracheostomy, the nose is no longer exposed to the regular movements of air associated with breathing, the mucous membranes become engorged and violaceous.

Hypertrophic Rhinitis

Vascular Atony

Chronic allergy and sinusitis causing stimulation of the vessels of the nose over a long period of time may lead to permanent vascular atony with continued nasal congestion, regardless of appropriate medical therapy. Surgical resection of grossly obstructive tissue may be required to establish an adequate airway. However, resection should be conservative to avoid creating the equivalent of atrophic rhinitis.

Compensatory Hypertrophic Rhinitis

Observed in patients with a deviated septum, this condition is the result of overgrowth of the nasal turbinates on the contralateral side, involving bone, mucosa, and/or vascular tissue. Any surgery to correct the septum must include correction of the turbinate overgrowth, or postoperative nasal congestion will result.

Paradoxical Nasal Obstruction

In the majority of the adult population each side of the nose normally goes through cycles of congestion and decongestion, alternating with the contralateral side, each cycle averaging about 2½ hours. Because total airway pressure remains constant, most individuals are unaware of this phenomenon. However, when a deviated septum leads to diminished airflow on one side, the patient will become aware of the congestive part of the cycle on the normal side because the contralateral side is unable to compensate and increase airflow.

Atrophic Rhinitis, Nasal Atrophy, and Ozena

The continuum of changes in this chronic degenerative disease complex has an insidious onset with early nasal atrophy. The nasal mucosa is usually first affected, showing a few thin and dry areas of metaplasia where the respiratory epithelium has lost its cilia, and small crusts and viscid secretions accumulate. Slight ulcerations and bleeding may occur. So-called rhinitis sicca observed in those who work in hot, dry and dusty surroundings fits into this early category. Patients with debilitating disorders—such as uncontrolled diabetes, uremia, and even mild endocrine or metabolic disturbances as seen in some postmenopausal women—show similar changes.

Moderate atrophy not only affects larger areas of the nasal mucosa but most prominently involves the blood supply of the nasal lining, gradually increasing the nasal space in all directions as the lining becomes thinner. Mucous glands atrophy and disappear, while fibrosis of the subepithelial tissues becomes gradually more generalized. Tissues surrounding the nasal mucosa become affected, including cartilage, muscle, and bone of the nasal skeleton. Eventually the dryness and crusting and irritation of the nasal mucosa extend to the lining of the nasopharynx, hypopharynx, and larynx. This can affect the patency of the eustachian tube, resulting in chronic middle ear effusion, and can cause adverse changes in the lacrimal apparatus, including keratitis sicca.

In the late changes of atrophic rhinitis, also referred to as ozena, extensive crusting may be accompanied by a loathsome fetor. While others around him cannot stand the odor, the patient is usually protected by anosmia. He complains of loss of taste and inability to sleep well or tolerate cold air. With his markedly widened airway he experiences progressively increased obstruction to his nasal breathing, mainly because the air baffles that regulate nasal pressure changes and convey sensory messages from the nasal mucosa to the central nervous system have moved farther and farther out of the picture.

Sensory disturbance and air flow changes may cause symptoms of obstruction in atrophic rhinitis.

Multiple theories exist for the cause of atrophic rhinitis and related degenerative disorders. Some authors emphasize hereditary factors. A causal relationship between the direct and indirect effects of trauma and tissue atrophy is almost universally recognized. The trauma may be accidental or iatrogenic, namely, the late effect of surgery. Radiation therapy to the nose most readily damages blood vessels and mucus-producing glands and almost always leads to atrophic rhinitis. Neurovascular changes, such as blood vessel deterioration mediated by insults to the autonomic nervous system, have been documented. Various infections, such as acute exanthemas, scarlet fever, diphtheria, and chronic infections, have been implicated as the cause of injury to the submucosal blood vessels. Environmental causes have also been suggested because of the increased incidence in lower socioeconomic populations.

Ozena is much more common in the countries around the Mediterranean Sea than in the United States. A drop in the incidence of measles, scarlet fever, and diphtheria in southern Europe since World War II appears to coincide with a similar sharp decline in the incidence of ozena.

To date, medical treatment of atrophic rhinitis has, at best, been palliative. It includes irrigations and cleansing of crust formation; local and systemic endocrine, steroid, and antibiotic therapy; vasodilators; the use of mild local tissue irritants such as alcohol; and lubricating ointments. The major treatment emphasis is surgical, all efforts being directed at narrowing the nasal passages again and by so doing improving the mucosal blood supply. Surgical techniques are divided into two major categories: (1) implants, through either an intra- or an extranasal approach and (2) operations, such as narrowing of the nasal lobule or infracture of the nasal bones.

Medical therapy in atrophic rhinitis is palliative.

NASAL MANIFESTATIONS OF SYSTEMIC DISEASE

Wegener's Granulomatosis

Wegener's granulomatosis is a potentially fatal, specific vasculitis of unknown etiology characterized by (1) focal necrotizing, granulomatous lesions in the upper and/or lower respiratory tracts, (2) systemic vascular focal necrosis, and (3) focal necrotizing glomerulitis. Affecting men and women equally, it is seen primarily in adults.

The patient will often present with a long-standing cold, recurrent sinusitis, epistaxis, progressive nasal obstruction, chronic otitis media, and hearing loss that are unresponsive to treatment. Although lesions may involve any area of the respiratory tract, nasal crusting and friable nasal mucosa are the norm, with eventual saddling a common sequela.

No specific laboratory test is diagnostic. A mild anemia is usually present, with an elevated erythrocyte sedimentation rate, and urinary abnormalities if there is kidney involvement. Diagnosis is dependent upon biopsy of the involved tissues for demonstration of necrotizing granulomas and extensive vasculitis. Multiple samples may be necessary to demonstrate the diagnostic lesion.

Multiple biopsies may be necessary to identify this potentially lethal disease.

Differential diagnosis includes polymorphic reticulosis, infectious granulomas, fungal and tuberculous infections, sarcoidosis, and other vasculitides.

Therapy in acute patients involves treatment with corticosteroids and cyclophosphamide. Some authors believe, however, that the addition of steroids to the cytotoxic medications provides symptomatic improvement without altering the course of the disease as when treated with cytotoxic medications alone.

Polymorphic Reticulosis

Polymorphic reticulosis is a rare disease characterized by local inflammation and destruction of the tissues of the midface. Fatal if untreated, it was originally called lethal midline granuloma, a term no longer considered appropriate.

The symptoms and clinical findings are very similar to those of Wegener's granulomatosis. Diagnosis is dependent upon a biopsy, with tissues characterized by a dense, mixed lymphoid infiltration. The absence of giant cells, vasculitis, and systemic involvement differentiates it from Wegener's granulomatosis, and the mixed population of cells differentiates it from lymphoma. This differential diagnosis is critical, since the only therapy shown to be effective is radiation therapy.

Relapsing Polychondritis

Relapsing polychondritis is a rare connective tissue disease of unknown etiology causing episodic inflammation and subsequent destruction of the cartilaginous structures of the body. Nasal involvement results in saddle-nose deformity with no involvement of the mucosa. No specific laboratory test is diagnostic; a biopsy helps provide the diagnosis. Corticosteroids have been found useful in severe cases, but in the majority of symptomatic cases, therapy with salicylates and nonsteroidal anti-inflammatory medications is indicated.

Sarcoidosis

Nasal sarcoidosis is usually associated with pulmonary manifestations.

Nasal sarcoidosis is generally associated with the more common pulmonary manifestations of this disease with world-wide distribution and unknown etiology. A generalized granulomatous disorder primarily affecting young adults, in the United States blacks are 10 times more likely to be affected than are Caucasians. Nasal findings include crusting and thickened mucosa on the inferior turbinate and septum.

A biopsy demonstrating noncaseating granulomas is characteristic, although not diagnostic. Other, systemic signs often include hypergammaglobulinemia and a reduction of serum albumin. Treatment of the symptomatic patient involves steroids, either systemically or in a topical nasal spray, aimed at reducing both nasal stuffiness and crusting. Local treatment with irrigation and moisturizing medication may also be helpful.

Osler-Weber-Rendu Syndrome

Also called hereditary hemorrhagic telangiectasia, this autosomally dominant syndrome is characterized by the formation of vascular lesions around the lips, oral cavity, and nose. One of the most common presenting manifestations is recurring epistaxis that requires multiple transfusions. Septal dermoplasty is one method designed to control the repeated epistaxis. The operative procedure involves careful removal of the mucosa of the anterior nasal septum, floor of the nose, and anterior portion of the inferior turbinate and replacement of this mucosa with a split-thickness skin graft (Fig. 12–13). The procedure is usually performed on one side only but may be repeated later on the opposite side. While it creates crust formation in the nose, it may be necessary in patients who have required multiple transfusions. Hormonal therapy has provided improvement for some patients, allowing them to avoid surgical intervention.

Recurring epistaxis occurs frequently in Osler-Weber-Rendu syndrome.

Sjögren's Syndrome

This disorder, consisting of dry eyes, dry mouth and nasopharynx, and a chronic arthritis, may also have some nasal manifestations. It is covered more fully in Chapter 17.

EPISTAXIS

Nasal hemorrhage is such a common problem that every physician should be prepared to handle the majority of such episodes. The keystone to proper treatment is the application of pressure to the bleeding vessel. Probably 90

Every physician should be able to control most episodes of epistaxis.

FIGURE 12–13. Septal dermoplasty. Nasal mucosa with numerous telangiectasias in Osler-Weber-Rendu disease can be replaced through (a) a lateral rhinotomy and (b) intranasal skin grafts when medical management fails.

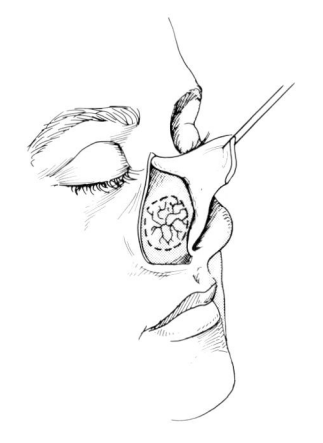

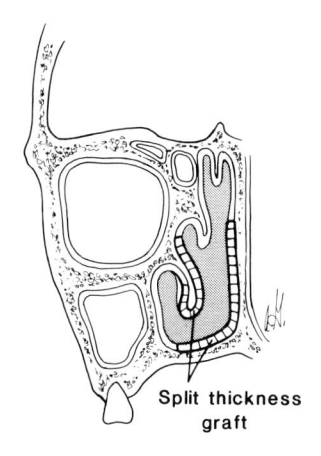

Split thickness graft

per cent of episodes of anterior epistaxis are easily treated by firm, continuous pressure applied to both sides of the nose just superior to the nasal alar cartilages, with the patient sitting in an upright position. This position reduces the vascular pressure, and the patient can more easily expectorate any blood in the pharynx. However, when it becomes apparent that control is not adequate, the patient's physician needs immediately to try another method. Only those methods available to the physician which can be applied to the majority of persistent cases of epistaxis will be dealt with here in detail. Other methods will be mentioned briefly.

Epistaxis—A Sign, Not a Disease

A brief, concise history and physical examination are obtained at the same time preparations are being made to control the epistaxis. Once the bleeding is stopped, an orderly evaluation is begun to determine the cause. A more complete history and physical examination, laboratory evaluations, routine x-ray examinations, and even angiography may be necessary at this time.

Blood Supply of the Nose

A detailed explanation of the vascular and nerve supply of the nose has been given in Chapter 10. Vessels are mentioned in this chapter only as they affect the site and control of active bleeding. Initially, one must note whether the bleeding source is on the right or the left side, in the front or the posterior part of the nose, and above or below the middle meatus, which roughly divides the blood supply from the two major contributors, the internal and external carotid arteries. The ophthalmic artery, deriving from the internal carotid artery, gives rise to the anterior and posterior ethmoid vessels. Together they supply the superior portion of the nose. The rest of the nasal vascular supply comes from the external carotid artery and its major divisions. The sphenopalatine artery brings blood to the lower half of the lateral nasal wall and the posterior part of the septum.

The ethmoid arteries are branches of the internal carotid.

All nasal vessels are connected by multiple anastomoses. A vascular plexus along the anterior portion of the cartilaginous septum incorporates many of these anastomoses and is referred to as Little's area or Kiesselbach's plexus (Fig. 12–14). Because of its vascular features and the fact that this area is subject to repeated physical and environmental trauma, it is the most frequent site for epistaxis.

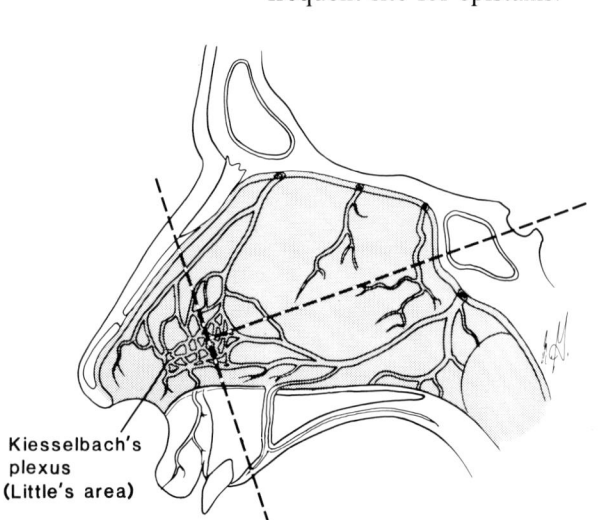

FIGURE 12–14. Blood supply of the nasal septum. Epistaxis originating superiorly in the nose usually originates from the ethmoid artery system, while posterior and inferior bleeding is from the internal maxillary artery and its branches. Kiesselbach's plexus is the most common site of bleeding and is fed from several vascular sources.

Kiesselbach's plexus (Little's area)

Management

History

Proper management of epistaxis will depend on a careful history. Important items include the following:

1. Previous bleeding episodes
2. Side of bleeding
3. Whether the flow of bleeding is primarily down the throat (posterior) or out the front of the nose (anterior) when the patient is sitting
4. Duration and frequency
5. Bleeding tendency
6. Familial history of bleeding disorders
7. Hypertension
8. Diabetes mellitus
9. Liver disease
10. Use of anticoagulants
11. Recent nasal trauma
12. Drugs, e.g., aspirin, phenylbutazone (Butazolidin)

Recurrent Minor Epistaxis

When first seen, the patient may not be actively bleeding but may give a history of recurrent epistaxis over the past few weeks. There have usually been several small episodes, but the last episode may have been frightening, causing the patient to seek help.

Nasal examination in this situation may reveal prominent vessels traversing the anterior septum, with small amounts of clotted blood noted in this area. Such vessels may be treated by chemical cauterization or electrocautery. The application of a topical anesthetic and vasoconstricting agent, such as 4 per cent cocaine solution or Xylocaine with epinephrine, is followed by cauterizing, for example, with a 50 per cent solution of trichloroacetic acid on the vessel (Fig. 12–15). If the vessels are prominent on both sides of the

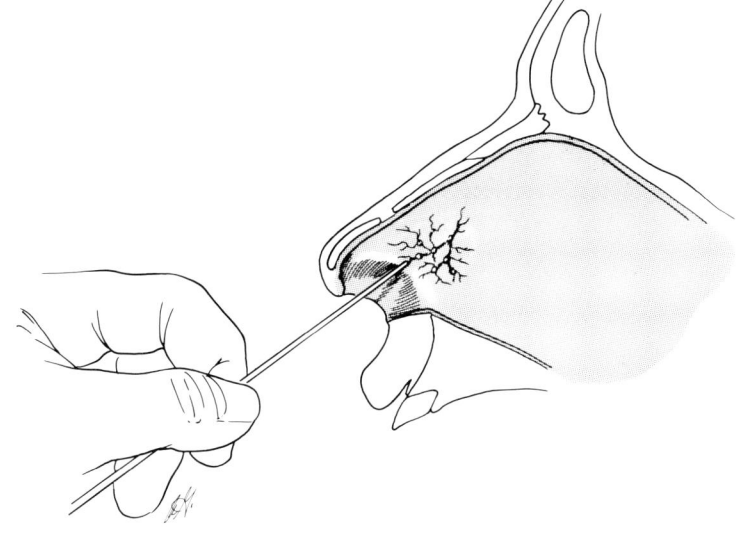

FIGURE 12–15. Nasal cautery. Superficial vessels can be chemically or electrically cauterized after a topical anesthetic has been applied.

Avoid cauterizing both sides of the septum.

septum, an effort should be made not to cauterize the same area on both sides. Even with very shallow penetration of the cauterizing agent, the surface area covered by cautery must be limited. Otherwise, as cilia are destroyed and squamous epithelium overlying scar tissue replaces normal respiratory mucosa, stowage points in the flow of the mucous blanket develop. As the flow of mucus slows or stops in those areas of previous cautery, crusts form on the septum. The patient then picks his nose to remove the crusts, injuring the lining, setting off a new nosebleed, and completing the vicious circle by returning to the doctor for another attempt at cautery.

Shallow penetration is also obtained with silver nitrate, which is fairly useful in children. Deeper penetration may be obtained with beads of chromic acid and even electrocautery. During very active bleeding, no method of cauterization of the nose is effective or safe. Repeated bleeding from a blood vessel over the septum may be resolved by locally elevating the mucosa and letting the tissues realign themselves or by reconstructing the underlying septal deformity to relieve the localized atrophy and mucosal tension spots.

With recurrent minor nosebleeds of unidentified nasal origin, the physician must rule out nasopharyngeal or paranasal sinus tumors that erode blood vessels. Chronic sinusitis is another possible cause. Finally, one should look for distant pathologic disturbances such as renal disease and uremia or systemic illness such as a coagulation disorder.

Active Anterior Hemorrhage—Minor

The patient who is actively bleeding from the front of the nose should be sitting upright and wearing a plastic apron and holding a kidney basin to protect clothing. Cotton pledgets moistened with 4 per cent cocaine are gently inserted into the nose. The physician, with head mirror on and a nasal speculum in one hand, holds a suction tip in the other for aspirating excess blood. Once the bleeding source is located, cautery may be tried if the vessel is small; otherwise, an anterior nasal pack is applied—unilateral if possible, bilateral in the face of severe bleeding or a poorly defined source of bleeding. The problem of localization of the bleeding source may be compounded in a patient with a marked septal deviation or a septal perforation. Packing is most easily made from sterile 72 × ½-inch Vaseline-impregnated gauze strips, layered from the nasal floor toward the nasal roof and extending throughout most of the length of the nasal cavity (Fig. 12–16). Prophylactic antibiotics are recommended by some physicians because the sinus ostia are obstructed by the packing, and a foreign body is present (the packing) along with the old blood, which provides an environment for bacterial growth. In addition, some physicians also impregnate the packing material with antibiotic cream or ointment to minimize bacterial growth and reduce odor formation. Nasal balloons of several different designs are now available and can be substituted for the nasal pack (Fig. 12–17). Similarly, nasal tampons that expand when placed in the nose can be substituted for a traditional nasal pack (Fig. 12–18). Both the balloons and nasal tampons are easier to place than are traditional packing materials and are better tolerated by most patients; however, they may not be as effective in controlling the bleeding and may need to be replaced by a traditional pack. With only an anterior nasal pack and no other underlying medical problem, the patient

An anterior nasal pack should fill the entire nasal fossa.

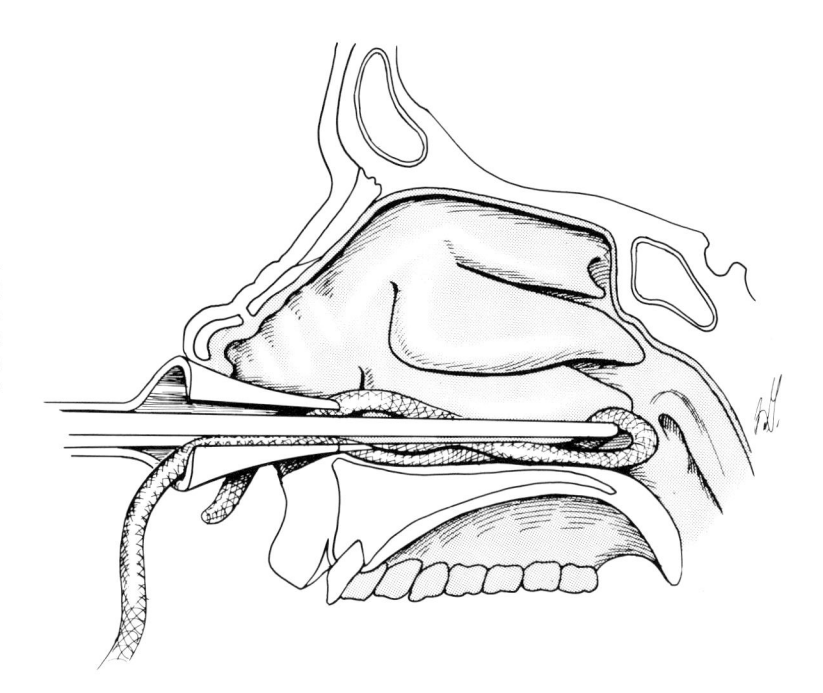

FIGURE 12–16. Anterior nasal packing. Layers of Vaseline-impregnated gauze are placed in the nose. It is important that the ends of the gauze be retained at the nares and that the packing be carefully layered and extend to the posterior choanae.

can be treated on an outpatient basis, being told to sit still most of the day and to slightly elevate the head at night. The pack may then be removed in the office after two to three days. Elderly or debilitated patients should be hospitalized.

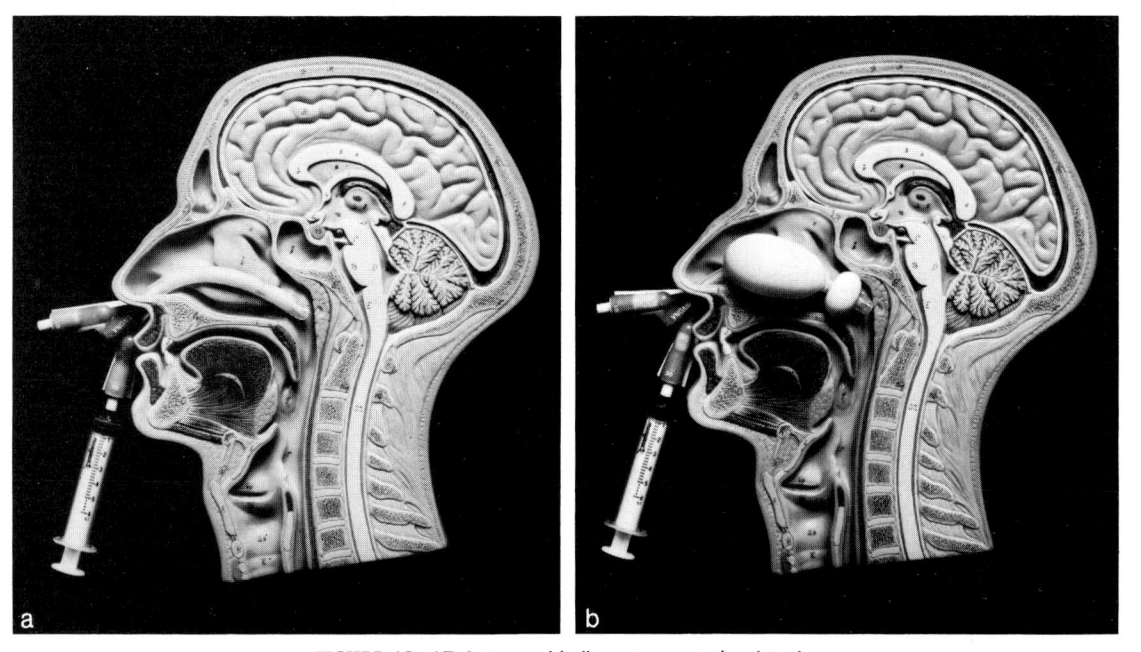

FIGURE 12–17. Intranasal balloon to control epistaxis.

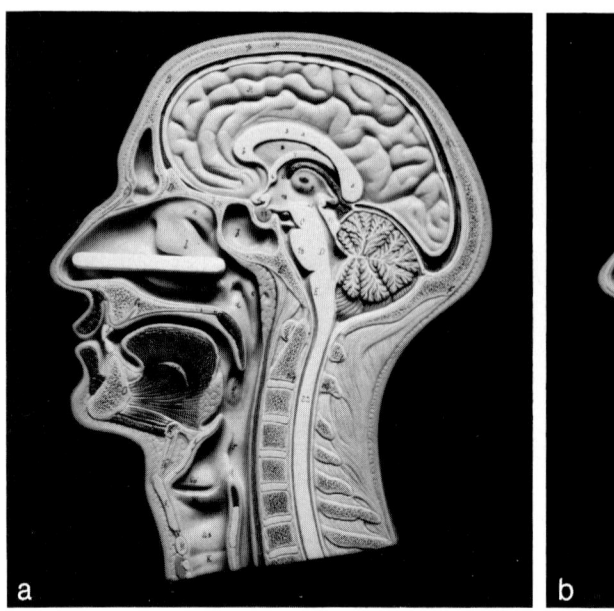

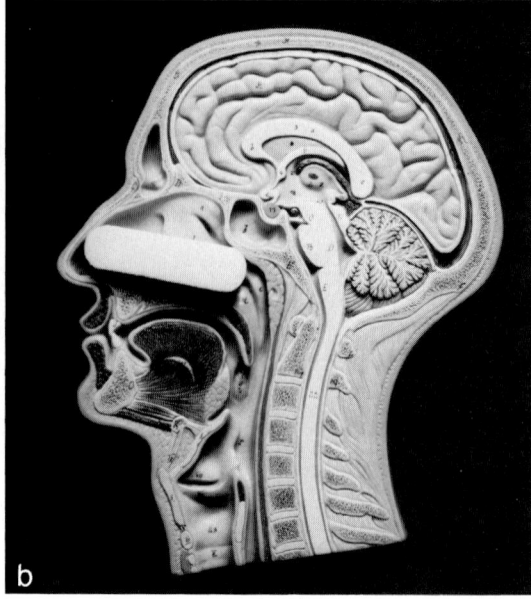

FIGURE 12–18. Intranasal tampons. A, Compressed tampon in nose. B, Tampon expanded to control hemorrhage.

Active Posterior Hemorrhage

Posterior epistaxis is believed to exist when (1) the majority of the blood loss is occurring into the pharynx, (2) an anterior pack fails to control the hemorrhage, or (3) it is evident from nasal examination that the hemorrhage is posterior and superior. This situation occurs commonly in elderly individuals who may have arteriosclerosis but may also occur in anyone after severe nasal trauma.

Sphenopalatine Ganglion Block. In the presence of posterior epistaxis some physicians recommend that a sphenopalatine block be given, which can be both diagnostic and therapeutic. Careful injection of 0.5 ml of Xylocaine, 1 per cent, with epinephrine, 1:100,000, into the greater palatine canal will cause vasoconstriction of the sphenopalatine artery. In addition to vasoconstriction, this injection provides anesthesia for the placement of a posterior nasal pack. Should the blood loss be from a division of the sphenopalatine artery, a decrease in the epistaxis will be noted within a few minutes. This decrease in bleeding may last only a short time until the Xylocaine is absorbed. Glycerin (2 per cent USP) and Xylocaine (2 per cent) can be injected for a more prolonged effect. When no effect is obtained from injection, the blood loss may be from the anterior or posterior ethmoid arteries. Because of possible ocular complications, this method is better reserved for the specialist.

Posterior Nasal Pack. A posterior pack placed through the mouth (Fig. 12–19) can be pulled by a catheter through the nose into the posterior choana. A 4- × 4-inch sponge rolled tightly and tied with No. 1 silk sutures makes an excellent pack. A topical antibiotic ointment is applied to reduce the incidence of infection. Tamponade by various commercially available preshaped nasal balloons passed anteriorly and then inflated is also possible.

FIGURE 12–19. Posterior choanal packing combined with an anterior nasal pack. *A*, Rubber catheter directed posteriorly through the nose and drawn into the mouth; two of the three strings attached to the pack are tied to the catheter, which is drawn back through the nose, pulling the pack securely into the postnasal position, *B*, Bilateral anterior pack of one-half inch Vaseline gauze impregnated with an antibiotic ointment is layered into position. *C*, Two strings attached to the posterior pack are tied firmly over a large 4- × 4-inch sponge. To facilitate the removal of the pack, a third string left attached to the postchoanal pack is brought out of the mouth or a short length is allowed to hang down into the pharynx.

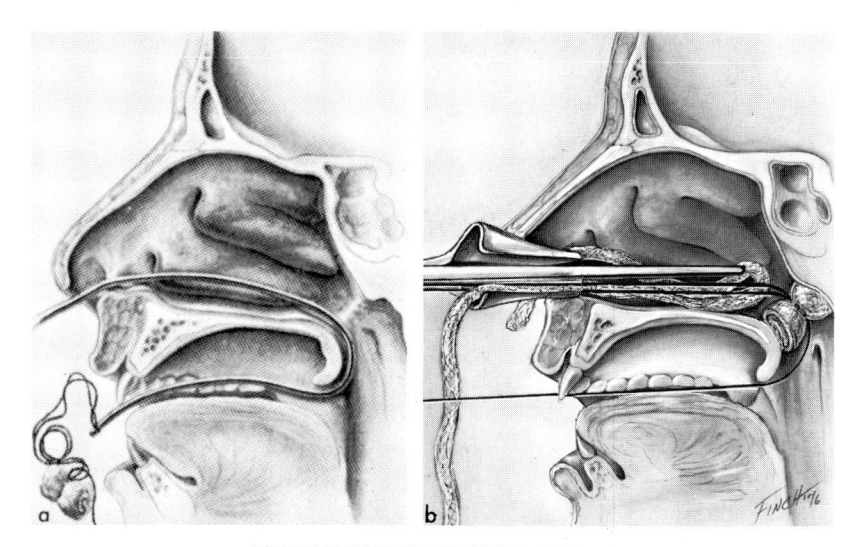

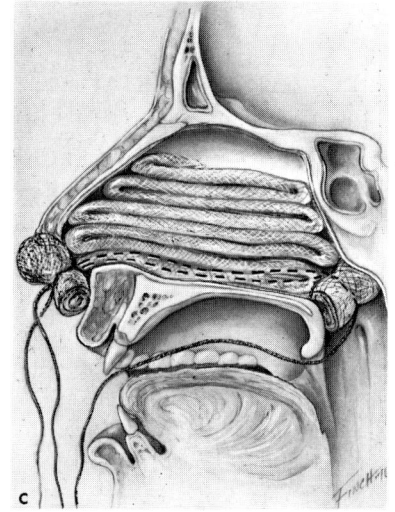

Some manufacturers make balloons with two separate chambers; one functions as an anterior pack, the other as a posterior pack. If a balloon is placed either anteriorly or posteriorly, it should be filled with saline, not air, because air will leak out and the tamponade will be lost. The common No. 14 Foley catheter with a 15-cc bag can also be inserted transnasally, inflated, and pulled firmly into the posterior choana. It can be secured in position with a padded umbilical clamp.

Most commonly, a catheter is passed all the way through the nose, grasped in the pharynx, and pulled out through the mouth. Two strings attached to a pack are tied to the catheter, which now protrudes through the mouth. A third string also attached to the pack will be allowed to lie in the pharynx to be utilized as a pullout string. The catheters are pulled out the anterior nose to position the pack in the choana. If necessary, the pack can be assisted into position above the soft palate by the physician's finger. The pack should be pulled firmly into position and should not depress the soft palate. While tension is held on the strings protruding from the anterior

The strings of a posterior pack should not be tied across the columella.

nose, the physician places the usual anterior pack between them and ties the two strings snugly in a bow over a roll of gauze. Both strings should be brought out through the same nostril and not tied over the columella—this can cause pressure necrosis of the soft tissues, a very unsightly deformity that is difficult to correct.

Patients with a posterior pack are admitted to the hospital.

Patients requiring a posterior pack are admitted to the hospital, with elderly patients or patients with underlying medical diseases placed in the intensive care unit. Consideration should include the following items when the patient is admitted:

1. Frequent monitoring of vital signs, including blood pressure, pulse, and respiration
2. Electrocardiogram (in a patient with significant medical illness, continuous monitoring with a cardiac monitor)
3. Use of oxygen as necessary (with caution in chronic obstructive lung disease) because of the possibility of complications secondary to sedation, acute blood loss, and a fall in arterial P_{O_2} associated with the pack
4. Monitoring of blood arterial gases
5. Hemoglobin and hematocrit at least every 12 hours
6. Studies (PT, PTT, platelet count) for any bleeding abnormality
7. All tests necessary to perform a sufficient medical evaluation of any possible underlying cause of the occurrence of the epistaxis, such as FBS, BUN, or creatinine
8. Intravenous fluids should be administered, as these patients will have a poor oral intake.
9. Pain medication, usually meperidine hydrochloride (Demerol) or codeine. (It is important to provide significant sedation and analgesia without causing respiratory depression.)
10. Clear liquid diet
11. Examination of the pharynx for active bleeding
12. Head elevated 45 degrees
13. Prophylactic broad-spectrum antibiotics because of interrupted drainage patterns from nose and sinuses
14. Type and cross-match for blood if significant blood loss has occurred

Hypoxia and hypercapnia are common when a posterior pack is present.

The posterior pack is generally kept in place for three to five days. During this period of time, the patient will be uncomfortable and will require sedatives and analgesics. Studies have shown that complete obstruction of the nasal airway in certain individuals may lead to an elevation of the P_{CO_2} and reduction of the P_{O_2}. This combination of events in a patient with a history of significant cardiac or pulmonary disease can lead to significant complications, e.g., myocardial infarction or cerebrovascular accident. It is often advisable to loosen a traditional pack or deflate a balloon prior to complete removal. If bleeding redevelops the tamponade can be re-established with less discomfort than if the packing needs to be replaced.

Specific Vessel Ligation

When posterior and anterior packs fail to control epistaxis, ligation of specific arteries is required. These include the external carotid artery, the internal maxillary artery with the terminal branch, the sphenopalatine artery, and the anterior and posterior ethmoidal arteries.

Ligation of the External Carotid Artery. Because of the numerous anastomoses present, ligation of the external carotid artery does not always control epistaxis. It is, however, a method that can be employed when necessary in almost all patients by physicians skilled in head and neck surgery. A transverse or longitudinal incision is made along the anterior border of the sternocleidomastoid muscle at the level of the hyoid bone. After elevation of the platysma muscle, the anterior border of the sternocleidomastoid muscle is identified. By gentle dissection, the carotid sheath, jugular vein, and vagus nerve can be identified. Further dissection will permit visualization of the carotid bulb. The internal and external carotid arteries must be specifically identified. Although named the external carotid artery, in the neck it actually lies medial to the internal carotid artery. Ligation is then performed by a single silk ligature above the level of the take-off of the lingual artery. The disappearance of temporal pulse should be verified as a double check before firming up the ligature. The wound may be closed in layers and a drain left in place for 24 hours.

Ligation of the external carotid artery is less effective than other techniques.

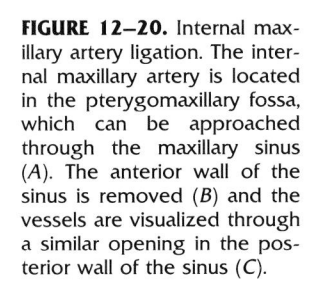

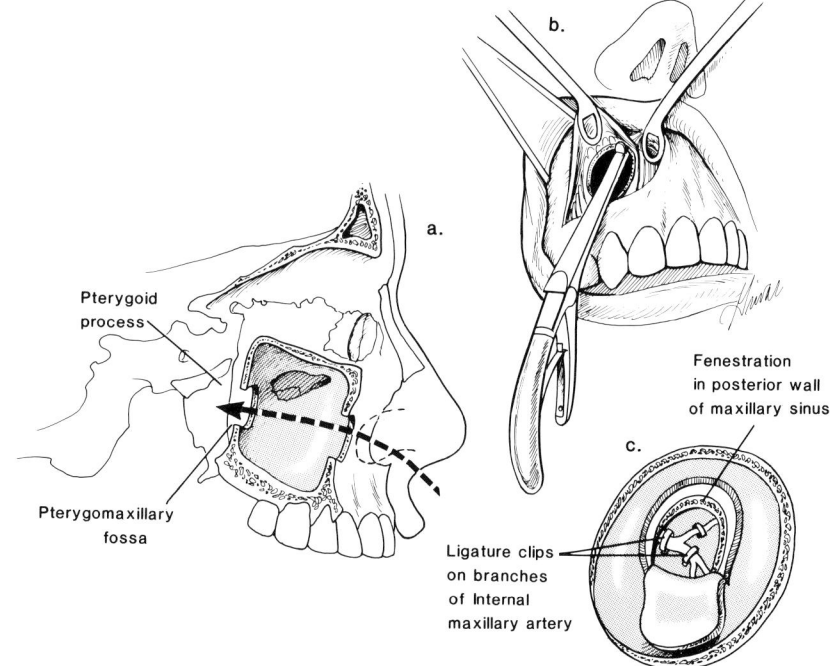

Ligation of the Internal Maxillary Artery. Ligation of the internal maxillary artery is generally performed by those skilled in the anatomical and surgical technique required to gain access to the pterygomaxillary fossa. This procedure may be performed under local or general anesthesia. Radiographs of the paranasal sinuses are obtained prior to the procedure. A Caldwell incision is made in the upper buccal gingival mucosa, extending from the midline to the area of the second maxillary molar. The mucoperiosteum is elevated from the anterior wall of the maxillary sinus, the maxillary sinus is entered, and the remaining anterior wall is removed while care is taken to preserve the infraorbital nerve. The bony posterior sinus wall is then carefully removed and the opening enlarged into the pterygomaxillary fossa. When the opening is sufficiently large, the operating microscope is employed for

FIGURE 12–20. Internal maxillary artery ligation. The internal maxillary artery is located in the pterygomaxillary fossa, which can be approached through the maxillary sinus (A). The anterior wall of the sinus is removed (B) and the vessels are visualized through a similar opening in the posterior wall of the sinus (C).

further dissection. Vessels are identified and metal clips placed on the internal maxillary, sphenopalatine, and descending palatine arteries (Fig. 12–20). The wound is closed and the posterior nasal pack removed. A lesser anterior nasal pack may still be required. If there is any evidence of an infection or fear that infection may develop, a nasal antral window is created during the procedure. Selective catheterization with embolization of branches of the external carotid artery is another approach that achieves the same objective as ligation.

Embolization is an alternative to ligation.

Ligation of the Anterior Ethmoid Artery. Hemorrhage from terminal branches of the ophthalmic artery occasionally requires ligation of the anterior ethmoid artery. The vessel is approached through a curved incision extending along the nose, midway between the dorsum and the medial canthal area. This incision is carried directly down to the bone, with the periosteum carefully elevated and the medial canthal ligament identified. The anterior ethmoidal artery always lies in the suture line between the ethmoid and frontal bone. A single ligature or hemostatic clip is applied to the vessel (Fig. 12–21). Because of the close approximation to the optic nerve, the ethmoid vessels are approached with care and gentle retraction on the globe.

Epistaxis Associated with Nasal Trauma

Epistaxis routinely occurs after any nasal and/or septal nasal fracture, is usually of short duration, and stops spontaneously. Occasionally such epi-

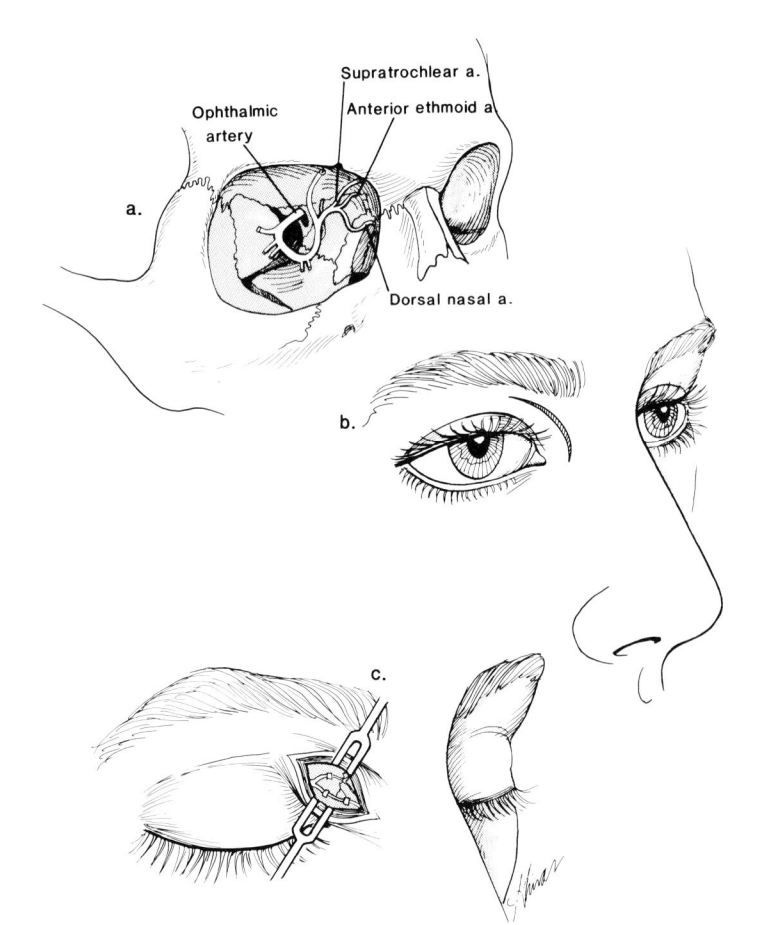

FIGURE 12–21. Ligation of the anterior ethmoid artery. *A,* The anterior ethmoid artery, a branch of the ophthalmic artery, is shown exiting the orbit at the level of the suture line between the ethmoid and frontal bones. *B,* The artery is exposed through an incision line beneath the brow and over the nasal bone. *C,* After the orbital contents are retracted, the artery is ligated with metallic clips. Occasionally ligation of both the anterior and posterior ethmoid arteries is necessary.

staxis begins again several hours later. It may, in fact, develop several days later in a nonreduced fracture when the swelling begins to subside. The best treatment in such circumstances is an immediate reduction of the nasal fracture. Failure to control the hemorrhage after fracture reduction may require any one of the various vessel ligation procedures previously described. If the septum has been fractured, the treating physician should investigate the area to rule out a septal hematoma.

Epistaxis Associated with Specific Bleeding Disorders

Epistaxis is frequently encountered in patients with hereditary hemorrhagic telangiectasia, a dominant syndrome characterized by the formation of vascular lesions around the lips, oral cavity, and nose. One of the most common presenting manifestations is recurring nasal epistaxis requiring multiple transfusions. Septal dermoplasty is one method designed to control the repeated epistaxis. The operative procedure involves careful removal of the mucosa of the anterior nasal septum, floor of the nose, and anterior portion of the inferior turbinate and replacement of this mucosa with a split-thickness skin graft. The procedure is usually performed on one side only but may be repeated later on the opposite side. While it creates crust formation in the nose, it may be necessary in patients who have required multiple transfusions.

When epistaxis occurs in patients with hemophilia, von Willebrand's disease, or other coagulopathies, it is generally best treated as conservatively as possible. This will involve placement of an anterior nasal pack when necessary with the concurrent transfusions of cryoprecipitated plasma, Factor VIII, or other clotting factors.

Epistaxis in Patients with Leukemia

Patients with acute or chronic leukemia or multiple myeloma, especially in the advanced stages, have repeated bouts of epistaxis due either to the basic disease process or to the treatment. Because severe infections develop more readily in these patients, the prolonged use of anterior and posterior nasal packing should be avoided. Although less dependable, topical thrombin on hemostatic substances such as Oxycel cotton or Gelfoam might be tried first. Even with only anterior packing of gauze, systemic antibiotics should be given. Correction of any underlying clotting defect, such as administration of platelet packs, should be performed simultaneously.

TRAUMA

Nasal fractures, along with other maxillofacial injuries, are discussed fully in Chapter 26. However, it is important to note here that nasal trauma is a frequent cause of nasal obstruction.

Although the patient may recall the incident leading to current obstructive symptoms, childhood injuries that are not remembered may have previously created significant anatomic alteration and obstruction. Moreover, what may have appeared to the patient or treating physician to be a "minor" injury can create enough deformity to be functionally significant.

Post-traumatic septal deformities are common sources of nasal obstruction.

The most common structural disturbance causing airway obstruction is a deflected or deviated nasal septum (Fig. 12–22). The normally straight

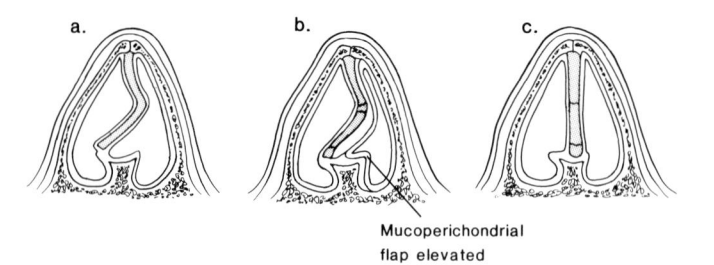

FIGURE 12–22. Septal deformity and septoplasty. *A*, A typical septal deformity is shown with deflection of the septum compromising both nasal fossae. *B*, Surgical correction is achieved by elevating the mucoperichondrium and excising deformed septal bone and cartilage, followed by replacing the septum in the midline. *C*, An adequate airway is re-created.

Minor trauma can cause significant septal deformities.

midline structure has, in almost all instances, been affected by trauma with its direct and indirect sequelae. Injuries to an individual during growth and development have more of an impact than similar insults suffered by an adult. The physiologic effect of the deformity depends not only on its relative structural complexity but also on its location. Moreover, other nasal pathology such as allergies, infections, neoplasm, or metabolic disorders can temporarily, recurrently, or permanently add to the severity of the obstructive symptoms. The injury may create a septal hematoma due to the collection of blood beneath the mucoperichondrium. The patient usually complains of severe obstruction, and intranasal inspection reveals boggy septal mucosa that does not shrink following application of topical decongestants. Immediate drainage is necessary, often followed by nasal packing to avoid the development of a septal abscess, as mentioned earlier in this chapter.

The structure of the external nose, both cartilaginous and bony portions, may be likened to a "pyramid" or a "tent" with a central support, the septum. Injuries may cause obstruction through one or more of the following mechanisms:

1. Collapse of the side wall medially, thus narrowing one nasal fossa (Fig. 12–23*A* and *B*). The fracture of a nasal bone often carries the attached upper lateral cartilage medially, resulting in obstruction.
2. Displacement of the septum. Unilateral displacement narrows one passage and enlarges the other, causing unilateral obstruction. Bilateral obstruction results if the septal fracture causes fragments to be displaced into each nasal fossa.
3. Fracture and displacement of both the nasal vault and septum, deviating the "pyramid." The fractures apparent on magnitude of the obstruction is dependent upon the degree of obstruction resulting from each component of the injury (Fig. 12–23*C*).

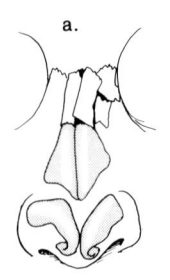

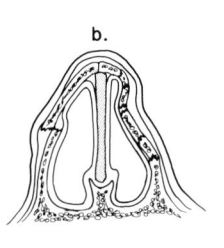

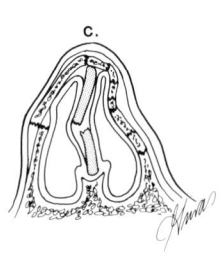

FIGURE 12–23. A nasal fracture is usually a comminuted and compound fracture that involves the nasal bones and ascending process of the maxilla. Often the upper lateral cartilage is displaced as well owing to its attachment to the nasal bone. *B*, Typically one nasal wall is displaced medially, narrowing the nasal airway, while the opposite wall is displaced laterally. *C*, Frequently the nasal septum is fractured as well as the nasal bones, further compromising the airway.

Because the cosmetic component, or external deformity, associated with a septal fracture is usually minor, the fracture often goes unnoticed. Because radiographs are of little use in detecting an injury of this sort, a thorough evaluation must include intranasal inspection and palpation before and after application of topical decongestants.

Septal fractures are rarely apparent on radiographs.

It is better, after acute injuries involving the septum, to perform an "open reduction"—namely, to explore the intraseptal space and return the fragments to their normal anatomic position—than to let the septum heal with any of the above-mentioned deformities and plan on a delayed septal reconstruction.

The results of closed nasal reduction are considered inadequate if any concomitant septal fracture is not addressed, because the septal deformity will cause persistent obstruction and result in redeviation of the external "tent" as the tissues heal. In essence, the "tent pole," the septum, will cause the "tent" to shift back to the preoperative position. The surgical procedure is reconstructive, not just aesthetic, and the cosmetic improvement is necessary if function is to be restored.

Deformity of the septum to one side of the midline often evokes a compensatory hypertrophy of the middle and inferior turbinates in the opposite nasal space (the wide side). After the septum is surgically straightened the hypertrophied soft tissues recede, and, in most instances, no further attention is needed for the turbinate. Gross or persistent hypertrophy may require reducing the size of the turbinate with electrocautery, cryosurgery, or partial resection (see Fig. 12–11). Aggressive reduction should be avoided to prevent iatrogenic atrophic rhinitis.

Surgery to correct obstructive septal injuries in children warrants gentle handling and conservative techniques. However, because of the potential for greater damage as changes occur with growth, children should not be denied needed surgical corrections on the basis of age.

Septal and nasal reconstruction are usually performed on an outpatient basis via incisions inside the nose. The adult is normally sedated and a local anesthetic applied to the area, although general anesthesia is preferred by some surgeons. When general anesthesia is used, as in small children, the patient is also given a local anesthetic to minimize the total amount of anesthetic agent needed and for the decongestant effect, which markedly reduces bleeding and therefore provides better operative visualization. Postoperative swelling normally resolves after several weeks, thus restoring the nasal airway.

NEOPLASMS

Neoplasms involving the nose and paranasal sinuses are discussed together owing to the intimate relationship of these structures. As a result of the diverse histologic make-up of the nose and paranasal sinuses, the variety of neoplasms that may occur is great. However, because most are found very infrequently, only those that are encountered with any regularity or are of special interest will be presented here. Malignant tumors are covered in Chapter 23.

Nasal neoplasms occur infrequently.

It is important for the physician to remember that the symptoms due to neoplasms of the nose and paranasal sinuses are not striking, the most common including nasal obstruction, epistaxis, and blood-tinged mucus. A nasal speculum is used to provide adequate examination of the nasal cavity, both before and after administration of either phenylephrine or a dilute cocaine solution. A mirror or other optical instrument is necessary to visualize the posterior choanae and nasopharynx.

Symptoms of nasal neoplasms are nonspecific.

While these steps will provide the physician with the location of abnormal tissue, imaging techniques such as radiographs, tomograms, computed tomographic (CT) scans, and magnetic resonance imaging (MRI) help determine the extent of the disease, whether surgery is a viable option, and, if so, the appropriate surgical approach.

Squamous Papilloma

Possibly of viral etiology, epithelial changes in squamous papilloma may range through various degrees of dyskeratosis. Lesions are often noted at the mucocutaneous junction in the anterior nose, especially on the anterior caudal margin of the septum. For both diagnosis and treatment the lesions are excised under local anesthesia. As most of them are small, no sutures are needed. Before closure of the larger ones, it is well to undermine skin and mucosa for a short distance.

Inverted Papilloma

Inverted papilloma may resemble a common nasal polyp but may contain areas of carcinoma.

A separate disorder from squamous papilloma, inverted papilloma inverts into the surface epithelium. Peculiar to the nose and paranasal sinuses, most originate on the lateral nasal wall and appear to be grossly similar to a typical nasal polyp. Although histologically benign, this neoplasm is aggressively treated like a premalignant tumor for two reasons: (1) locally invasive, at times it involves extensive bone erosion, and, if conservatively removed, shows a high incidence of local recurrence; and (2) focal areas of squamous cell carcinoma are found within the papilloma in approximately 10 per cent of the cases. It is therefore essential that the pathologist section the entire surgical specimen and look for islands of malignancy.

Treatment consists of wide surgical excision, with the selected approach having the capability of further extension to provide wide exposure to the paranasal sinuses when required. The most often chosen route is a lateral rhinotomy approach, which starts with an incision in the nasal-alar fold and can be carried upward along the nasal-facial groove.

Extramedullary Plasmacytoma

Evaluation for systemic disease is important.

As its name implies, extramedullary plasmacytoma is a primary tumor of lymphoid tissue histologically similar to plasma cell myeloma. It may, however, present a solitary mass confined to soft tissues. A patient with this tumor should be evaluated for possible systemic disease. Tests include serum protein electrophoresis and urinalysis for Bence Jones protein. A hematologic consultation is necessary and will generally involve a bone marrow biopsy. Solitary lesions can be treated surgically and/or with radiation therapy. Regardless of treatment, recurrences are common; therefore, all

Fibrous Dysplasia

Fibrous dysplasia refers to nonencapsulated fibro-osseous tumors involving the facial bones with frequent impingement on the paranasal sinuses of the nose (Fig. 12–24). The etiology is unknown.

A slow-growing tumor, it is rarely associated with pain and tends to appear around the time of puberty, with the patient presenting for cosmetic reasons due to facial asymmetry. Because growth of this tumor again slows with age, the need for treatment is dependent upon the degree of deformity or the presence of pain. Although complete resection is desirable owing to the slow growth of the tumor, in the majority of patients only sufficient tumor is removed to restore normal facial contours and function.

In a small proportion of patients malignant degeneration of the tumor has been reported. The majority of these reports involved patients treated with radiation for the fibrous dysplasia. It is imperative, therefore, that radiation therapy be avoided unless there are no other alternatives and that patients with fibrous dysplasia be followed closely to detect any changes.

Juvenile Nasopharyngeal Angiofibroma

Covered more fully in Chapter 17, juvenile nasopharyngeal angiofibroma is a benign tumor that often originates in the nasal chambers near the sphenopalatine foramen. This diagnosis should be considered when the patient is a young boy with a long history of epistaxis and nasal obstruction.

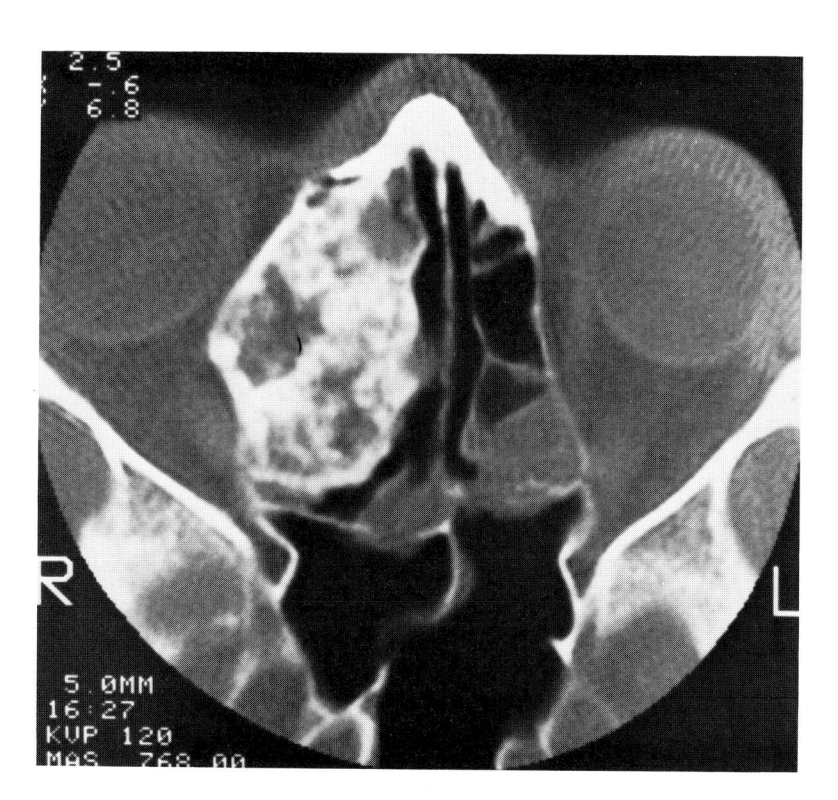

FIGURE 12–24. Fibrous dysplasia. Irregular calcification in ethmoid air cells characteristic of fibrous dysplasia.

MISCELLANEOUS

Septal Perforation

Until the advent of penicillin, tertiary lues was the most common cause of perforations of the nasal septum. As the incidence of syphilis decreased, the most common cause shifted to the large number of patients who had had excessive septal injury. Other causes include acute as well as chronic trauma like nose-picking; infected septal hematomas, tuberculosis, leprosy, and other infections; and the illicit use of cocaine, with accompanying frequent intranasal manipulation, mucous alterations, ischemia, and septal necrosis.

Nasal crusting and whistling are frequent symptoms of septal perforations.

The symptoms of nasal perforations can be annoying to the patient. There may be a whistling sensation through the nose during speech. Small perforations frequently tend to have more of a whistling sensation than very large perforations. The edges of the perforations tend to crust, resulting in obstruction. As the crusts break off, bleeding occurs (Fig. 12–25). The resultant epistaxis may be difficult to control and will require packing of both sides to apply adequate pressure.

Surgical repair is difficult.

Repair of anything other than small perforation of the nose is difficult. Both homogeneous and autogenous tissues of various types have been utilized to replace the absent cartilaginous support. The mainstay of the repair requires development of mucoperichondrial flaps, which are then swung to close the defect. A flap is developed on each side in such a manner as not to expose cartilage in the same place on the opposite side. These flaps are then sutured into position and held there by stents. Silastic prostheses that obturate the defect are an alternative to surgery and are preferred by some patients.

Foreign Bodies

Foreign bodies as a cause of nasal obstruction are practically always encountered in children. Children at play tend to place small objects in the

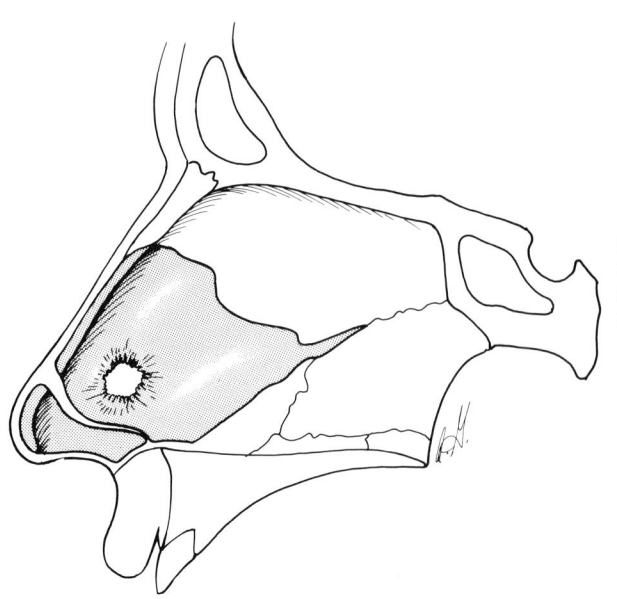

FIGURE 12–25. Septal perforation. Perforation most often occurs in the cartilaginous septum.

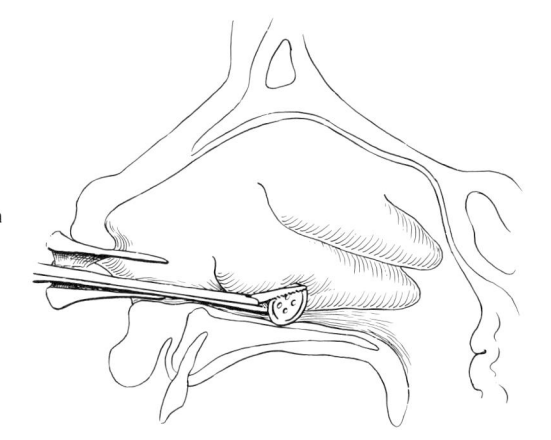

FIGURE 12–26. Removal of a foreign body by use of alligator forceps.

nasal passages. Common foreign bodies found in children are beads, buttons, erasers, marbles, peas, beans, stones, and nuts. Recently inserted objects give little or no discomfort unless they are sharp or very large. The usual symptoms are unilateral obstruction and discharge with odor. The majority of foreign objects are found either in the anterior part of the vestibule or in the inferior meatus along the floor of the nose. None should be allowed to remain in the nasal passages because of the danger of producing necrosis and secondary infection and the potential for aspiration into the lower respiratory tract. Removal can be accomplished in the cooperative child in the clinic after applying a topical anesthetic and vasoconstrictor, such as cocaine. A blunt, bent hook inserted behind the object or a small alligator forceps is helpful (Fig. 12–26). Occasionally, general anesthesia will be needed.

Foreign bodies often present as unilateral obstruction and rhinorrhea.

Rhinoliths

Rhinoliths are considered to be a special type of foreign body usually observed in adults. Insoluble salts of the nasal secretions form a calcareous mass about any long-retained foreign body or blood clot. A chronic sinus discharge may initiate such a mass to form in the nasal passages.

Rhinophyma

Rhinophyma is a red thickening of the nasal tip with hypertrophy of the sebaceous glands associated with acne rosacea. Occurring most commonly in men, its exact etiology has not yet been determined. Treatment becomes necessary when the rhinophymatous tissue causes an obvious cosmetic deformity or when the bulk of tissue compromises the airway. Surgical correction can be performed under local anesthesia. One of the more frequently used procedures is to carefully carve down the excessive tissue with a sharp blade. Reduction via dermabrasion and laser excision are also treatment options. Care is taken not to expose the underlying cartilage and to leave sufficient epithelium to permit re-epithelialization and healing. In severe cases relining with full-thickness or split-thickness skin grafts is necessary.

References

Anderson TW, et al: The effect on winter illness of large doses of vitamin C. Can Med Assoc J 111:31, 1974.

Andrewes CH: Rhinoviruses and common colds. Ann Rev Med 17:361–370, 1966.

Barton RPE: Clinical manifestations of leprous rhinitis. Ann Otol Rhinol Laryngol 85:74–82, 1976.

Bernstein L, et al: The nasal cavities. Otol Clin North Am 6:609–874, 1973.

Dykes, MH, Meier P: Ascorbic acid and the common cold. JAMA 231:1073, 1975.

Karlowski TR, et al: Ascorbic acid for the common cold. JAMA 231:1038, 1975.

Luke M, Mehrize A, Folger F, Rowe R: Chronic nasopharyngeal obstruction causing cor pulmonale. Pediatrics 37:762–768, 1966.

McDonald TJ, DeRemee RA, Kern EB, Harrison EG: Nasal manifestations of Wegener's granulomatosis. Laryngoscope 84:2101–2112, 1974.

Meyer HM: The control of viral diseases. J Pediatr 73:653, 1968.

Ogura J, Togawa K, Dammkeohler D, et al: Nasal obstruction and the mechanics of breathing. Arch Otolaryngol 83:135–150, 1966.

Pauling L: Ascorbic acid and the common cold. Scott Med J 18:1–2, 1973.

Riggs RH: Some congenital nasal anomalies including dermoid cysts. J Louisiana State Med Soc 118:1–4, 1966.

Schaeffer JP: The Nose, Paranasal Sinuses, Nasolacrimal Passageways and Olfactory Organ in Man. New York, Blakiston, 1920.

Settipane GA: Allergic rhinitis—update. Otolaryngol Head Neck Surg 94:470–475, 1986.

Sooknundun M, Deka RC, Kacker SK, Kapila K: Congenital mid-line sinus of the dorsum of the nose. Two case reports with a literature survey. J Laryngol Otol 100:1319–1322, 1986.

Stahl RH: Allergic disorders of the nose and paranasal sinuses. Otolaryngol Clin North Am 7:703–718, 1974.

Stoksted P, Neilsen J: Rhinometric measurements of the nasal passages. Ann Otol Rhinol Laryngol 66:187–197, 1957.

13
DISEASES OF THE PARANASAL SINUSES

by Peter A. Hilger, M.D.

For a physician one of the most common daily occurrences is the visit by a patient who declares that he or she has "sinus problems." The lay public blames the paranasal sinuses for more symptoms than almost any other single anatomic structure in the body. However, it is an undeniable fact that sinus infection, as we know it today, is much less frequent than in the preantibiotic era. Patients still attribute to dysfunction of the sinuses such symptoms as headache, nasal obstruction, postnasal drainage, fatigue, halitosis, and dyspepsia. Sinus disease, however, produces a set of rather characteristic symptoms which varies only with the severity of the disease and its location. It is the purpose of this chapter to describe the usual clinical picture of various acute and chronic diseases of the paranasal sinuses. The information in this chapter and in the chapters on tumors of the nose and sinuses and on diseases of the nose should clarify diagnosis of true sinus disorders and indicate the appropriate management for each.

INFLAMMATORY SINUS DISEASE

Infectious Sinusitis

General Considerations

The most important concept in dealing with sinus infection is to realize that the nose and paranasal sinuses are only a part of the total respiratory system. Diseases that can affect the bronchi and lung can also affect the nose and paranasal sinuses. In relation to the infective process, therefore, the whole of the respiratory tree with its anatomic extensions should be considered as one entity. The infection may initially affect the entire respiratory system, but in varying degrees, and the subsequent pathologic change or clinical condition is determined by the predominance of the infection in a particular area, leading to sinusitis, laryngitis, pneumonitis, and so on. This relationship between the upper and lower respiratory tracts is responsible for the so-called sinobronchial syndrome.

The sinobronchial syndrome refers to concurrent exacerbation of sinus and pulmonary disease.

The anatomy of the sinuses is described in Chapter 10; however, it is important to remember when the different sinuses develop during childhood and adolescence and, therefore, when they become susceptible to infection. The maxillary and ethmoid sinuses are present at birth and are usually the only sinuses that are involved in childhood sinusitis. The frontal sinuses start to develop from the anterior ethmoid sinuses at about 8 years of age and

The maxillary and ethmoid sinuses are the only sinuses present at birth.

become clinically important by 12 years of age, continuing to develop until 25 years of age. Acute frontal sinusitis usually occurs in young adults. In about 20 per cent of the population, the frontal sinuses are absent or only rudimentary and, therefore, of no clinical significance. The sphenoid sinus starts pneumatizing at about 8 to 10 years of age and continues developing into the late teens or early twenties.

It is well known that a great variety of physical, chemical, nervous, hormonal, and emotional factors will influence the nasal mucosa and, to a lesser extent, simultaneously affect the sinus mucosa. In general, chronic sinusitis is more common in cold, wet climates. Nutritional deficiency, fatigue, poor physical fitness, and general systemic disease are important considerations in the etiology of sinusitis. Changes in environmental factors, such as cold, heat, humidity, and dryness, as well as atmospheric pollutants, including tobacco smoke, may predispose to infection. In this list of general predisposing factors, exposure to previous infection such as the common cold must be included.

Certain local factors also may predispose to sinus disease. These factors will be described for each specific sinus infection, but, in general, consist of skeletal deformities, allergies, dental conditions, foreign bodies, and neoplasms.

The etiologic agents in sinusitis may be viral, bacterial, or fungal.

Viral. Viral sinusitis usually occurs during an upper respiratory tract infection; the viruses that commonly affect the nose and nasopharynx also affect the sinuses. The mucosa of the paranasal sinuses is contiguous with the nose, and one should expect that viral illnesses involving the nose may also extend into the sinuses.

Bacterial. The edema and loss of normal ciliary function associated with viral infections provide an environment suitable for the development of a bacterial infection. Frequently, more than one bacterium may be involved. Acute sinusitis shares many of the same causative organisms as otitis media. Those most frequently seen, in descending order of frequency, are *Streptococcus pneumoniae*, *Haemophilus influenzae*, the anaerobes, *Branhamella catarrhalis*, the alpha streptococci, *Staphylococcus aureus*, and *Streptococcus pyogenes*. During an acute phase, chronic sinusitis may be caused by the same bacteria as those involved in acute sinusitis. However, because chronic sinus disease is associated with either inadequate drainage or compromised mucociliary function, the infectious agents involved tend to be opportunistic, with a high proportion of anaerobic bacteria. As a result, routine cultures are inadequate and careful anaerobic sampling is required. Aerobic bacteria frequently seen, in decreasing order of frequency, include *Staphylococcus aureus*, *Streptococcus viridans*, *Haemophilus influenzae*, *Neisseria flavus*, *Staphylococcus epidermidis*, *Streptococcus pneumoniae*, and *Escherichia coli*. Anaerobic bacteria include *Peptostreptococcus*, *Corynebacterium*, *Bacteroides*, and *Veillonella*. Mixed infections of both aerobic and anaerobic organisms occur frequently.

Streptococcus pneumoniae is most often the cause of acute sinusitis.

Mixed infections occur frequently in chronic sinusitis.

Acute Sinusitis

Maxillary Sinusitis

Acute maxillary sinusitis usually follows a mild upper respiratory tract infection. Chronic nasal allergies, foreign bodies, and deviated nasal septum are among the most common predisposing local factors. Maxillofacial deformity, particularly cleft palate, can cause considerable problems in children. These children tend to suffer from chronic nasopharyngeal and sinus infections at a much higher rate. Dental conditions account for approximately 10 per cent of all acute maxillary sinus infections.

The symptoms of acute maxillary sinus infection consist of fever, malaise, and a vague headache that is usually relieved with simple analgesics such as aspirin. There is a feeling of fullness in the face, and pain in the teeth may be felt during sudden movements of the head, such as when going up and down stairs. Often there is some degree of characteristic dull, throbbing cheek pain with tenderness to pressure and percussion. Mucopurulent secretions may emanate from the nose and are sometimes malodorous. Frequently, an irritative, nonproductive cough is present. During acute maxillary sinusitis, physical examination may reveal pus in the nose, usually from the middle meatus, or pus or mucopurulent secretions in the nasopharynx. There is tenderness upon palpation and percussion of the maxillary sinuses. Transillumination is decreased if the sinus is full of fluid. The radiologic appearance of acute maxillary sinusitis may be that of mucosal thickening initially, followed by complete opacification of the sinus due to severe mucosal swelling or to an accumulation of fluid filling the sinus (Fig. 13–1*A*). Finally, the characteristic air-fluid level due to accumulation of pus is seen in the upright views of the maxillary sinus (Fig. 13–1*B*). Therefore, sinus radiographs should include the supine and upright views, the most advantageous for detecting maxillary sinusitis. A-mode ultrasound screening has also been mentioned as a safe, noninvasive diagnostic method. Further investigations might require a complete blood count and nasal culture. A strong word of caution must be issued with regard to interpretation of nasal cultures. Cultures from the maxillary sinus would be valid; however, this pus is loculated within a bony cavity. An anterior nasal culture, on the other

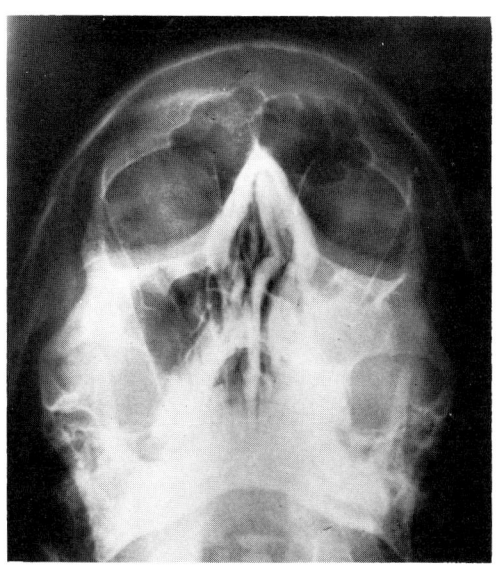

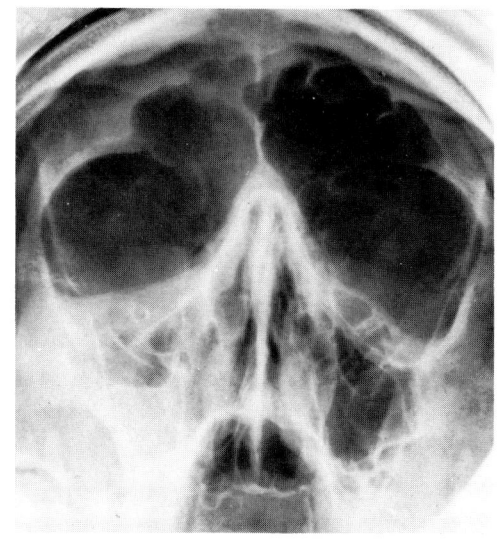

FIGURE 13–1. *A*, X-ray (Waters' view) of maxillary sinus showing an opaque sinus and a grossly deviated bony nasal septum. *B*, An x-ray view (Waters-Waldron position) of a pansinusitis involving the right maxillary, ethmoid, and frontal sinuses. There is a fluid level visible in the involved maxillary sinus.

Anterior nasal cultures are unreliable in sinusitis.

hand, will reveal all the organisms within the nasal vestibule, including the normal inhabitants, such as *Staphylococcus* and several other gram-positive cocci, which bear no relationship to the bacteria that may be causing the sinusitis. Therefore, the bacterial nasal culture taken from the anterior part of the nose is of little value in interpreting the bacteria within the maxillary sinus and may even give false information.

A culture from the posterior aspect of the nose or the nasopharynx would be much more accurate but, technically, this is extremely difficult to obtain. Specific cultures of the bacteria concerned with sinusitis are obtained using maxillary irrigation. Most frequently, an appropriate antibiotic is given to cover the more common organisms involved in this disease (*Streptococcus pneumoniae, Haemophilus influenzae,* anaerobes, *Branhamella catarrhalis*).

Acute maxillary sinusitis is generally treated with a broad-spectrum antibiotic such as amoxicillin, ampicillin or erythromycin plus sulfonimide, with other alternatives being amoxicillin/clavulanate, cefaclor, cefuroxime, and trimethoprim plus sulfonamide. Decongestants such as pseudoephedrine are useful, and potent nose drops such as phenylephrine (Neo-Synephrine) or oxymetazoline may be used during the first few days of the infection but then should be discontinued. Hot packs to the face and analgesics such as aspirin and acetaminophen are useful for symptomatic relief. The patient usually shows some signs of improvement within two days, and the disease process is often completely resolved within 10 days, although radiologic confirmation of complete resolution may take two or more weeks. Failure to resolve on active therapy would indicate either that the organisms are not sensitive to the antibiotics or that the antibiotics are failing to reach the loculated infection. In this instance, the sinus ostium may be so edematous that the sinus cannot drain freely and a true abscess is formed. In this instance, prompt antral irrigation is indicated. The route of insertion of the trocar for maxillary antral irrigation is usually beneath the inferior turbinate after initial cocainization of the mucous membrane (Fig. 13–2). An alternate route is the sublabial approach, in which a needle is passed through the gingival buccal sulcus through the incisive fossa (Fig. 13–3). Warm saline is irrigated into the maxillary antrum via this route, and the pus is flushed out through the natural ostium. Either method is acceptable, provided that the clinician has the skill and experience necessary to perform the procedure.

Radiologic changes lag behind clinical improvement.

Pus in Maxillary sinus

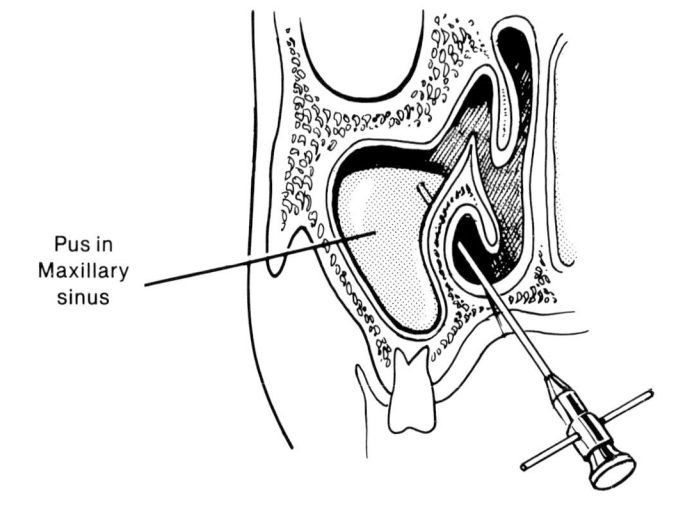

FIGURE 13–2. Antral irrigation. Purulent secretions in the maxillary sinus can be irrigated by passing a needle through the inferior meatus.

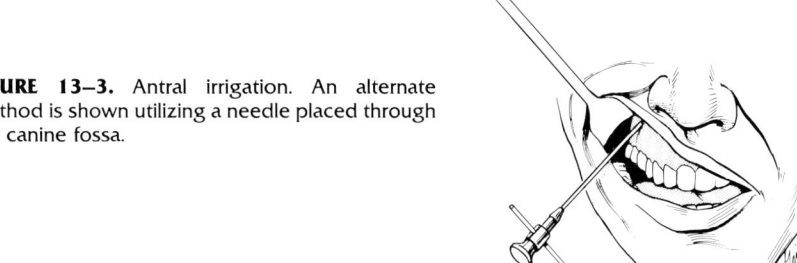

FIGURE 13–3. Antral irrigation. An alternate method is shown utilizing a needle placed through the canine fossa.

Maxillary Sinusitis of Dental Origin. This particular form of maxillary sinusitis occurs following dental problems. The most common cause is the extraction of a molar tooth, usually the first molar, during which a small piece of bone lying between the apex of the tooth and the maxillary sinus is removed (Fig. 13–4). It was Nathaniel Highmore in 1651 who described the thin membrane of bone that separates the teeth from the sinus. He stated, "The bone which encloses the maxillary antrum and which separates it from the socket of the teeth does not much exceed a piece of wrapping paper in thickness." The maxillary antrum is frequently called the antrum of Highmore. Other dental infections such as apical abscess or periodontal disease may cause a similar condition. The bacteriologic picture of sinusitis of dental origin is predominantly that of the gram-negative infection. This leads to a particularly foul-smelling pus and, consequently, foul odor from the nose. Antibiotics, irrigation of the sinus, and correction of the dental problem are the mainstays of therapy.

Dental disease is responsible for 10 per cent of sinusitis cases.

Predisposing Local Factors. Other local predisposing causes of acute maxillary sinusitis are a foreign body in the nose and a deviated nasal septum. Surgical removal of the foreign body is obviously mandatory, and surgical correction of the deviated nasal septum is usually performed after the acute phase has resolved completely. Since sinusitis may also follow packing of the nose for epistaxis, it is common practice to prescribe a prophylactic antibiotic in any nasal packing. Facial fractures can disturb the normal physiologic drainage of the sinus and lead to infection. Barotrauma causes mucosal edema and occlusion of the sinus ostium, leading to an accumulation of sinus secretions and subsequent infection.

FIGURE 13–4. Oroantral fistula and chronic suppurative maxillary sinusitis. Infection in the maxillary sinus must be resolved before closure of the fistula is feasible. Note the high position of the maxillary ostium.

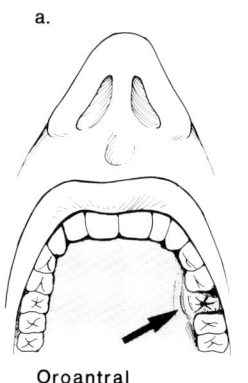

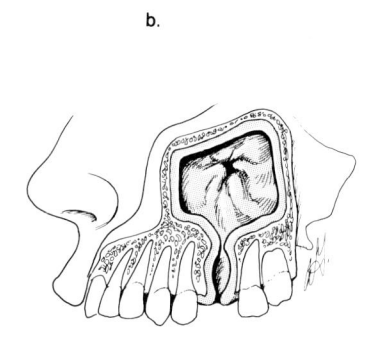

Oroantral fistula

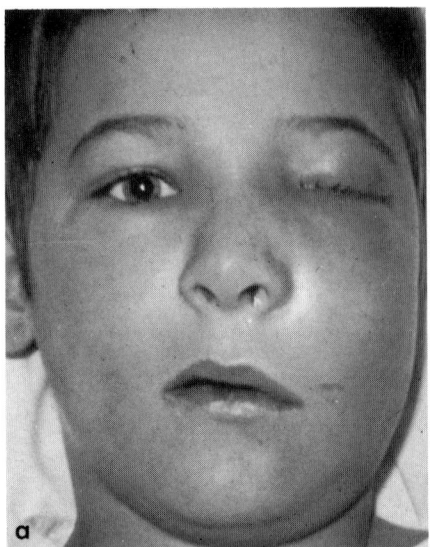

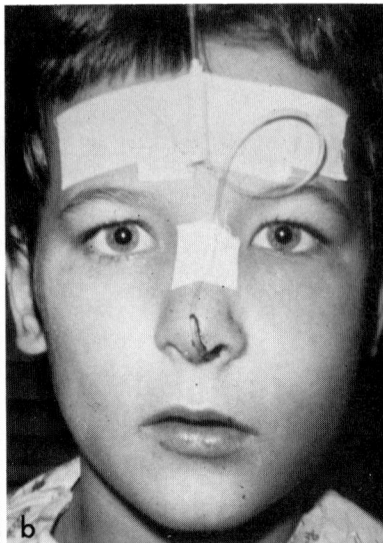

FIGURE 13–5. Complicated ethmoid sinusitis. *A,* Appearance on admission. There is a tense swelling of the left half of the face and mucopus in the left nostril. *B,* Appearance of the same child on the fifth hospital day. Swelling has almost subsided, and the catheter into the maxillary antrum is shown. (From Quick CA, Payne E: Complicated acute sinusitis. Laryngoscope 82:1253, 1972.)

Ethmoid Sinusitis

Isolated acute ethmoid sinusitis is more common in children, frequently presenting as orbital cellulitis. In adults it often accompanies maxillary sinusitis and must be regarded as an inevitable accompaniment of frontal sinusitis. Symptoms include pain and tenderness between the eyes and over the bridge of the nose, nasal drainage, and nasal obstruction. In children, the lateral wall of the ethmoid labyrinth, the lamina papyracea, is often dehiscent, and orbital cellulitis is therefore more likely to occur (Fig. 13–5). Treatment of ethmoid sinusitis involves the use of systemic antibiotics, nasal decongestants, and topical vasoconstrictor sprays and drops. Development of impending complications and inadequate improvement are indications for an ethmoidectomy (Fig. 13–6).

Frontal Sinusitis

Acute frontal sinusitis is almost always associated with anterior ethmoid infection. The frontal sinus develops from the anterior ethmoid air cells, and the tortuous frontal nasal duct runs in close relationship to these cells. The predisposing factors of acute frontal sinus infection are similar to those for other sinus infections. The disease is seen predominantly in adults, and, apart from the usual general symptoms of any infection, frontal sinusitis is

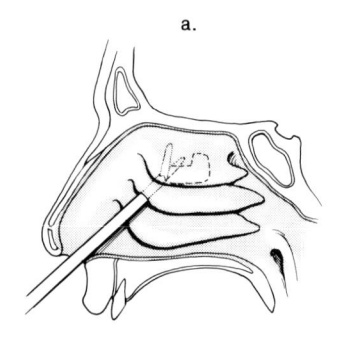

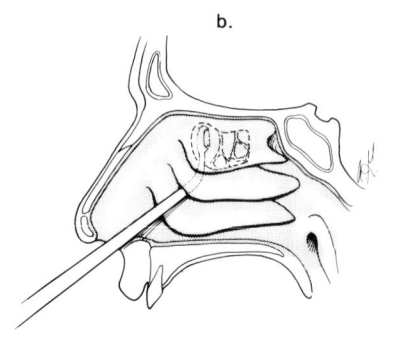

FIGURE 13–6. Intranasal ethmoidectomy. *A,* Biting forceps remove the partition between the anterior ethmoid air cells, converting them into one large cell that opens into the middle meatus. *B,* A curette can be used to accomplish the same objective.

FIGURE 13–7. Frontal sinus trephination. *A*, A small drill is used to create a hole in the thin bone of the floor of the frontal sinus. *B*, A catheter placed into the sinus allows drainage of pus and irrigation of the sinus. The catheter can be removed when the irrigant flows into the nose, demonstrating patency of the nasofrontal duct.

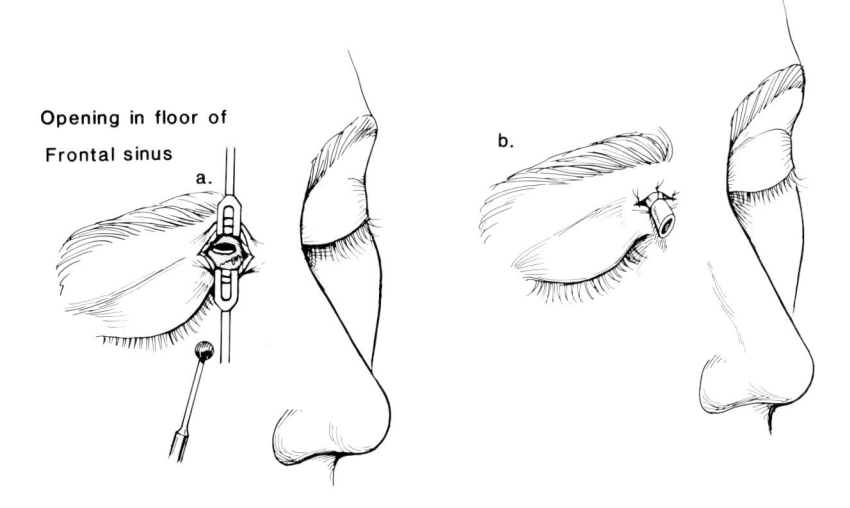

associated with a characteristic head pain. The pain is situated above the eyebrows, is present usually in the morning, becomes worse by midday, and then gradually lessens during the remainder of the waking hours. The patient will usually state that the forehead is tender to the touch, and there may be supraorbital swelling. The pathognomonic sign is excruciating tenderness to pressure and percussion over the infected sinus. Transillumination may be impaired, and sinus radiographs will confirm either periosteal thickening, generalized opacity of the sinus, or an air-fluid level. The treatment consists of appropriate antibiotics as described previously, decongestants, and vasoconstrictor nasal drops. Failure to resolve quickly or the onset of complications would require drainage by frontal sinus trephine technique (Fig. 13–7).

Sphenoid Sinusitis

Acute isolated sphenoid sinusitis is exceptionally rare. It is supposed to be characterized by headache directed to the vertex of the skull. Much more commonly, it forms part of a pansinusitis, and, therefore, its symptoms are intermingled with those of other sinus infections. Sphenoid sinus trephination was performed with some frequency in the preantibiotic era but now has become almost an extinct procedure.

Chronic Sinusitis

By definition, chronic sinusitis lasts several months or years. In acute sinusitis, pathologic changes of the mucous membrane consist of polymorphonuclear infiltrates, vascular congestion, and desquamation of the surface epithelium, all reversible changes. The pathologic picture of chronic sinusitis is complex and irreversible. The mucosa is generally thicker, thrown into folds or pseudopolyps. The surface epithelium may show areas of desquamation, regeneration, metaplasia, or simple epithelium in varying amounts on the same histologic section. Microabscess formation, granulation tissue, and healing by scar tissue are intermingled. Overall, there is a round cell and polymorphonuclear infiltrate in the submucosal layers.

The etiology and predisposing factors of chronic sinusitis are quite varied.

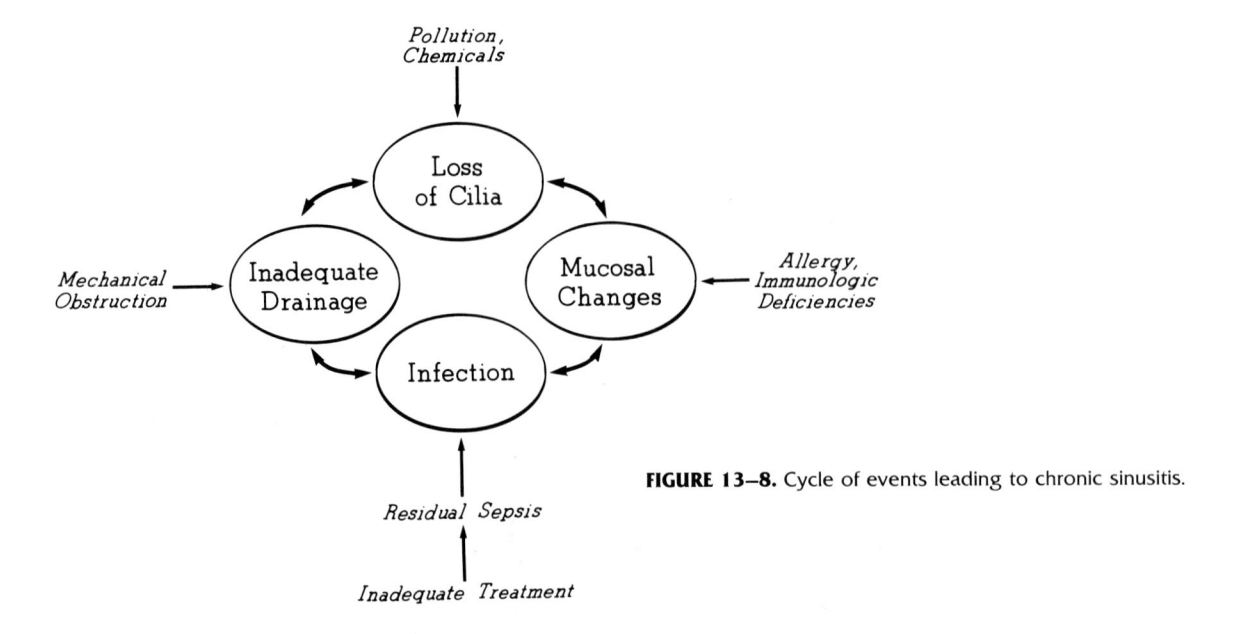

FIGURE 13–8. Cycle of events leading to chronic sinusitis.

In the preantibiotic era, chronic hyperplastic sinusitis was a result of repeated acute sinusitis with incomplete resolution. In the pathophysiology of chronic sinusitis, several factors may contribute to the recurring cycle of events (Fig. 13–8).

The mucoperiosteal lining of the paranasal sinus has a tremendous resistance to disease as well as ability to heal itself. Fundamentally, the local factors that allow healing of infected mucosa in the sinus are drainage and good ventilation. If anatomic and physiologic factors cause failure of paranasal sinus ventilation and drainage, a favorable medium exists for further infection by microaerophilic or anaerobic cocci, and a vicious circle of edema, obstruction, and infection results.

Failure to adequately treat acute or recurrent sinusitis will lead to an incomplete regeneration of the surface ciliated epithelium, resulting in a failure to remove sinus secretions and, therefore, predisposing to further infection. Drainage obstruction may also be caused by structural changes of the sinus ostium or by lesions in the nasal passages, such as adenoid hypertrophy, tumors of the nose and nasopharynx, and a deviated septum. The most common predisposing factor, however, is nasal polyposis resulting from allergic rhinitis; polyps can fill the nasal cavity and completely occlude the sinus ostium.

A peculiar form of nasal polyp is the antrochoanal polyp, which arises from the mucosa near the maxillary sinus ostium (Fig. 13–9). This polyp occludes the ostium and grows by proliferation and edema into a "bilobed structure." One lobe remains in the sinus and the other enters the nose and passes into the nasopharynx. Complete removal of the antrochoanal polyp usually fully resolves the problem, and recurrence is rare.

Nasal allergies predispose to sinus infection.

Allergies, by causing edematous mucosa and hypersecretion, may also predispose to infection. The swollen sinus mucosa may occlude the sinus ostium and impair drainage, leading to further infection, which, in turn, destroys the surface epithelium, and hence the cycle of events continues.

The symptoms of chronic sinusitis are vague. During an acute exacerbation

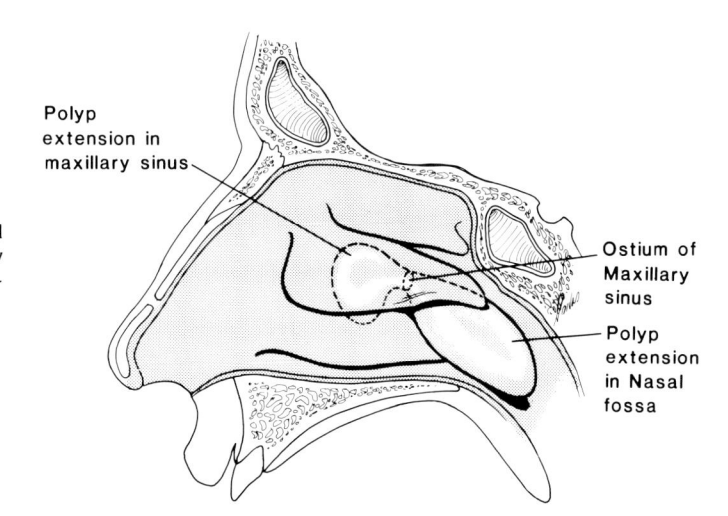

FIGURE 13–9. Antrochoanal polyp. A bilobed polyp is shown with one lobe in the maxillary sinus and the other in the nose and nasopharynx.

of chronic sinusitis the symptoms are similar to those of acute sinusitis; however, for the remainder of the time, the symptoms include a feeling of fullness in the face and nose and hypersecretion that is often mucopurulent. Headache is sometimes present, but this has been greatly overrated as a symptom of sinus disease. There is usually some nasal obstruction, and, of course, the symptoms of the predisposing factors, such as perennial allergic rhinitis, are prominent components of the complaints. A chronic cough with chronic mild laryngitis or pharyngitis often accompanies chronic sinusitis, and these may be the particular symptoms that bring the patient to the physician.

Treatment must consist of simultaneously treating the infection and the factors that led to the infection. In addition to adequate medical therapy with decongestants and antibiotics, attention must be paid to the predisposing obstructive abnormalities and to any allergies that may be present. Allergies may be treated by methods discussed in the chapter on nasal diseases (Chapter 12) and the chapter on allergy (Chapter 11). For chronic maxillary sinusitis the simplest surgical intervention consists of creating an adequate drainage opening. The most common procedure is termed nasoantrostomy, or the formation of a nasoantral window (Fig. 13–10).

FIGURE 13–10. Nasoantral window. An opening is made into the maxillary sinus, usually through the inferior meatus as shown.

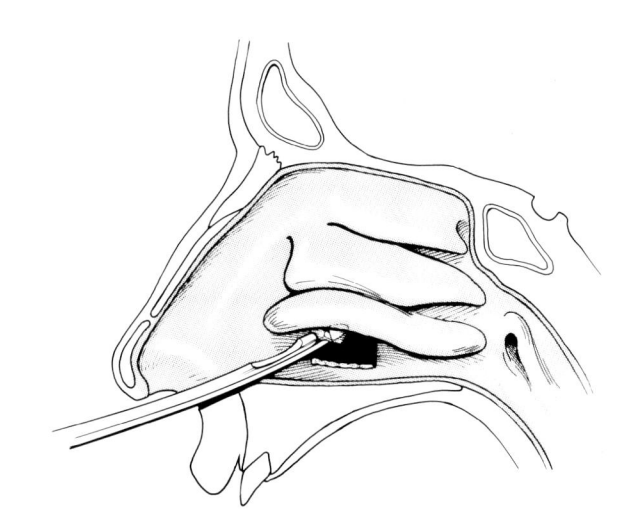

A large piece of the medial wall of the inferior meatus is removed to allow gravitational drainage and ventilation, and possibly, therefore, to allow regeneration of healthy mucous membrane within the maxillary sinus. A more radical procedure bears the name of two surgeons who popularized it—the Caldwell-Luc operation (Fig. 13–11). In this surgical procedure, the epithelium of the maxillary sinus cavity is removed completely and a drainage antrostomy is performed at the termination of the procedure in a manner similar to that described previously. The end result is satisfactory, since the active diseased mucous membrane has been either replaced with normal mucosa or filled with inert scar tissue.

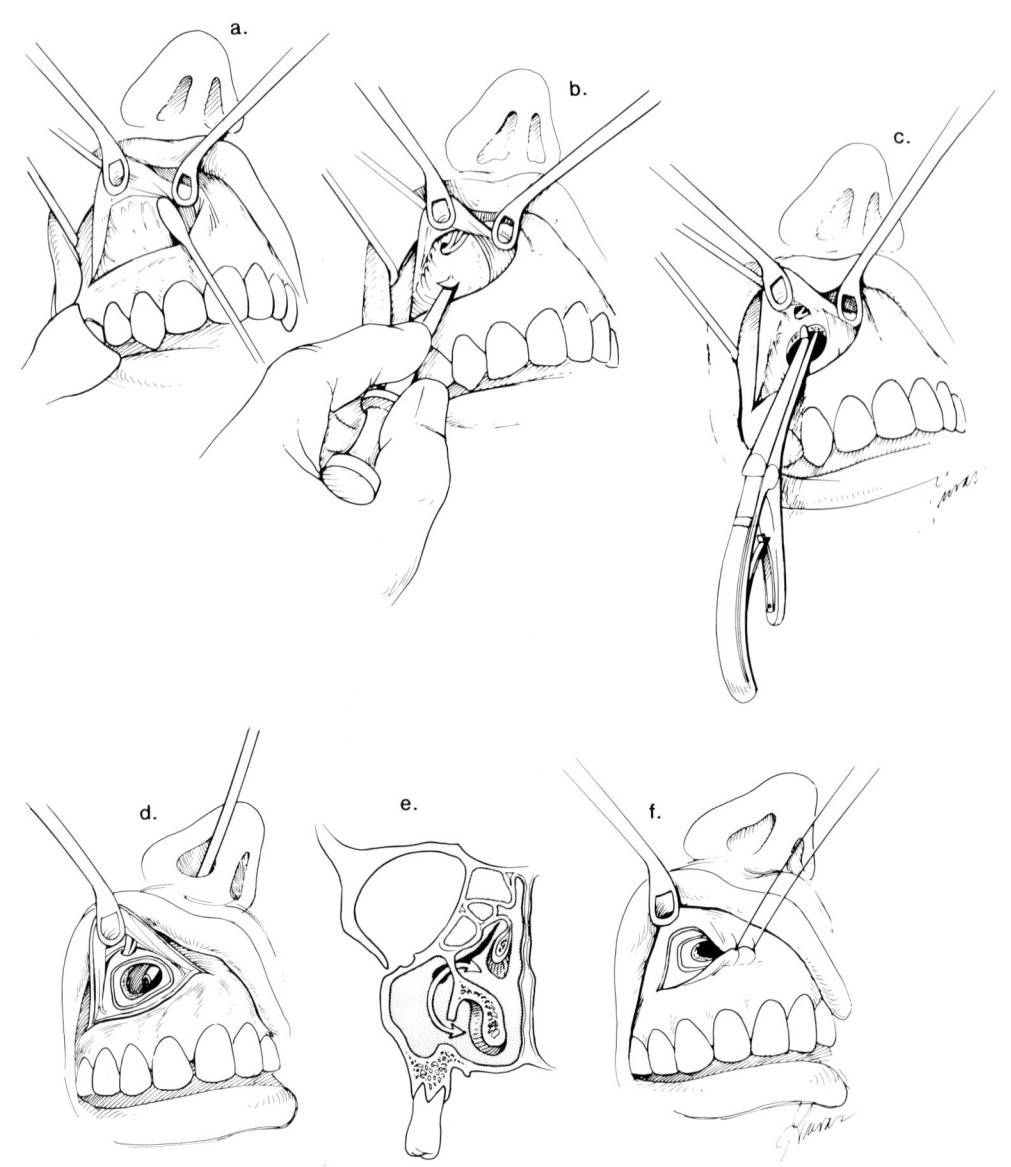

FIGURE 13–11. Caldwell-Luc procedure. Irreversible maxillary sinus disease can be treated surgically by (A) an incision in the canine fossa and (B) removing a portion of the bone of the anterior wall of the sinus. The opening can be enlarged (C) with a biting forceps. An opening (D) into the inferior meatus similar to a nasoantral window is made to replace the compromised natural ostium. Ventilation and drainage of the sinus can then occur through (E) the inferior meatus or the natural ostium if resolution of the sinus disease opens the natural ostium. The operation is completed by (F) closure of the oral incision.

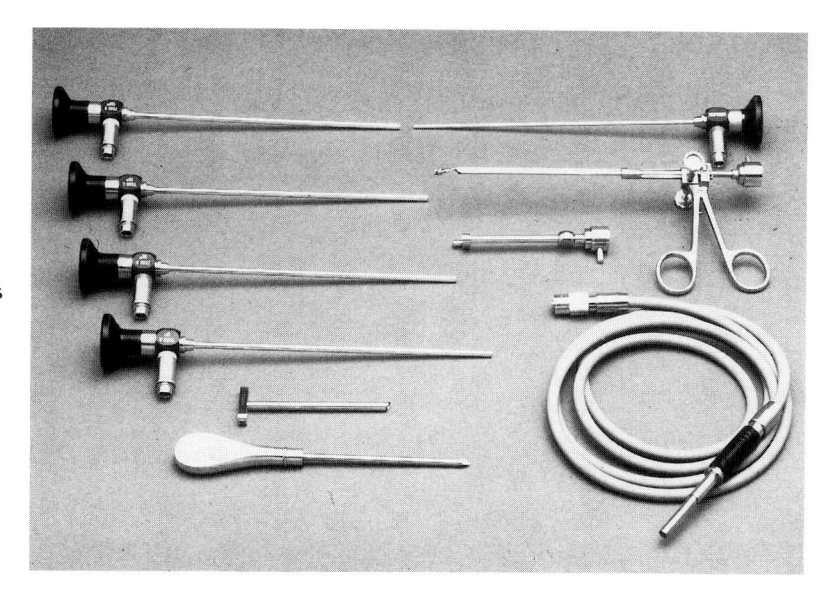

FIGURE 13-12. Endoscopic sinus surgery instruments.

Endoscopic sinus surgery, a technique that allows the surgeon excellent visualization and magnification of the nasal anatomy and normal sinus ostia, has been popularized in the recent past (Fig. 13-12).

Sinusitis is primarily rhinogenic. In chronic sinusitis the source of the recurrent infection tends to be a stenotic area, usually the ethmoid infundibulum and the frontal recess. Because inflammation causes the apposing mucosae in these narrowed spaces to press together, interference with normal mucociliary transport is the result, causing mucous retention and enhanced viral or bacterial growth. The infection then spreads to the adjacent sinuses. Since the cilia of the maxillary sinus sweep toward the natural ostium even if an opening in the inferior meatus has been created, enlarging the natural ostium and removing persistently inflamed or anatomically defective tissue on the limited basis permitted by this technique has the advantage of re-establishing normal mucociliary clearance. Other advantages include improved diagnosis, a clearer operative visualization, and less surgical alteration to normal anatomy. The improved diagnostic ability provided by functional endoscopy is enhanced by the complementary use of computed tomography (CT) scans, which have proven to be a real asset in evaluating chronic sinus diseases. Chronic ethmoiditis is almost always associated with chronic maxillary or chronic frontal disease and may require surgical treatment along with these other diseases. Chronic ethmoiditis can accompany chronic nasal polyposis, and, of course, the treatment will include removal of the nasal polyps. Removal of the tissues from which the polyps originate reduces the rate of recurrent diseases. This procedure, known as an ethmoidectomy, may be done by the intranasal, transantral, or external route (Fig. 13-13). Endoscopic sinus surgery is an asset in this situation, too. The directed surgery with excellent visualization allowed by this technique permits the surgeon to remove more diseased tissue and less of the normal tissue. Preoperative CT scans are an invaluable study before endoscopic surgery (Fig. 13-14).

Functional endoscopy has enhanced both the diagnosis and treatment of sinus disease.

The etiologic factors of chronic frontal sinusitis are similar to those of all forms of chronic sinusitis. The clinical features consist of frontal head pain of a constant nature and puffiness and tenderness of the skin over the sinus.

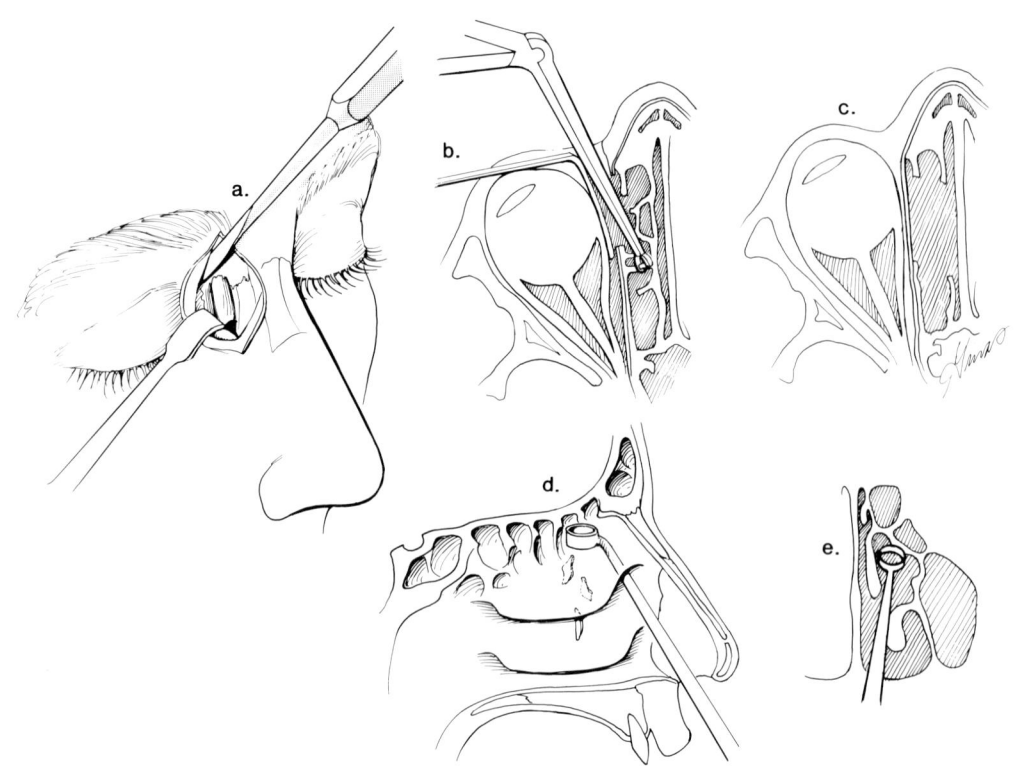

FIGURE 13–13. Ethmoidectomy. Two methods to remove diseased ethmoid air cells are demonstrated. An external ethmoidectomy is performed through (A) an incision on the lateral side of the nose. The soft tissues and periosteum, including the lacrimal sac and medial canthus, are elevated. Biting forceps and curettes are used to (B) remove the diseased air cells. At the completion of the procedure, the ethmoid air cells have been replaced by one large cell that opens into the nose (C). An intranasal ethmoidectomy accomplishes the same objective but is performed with instruments that reach the ethmoid cells through the nares and middle meatus (D and E).

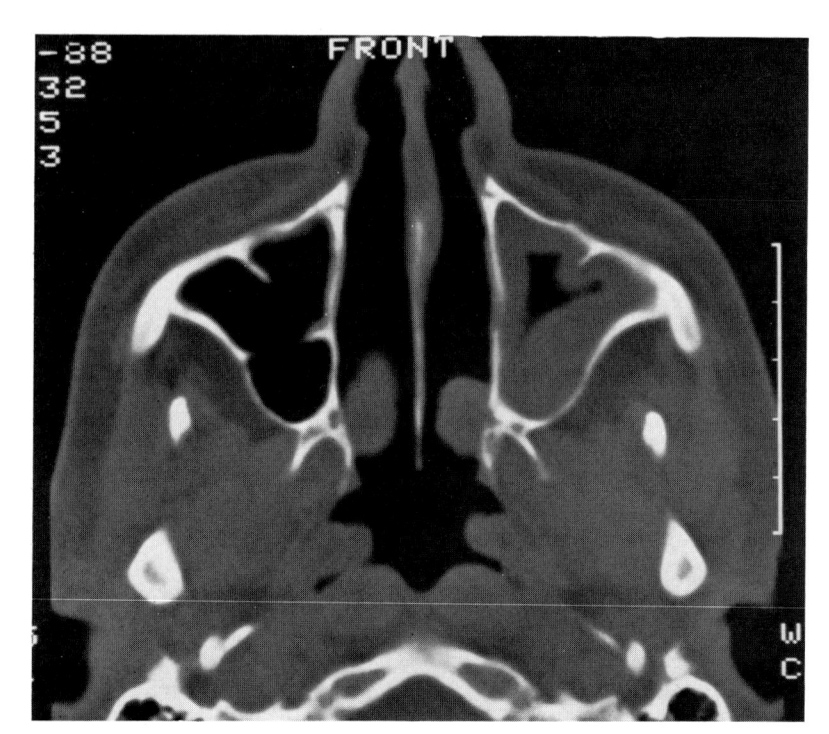

FIGURE 13–14. Computed tomography demonstrating sinus mucosal thickening characteristic of chronic sinusitis.

Complications such as subperiosteal abscess, osteitis, and osteomyelitis occur more readily in frontal sinusitis and will be discussed subsequently. Treatment of chronic frontal sinusitis often requires surgical intervention after the acute infection and other factors have been treated. The frontonasal duct is usually irreparably obstructed, and surgical techniques have been devised to create new frontonasal ducts or obliterate the sinuses.

An external frontoethmoidectomy provides access to the frontal sinus for removal of diseased mucosa and excision of ethmoid air cells and permits the creation of a new frontonasal duct, which is allowed to form around a plastic drainage tube left in place about two months (Fig. 13–15). A more radical surgical procedure is the obliteration procedure. In this operation, all of the mucous membrane, including the remnant of the frontonasal duct, is excised from the sinus, which is then filled with an inert fatty tissue graft (Fig. 13–16). The surgical incision procedure can be made through both

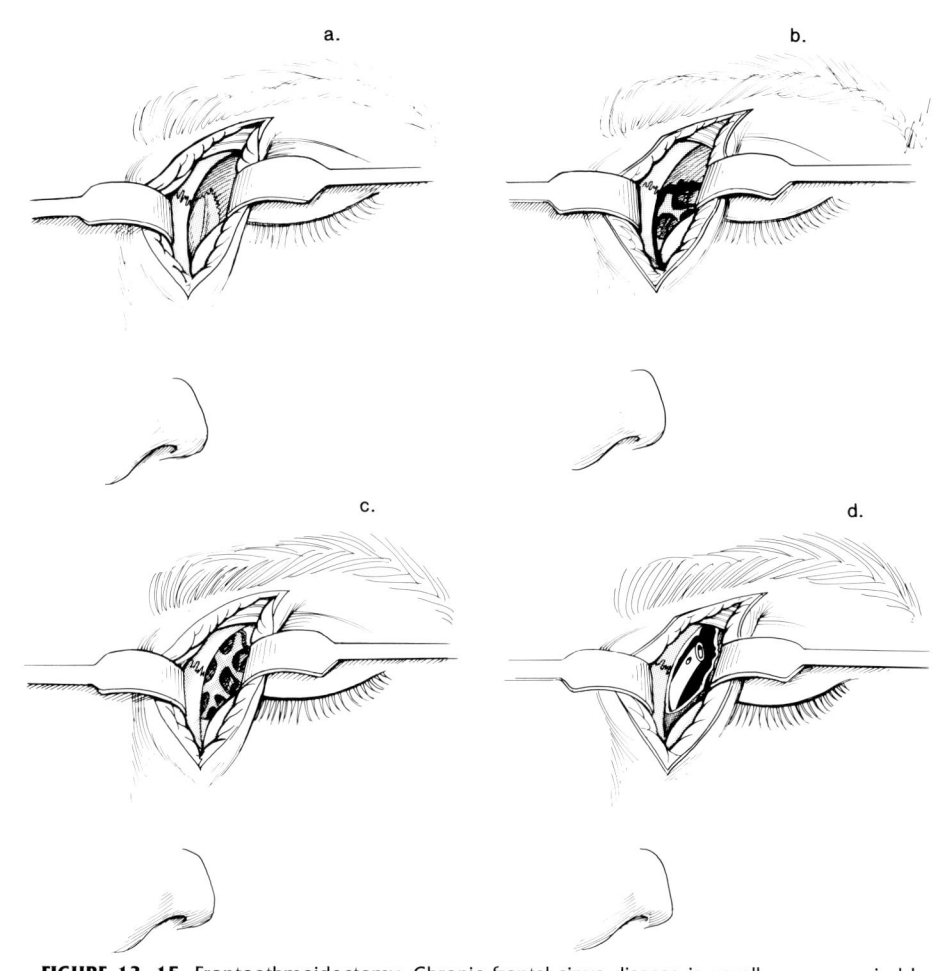

FIGURE 13–15. Frontoethmoidectomy. Chronic frontal sinus disease is usually accompanied by ethmoid sinusitis and a compromised nasofrontal duct. A frontoethmoidectomy addresses disease in both areas. The procedure is accomplished through (A) an incision on the lateral aspect of the nose. The soft tissues are elevated and the ethmoid air cells are removed in an external ethmoidectomy (B and C). The nasofrontal duct is enlarged (D) and a tube stent is placed from the nose into the frontal sinus. The tube helps maintain the patency of the newly created duct and may be left in place for several weeks.

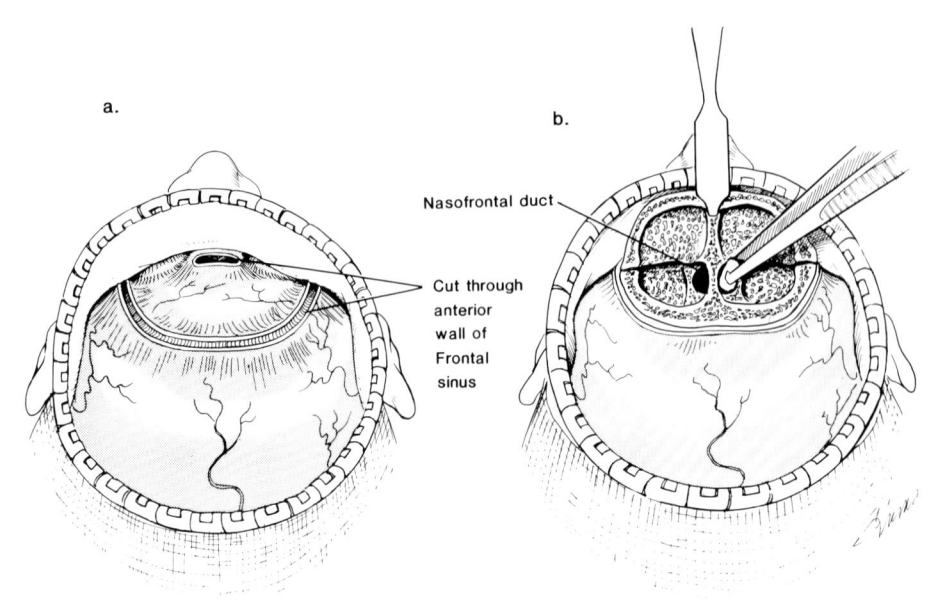

FIGURE 13–16. Frontal sinus obliteration. Chronic frontal sinus disease can be treated by eliminating the sinuses altogether. The procedure can be performed through a brow incision or a coronal incision. The anterior wall of the sinus is incised (A). The sinus mucosa is removed (B), the nasofrontal ducts are plugged, and the sinus is filled with fat.

eyebrows or coronally, through the scalp. A template of the sinus, patterned from the radiographs, is then placed on the skull, and the anterior wall of the sinus is outlined. The anterior wall may be incised and reflected forward but is hinged at the inferior edge by its attachment to the periosteum.

Chronic sphenoid sinusitis is usually part of chronic ethmoid and frontal infections, and the surgical procedures used to alleviate these diseases can easily include a sphenoid exploration.

Sinusitis in Children

The ethmoid and maxillary sinuses are present at birth, with the remaining sinuses developing during late childhood and adolescence. Until the second decade of life the ethmoid and maxillary sinuses are the only clinically important sinuses.

Children of all ages are particularly prone to upper respiratory tract viral infections as well as allergies. Common sequelae of these conditions include mucosal edema and loss of cilia with viral infections, resulting in occlusion of the sinus ostia. Once the ostium is closed, the air within the sinus is absorbed and replaced by an effusion that easily becomes infected secondarily by bacteria.

Mechanical factors such as adenoid hypertrophy, foreign bodies, choanal atresia, and stenosis may contribute significantly to poor airway physiology and stasis of secretions.

Congenital immunologic defects, Kartagener's syndrome, Down's syndrome, Hurler's syndrome, and the various dysglobulinemias are associated with sinusitis in children, as are the acquired immunodeficiencies of leukemia and immunosuppression by drugs. Nasal polyps occur in approximately 50 per cent of children with cystic fibrosis. Sinusitis in these children is common.

Bacteriology. As stated in the preceding paragraphs, although the preliminary infection may be viral and transitory, the resulting physical circumstances provide a means whereby bacteria can flourish. The bacteriology of sinusitis in children differs only slightly from that in adults, the main difference being that *H. influenzae* is more frequent in sinusitis of children of all ages.

Symptoms. All symptoms of sinusitis described previously occur in children, but children seem less concerned with pain and tenderness than do their adult counterparts. The symptoms of persistent mucopurulent nasal drainage should alert the physician to the possibility of sinusitis. Recurrent or persistent laryngitis and chronic cough, particularly a nocturnal cough, are common presenting symptoms of sinusitis in children. The complications of sinusitis, particularly cellulitis of the face and orbit, occur more frequently in children than in adults and may develop with surprising rapidity. Because of the anatomic proximity, similar histologic make-up, and sinus drainage into the nasopharynx, otitis media may also be seen with childhood sinus disease. Therefore, both the sinuses and middle ears should be assessed in a child with symptoms in either area.

Facial cellulitis of sinus origin occurs more frequently in children than adults.

Treatment. The mainstay of treatment of acute childhood sinusitis is antibiotics—amoxicillin, ampicillin or erythromycin plus sulfonamide, with other alternatives being amoxicillin/clav, cefaclor, cefuroxime, and trimethoprim plus sulfonamide. Surgical drainage is reserved for complications or unresolved infections. The importance of adequate treatment for sinusitis in children cannot be overemphasized. Failure to treat the infection adequately can result in chronic sinusitis and complications in the lower respiratory tract.

COMPLICATIONS OF SINUSITIS

Computed tomography (CT) scans are a great asset in defining the extent of the sinus disease and the extent of infection outside the sinuses—into the orbit, soft tissues, and cranium. This type of investigation should be routine in refractory, chronic, or complicated sinusitis.

Orbital Complications

The ethmoid sinuses are predominantly responsible for orbital complications. Orbital swelling may also be the presenting sign of acute ethmoiditis; however, both the frontal sinuses and the maxillary sinuses lie in close proximity to the orbit and may also cause infection of the orbital contents. There are five stages:

1. Mild inflammatory or reactionary edema (Fig. 13–17A). This can occur in the orbital contents as a result of the proximity of infection in the ethmoid sinuses. As stated previously, this is particularly seen in children because the lamina papyracea that separates the orbit from the ethmoid sinuses is frequently dehiscent in this group.
2. Orbital cellulitis. Edema is diffuse and bacteria have actively invaded the orbital contents, but pus formation does not occur (Fig. 13–17B).

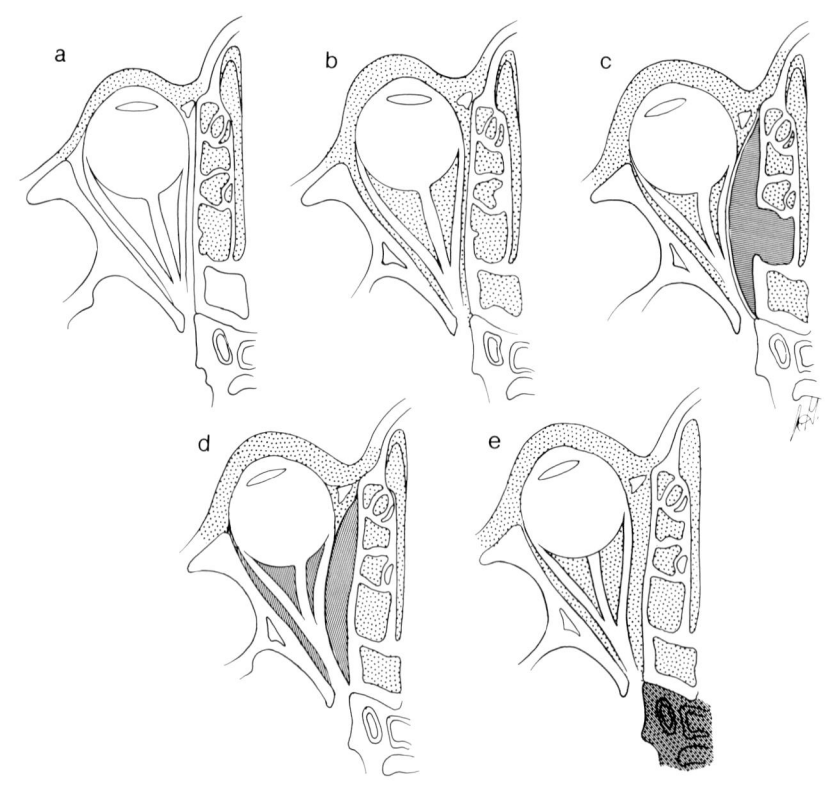

FIGURE 13–17. Orbital complications of sinus disease. (*A*) Ethmoiditis and preseptal cellulitis; (*B*) orbital cellulitis; (*C*) subperiosteal abscess; (*D*) orbital abscess; (*E*) cavernous sinus thrombosis.

3. Subperiosteal abscess. Pus collected between periorbital and bony orbital wall causes proptosis and chemosis (Fig. 13–17*C*).
4. Orbital abscess. At this stage pus has broken through the periosteum and has intermingled with the orbital contents (Fig. 13–17*D*). This stage is associated with the more serious unilateral sequelae of optic neuritis and blindness. Diminished extraocular movements of the involved eye(s) and chemosis of the conjunctiva are characteristic signs of orbital abscess along with increased proptosis.
5. Cavernous sinus thrombosis (Fig. 13–17*E*). This complication is due to the spread of bacteria through the venous channels to the cavernous sinus, where a septic thrombophlebitis develops. Pathognomonically, cavernous sinus thrombosis consists of total ophthalmoplegia, chemosis of the conjunctiva, severe impairment of vision, patient prostration, and signs of meningitis due to the proximity of the cavernous sinus to cranial nerves II, III, IV, and VI as well as to the brain (Fig. 13–18 and 13–19).

Treatment of the orbital complications of sinusitis consists of large doses of intravenous antibiotics and specialist surgical approaches to release the pus from the abscess cavities. The question of anticoagulant therapy in cavernous sinus thrombosis has not yet been resolved. In cases of septic thrombophlebitis, it seems logical that anticoagulant therapy would only disseminate the infected thrombus. It must be remembered that the mortality

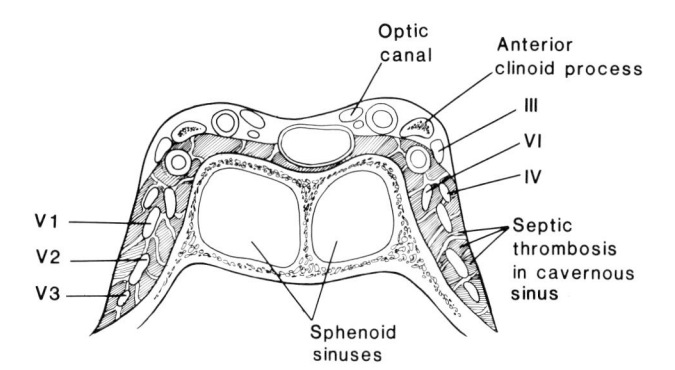

FIGURE 13-18. A coronal section through the sphenoid sinuses, demonstrating how cavernous sinus thrombosis can affect multiple cranial nerves.

rate following cavernous sinus thrombosis may be as high as 80 per cent. In the survivors, the morbidity is usually in the range of 60 to 80 per cent, and the most common sequela from cavernous sinus thrombosis is optic atrophy.

Mucocele

A mucocele is a mucus-containing cyst found in the sinuses. These cysts are most frequently seen in the maxillary sinus, are often referred to as mucous retention cysts, and are quite innocuous. In the frontal, sphenoid, and ethmoid sinuses these cysts may enlarge and, by pressure atrophy, erode the surrounding structures. They may, therefore, present as swelling of the forehead or nasal bridge or may displace the eye laterally. In the sphenoid sinus they may cause diplopia and impairment of vision by pressure on the neighboring nerves.

A pyocele is an infected mucocele. The symptoms of a pyocele are quite similar to those of a mucocele, although more acute and more severe.

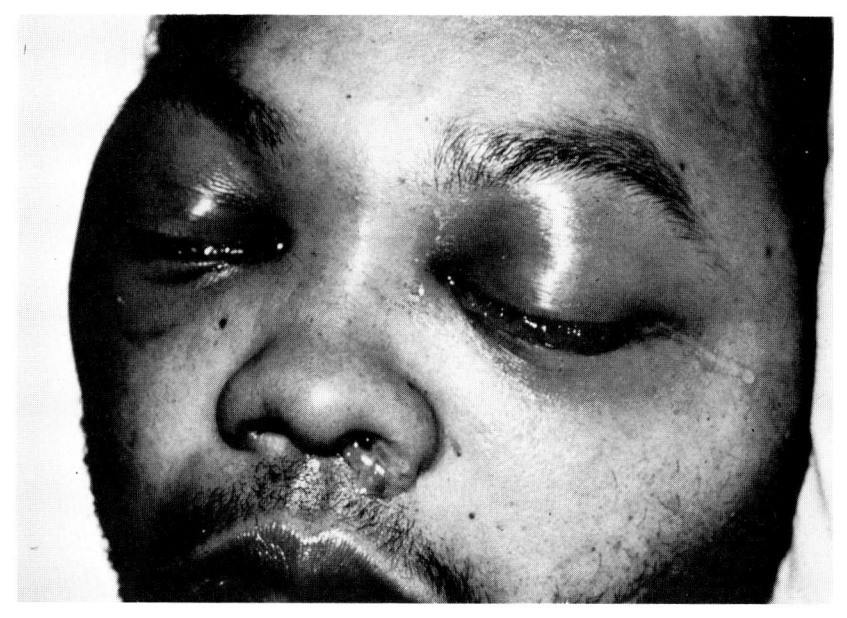

FIGURE 13-19. Cavernous sinus thrombosis. Appearance on admission. Swollen conjunctiva is protruding through swollen eyelids. Mucopus is present in the left nostril. (From Quick CA, Payne E: Complicated acute sinusitis. Laryngoscope 82:1257, 1972.)

Surgical exploration of the sinus for removal of all diseased and infected mucosa and re-establishment of good drainage or obliteration of the sinus are the mainstays of treatment.

Intracranial Complications

Acute Meningitis. Apart from cavernous sinus thrombosis, which has previously been described, one of the most severe complications of sinusitis is acute meningitis. Infection from the paranasal sinuses may spread along the preformed venous channels or directly from the neighboring sinuses, such as through the posterior wall of the frontal sinus or through the cribriform plate near the ethmoid air cell system (Fig. 13–20).

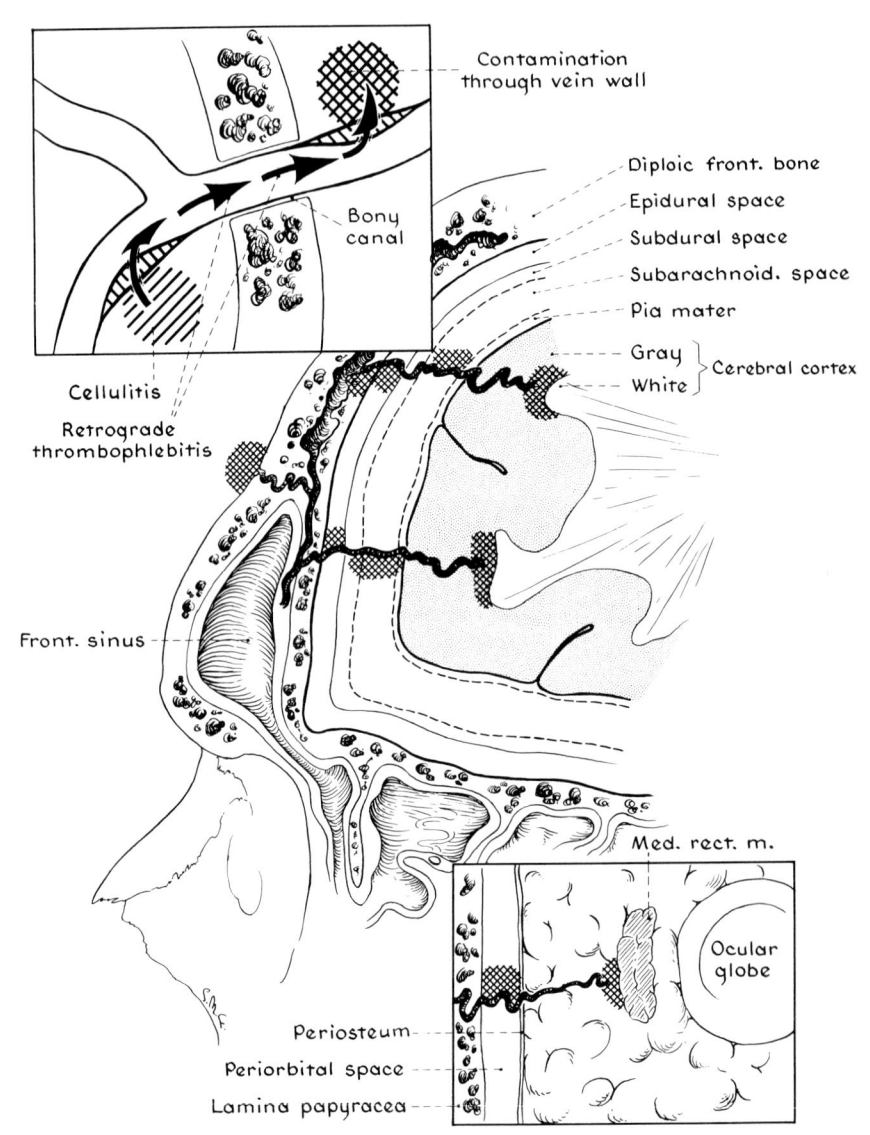

FIGURE 13–20. Diagrammatic representation of the venous system as the "highway" of extension of suppuration from the sinus mucosa to adjoining structures. Note the depth at which brain abscess develops because of the venous anatomy of the cerebral cortex.

Dural Abscess. An extradural abscess is a collection of pus between the dura and internal table of the skull; it most commonly follows frontal sinusitis (Fig. 13–20). The process may be so insidious in nature that the patient will present only with headache, and, until the collection of pus is sufficient to cause a rise of intracranial pressure, other neurologic symptoms may be absent. A subdural abscess is the collection of pus between the dura mater and arachnoid or the surface of the brain (Fig. 13–20). Similarly, the symptoms of this condition are intractable headache and spiking fevers, with some signs of meningeal irritation. The major symptoms may not present until intracranial pressure has increased or the abscess ruptures into the subarachnoid space.

Brain Abscess. Once the venous system in the mucoperiosteum of a sinus is infected, it is conceivable that hematogenous metastatic extension may occur anywhere in the brain. However, brain abscess usually develops by directly extending thrombophlebitis. Hence, the usual site of formation is at the termination of the involved perforating veins which extend through the dura and arachnoid mesh to the juncture between the gray and white substance of the cerebral cortex (Fig. 13–20). It is at this point that the terminals of the venous drainage to the surface of the brain approximate the terminals draining centrally into the cerebral veins.

The contamination of the brain substance may occur at the peak of a severe suppurative sinusitis, and the process of brain abscess formation may continue as the sinus involvement progresses satisfactorily through the stages of normal resolution. The possibility of brain abscess, therefore, must be considered in all cases of severe acute suppurative frontal, ethmoidal, or sphenoidal sinusitis attended in the acute phase by the sharp rise in temperature and chill characteristic of intravenous infection. A case of this type must be observed for several months. Lack of appetite, loss in weight, moderate cachexia, low-grade afternoon fever, recurring headache, and occasional unexplained nausea and vomiting may be the only signs of infection that is localizing in the cerebral hemisphere.

In no way must it be construed that these intracranial complications usually follow a logical sequence from meningitis to frontal lobe abscess. Any one of the complications may occur at any time with little or no involvement of the other varieties. Treatment of a severe intracranial suppurative infection is, again, intensive antibiotic therapy, surgical drainage of abscessed cavities, and prevention of spread of the infection.

Osteomyelitis and Subperiosteal Abscess

The most common source of osteomyelitis and subperiosteal abscess of the frontal bone is frontal sinus infection. Localized forehead pain and tenderness are extreme. Systemic symptoms of malaise, fever, and chills are usual. Swelling over the eyebrows is usual but becomes more extensive if a subperiosteal abscess occurs, in which case supraorbital edema develops and the eye may close. Fluctuation is seen, and the bone is extremely tender. Radiographs may show an erosion of the bony margins and loss of the intrasinus septa in an opacified sinus. In the advanced stages radiographs will show a "moth-eaten" appearance of the margins of the sinus, indicating that the infection has spread beyond the sinus. Bony destruction and soft tissue swelling as well as fluid or swollen sinus mucosa can best be seen on a CT scan. Prior to antibiotic use, this spread of infection into the calvarium would elevate the pericranium and lead to the classic description of Pott's puffy tumor. Treatment of this complication includes large doses of antibiotics given intravenously, followed by prompt incision of the periosteal abscess and trephination of the frontal sinus to provide drainage. A drainage tube or catheter is sutured into the sinus until the acute infection has completely subsided and the frontonasal duct is functioning well. If the frontonasal duct has been irreparably damaged by the process, a subsequent procedure will be necessary to re-create a new frontonasal duct. In spreading osteomyelitis of the calvarium, wide debridement and massive antibiotic therapy are mandatory. Fortunately, this complication is now rare.

Other Sinus Problems

Fungal infections of the sinus, sinus manifestations of systemic disease, and other infections that may also involve the sinuses as well as the nose, e.g., sarcoidosis, leprosy, etc., are covered in Chapter 12.

NONINFECTIOUS SINUSITIS

Barosinusitis

Ostial compromise is a precursor of barosinusitis.

Paranasal sinus homeostasis is dependent upon ostial integrity. Any pathologic condition that causes edema of the mucosa near a sinus ostium predisposes a patient to the development of barosinusitis. As the environmental atmospheric pressure changes, the compromised ostium prevents pressure equilibration in the adjacent sinus. When environmental alteration produces significant negative intrasinus pressure, as noted in scuba diving or the descent from altitude in an airplane, fluid transudation or hemorrhage occurs in the sinus. Pain and pressure usually accompany the change and occasionally mild epistaxis occurs. A sinus with an incompetent ostium and fluid is an ideal environment for the development of acute suppurative sinusitis. Radiography may reveal complete opacification or an air-fluid level. Treatment includes the use of topical and systemic decongestants, antibiotics in many cases, and the avoidance of environmental pressure changes until sinus ostial function is re-established.

Allergic Sinusitis

The changes occurring in the sinuses are the same as those observed in the nose. Polyps presenting in the nose usually originate in the sinuses and may also fill the sinuses. Polypoid changes alter the normal homeostatic mechanism of the sinuses and predispose the sinuses to acute and chronic sinusitis, e.g., osteal obstruction, loss of normal ciliary epithelium. Acute and chronic infections are treated as noted earlier in this chapter. Polypoid changes may require medical therapy, as noted in the section on allergic rhinitis, with steroids (topical and systemic), decongestants, and antihistamines. Polyps need resection if they obstruct the nasal airway or sinus ostia. Extensive or recurrent polypoid diseases are an indication for additional sinus surgery, such as a nasal-antral window and, occasionally, frontal sinus surgery. If the polypoid disease involves the turbinates, partial turbinectomy, cryosurgery, or diathermy may be necessary to reduce the bulk of the turbinate.

CONGENITAL SINUS DISEASE

Size Variation. A variation in sinus size with asymmetry is seen occasionally; sinuses may even fail to develop. Most frequently, a frontal sinus may be absent or represented by a small air cell. Occasionally this occurrence is also seen in the sphenoid sinus.

Kartagener's Syndrome. Apparently inherited as an autosomal recessive trait, Kartagener's syndrome is classically expressed as situs inversus, bronchiectasis, and sinusitis, although other phenotypic variations exist. Other expressions include absence or hypoplasia of one or more of the sinuses, recurrent infection, and nasal polyposis. Hearing loss secondary to repeated infections has also been reported by some authors as well as infertility in males. Electron microscopy has demonstrated cilia and spermatozoa with missing or shortened dynein arms in addition to oddly numbered and unusual microtubule orientation. These ultrastructural changes and the associated ciliary dysfunction are postulated to be related to chronic respiratory tract symptoms.

Sinusitis and bronchiectasis are seen in Kartagener's syndrome.

Cystic Fibrosis. Cystic fibrosis, transmitted as an autosomal recessive trait, has protean expressions and complications, with involvement of many of the mucus-secreting glands of the respiratory and alimentary tracts. Also termed mucoviscidosis, the abnormally viscid mucus produced along with the resultant respiratory obstruction leads to secondary infection. In addition to nasal obstruction caused by the mucus, the nasal mucosa also becomes chronically thickened and nasal polyps are common. Chronic sinusitis is frequently seen. The majority of deaths are due to chronic pulmonary infections and pulmonary insufficiency caused by the combination of sticky mucus and the products of the infectious processes.

Cystic fibrosis should be suspected in any child with chronic or recurrent upper or lower respiratory tract symptoms, as well as those appearing to have pancreatic insufficiency or malabsorption. The range of symptoms and age of onset are highly variable. The most reliable diagnostic test is the sweat test, with a characteristic three- to six-fold elevation of sodium and chloride in eccrine sweat present from birth in 99 per cent of the individuals with this disease.

With the advent of new antibiotics and other supportive therapy the life-span of individuals with this disease has increased to the point where some have finished college, married, and had children. Prognosis is dependent in a large part upon the degree to which the pulmonary deterioration can be prevented. Early diagnosis and awareness of the various clinical expressions of this disease will allow a greater degree of clinical support before advanced, irreversible changes have occurred.

TRAUMATIC SINUS DISEASE

Specific fractures of the facial skeleton are mentioned in Chapter 26. It is worthwhile to note, however, that frontal sinus fractures, nasoethmoid fractures, most malar fractures, and all maxillary fractures communicate with the paranasal sinuses and are, therefore, compound fractures. Post-traumatic mucosal swelling can compromise the sinus ostia, and this, in combination with blood in the sinuses, predisposes the patient to acute infection. Many surgeons advocate the use of antibiotics in these fractures to prevent such infections.

Chronic sinus disease in the form of chronic sinusitis or mucocele can occur as a result of fractures that alter the normal sinus ostial architecture. These conditions should be treated as discussed in the section on inflammatory diseases.

NEOPLASTIC SINUS DISEASE

Benign tumors that are seen in the sinuses are the same as those noted in the nose. They are discussed in Chapter 12.

One additional tumor that deserves mention is the osteoma, a benign tumor that can develop within the sinuses—most frequently the frontal sinus. Its clinical significance lies in the potential for the tumor to obstruct the sinus ostium as it enlarges. This can then set the stage for the development of sinusitis. When an osteoma encroaches upon the sinus ostium it should be resected or the sinus obliterated if a frontal sinus is involved.

Malignant tumors are covered in Chapter 23.

References

Chandler JD, Langenbrunner DJ, Stevens ER: The pathogenesis of orbital complications in acute sinusitis. Laryngoscope 80:1414–1428, 1970.
Dawes JDK: The management of frontal sinusitis and its complications. J Laryngol Otol 75:297–344, 1961.
Eavey RD, Nadol JB, Holmes LB, et al: Kartagener's syndrome. A blinded, controlled study of cilia ultrastructure. Arch Otolaryngol Head Neck Surg 112:646–650, 1986.
Eliasson R, Mossberg B, Cammer P, et al: The immotile-cilia syndrome: A congenital ciliary abnormality as an etiologic factor in chronic airway infections and male sterility. N Engl J Med 297:1–6, 1977.
Fairbanks DNF: Antimicrobial Therapy in Otolaryngology—Head and Neck Surgery. American Academy of Otolaryngology—Head and Neck Surgery Foundation, 1987.
Fearon B, Edmonds B, Bird R: Orbital facial complications of sinusitis in children. Laryngoscope 89:947–953, 1979.
Hawkins DB, Clark RW: Orbital involvement in acute sinusitis. Clin Pediatr 16:464–471, 1977.
Imbrie JD: Kartagener's syndrome: A genetic defect affecting the function of cilia. Am J Otolaryngol 2:215–222, 1981.
Jarsdoerfer R, Feldman P, Rubel E, et al: Otitis media and the immotile cilia syndrome. Laryngoscope 89:769–777, 1979.
Kennedy DW, Zimreich SJ, Rosenbaum AE, Johns ME: Functional endoscopic sinus surgery. Theory and diagnostic evaluation. Arch Otolaryngol 111:576–582, 1985.
Kennedy DW: Functional endoscopic sinus surgery: Technique. Arch Otolaryngol 111:643–649, 1985.
Quick CA, Payne E: Complicated acute sinusitis. Laryngoscope 82:1248–1263, 1972.
Schramm VL, Meyers EN, Kennerdell JS: Orbital complications of acute sinusitis: Evaluation, management and outcome. ORL J Otorhinolaryngol Relat Spec 86:221–230, 1978.
Shahin J, Gullane PJ, Dayal VS: Orbital complications of acute sinusitis. J Otolaryngol 16:23–27, 1987.
Shapiro ED, Wald ER, Brozanski BS: Periorbital cellulitis and paranasal sinusitis: A reappraisal. Pediatr Infect Dis 1:91–94, 1982.
Stammberger H: Endoscopic endonasal surgery—Concepts in treatment of recurring rhinosinusitis. Part I. Anatomic and pathophysiologic considerations. Head Neck Surg 94:143–147, 1986.
Stammberger H: Endoscopic endonasal surgery—Concepts in treatment of recurring rhinosinusitis. Part II. Surgical technique. Head Neck Surg 94:147–156, 1986.

PART FOUR

THE ORAL CAVITY AND PHARYNX

14

EMBRYOLOGY, ANATOMY, AND PHYSIOLOGY OF THE ORAL CAVITY, PHARYNX, ESOPHAGUS, AND NECK

by Stephen L. Liston, M.D.

An understanding of the embryologic development of the oral cavity and pharynx permits the clinician to appreciate the pathophysiology of many of the congenital anomalies that occur in the region. Some anomalies, like branchial cleft cysts, thyroglossal duct cysts, or cleft palate, are fairly common. Others, such as Treacher Collins syndrome or congenital conductive hearing loss, occur infrequently. If not recognized early, some congenital anomalies, such as Pierre Robin syndrome, can lead to intermittent attacks of airway obstruction with possible episodes of anoxia and brain damage. This chapter will provide basic embryologic information that will help with the management of these deformities when they occur.

EMBRYOLOGY

The oral cavity, pharynx, and esophagus are derived from the embryonic foregut. The foregut also gives rise to the nasal cavity, teeth, salivary glands, anterior pituitary, thyroid and larynx, trachea, bronchi, and alveoli of the lungs. The mouth forms when the primitive stomodeum, a fusion of the ectoderm and endoderm, breaks down. The upper lips are formed by elements of the medial and lateral nasal processes and the maxillary processes. Cleft lips are usually not midline but lateral to the medial nasal process, which forms the premaxilla. The lower lip develops from elements of the mandibular processes. The muscles of the lip are derived from the second branchial region and supplied by the facial nerve. The vermilion border of the lips has a characteristic bowed appearance; a notch in this bow is a very noticeable cosmetic defect.

The teeth are derived from the dental lamina, which gives rise to the cementum and enamel of the definitive teeth. The development of the human dentition through the milk teeth to the final eruption of the adult third molar corresponds to the age of the patient, and charts are available to follow the normal eruption of the dentition. There are a variety of benign and malignant cysts and tumors that derive from remnants of the dental lamina. The teeth are supplied by branches from the maxillary and mandibular branches of the trigeminal nerve. In the upper jaw, there is some variation and overlap in the regions of supply of the branches of the maxillary nerve.

The palate is formed in two parts: the premaxilla, containing the incisor teeth and derived from the medial nasal process, and the posterior palate, both hard and soft palate, formed by fusion of the palatal shelves. A cleft palate, therefore, will be midline posteriorly but will swing to the side of the premaxilla anteriorly. At one stage, the palatal plates are lateral to the tongue and if the tongue does not descend, the palatal plates cannot fuse. This is the basis of the cleft palate associated with the micrognathia of the Pierre Robin syndrome.

> The lingual nerve provides general sensation to the tongue; the mental nerve, which transverses the mandible and exits through the mental foramen, provides sensation to the lower lip region.

The tongue is formed from several epithelial eminences in the floor of the mouth. The anterior tongue is derived mainly from the first branchial region and supplied by the lingual nerve, with the chorda tympani branch of the facial nerve supplying the taste buds and the secretomotor supply of the submandibular gland. The glossopharyngeal nerve supplies all the sensation to the posterior third of the tongue. The muscles of the tongue are derived from postbranchial myotomes that migrate forward, bringing with them the hypoglossal nerve. This migration of the hypoglossal nerve is responsible for its having a predictable relationship to branchial fistulas. The thyroid arises from the foramen cecum in the posterior part of the tongue and migrates along the thyroglossal duct into the neck. If this migration does not occur, the result is a lingual thyroid. Remnants of the thyroglossal duct may persist, and these may be tucked up behind the body of the hyoid bone.

The salivary glands grow as outpouchings of the epithelium of the mouth and come to lie in close proximity to important nerves. The submandibular duct is crossed by the lingual nerve. The facial nerve comes to be embedded in the parotid gland.

ANATOMY

The oral cavity and the pharynx are somewhat arbitrarily divided into regions. The oral cavity is anterior to the free margin of the soft palate, the anterior tonsillar pillar, and the base of the tongue. The nasopharynx extends

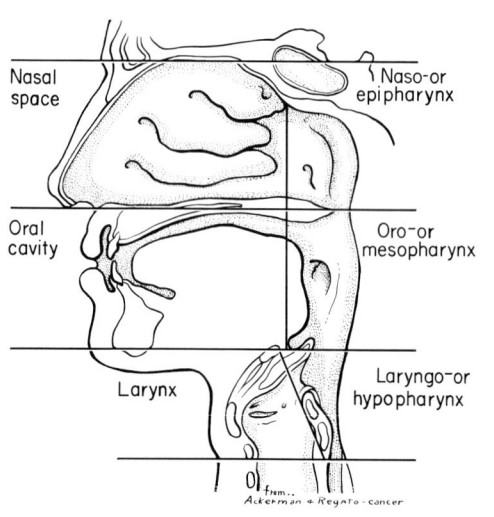

FIGURE 14–1. Divisions of the pharynx.

from the base of the skull to the level of the soft palate. The oropharynx extends from this level to the level of the epiglottis, while below this line is the laryngopharynx, or hypopharynx (Fig. 14–1).

The Oral Cavity

The lips and cheeks are composed mainly of the bulk of the orbicularis oris muscle supplied by the facial nerve. The vermilion is red due to a thin squamous epithelial covering. The region between the internal mucosa of the cheek and the teeth is the vestibule of the mouth. The parotid duct opens opposite the upper second molar.

The teeth are supported by the mandibular alveolar ridge inferiorly and the maxillary alveolar ridge superiorly. The infant dentition consists of two incisors, one canine tooth, and two molar teeth. The adult dentition consists of two incisors and one canine, two premolar, and three molar teeth. The occlusal areas of the incisor teeth are chisel-like and the canine teeth are pointed, while the premolars and molars have flattened occlusal areas. The area between the upper and lower posterior molars is known as the retromolar trigone.

The palate is made up of the bone of the hard palate anteriorly and the highly muscular soft palate posteriorly. The soft palate can be raised to seal the nasal pharynx from the oral cavity and oropharynx. The inability to make such a seal results in abnormal speech (rhinolalia aperta) and difficulty in swallowing. The floor of the mouth between the tongue and the teeth contains the sublingual and part of the submandibular salivary glands. The submandibular ducts open anteriorly on either side of the lingual frenulum. Failure of the salivary glands to secrete saliva causes a dry mouth, or xerostomia. This is a very distressing complaint to any patient.

The tongue is a mobile muscular organ. The anterior two thirds can be moved, while the base is fixed. The muscles of the tongue are supplied by the hypoglossal nerve. Common sensation is supplied by the lingual nerve on the anterior two thirds and the glossopharyngeal nerve on the posterior one third of the tongue.

The chorda tympani supplies taste to the anterior two thirds of the tongue, while the glossopharyngeal nerve supplies the posterior one third. Tastes are distributed somewhat in specific regions of the tongue. For example, bitterness is appreciated on the posterior part of the tongue. The superior surface of the tongue is separated into the anterior two thirds and posterior one third by a V-shaped line of circumvallate papillae. The foramen cecum at the apex of the V is the site of origin of the thyroglossal duct. The tongue functions in speech and it moves the food bolus in chewing and swallowing.

The chorda tympani nerve, which passes through the middle ear, provides taste sensation to the anterior two thirds of the tongue. It also carries parasympathetic fibers to the submandibular gland.

The Pharynx

Behind the mucosa of the posterior wall of the pharynx is the basisphenoid and basiocciput superiorly, then the anterior portion of the atlas and the bodies of the axis, and then the other cervical vertebrae. The nasopharynx opens anteriorly into the nose via the posterior choanae. Superiorly, the adenoid lies on the mucosa of the roof of the nasopharynx. Laterally, the opening of the cartilaginous eustachian tube occupies a region anterior to a recess called the fossa of Rosenmüller. Both these structures pass above the

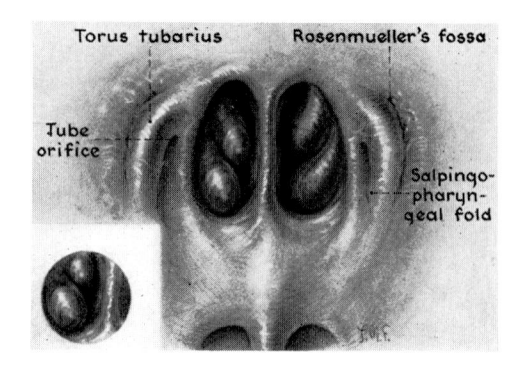

FIGURE 14–2. The nasopharynx as viewed through a nasopharyngeal mirror inserted into the throat through the mouth. The amount of the nasopharynx seen in the mirror at one time is indicated in the small inset. By moving the mirror, the entire nasopharynx can be examined, and information on all parts of the nasopharynx shown in the larger figure can be obtained.

free border of the superior constrictor. The tensor veli palatini, the muscle that tenses the palate and opens the eustachian tube, enters the pharynx via this space. This muscle forms a tendon that hooks around the bony hamulus to enter the soft palate. The tensor veli palatini is supplied by the mandibular nerve via the otic ganglion (Fig. 14–2).

The oropharynx communicates anteriorly with the oral cavity. The pharyngeal tonsil within its capsule lies on the mucosa on the lateral wall of the oral cavity. Anterior to the tonsil, the anterior tonsillar pillar is composed of palatoglossus muscle, and posteriorly the posterior tonsillar pillar is composed of the palatopharyngeus. These muscles help close the posterior oropharynx. They are innervated by the pharyngeal plexus of nerves.

The tonsil is composed of lymphoid tissue covered by squamous epithelium containing many crypts (Fig. 14–3). There appears to be no documentable

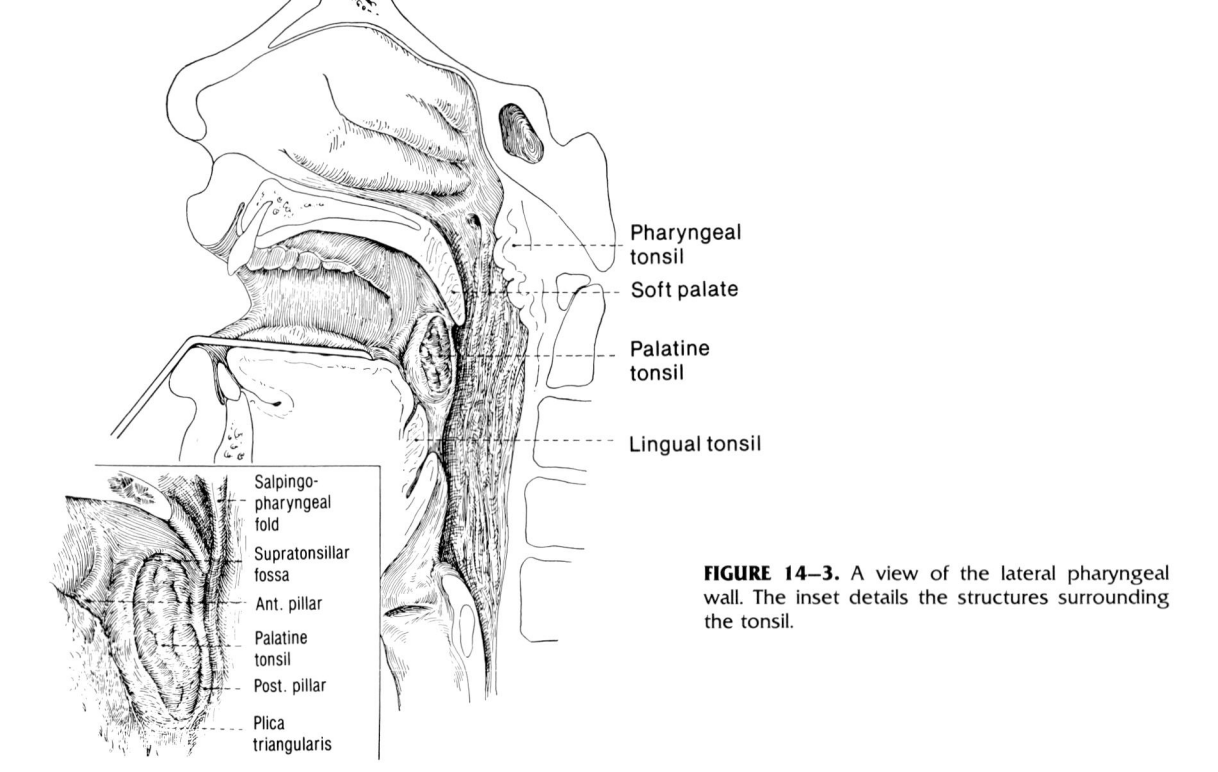

FIGURE 14–3. A view of the lateral pharyngeal wall. The inset details the structures surrounding the tonsil.

immune deficit caused by removing the tonsils (or adenoids). The cleft above the tonsil represents the remnant of the endodermal opening of the second branchial arch; this is where a second branchial fistula or internal sinus will open. Infection may collect between the capsule of the tonsil and the loose surrounding tissues and may track up toward the base of the soft palate as a peritonsillar abscess.

The hypopharynx opens anteriorly into the introitus of the larynx (Fig. 14–4). The epiglottis is attached to the base of the tongue by two lateral and one midline frenulum. These produce two valleculae on either side. Below the valleculae is the laryngeal surface of the epiglottis. Below this is the opening of the glottis medially, and laterally there is a space called the piriform sinus between the aryepiglottic folds and the thyroid cartilage. More inferiorly are the muscles of the cricoid lamina, and below this the opening of the esophagus.

The cervical esophagus runs more or less in the midline of the neck behind the trachea and anterior to the vertebral bodies. The recurrent laryngeal nerves lie in the groove between the esophagus and trachea. The common carotid artery and the contents of the carotid sheath lie lateral to the esophagus. There is a triangular weakness in the muscular coat of the pharynx above the cricopharyngeus muscle which arises from the cricoid and encircles the upper esophagus. A diverticulum, called Zenker's diverticulum, can project through this weak area and interfere with swallowing.

A Zenker's diverticulum develops through the posterior pharyngeal wall below the inferior constrictor and above the cricopharyngeus.

The pharynx is an area in which the air passages from the nose to the larynx cross the food passages from the mouth to the esophagus. Hence, any dysfunction of the pharyngeal musculature, mainly composed of the three pharyngeal constrictors, will cause difficulty in swallowing and usually also aspiration of saliva or food into the tracheobronchial tree.

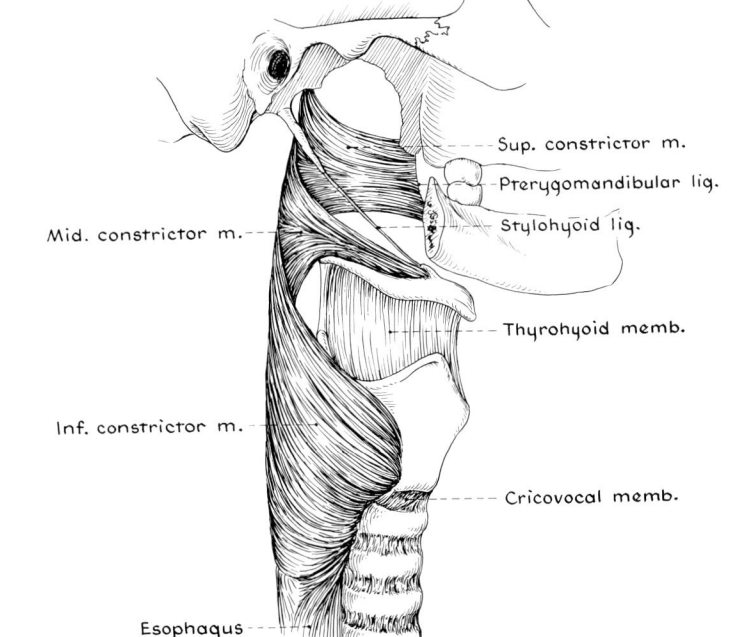

FIGURE 14–4. The relative size, position, and attachments of the three constrictor muscles of the pharynx. (Adapted from Grant.)

The Neck

In the early embryo there is no well-defined neck separating the thorax from the head. The neck is formed as the heart, which is originally below the foregut, migrates into the thorax and the branchial apparatus develops its final form. The migration of the heart is the reason why many of the structures of the neck migrate caudally. In the early embryo there are ridges along the side of the foregut which are also visible externally. These ridges are the branchial apparatus.

Although there are phylogenetically six branchial arches, the fifth arch never develops in man, and its only derivative is the ligamentum arteriosum. Only four arches are ever visible externally. Each branchial arch has a cartilaginous bar; associated with this bar is an arterial arch, a nerve, and some mesenchyma that will form muscle. Behind each arc is an external groove consisting of ectoderm and an internal pouch consisting of endoderm. The area between the ectoderm and endoderm is known as the closing plate.

Each of the four branchial arches contains a cartilaginous bar, an artery, a nerve, and some mesenchyma that will form muscle.

Parts of these structures named above develop into definitive adult structures. Other parts that normally disappear may persist and form abnormal structures in the adult. The normal derivatives of the branchial apparatus are listed in Table 14–1. It should be noted that the ectodermal cleft and endodermal pouch are located posterior to the cartilaginous arch, artery, and nerve.

Abnormal persistence of parts of the branchial apparatus can lead to a variety of cysts, sinuses, and fistulas. Persistence of the ectoderm of the first branchial arch may result in a cyst or sinus lying parallel to and even reduplicating the external ear canal. A different type of persistence may lead to cysts, sinuses, or fistulas running in a line from deep in the external ear canal through the parotid gland to the angle of the mandible anterior to

Excision of a first branchial cleft cyst requires identification and dissection of the facial nerve.

TABLE 14–1. DERIVATIVES OF THE BRANCHIAL APPARATUS

	I	II	III	IV	V
Cartilage	Malleus Incus Sphenomandibular ligament Mandible (in membrane around cartilage)	Stapes Styloid Stylohyoid ligament Body of the hyoid	Greater cornu Lower body hyoid	Thyroid	Cricoid
Artery	Middle meningeal	Stylomastoid branch of postauricular Persistent stapedial	Common and internal carotid	Aortic arch Ligamentum arteriosum Right subclavian	Pulmonary arteries
Nerve	Mandibular	Facial	Glosso-pharyngeal	Superior laryngeal	Recurrent laryngeal
Muscle	Mastication Tensor tympani Tensor veli palatini Mylohyoid Anterior digastric	Facial expression Stapedius Auricular Stylohyoid Posterior belly digastric	Stylopharyngeus	Cricothyroid	Intrinsic muscles of the larynx
Ectoderm	Exterior canal External tympanic membrane	—	—	—	—
Endoderm	Eustachian tube Middle ear Mastoid air cells	Cleft above tonsil	—	—	—

the sternocleidomastoid. Such first-arch remnants may pass anterior to, posterior to, or even through the branches of the facial nerve.

The bony derivatives of the first arch may be abnormal in the Treacher Collins syndrome. The artery of the second arch may form a persistent stapedial artery that passes through the crura of the stapes. In the presence of such an artery, it is not possible to perform a stapedectomy.

The ectoderm and endoderm of the second and third arches may also form cysts, sinuses, and fistulas. Normally the external openings of the second, third, and fourth arches are covered over by growth of an area called the epipericardial ridge. The nerve of this region is the spinal accessory nerve, and its mesenchyma forms the sternocleidomastoid and trapezius. The epicardial ridge fuses with the second branchial arch, burying the opening of the second, third, and fourth branchial grooves as an ectodermal cyst, the cervical sinus of His, which normally degenerates. Also, the tongue muscles, which are derived from postbranchial myotomes, migrate to the floor of the mouth, passing behind the branchial derivatives. Therefore any external opening of a persistent branchial derivative must open anterior to the sternocleidomastoid and the tract must pass superior to the hypoglossal nerve. It is therefore possible to accurately predict the line of second and third branchial cysts, sinuses, and fistulas.

The tract of a branchial cleft cyst must pass superior to the hypoglossal nerve.

A second branchial fistula will open anterior to the sternocleidomastoid, pass into the neck anterior to the common and the internal carotid artery, usually between the internal and external carotid arteries, and then above the glossopharyngeal and hypoglossal nerves to reach the tonsil. A third branchial fistula will open anterior to the sternocleidomastoid, pass posterior to the common and the internal carotid artery and above the hypoglossal nerve but below the glossopharyngeal nerve and stylopharyngeus, to enter the pharynx above the region supplied by the superior laryngeal nerve. There is some evidence that a remnant of the fourth branchial pouch may persist as a tract from the inferior pharynx to the region of the thyroid and may occasionally be a cause of suppurative thyroiditis.

Another interesting anomaly of the branchial apparatus occurs when the right subclavian artery has an anomalous origin and the right recurrent laryngeal nerve runs straight from the skull base to the larynx. The thyroid gland may not migrate from the foramen cecum, forming a lingual thyroid. Remnants or all of the thyroglossal duct may persist. Total removal of this duct involves also excising the body of the hyoid. The parathyroid glands are quite variable in their positions, and parathyroid tissue may even migrate with the thymus into the anterior mediastinum.

Blood Supply, Innervation, and Lymphatic Drainage

The pharyngeal blood supply derives from various branches of the external carotid system. Many anastomoses exist not only on each side but between vessels from opposite sides. Terminal branches of the internal maxillary artery, the tonsillar branch of the facial artery, the dorsal lingual branch of the lingual artery, a branch of the superior thyroid artery, and the ascending pharyngeal artery all contribute to a vast anastomotic network. The motor nerve supply has been discussed. The sensory supply to the nasopharynx and oropharynx, as well as to the base of the tongue, is essentially via the pharyngeal plexus of the glossopharyngeal nerve. Lower in the pharynx there is an increasing sensory involvement of the vagus via the superior laryngeal nerve. The pharyngeal lymphatic drainage may involve the retropharyngeal and lateral pharyngeal chains with subsequent passage into the deep cervical nodes. Nasopharyngeal malignancies often metastasize into the posterior cervical chain.

PHYSIOLOGY OF THE PHARYNX

The pharynx functions chiefly in respiration, deglutition, voice resonance, and articulation. Three of these functions are obvious. The function of deglutition merits detailed description.

Deglutition

Disorders of swallowing are best demonstrated on a modified video esophagram.

Deglutition may be divided into three stages. The first is the voluntary movement of food from the mouth into the pharynx. The second stage, the transport of the food through the pharynx, and the third stage, the passage of the bolus through the esophagus, are both involuntary. The actual steps of deglutition are as follows: Following mastication food is positioned on the middle third of the tongue. Elevation of both the tongue and soft palate forces the bolus into the oropharynx. The suprahyoid muscles contract, elevating the hyoid bone and larynx and thus opening the hypopharynx and the piriform sinuses. Simultaneously the intrinsic laryngeal muscles contract in a sphincter-like fashion to prevent aspiration. A strong motion of the tongue posteriorly plunges the food inferiorly through the oropharynx, a movement aided by the contraction of the superior and middle pharyngeal constrictors. The bolus is guided through the esophageal introitus when the inferior pharyngeal constrictor contracts and the cricopharyngeus muscle relaxes. Peristalsis, assisted by gravity, moves the food down the esophagus and into the stomach.

THE FASCIAL SPACES

Initially, abscesses are confined to potential spaces formed by cervical fascia.

The fascial spaces of the head and neck are areas of loose connective tissue that may be the sites of abscess formation as well as pathways by which infection may spread. These spaces are surrounded by fascial sheaths, which are layers of thickened connective tissue enclosing the muscles and organs. The function of these sheaths is to offer some protection as well as to allow the movement of the structures against one another.

Fascial spaces are not completely closed spaces, and abscess can extend from one space to the other and even to the opposite side of the neck.

The superficial cervical fascia encircles the scalp, face, and neck subcutaneously to enclose the muscles of facial expression and the platysma. The deep cervical fascia has been described as having two or three components, and the nomenclature is often confusing. For practical purposes, there is a superficial, a middle, and a deep component to the deep cervical fascia (Fig. 14–5). The superficial component is also called the investing layer; the middle component is termed the pretracheal (or visceral) layer; and the deep component is referred to as the vertebral (or prevertebral) layer. The superficial (investing) component of the deep fascia encircles the neck, attaching only to the nuchal ligament of the vertebrae posteriorly. It splits to enclose the trapezius and sternomastoid muscles but lies anterior to the strap muscles. The pretracheal layer is limited to the anterior neck below

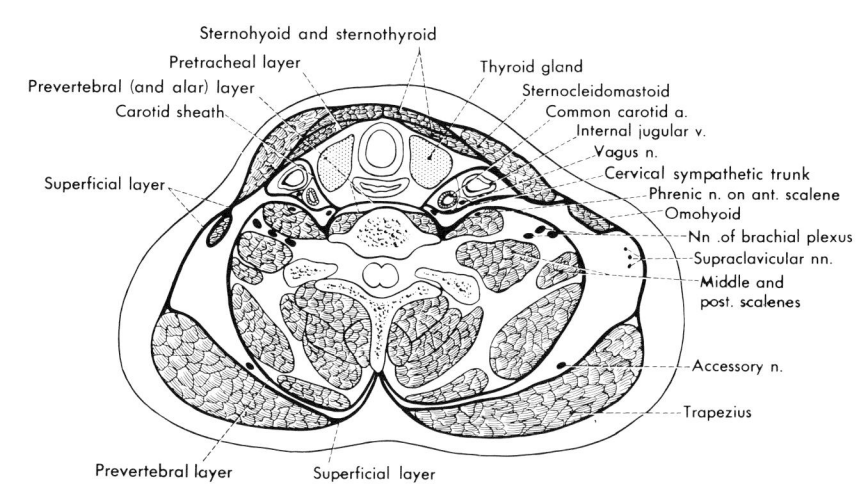

FIGURE 14–5. Chief layers of the cervical fascia below the hyoid bone. Note the relations of the various nerves. The fascias and fascial spaces are, of course, schematically shown and exaggerated. (From Hollinshead WH: Anatomy for Surgeons. Vol. 1: The Head and Neck. New York, Hoeber Medical Division, Harper & Row, 1982, p 271.)

the hyoid bone. It attaches to the superficial layer at the lateral border of the strap muscles on each side, extends posterior to these muscles in front of the larynx and trachea, and encircles the thyroid gland. From it arises a thin fascial tissue that encircles the hypopharynx and esophagus and is sometimes considered part of the pretracheal layer. Below, this layer is continuous with the pericardium. The vertebral layer of the deep cervical fascia, like the superficial layer, also attaches to the nuchal ligament and encircles the neck, but at a deeper level. It covers the vertebral bodies and the scalene muscles anteriorly and the paraspinous and deep neck muscles laterally. Over the front of the vertebral bodies it splits to form two layers, an alar part anteriorly and a true prevertebral part posteriorly. The space between these two parts is considered a "danger space," through which an infection may spread downward to the chest. Between the prevertebral layer and the pretracheal layer on each side is a tube of fascia encircling the carotid artery, vagus nerve, and jugular vein called the carotid sheth. Above the hyoid bone, the superficial and pretracheal layers change. The superficial layer of the deep cervical fascia becomes external to the suprahyoid musculature but then splits to enclose the mandible and muscles of mastication and also forms the capsules of the submandibular and parotid glands. The pretracheal layer extends above the hyoid bone posteriorly only as the layer encircling the pharyngeal muscles. The vertebral layer is unchanged above the level of the hyoid, but the carotid sheath at this level is less easily identified.

Infections that can involve these potential spaces are discussed in Chapter 17.

References

Davies J: Embryology and anatomy of the head, neck, face, palate, nose, and paranasal sinuses. *In* Paparella MM, Shumrick DA (eds): Otolaryngology, Ed 2, Vol 1. Philadelphia, WB Saunders Co, 1980, pp 63–123.

Hollinshead JW: Anatomy for Surgeons, Vol I: The Head and Neck. New York, Harper & Row, 1968.

15

DISEASES OF THE ORAL CAVITY

by Robert J. Gorlin, DDS, MS, DSc

Diseases of the oral cavity are of interest to both physicians and dentists. These diseases may represent a localized disease entity or a manifestation of a systemic illness. Diagnosis and treatment of oral lesions can be puzzling to the medical student and primary care physician, who may have had limited experience in this area. While it is not the intention of the authors to catalogue the many and varied conditions that may present in the oral cavity, it is believed that an overview of these conditions, including some common dental disorders, will provide a framework for differential diagnosis and management.

DEVELOPMENTAL ANOMALIES OF THE FACE, JAWS, AND MOUTH

Oral Tori

Torus palatinus (Fig. 15–1) is characterized by a nodular or lobular bony growth in the midline of the hard palate. Like its mandibular counterpart, it is rare in infants and is usually not manifest until puberty. In the adult population, it is noted in 25 per cent of females and 15 per cent of males. Surgical removal may be indicated for maxillary denture construction.

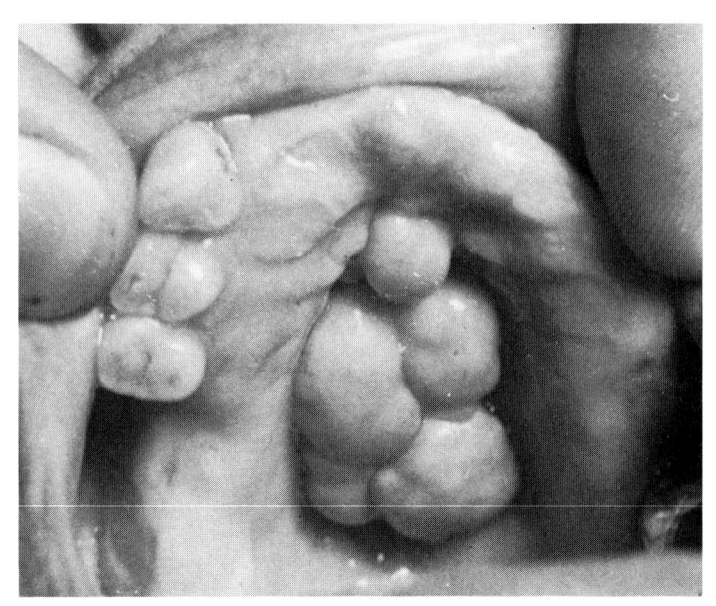

FIGURE 15–1. Torus palatinus. This developmental anomaly occurs approximately twice as frequently in females. Rarely does it arise prior to puberty.

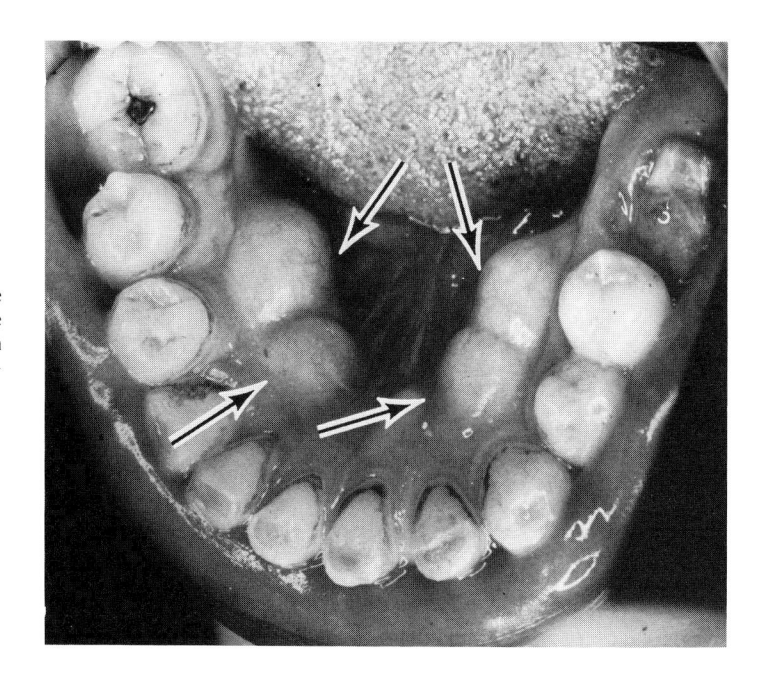

FIGURE 15–2. Torus mandibularis. Note multiple tori located in the region of the canine and premolar tooth. This is seen in about 7 per cent of the population. (Courtesy of I. Scopp, Chicago, IL.)

Torus mandibularis (Fig. 15–2) is represented by single or multiple, unilateral or bilateral bony growths on the lingual aspect of the mandible in the region of the premolars. It usually becomes evident at puberty or later. By adulthood, as much as 10 per cent of the population manifests this condition. The growth is of no significance unless it interferes with a dental prosthesis. Treatment, if indicated, consists of surgical removal.

Micrognathia

Micrognathia may be congenital or acquired (e.g., as a sequel to trauma, infection, or juvenile rheumatoid arthritis). Although the term is rather nonspecific in that it may refer to diminution in size of either jaw, common usage has essentially limited it to the mandible.

Whatever the association, the ultimate diminution in size of the mandible is due to a failure at the growth center in the condyle. Trauma or infection of the area of the condyle, almost always unilateral, will produce unilateral reduction of the mandible.

Mandibular micrognathia is usually an isolated polygenic trait but has been noted in association with a plethora of syndromes. Maxillary micrognathia is seen in craniofacial dysostosis, in acrocephalosyndactyly, and in trisomy 21. Mild occlusal deformities may be corrected by the orthodontist. Surgical correction of severe maxillary or mandibular hypoplasia is usually carried out by the maxillofacial or oral surgeon after growth of the jaws is complete.

Robin Anomaly

The combination of cleft palate, micrognathia, and glossoptosis is nonspecific, being seen as an isolated finding or in association with several syndromes.

This anomaly appears to represent arrested intrauterine development.

Pierre Robin: (1) micrognathia (mandibular hypoplasia), (2) glossoptosis, (3) posterior cleft palate.

During the tenth to twelfth week in utero, the maxilla grows rapidly, and by the fourth to fifth month the disparity between the upper and lower jaws is quite apparent.

The "Andy Gump" facies is quite distinctive. Dyspnea and periodic cyanotic attacks associated with recession of the sternum and ribs are in evidence during the inspiratory phase of respiration, especially when the infant is in the supine position. The difficulty is usually noted at birth. If the infant survives the initial period, mandibular growth subsequently catches up so that a normal profile is achieved by four to six years of age.

The exact physiologic mechanism by which the syndrome is produced is not known, but most investigators have suggested that the symmetric lack of mandibular growth (micrognathia) prevents adequate support of lingual musculature, allowing the tongue to fall downward and backward (glossoptosis). This obstructs the epiglottis, permitting egress of air but preventing inhalation, much like a ball valve.

Airway is maintained by forward traction on the tongue.

Patient is kept in prone position to keep tongue from falling back and causing airway obstruction. Tracheostomy is required in the more severe cases.

Treatment, in the mild case, consists of keeping the infant in a prone position, at times suspending the head by means of a stocking cap. In the severe case, the tongue tip is sutured to the anterior mandible or lower lip.

Prognathism

Enlargement or anterior placement of the lower jaw may be absolute or relative and is a multifactorial hereditary trait. After the jaws have ceased to grow (usually by 16 to 17 years), the patient is referred to an orthodontist and oral or maxillofacial surgeon for correction. Many successful surgical techniques are available.

Malocclusion

Various types of disturbed development of the face and jaws may result in malocclusion. Underdevelopment of the maxilla or mandible or overdevelopment of the mandible may require special surgical procedures after puberty. Incompatibility of tooth size and jaw size may result in spacing, crowding, or irregularity of teeth. Prolonged retention of primary teeth may result in delayed eruption of permanent teeth. Neglected primary or permanent teeth may be lost prematurely. Early consultation with an orthodontist is indicated to resolve problems associated with malocclusion.

Macroglossia

CO_2 and Yas laser surgery can be effective in removal of limited lesions.

An enlarged tongue may be relative or absolute and may result in abnormal speech. Most congenital cases are due to lymphangioma or hemangiolymphangioma. Cystic hygroma may also be present. The tongue surface is most often irregular or papillary, with 1- to 3-mm blister-type nodules. The most successful treatment is a combination of sclerosing agents and corrective surgery.

The tongue may also be enlarged in the macroglossia-omphalocele syndrome. In the adult, macroglossia may be seen with primary amyloidosis.

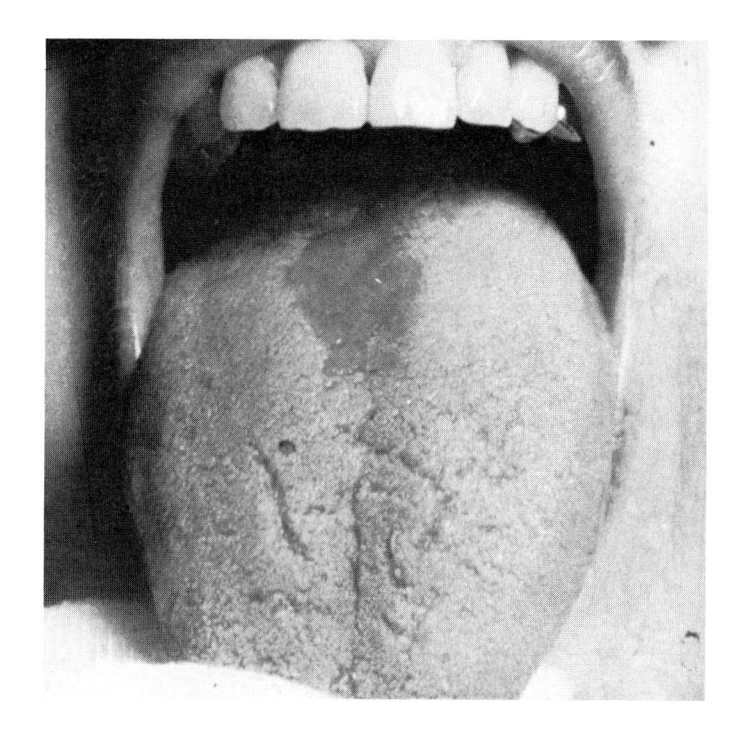

FIGURE 15–3. Median rhomboid glossitis. Note the bald, lozenge-shaped area on the mid-dorsum of tongue, just in front of the circumvallate papillae.

Median Rhomboid Glossitis (Fig. 15–3)

This entity is not truly a glossitis. Some have considered it to be caused by embryonal failure of the tuberculum impar to submerge, that is, to be covered by the lateral lingual tubercles. Others have suggested that it is a form of candidosis and is associated with diabetes. Nevertheless, it is innocuous. Its incidence is about 1 in 400 persons with a 3:1 male predilection. Classically, it is characterized by a smooth to nodular, elevated or depressed area void of papillae, located just anterior to the circumvallate papillae on the dorsum of the tongue. No treatment is required.

Lingual Thyroid (Fig. 15–4)

This condition is due to partial or complete embryologic failure of the thyroid gland to descend from the foramen cecum to its normal position in

FIGURE 15–4. Lingual thyroid. Arrow points to a mass rising above the dorsum of the tongue in the region of the foramen cecum.

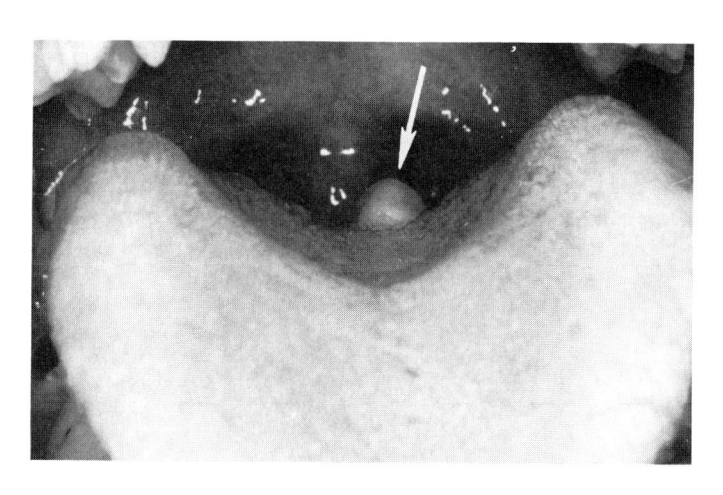

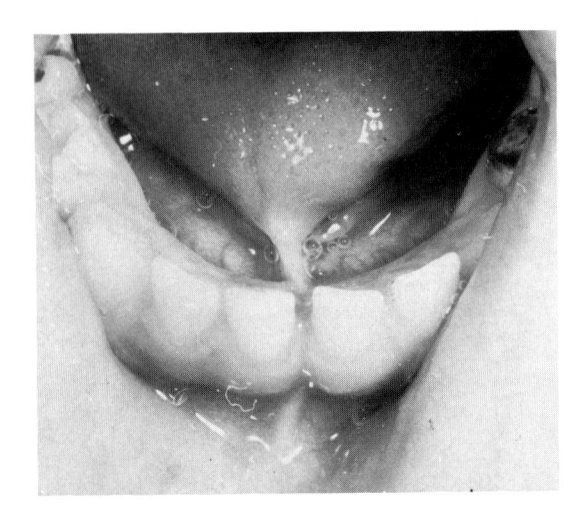

FIGURE 15–5. Ankyloglossia. Note attachment of the tongue tip to the floor of the mouth and gingiva.

the neck. It is characterized by multiple nodules of thyroid tissue on the dorsum of the tongue in the area of the foramen cecum and within the body of the tongue. In rare cases all the thyroid tissue remains in the tongue. Some ectopic thyroid tissue is seen post mortem in approximately 10 per cent of the population, the amount varying from a few acini to nodules 1.0 cm in diameter. No treatment is required for small discrete lesions. Larger lesions that may by position become traumatized should be removed surgically. However, no lingual thyroid tissue should be removed until the presence of thyroid tissue elsewhere is ascertained.

Before considering surgical removal, make certain that this is not the only thyroid tissue present.

Ankyloglossia (Fig. 15–5)

This condition has been arbitrarily defined as the inability to elevate the tongue tip above a line extending through the commissures of a congenitally short lingual frenum. From a speech standpoint, no treatment is generally required if the tongue tip can be elevated, independently of the mandible, to the alveolar ridge during the production of the speech sounds *a*, /d/, and /n/. In extremely severe forms, the frenulum should be clipped in infancy. A preferred treatment may be a Z-plasty performed in such a manner as to produce more freedom of tongue mobility.

CLEFT LIP AND CLEFT PALATE

Clefts of the primary and secondary palates are among the more common congenital anomalies. A vast amount of data has been gathered about facial clefts, only a small portion of which can be presented here.

Clinically, there is great variability in the degree of cleft formation (Fig. 15–6). The minimal degrees of involvement include such anomalies as bifid uvula, linear lip indentations, so-called intrauterine healed clefts, and submucous cleft of the soft palate. A cleft may involve only the vermilion border of the upper lip or may extend to involve the nostril and the hard and soft palates. Isolated palatal clefts may be limited to the uvula (bifid uvula), or they may be more extensive, cleaving the soft palate or both the soft and hard palates.

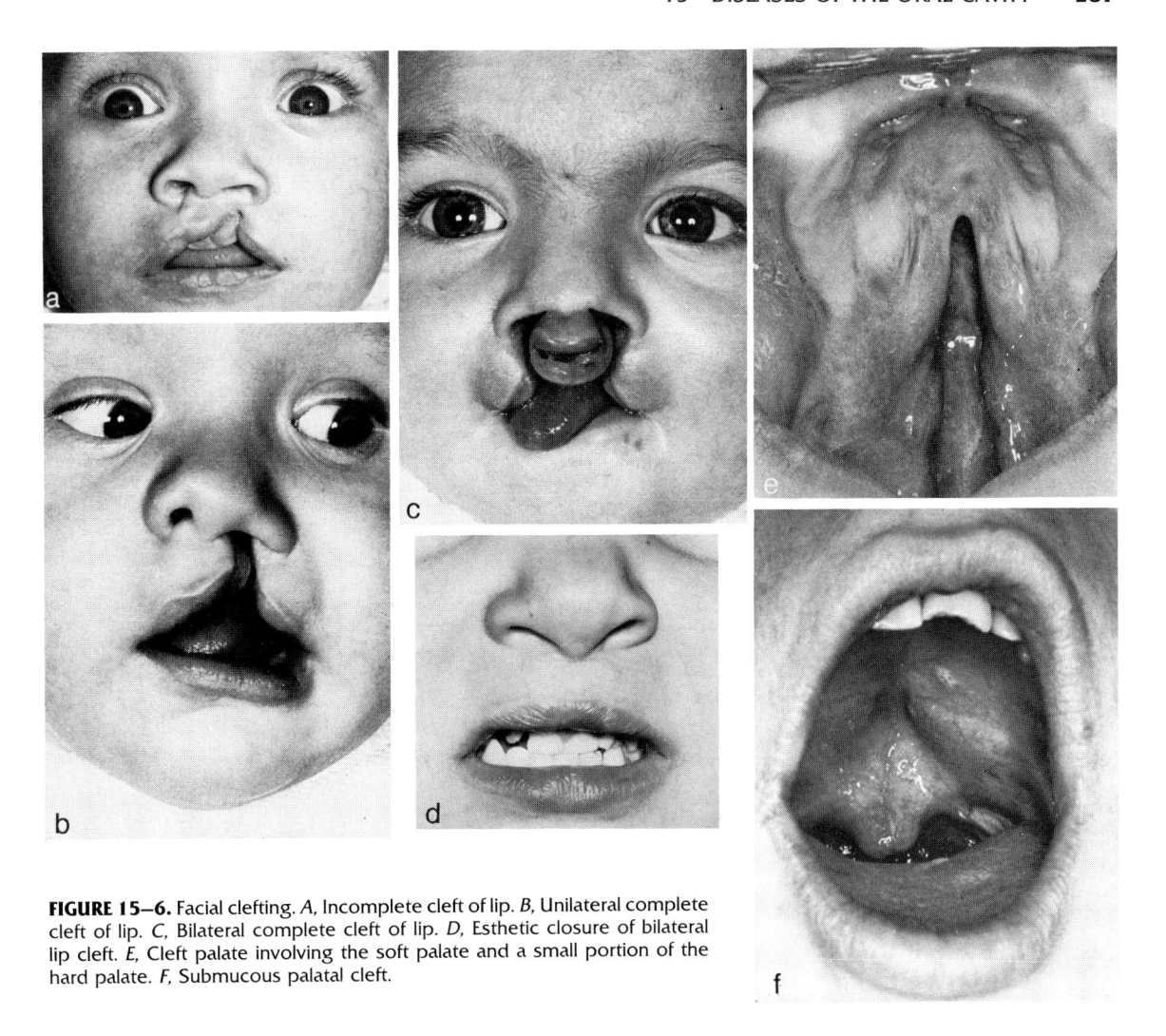

FIGURE 15–6. Facial clefting. *A,* Incomplete cleft of lip. *B,* Unilateral complete cleft of lip. *C,* Bilateral complete cleft of lip. *D,* Esthetic closure of bilateral lip cleft. *E,* Cleft palate involving the soft palate and a small portion of the hard palate. *F,* Submucous palatal cleft.

Of all maxillofacial clefts, the combination of cleft lip and cleft palate comprises about 50 per cent of the cases, with isolated cleft lip and isolated cleft palate each accounting for about 25 per cent, irrespective of race.

Cleft lip, with or without cleft palate, occurs in about 1 (range, 0.6 to 1.3) per 1000 white births. The incidence appears to be increasing, probably as a result of declining postnatal mortality, decreasing operative mortality, steadily improving operative results, and attendant increases in marriage and childbearing. The prevalence is higher in Orientals (about 1.7 per 1000 births) and lower among blacks (approximately 1 per 2500 births).

Isolated cleft lip may be unilateral or bilateral (approximately 20 per cent). When unilateral, the cleft is more common on the left side (about 70 per cent of cases), although no more extensive. Lips are somewhat more frequently cleft bilaterally (approximately 25 per cent) when combined with cleft palate. Cleft lip–cleft palate is more common in males. About 85 per cent of bilateral cleft lips and 70 per cent of unilateral cleft lips are associated with cleft palate.

The development of *isolated cleft palate* appears to be quite separate from that of cleft lip with or without cleft palate. It has been demonstrated that siblings of patients with cleft lip, with or without cleft palate, have an increased frequency of the same anomaly but not of isolated cleft palate, and vice versa. Children with isolated cleft palate not uncommonly (about 30 per cent) have associated congenital anomalies.

The incidence of isolated cleft palate among whites and blacks appears to be 1 per 2000 and 1 per 2500 births, respectively, and may be somewhat more frequent among Orientals. It is more common in females. Breakdown of cleft palate according to extent clearly indicates that whereas a 2:1 female predilection exists for complete clefts of the hard and soft palates, the male:female ratio approaches 1:1 for clefts of the soft palate or uvula only.

Complete clefts are more common in females.

The recurrence risk for cleft lip with or without cleft palate, if both parents are normal, is 3 to 4 per cent. The corresponding figure for cleft palate is about 2 per cent. Essentially the same risk data can be applied to the offspring of an affected person.

A cleft uvula can be a sign of a submucosal cleft of the palate. Adenoidectomy is contraindicated in the presence of a submucosal cleft.

Cleft uvula appears to be an incomplete form of cleft palate. The incidence of cleft uvula is about 1 per 80 whites. The frequency of cleft uvula among various American Indian groups is quite high, ranging from 1 per 9 to 1 per 14 individuals. In blacks it is comparatively rare (1 per 300 births).

Treatment

Treatment of cleft lip–cleft palate is complex and involves several disciplines. The best treatment is provided by a "team approach." The team comprises a maxillofacial surgeon, otolaryngologist, pedodontist, orthodontist, prosthodontist, speech pathologist, human geneticist, psychologist, and social worker. A considerable overlap of interest and concern for this clinical problem related to structure, function, and well-being of the patient demands the diagnostic and treatment skills of all these specialists for an extended period of time.

Otitis media is almost universal in infants under age two with unrepaired clefts.

The development of adequate speech and language skills is an important concern. Speech and language are learned primarily through audition. Since there is a relatively high incidence of ear disorders and consequent hearing loss (primarily conductive) in the child with cleft palate, early identification and treatment are important to ensure optimal hearing function during speech and language developmental years.

Surgical closure of the lip is usually performed within the first few months of life, whenever body weight exceeds 10 pounds. The ideal time for surgical closure of the palate has been debated, but in the United States at least 80 per cent of the surgeons prefer some time between the first and second years of life. Various techniques have been used in lip closure, but those employing angular rather than linear incision lines are preferred because of late postoperative shortening of the upper lip on the operated side following the linear techniques. In the case of bilateral clefts, lip closure is much more difficult owing to anterior displacement of the primary palate and is often accomplished in two stages.

Early closure of the palatal cleft provides a better mechanism with which to produce speech. Surgical closure of the secondary palate can be performed with a variety of techniques, most notably the bridge flap technique of von Langenbeck and the pedicle flap technique of Veau. The primary goal of surgery is to achieve complete closure of the hard and soft palates and to provide a soft palate that has sufficient length and mobility. Lengthening of the soft palate is ordinarily accomplished by a so-called push-back procedure.

Attainment of adequate length and mobility of the soft palate becomes important in the processes of deglutition and speech. Both these functions require velopharyngeal closure, that is, the ability to seal off the nasal cavity from the oral cavity. Although velopharyngeal closure for speech and certain nonspeech activities, such as deglutition and blowing, is sphincteric in nature, involving movements of palatal and pharyngeal structures, the soft palate is considered the prime mover in accomplishing closure.

If velopharyngeal closure is not achieved following the initial surgical procedures, foods and liquids may be directed into the nasopharynx during deglutition. Similarly, speech may be characterized by excessive air escape through the nose during pronunciation of consonants that require intraoral pressure for their production and by excessive nasal resonance perceived as hypernasality.

Although the primary evidence of the adequacy of the velopharyngeal closure mechanism for speech is the speech product itself, other evaluation techniques involve direct oral-pharyngeal-nasal observations, radiography, and air pressure–air flow instrumentation.

Secondary procedures to correct the velopharyngeal inadequacy for speech may be indicated. Such procedures may include a surgical pharyngeal flap, prosthodontic speech appliances (speech bulb or palatal lift), or a pharyngeal implant. Because treatment choice depends upon a number of surgical-dental-speech considerations and because the inadequacy of velopharyngeal mechanisms for speech may be due to several anatomic and physiologic variations, complete diagnosis and evaluation are required by all members of the cleft palate team.

In some persons with cleft lip–cleft palate, velopharyngeal closure may be achieved with the aid of tonsillar or adenoidal tissue. Decision as to the complete removal of such tissues in these patients should be made with caution, since persistent hypernasality and audible nasal air emission may result.

It should be pointed out that velopharyngeal inadequacy for speech is not limited to persons with cleft lip–cleft palate but may occur with a number of other congenital anomalies and syndromes involving the craniofacial complex.

Dental observation and treatment for the patient with clefts are important, since they relate to occlusion, appearance, adequate oral functions (mastication, deglutition, speech), and good oral hygiene. The status of the dentition can make an important difference in treatment choice.

Cleft palate teams are currently broadening their interest to include diagnostic and treatment services for a variety of developmental anomalies of the face, jaws, and mouth, some of which are presented in the following section.

Associated Developmental Anomalies

Facial Clefts. *Lateral facial cleft* (macrostomia, transverse or horizontal facial cleft) is caused by failure of penetration of ectomesenchyme between the embryonic maxillary and mandibular processes. The cleft may be unilateral or bilateral, partial or complete (rare), extending from the angle of the mouth toward the ear. In many cases, the cleft extends above or below the tragus.

It appears to be more common in males and, when unilateral, more often involves the left side. It may be an isolated phenomenon but more frequently is associated with other malformations. There does not appear to be a genetic basis for this anomaly.

Lateral facial cleft may be found with the first and second branchial arch syndrome (hemifacial microsomia, that is, hypoplasia of the ascending ramus and condyle of the mandible, ear tags, and microtia), oculoauriculovertebral dysplasia (essential hemifacial microsomia with epibulbar dermoids and hemivertebra), and rarely, mandibulofacial dysostosis.

Oblique facial cleft is extremely rare and is variable in appearance. Most commonly it is associated with cleft lip and extends to the inner canthus of the eye. In some cases, the cleft runs lateral to and does not involve the ala of the nose, passing near the outer canthus into the temporal region. It may be superficial but more often separates the underlying bone. If the cleft reaches the orbital margin, the eyelid may be involved. It is thought that the cleft is due to failure of ectomesenchymal penetrance between the maxillary, median nasal, and lateral nasal processes or failure of coverage of the nasolacrimal groove. The oblique facial cleft often fails to follow the epithelial grooves especially with amniotic disruption sequence.

The oblique cleft may be unilateral or bilateral and is nearly always associated with cleft lip, cleft palate, or lateral facial cleft. There does not appear to be any evidence of a genetic role.

Acrocephalosyndactyly (Apert Syndrome). This syndrome is characterized by turribrachycephaly associated with syndactyly of the hands and feet. Often the anterior fontanel fails to close, whereas other cranial sutures, especially the coronal, tend to close prematurely. On radiographic examination of the skull, increased digital markings are seen. Since the mental retardation and physical appearance of these patients discourage marriage and procreation, nearly all cases are sporadic, although the disorder, in fact, has autosomal dominant inheritance.

Apert syndrome: (1) craniosynostosis leading to turribrachycephaly and syndactyly; (2) progressive synostoses of hands, feet, spine; (3) some mental retardation; (4) case reports of conductive deafness.

Usually there is midfacial hypoplasia with resultant distorted nose. Proptosis of the eyeballs, downward slanting of the palpebral fissures, and ocular hypertelorism occur in most cases.

A mid-digital hand mass is present, consisting of osseous and soft tissue syndactyly of the second, third, and fourth digits. In some cases the first and fifth digits may be fused to the second and fourth, respectively. Fingernails of the mid-digital hand mass are continuous or partially continuous with some degree of segmentation. Soft-tissue fusion of the toes is also a feature.

The hard palate is Byzantine arch–shaped. Cleft soft palate is present in over 30 per cent of patients.

Mild conduction hearing loss due to fixation of the footplate of the stapes has been demonstrated.

Major maxillofacial surgery is required to correct acrocephalosyndactyly.

Craniofacial Dysostosis (Crouzon Syndrome). In craniofacial dysostosis the skull tends to be high, domelike, and thin, with obliterated coronal, sagittal, and lambdoid sutures. The anterior fontanel remains open and wide. A crest of bone may be present along the sagittal suture.

Crouzon syndrome: (1) craniosynostosis, (2) hypoplasia of midface, (3) relative mandibular prognathism, (4) ocular proptosis, (5) hypertelorism, (6) conductive hearing loss.

Typically, the facies is characterized by underdevelopment or flattening of the middle of the face associated with relative mandibular prognathism and a beaklike nose. The maxillary teeth are crowded, and the arch is V-shaped. Exophthalmos is a constant feature. Optic atrophy and divergent strabismus are present in some patients. Intelligence is usually normal. The disorder has an autosomal dominant inheritance pattern.

About one third of patients with this syndrome have hearing loss, mostly conductive. Occasionally there is atresia of the external auditory canals. Deformity of the ossicles or fixation of the footplate of the stapes has been found on postmortem examination. Craniofacial dysostosis may be corrected by major maxillofacial surgery.

Mandibulofacial Dysostosis (Treacher Collins Syndrome). This autosomal dominantly inherited syndrome is characterized by (1) anomalies of the eye, such as antimongoloid obliquity of the lids and coloboma of the lower lids with lack of cilia, (2) abnormalities of the external and middle ears, and (3) hypoplasia of the mandible and malar bones.

The facies is remarkably striking. The palpebral fissures slope laterally downward, and often there is a coloboma in the outer third of the lower lid with a deficiency of cilia medial to the coloboma. The pinna is often deformed, and there may be absence of the external auditory canal and abnormalities within the middle ear cleft, such as agenesis or malformation of the ossicles with resultant conduction deafness. Ear tags and blind fistulas may occur anywhere between the tragus and the angle of the mouth.

Conductive hearing loss is secondary to ossicular malformation.

The mandible is always hypoplastic. The angle is more obtuse than normal, and the undersurface of its body is markedly concave. The palate is high or cleft in over 40 per cent of reported patients. Dental malocclusion is frequent.

Connective tissue may fill middle ear cleft. Deafness is not progressive.

CYSTS OF THE JAWS AND ORAL FLOOR

A true cyst is defined as a cavity lined by epithelium. It may be situated entirely within soft tissues or deep within bone or may lie on the bony surface, producing a saucerization (Table 15–1). Within the jaws, the epithelium may have its origin in odontogenic epithelium (i.e., from the remnants of the dental lamina or from the enamel organs of the teeth). Proliferation and cystic degeneration of this epithelium would give rise to odontogenic cysts. Considered within this category are the dentigerous cyst, radicular cyst, and odontogenic keratocyst. Nonodontogenic cysts are derived from epithelial remnants of the tissue covering the embryonal processes that participate in the formation of the face and jaws. These so-called fissural cysts include the nasoalveolar cyst, dermoid and epidermoid cyst, and palatal cyst of newborn infants. Nonodontogenic cysts may arise also from the

TABLE 15–1. CYSTS OF THE JAWS AND ORAL CAVITY

Odontogenic cysts
  Dentigerous cyst
  Eruption cyst
  Gingival cyst of newborn infants
  Radicular cyst
  Keratocyst
Nonodontogenic and fissural cysts
  Nasoalveolar cyst
  Nasopalatine or incisive canal cyst
  Palatal cyst of newborn infants
  Dermoid and epidermoid cyst
  Submental or geniohyoid dermoid cyst
  Retention cyst

remains of the nasopalatine duct, which gives rise to the nasopalatine cyst. Grouped as pseudocysts of the jaws are the aneurysmal bone cyst, static bone cyst, and solitary bone cyst. None of these is epithelium-lined. The static bone cyst appears to be a congenital bone defect; trauma has been suggested as the etiologic agent in both the aneurysmal bone cyst and the solitary bone cyst. Some of the more common cysts are considered separately.

Odontogenic Cysts

Dentigerous Cyst (Fig. 15–7). The dentigerous cyst surrounds the crown of an unerupted tooth of either the regular (in approximately 95 per cent of all cases) or the supernumerary dentition. It probably arises through alteration of the reduced enamel epithelium after the crown has been completely formed. Fluid accumulates either between layers of the enamel epithelium or between the epithelium and the tooth crown. The cyst may arise, however, from cystic degeneration of remnants of the dental lamina.

The teeth usually involved are the mandibular third molar, maxillary canine, maxillary third molar, and second mandibular premolar, although the cyst may occur about any unerupted tooth. The crown of the tooth projects into the lumen of the cystic cavity. The cyst may be of any size, ranging from a subtle dilatation of the pericoronal sac to a space occupying the entire body and ramus of half the jaw. Possibly because of the anatomy of the upper and lower jaws, the larger cysts involve the mandible. Although the cyst develops in relationship to a single tooth, it may include the crowns of several adjacent teeth as it enlarges. Furthermore, it may displace teeth to positions remote from their normal sites, especially in the maxilla.

Dentigerous cysts are usually solitary. When multiple, however, possible association with nevoid basal cell carcinoma syndrome should be ruled out.

Eruption Cyst. The eruption cyst is an uncommon type of dentigerous cyst associated with erupting deciduous or rarely permanent teeth. It represents the accumulation of tissue fluid or blood in a dilated follicular space about the crown of an erupting tooth. It may be unilateral or bilateral, single or multiple, and may be present at birth.

Gingival and Palatal Cysts of Newborn Infants. Nearly all human fetuses after their fourth month in utero and at least 80 per cent of newborn infants have small nodules or cysts (Epstein's pearls, Bohn's nodules) at the junction of the hard and soft palates near the median raphe. The nodules, usually several, are white to yellowish white small epithelial inclusion cysts, probably

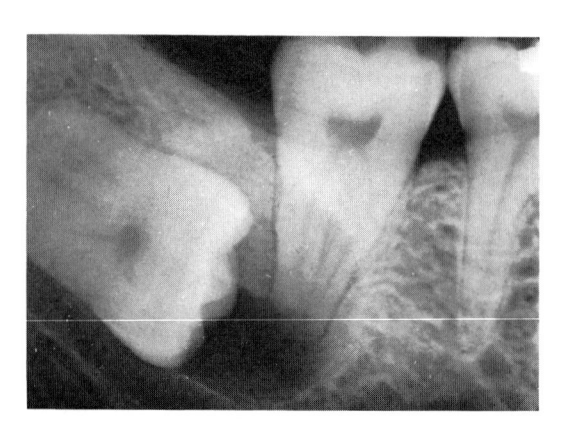

FIGURE 15–7. Dentigerous cyst. Note the radiolucency surrounding the crown of the unerupted molar.

resulting from incorporation of epithelium during the embryonic process of palatal fusion. These cysts become superficial and rupture, usually within the first few weeks of life. Gingival cysts represent degeneration of dental lamina remnants.

Radicular Cyst (Fig. 15–8). Certainly the most common of oral cysts, the radicular (periapical) periodontal cyst is inflammatory in origin. It occurs as a sequela of dental caries.

With the spread of the inflammatory process from the pulp to the periapical area of the tooth, a mass of chronic inflammatory tissue is formed, called an

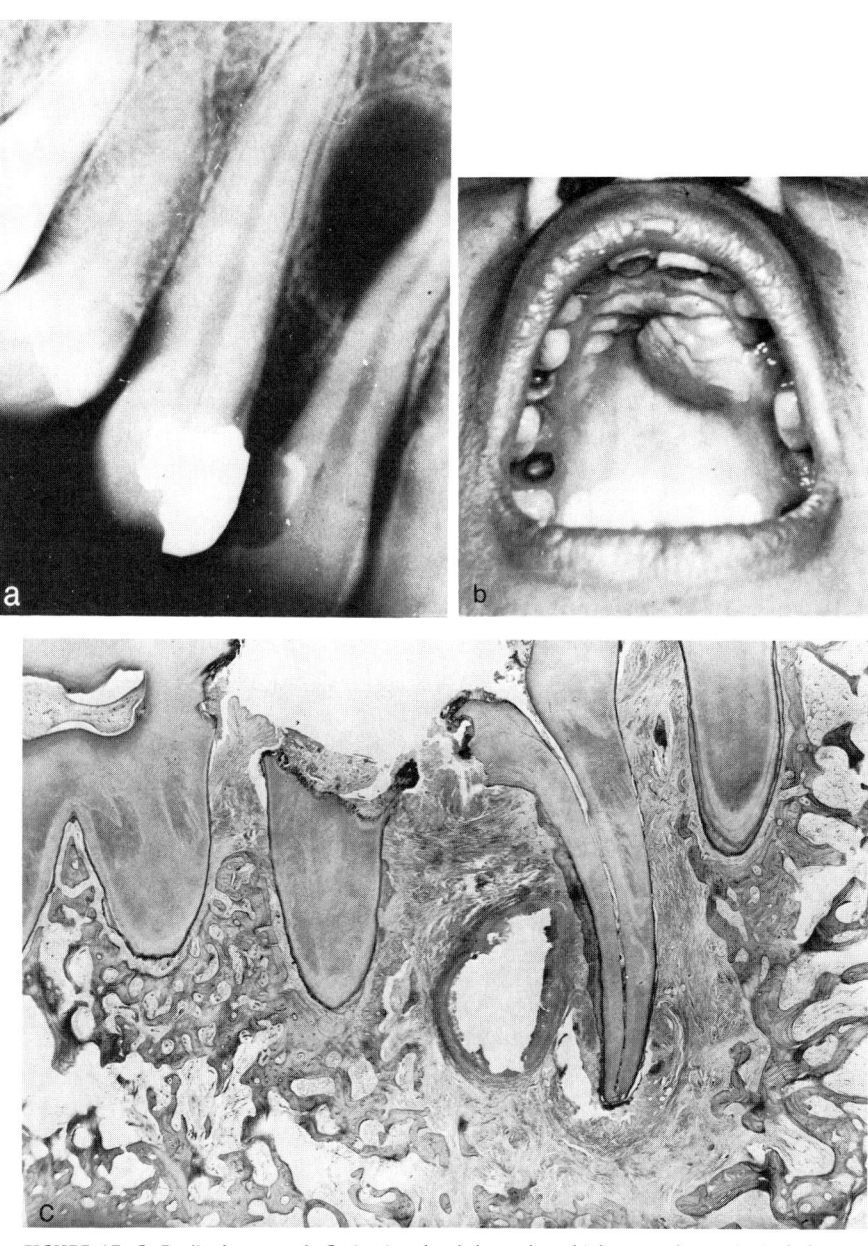

FIGURE 15–8. Radicular cyst. *A*, Caries involved the pulp, which caused a periapical abscess surrounding the root of the maxillary lateral incisor. *B*, Clinical appearance. Note swelling extending to the palate. *C*, Observe extensive destruction of the crown.

apical granuloma. Within this mass, epithelial rests of Malassez normally present in the periodontal ligament proliferate extensively. These epithelial islands coalesce and become cystic, giving rise to the radicular cyst.

The cyst is often symptomless and is diagnosed on routine dental radiographs. The associated tooth is nonvital and usually manifests dental caries. However, in some cases, a history of trauma to the area is obtained. The radicular cyst tends to remain small and does not produce jaw expansion. One cannot differentiate radiographically between an apical granuloma and a radicular cyst. The cyst that remains in place after the extraction of the responsible tooth is known as a residual cyst. Rarely does a radicular cyst exceed 0.6 cm in diameter.

Nevoid Basal Cell Carcinoma Syndrome. The association of multiple keratocysts with multiple cutaneous nevoid basal cell carcinomas and numerous skeletal and other abnormalities is a well-recognized syndrome. The syndrome probably occurs in 1 in 200 individuals with cutaneous basal cell carcinoma. It has autosomal dominant inheritance with complete penetrance and extremely variable expressivity.

(1) basal cell carcinoma
(2) multiple keratocysts
(3) skeletal abnormalities

The skin is involved with numerous basal cell carcinomas, some of which become aggressive. They usually appear early in life and often are in areas not exposed to sunlight.

Bifurcated and splayed ribs, kyphoscoliosis, fusion of vertebrae, and cervicothoracic spina bifida occulta are common. Lamellar calcification of the falx cerebri, bilateral calcified fibromas of the ovary, and medulloblastoma and meningioma are seen.

Scattered throughout the jaws are numerous cysts that vary in size from microscopic to several centimeters in diameter. These odontogenic keratocysts are lined by epithelium that ranges from a simple to a thinly keratinized stratified squamous variety. They may appear for the first time as early as the age of seven or eight years or as late as the thirties. There is a marked tendency for these cysts to recur, possibly from adjacent microcysts, in spite of thorough curettement.

Nonodontogenic and Fissural Cysts

Nasopalatine or Incisive Canal Cyst (Fig. 15–9). The incisive canal cyst is a closed, epithelium-lined intrabony sac. When it is located below the incisive foramen, it is called a cyst of the palatine papilla.

Embryologically, the incisive canal joining the nasal and oral cavities is formed when the maxillary palatine processes fuse with the primary palate, leaving two passageways, one on each side of the nasal septum. Within each canal is an epithelial nasopalatine duct or cord of epithelial cell remnants.

The type of epithelium composing the nasopalatine duct or its remnants depends upon location: respiratory epithelium is formed nearest the nasal cavity, then the cuboidal type is seen, and finally stratified squamous epithelium appears as the oral cavity is approached.

Most patients in whom the cyst becomes clinically evident are in the fourth to sixth decades of life. Generally, nasopalatine cysts are painless unless they become infected.

Clinically there is often enlargement at the anterior midline of the palate. Swelling occurs in about half the patients with incisive canal cysts and in those with cysts of the palatine papilla. Drainage is a common sequela.

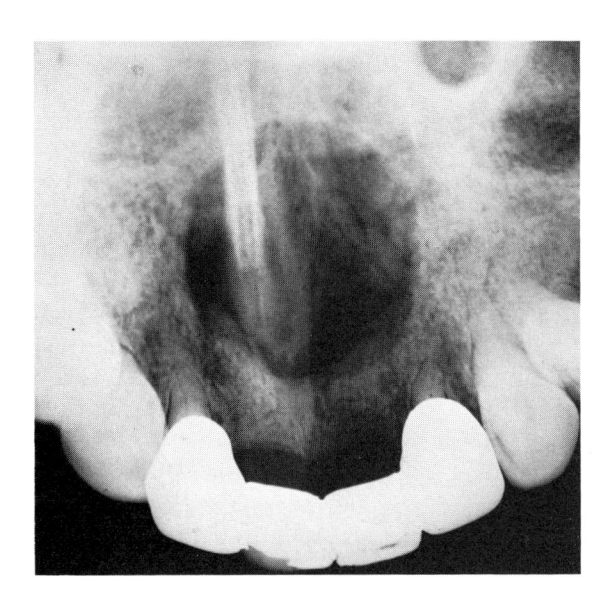

FIGURE 15–9. Nasopalatine cyst. Note extensive radiolucency in the area of the nasopalatine duct.

Nasoalveolar Cyst. The nasoalveolar (nasolabial) cyst has also been called Klestadt's cyst. It probably arises from epithelial rests located at the junction of the globular, lateral nasal, and maxillary processes.

The cyst is situated at the attachment of the ala of the naris, i.e., near the base of the nostril. It is not located within bone. The nasoalveolar cyst may cause enough facial swelling to obliterate the nasolabial fold on the involved side. Bilateral involvement is noted in about 10 per cent of the patients. Ordinarily the cyst swells into the floor of the nasal vestibule, projecting beneath the anterior end of the inferior turbinate. At times, this causes nasal obstruction. Intermittent pain is experienced by about one third of the patients. Blunt dissection of the cyst has indicated that it is attached to the nasal mucosa. It can be clearly demonstrated with the use of a radiopaque material.

The nasoalveolar cyst occurs predominantly (about 75 per cent of all cases) in women and appears to occur more often in blacks.

Dermoid and Epidermoid Cysts. The term "dermoid cyst" will be used here to denote a developmental cyst lined by epidermis and cutaneous appendages. It probably results from incorporation of ectoderm at the time of closure of embryonic fissures during the third and fourth weeks in utero.

Oral dermoid cysts most commonly arise in the floor of the mouth and have been classified into median (midline) and lateral dermoid cysts. They probably always originate above the mylohyoid muscle, although they may penetrate through a developmental hiatus. They usually become evident between 12 and 25 years of age.

The cyst, if located above the geniohyoid muscle (sublingual or genioglossal dermoid cyst), causes elevation and displacement of the tongue, producing difficulty in speaking, eating, and even breathing due to pressure exerted upon the epiglottis. If the cyst is deeper (between the geniohyoid and mylohyoid muscles), it may bulge into the submental area.

The submental or geniohyoid dermoid cyst is manifested by a slow painless swelling in the submental region. It extends from the mandible to the hyoid bone, giving the appearance of a double chin. As it enlarges, it may push the larynx down and by upward growth causes a bulge in the oral floor. The cyst varies in size but may approach several centimeters in diameter. It usually feels doughy but may be more fluctuant.

Microscopically, the lining of the cyst is a keratinized stratified squamous epithelium. One or more skin appendages such as hair follicles, sweat glands, or sebaceous glands are present. In the absence of skin appendages, it is not considered a dermoid cyst; the term *epidermoid cyst* is used to describe such lesions.

Retention "Cysts" (Mucocele). Mucous retention "cysts" result from rupture of a duct of a minor salivary gland, allowing the mucus to spill into the connective tissue where it is treated as a foreign substance by the body. The mucocele occurs most often on the mucosal surface of the lower lip. It may also appear on the buccal mucosa, oral floor, or ventral surface of the tip of the tongue (cyst of Blandin-Nuhn). If it is large and involves the sublingual salivary gland, it is called a ranula. Treatment consists of complete excision of the mucocele and the offending group of minor salivary glands and duct. Incision and drainage yield temporary improvement only.

DENTAL AND PERIODONTAL DISORDERS

Dental Caries and Sequelae

Dental caries is a disease of the enamel, dentin, and cementum that produces progressive demineralization of the calcified component and destruction of the organic component with the formation of a cavity in the tooth. Microorganisms are present at all stages of the disease and from the results of animal experiments appear to be essential etiologic factors.

Tooth decay commonly is stated to be the most frequent disease of civilized man. Once a carious cavity has formed, the defect is permanent.

After the introduction of fluoride to the drinking water (1 ppm), the DMF* rate has generally decreased over a period of years by more than 60 per cent. An optimal amount of fluoride built into the apatite crystal during tooth formation decreases the acid solubility of enamel. Topical applications of fluoride solutions to recently erupted tooth surfaces and brushing the teeth with dentifrices containing fluoride appear to be effective in reducing susceptibility to dental caries. Bonding agents applied prophylactically to pits and fissures are also efficacious.

Caries occurs in areas on tooth surfaces where saliva, food debris, and bacterial plaque accumulate. These areas are chiefly the cervical portion of the tooth, interproximal surfaces, and pits and fissures. Surfaces that are self-cleansing by the excursion of food and the action of the tongue and cheeks are usually free of caries.

The formation of bacterial plaques in areas of stagnation precedes cavity formation. Acidogenic and aciduric bacteria, together with filamentous forms, are present in such plaques. Once a cavity has been produced in the enamel with exposure of the underlying dentin, proteolytic microorganisms complete the destruction of the decalcified tooth structure. Caries spreads laterally at the dentinoenamel junction, weakening and undermining the

---

*DMF = decayed, missing, filled teeth.

enamel. It also progresses along dentinal tubules and especially in the young may rapidly lead to exposure of the underlying pulp tissue.

Inflammatory processes in the tooth pulp may be infected or noninfected. Trauma to the tooth from a blow (which may or may not fracture the tooth), from dental operations, or from excessive thermal changes may induce inflammation. Since the rigid walls of the tooth do not permit expansion of the inflamed pulp, the circulation may be cut off and the pulp may become an infarct that is later replaced by fibrous connective tissue. Bacterial infection is the common sequel to dental caries or to mechanical exposure of the tooth pulp.

Pulpitis may be acute or chronic. In acute pulpitis pain is usually severe and is increased by heat or cold. It is often aggravated by lying down (increased vascular pressure) and may be accompanied by a mild fever and leukocytosis. Characteristically, the purulent process spreads to involve the entire pulp and, unless the tooth is opened to establish drainage, the periapical tissues become involved in an acute alveolar abscess. Once the tissues about the root apex become involved, the tooth becomes sensitive to percussion.

Acute alveolar abscess is usually the result of suppurative infection spreading from the tooth pulp through the root canals to the periodontal ligament about the tooth root ends. The inflammation characteristically follows the blood vessels into the bone marrow spaces. Suppuration follows pathways determined by the location of the tooth roots and the characteristics of adjacent structures. Usually the periosteum overlying the tooth root end is destroyed, and eventually pus is drained through a fistula (gum boil). In maxillary teeth, drainage may occur into the antrum or into the palate. Occasionally the soft tissues are extensively involved, and, if they are not treated, drainage to the surface of the skin of the face or neck may occur. Osteomyelitis, cavernous sinus thrombosis, and Ludwig's angina are serious complications.

A much more common sequel to dental pulp infection is the dental granuloma. Clinically this may be completely symptomless. Radiographic examination frequently discloses an area of bone rarefaction about a tooth root apex, with a chronically infected or partially obliterated root canal. This area is usually spherical and well demarcated.

A granuloma represents a balance between the defense forces of the body and a chronic area of necrotic tissue in the tooth root that is acting as an infected sequestrum. If the tooth is extracted, the granulation tissue usually disappears during the healing process. Occasionally a granuloma may persist as an area of "residual infection" after the tooth is extracted. Common oral organisms, chiefly *Streptococcus* and *Staphylococcus,* have been demonstrated in many dental granulomas, although some lesions appear to be sterile.

Gingivitis and Periodontitis (Fig. 15–10)

Inflammatory and degenerative processes that develop at the gingival margin and progress until the tooth-supporting structures are lost have much in common with periapical periodontal disease. In both instances, chronic asymptomatic infection by the common oral pathogens is usual, although

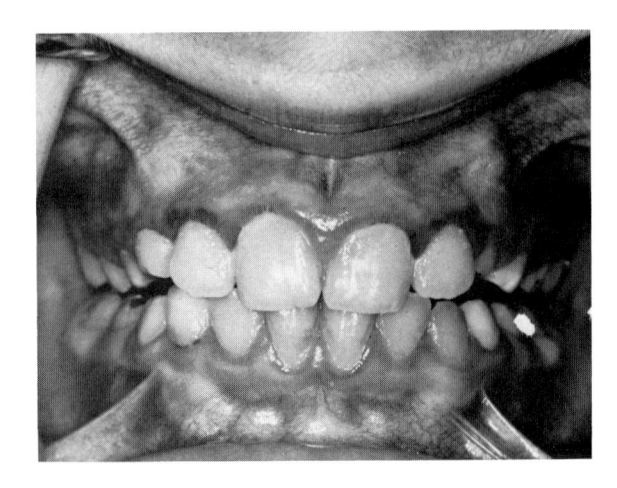

FIGURE 15–10. Gingivitis.

episodes of acute suppuration may occur. The reactions in both cases consist of a walling-off process with a marked chronic inflammatory cell infiltration. In periodontal disease this represents an attempt to cover the surface of the chronic ulcer that develops about the involved tooth root area.

The disease commonly begins as gingivitis. Plaque and calculus deposited upon the tooth surfaces, impaction of food, decayed teeth, overhanging margins of dental restorations, and ill-fitting dental appliances are among the local causes. Once a "pocket" has been established below the gingival margin, calcified deposits form on the tooth root surfaces and act as infected foreign bodies, thus prolonging and promoting the inflammatory process with progressive resorption of the fibrous and bony tooth-supporting structures. Proliferation of epithelium that lines the pocket occurs concomitantly with the loss of tissue. Periodontal disease is more common in older individuals, and after middle age, it becomes the chief cause of tooth loss.

Patients with diabetes mellitus are especially susceptible to periodontal disease, and an alert clinician should suspect this condition if there are oral signs and symptoms.

Pregnancy, with its change in endocrine balance, frequently is accompanied by gingivitis and hyperplastic inflammatory responses. Gingivitis may be somewhat more frequent during puberty.

Necrotizing Ulcerative Gingivitis (Vincent's Infection) (Fig. 15–11). This condition is extremely rare in children, occurring far more commonly in

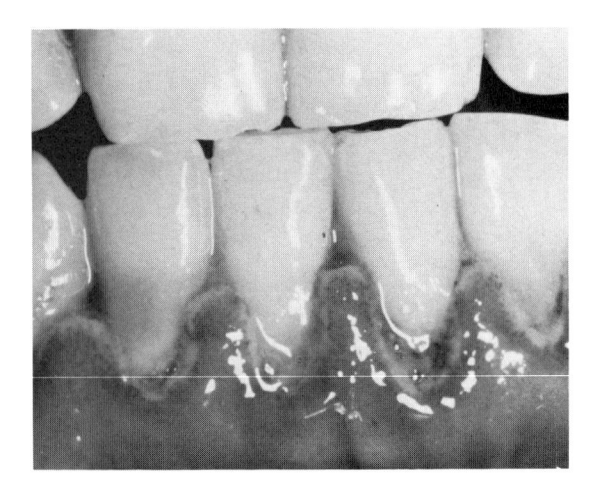

FIGURE 15–11. Necrotizing ulcerative gingivitis. Note destruction of the interdental papillae.

young adults. It is infectious but not contagious. (Most cases of so-called Vincent's infection in children are actually acute herpetic gingivostomatitis.) The condition seems to be associated with lowered resistance and invasion of the oral tissues by organisms normally present in the mouth, principally *Borrelia vincentii* and fusiform bacilli. The interproximal gingival papillae are destroyed, and a pseudomembrane covers the marginal gingiva. The gingiva bleeds easily and is painful, and not uncommonly, associated symptoms include malaise, fever, loss of appetite, and a fetid odor in the mouth.

The disease is treated by debridement, subgingival curettage, and dilute (3 per cent) hydrogen peroxide mouthwashes. In addition, if the process is accompanied by systemic symptoms such as fever, oral administration of penicillin V is indicated, 25,000 to 50,000 units per kilogram of body weight per 24 hours divided into four doses. Ordinarily the process, if treated, subsides within 48 hours. It is important that dental consultation be recommended for a thorough cleaning of the teeth to prevent recurrence or for correction of damage to the periodontium.

Gingival Fibromatosis (Fig. 15–12)

Generalized enlargement of the gingiva is often inherited as an autosomal dominant characteristic. The gingiva seems to enlarge until the permanent teeth are covered by a hard, firm, painless gingiva that may displace the teeth. Therapy consists of surgical removal of the hyperplastic tissue. Recurrence within a year is not uncommon, and repeated gingivectomies may be required.

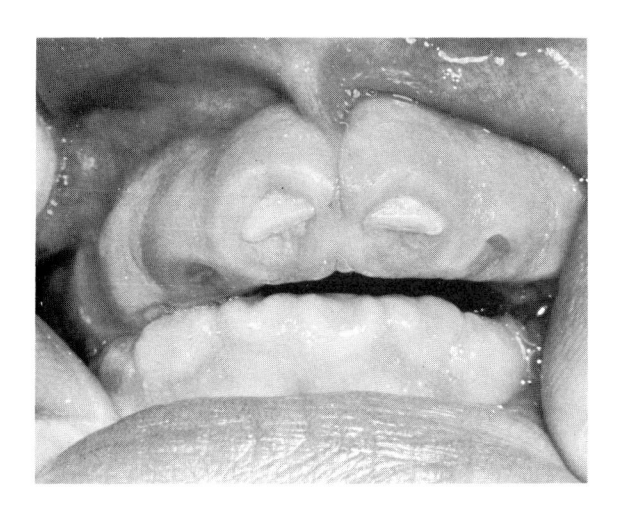

Dilantin Gingival Enlargement (Fig. 15–13)

A generalized, painless hyperplasia of the gingiva is associated with prolonged therapeutic use of Dilantin sodium. In some patients, the gingiva may actually cover the teeth. The degree of hyperplasia appears to be most closely related to oral hygiene: the poorer the hygiene, the more pronounced the enlargement. Gingival surgery may be indicated for severe hyperplasia. Vigorous tooth brushing and gingival massage, either manual or preferably with an electric toothbrush, are indicated. Similar enlargement may occur with cyclosporine A and nifedipine therapy.

FIGURE 15–12. Gingival fibromatosis. This disorder is frequently inherited as an autosomal dominant trait. In some patients, the teeth are completely covered by extremely hard fibrous tissue.

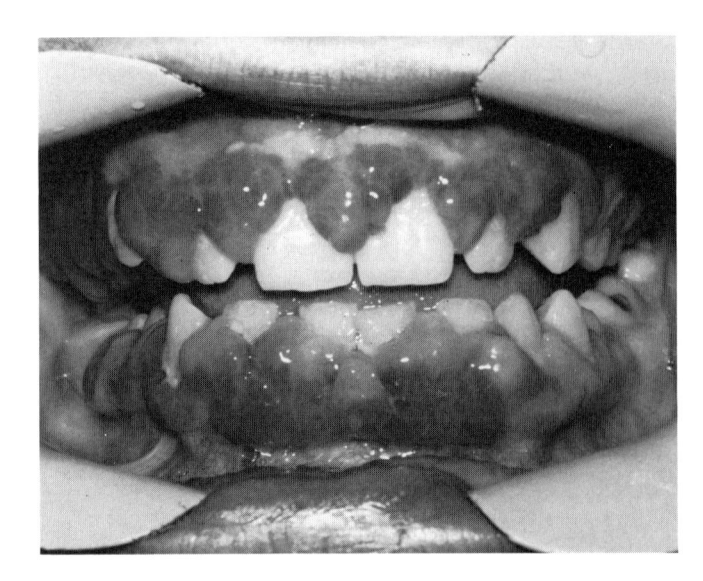

FIGURE 15–13. Dilantin gingivitis.

Tetracycline Side Effects

Yellow-gray, bright yellow, gray-brown, or darker discoloration of teeth which may or may not be accompanied by hypoplasia of the enamel has been traced to tetracycline therapy during the period of tooth formation. Tetracyclines have caused tooth defects in children when administered to mothers in the last trimester of pregnancy, as well as when administered to the child. The effects are dosage-dependent. Although individual susceptibility varies, tetracyclines used during periods of tooth formation at levels exceeding 75 mg/kg of body weight nearly always cause enamel hypoplasia.

As many as 35 per cent of children in a pediatric medical practice have been noted to demonstrate such changes. Diagnostically, a yellow to yellow-brown fluorescence is noted under ultraviolet light, peaking at 340 to 370 nm. Although no treatment is usually necessary, severe hypoplasia may require dental restoration of teeth. Jacket crowns may be desirable in cases of severe staining. Acid etching of the enamel and resin application may be employed to esthetically restore the teeth.

In addition to the previously mentioned causes, many systemic conditions may interfere with matrix formation and calcification. These include rickets, hypoparathyroidism, and various disorders accompanied by high fever.

Disorders in Tooth Eruption

Primary teeth erupt prematurely about once in 3000 live births. They may be present at birth (natal teeth) or may erupt within the first month (neonatal teeth). This disorder may be associated with syndromes such as pachyonychia congenita, Ellis–van Creveld syndrome, or oculomandibulodyscephaly. If the teeth are loose or interfere with nursing, they should be gently extracted.

The most common disturbance in the eruption of teeth is caused by premature loss or extraction of neglected permanent or primary teeth. Loss of a first permanent molar without subsequent space maintenance may result in serious malocclusion. Early, premature loss of a primary tooth impairs mastication and may result in improper eruption or impaction of the permanent tooth.

Premature Periodontal Destruction

Inflammation of supporting tissues and structures of the teeth such as gingiva, bone, and periodontal ligament is so rare in children that the clinician should be alert to its frequently systemic implications. It is seen in more than 90 per cent of children with Down's syndrome (trisomy 21). Not uncommonly in these children there is loss of mandibular incisors because of alveolar bone loss. Meticulous oral care must be given to children with this condition. Early loss of anterior deciduous teeth—the permanent dentition is almost always spared—is seen in hypophosphatasia due to lack of cementum.

Severe periodontal destruction occurs about both deciduous and permanent teeth in the Papillon-Lefèvre syndrome. This is a rare autosomal recessive condition associated with infantile palmar and plantar hyperkeratosis. Histiocytosis X is frequently associated with periodontal destruction and early individual tooth loss, especially in the molar areas of the primary teeth. Most important, children with leukemia or agranulocytosis frequently present with oral signs resembling periodontitis. This may take the form of engorged, edematous gingival tissue or periodontitis. The gingiva rapidly becomes necrotic, with associated exfoliation of teeth.

DISORDERS OF THE ORAL MUCOSA

Geographic Tongue (Fig. 15–14)

This condition is noted in 1 to 6 per cent of the population and, in most cases, is asymptomatic. The dorsum of the tongue shows characteristic smooth, shiny, erythematous areas that are slightly depressed below the surrounding normal papillae. These patches disappear and reappear in different areas and at different times throughout the person's life. There appears to be no treatment for this condition except to reassure the parent or patient that the disorder is not serious.

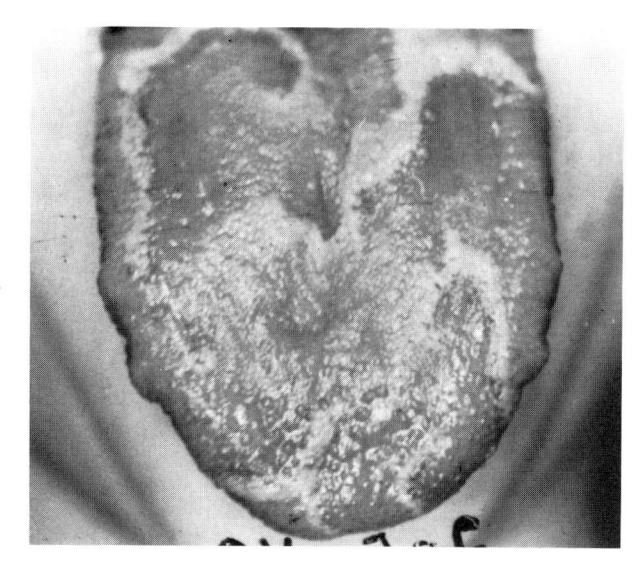

FIGURE 15–14. Geographic tongue.

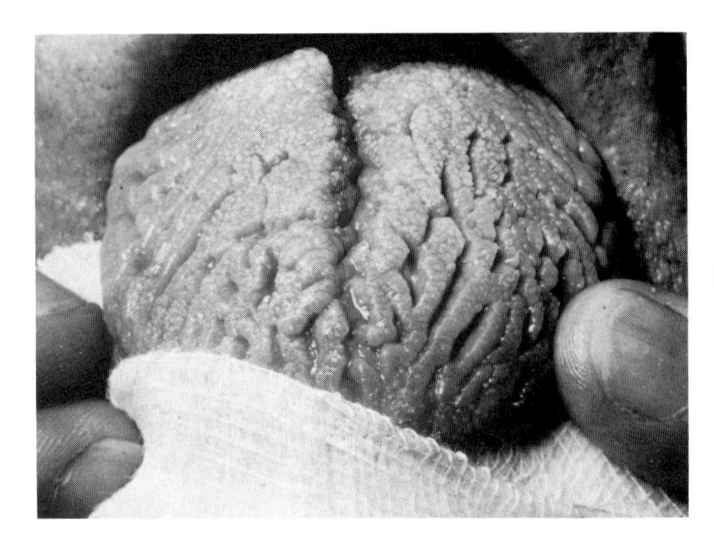

FIGURE 15–15. Fissured or scrotal tongue.

Scrotal Tongue (Fig. 15–15)

This condition is characterized by tongue papillae divided into groups and clumps by small fissures that may not be apparent until the tongue is folded. There seems to be a linear progression in the prevalence of this entity with age, being seen in 1 per cent of infants and approximately 2.5 per cent of children and in 4 per cent of young adults. Scrotal tongue may also be part of the Melkersson-Rosenthal syndrome and is also found frequently in trisomy 21. The condition does not adversely affect the patient, and no treatment is recommended.

Black Hairy Tongue (Fig. 15–16)

This entity is characterized by an elongation of the filiform papillae and concurrent growth of a black pigment-producing fungus. The development

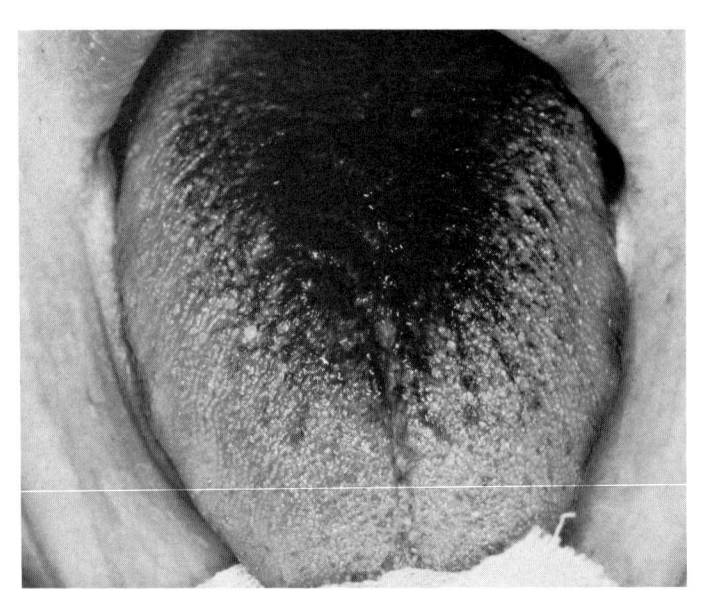

FIGURE 15–16. Black hairy tongue.

of black hairy tongue is often associated with antibiotic therapy. The condition is harmless and usually disappears spontaneously. Although treatment is not necessary, frequent application of 20 per cent aqueous caprylate or 0.25 per cent triamcinolone acetonide in an adhesive base is effective. In addition, the patient should brush the dorsum of the tongue two or three times daily.

Herpes Simplex (Fig. 15–17)

Distinction should be made between primary and secondary (recurrent) disease usually due to herpes simplex, type 1 virus. The type 2 virus is occasionally the agent in primary oral disease in adults. In the former, herpetic gingivostomatitis and inoculation herpes simplex are the most common manifestations. Recurrent herpetic lesions occur in various locations, there being a predilection for transitional zones from skin to mucosa (herpes simplex labialis) and on the fixed gingiva or hard palate.

Primary Herpes Simplex. *Primary herpetic gingivostomatitis* usually occurs between one and five years of age and has been estimated to occur in less than 1 per cent of the population. The incubation period is variable (2 to 20 days) but averages about 6 days. It is rarely observed in adults. As with primary inoculation herpes, the acute vesicular lesions last from 5 to 7 days and are accompanied by high fever, dehydration, malaise, nausea, and even somnolence and convulsions. Initially, the gingiva becomes swollen, with associated salivation, fetor oris, dysphagia, and painful lymphadenopathy.

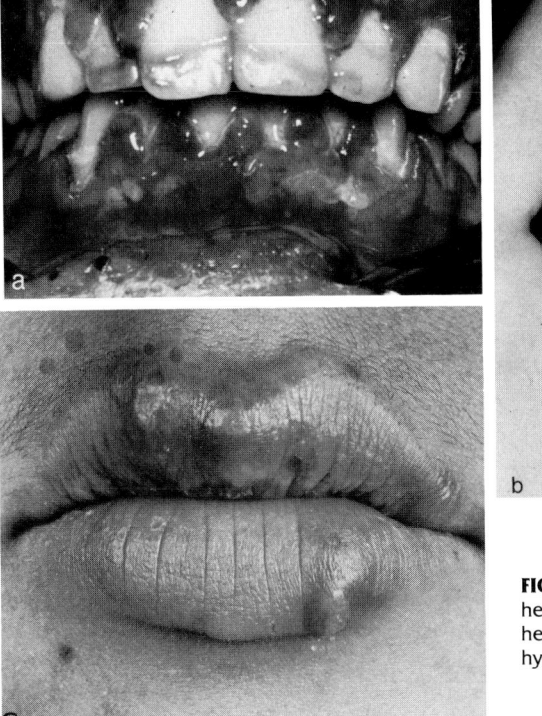

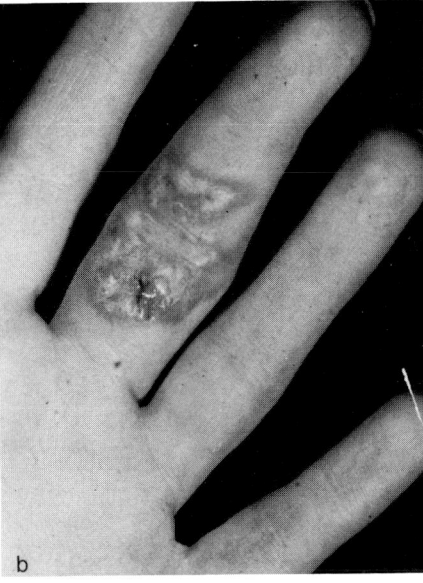

FIGURE 15–17. Herpes simplex. *A,* Acute herpetic gingivostomatitis. *B,* Inoculation herpes simplex on the finger of a dental hygienist. *C,* Recurrent herpes simplex.

The oral mucous membranes, especially those of the gingiva and tongue, are sites of round to oval, sharply demarcated, disseminated vesicles or erosions. The individual lesions are 2 to 4 mm in diameter, painful, covered by a yellowish pseudomembrane, and surrounded by a red margin. The intact vesicle rarely lasts for more than 24 hours.

After about 10 to 14 days, the primary infection subsides without scar formation. Following a latent period of varying length, often not until after puberty, secondary or recurrent herpes simplex may develop. Immunocompromised patients may suffer a severe primary infection.

Treatment consists largely of supportive therapy, topical anesthetics such as 5 per cent Xylocaine (lidocaine) ointment, and enriched liquid diet. Topical acyclovir (Zovirax) is of limited efficacy.

Inoculation herpes simplex is not uncommon among physicians, dentists, and dental hygienists, the virus in the saliva of a patient penetrating through an abrasion of the skin.

Regardless of whether the primary infection is clinical or subclinical, recurrent herpetic lesions develop later in many persons, being precipitated by many different factors. Not all individuals suffer from recurrent herpes simplex. It has been estimated that from 70 to 90 per cent of the population are carriers of the virus after 14 years of age.

Secondary (Recurrent) Herpes Simplex. The most common form of herpetic infection, secondary herpes simplex, possibly affects 25 to 50 per cent of the adult population. After a prodromal period of 24 to 48 hours, marked by a burning, itching, or tingling sensation in the region of the forming lesions, the eruption appears. This consists of groups of small clear vesicles that soon become transformed into pustules or crusted confluent erosions located most often on the vermilion or mucocutaneous junction of the upper or lower lip. The infection generally recurs at the same sites. Secondary herpes simplex may very rarely involve the oral cavity proper where, in contrast to primary gingivostomatitis, it affects only circumscribed areas such as the hard palate and fixed gingiva. They appear as grouped small (1 to 2 mm) ulcers.

A variety of stimuli may precipitate recurrent herpes simplex. These include fever, sunlight, food allergy, colds, menstruation, mechanical trauma, and possibly even psychosomatic factors.

Subjective complaints extend from mild itching or burning to severe pain in addition to the cosmetic inconveniences involved. After four to ten days, the crusted lesions heal without scarring.

Identification of the herpes simplex virus in either the primary or recurrent form can be done by viral isolation, fluorescent antibody examination, or cytologic study (Giemsa smears).

Treatment is largely ineffective. The immunosuppressed patient should be treated with oral or intravenous acyclovir.

Recurrent Aphthous Stomatitis

Aphthous stomatitis is a non-viral recurrent ulceration of the oral cavity and lips.

Recurrent aphthous stomatitis (aphthae, canker sores) is a disorder that affects about 20 per cent of the population. It appears to be at least twice as prevalent among professional school student personnel as among the general population. The disorder is of unknown etiology, although a host of causes has been blamed, most recently the pleomorphic transitional L form of alpha-hemolytic streptococci. It is definitely not of viral origin.

Trauma may play some role, since typical aphthae may arise at the site of injury (needle puncture, "cotton roll" stomatitis). It has been recently suggested that recurrent aphthous stomatitis represents a form of autoimmunity, since autoantibodies to oral mucosal homogenates are found in 70 to 80 per cent of those with recurrent aphthous stomatitis as opposed to 10 per cent of controls. After a burning sensation in the affected mucosa during the prodromal stage, the mucosa becomes focally erythematous and necrotic, with formation of single or multiple, round to oval ulcerations usually 2 to 10 mm in diameter, with about 10 per cent being larger than 1 cm. The ulcer is covered by a grayish white fibrinous exudate and surrounded by a bright red halo. It usually persists for one or two weeks and heals without scarring. Xylocaine ointment (5 per cent) is effective in reducing discomfort. Tetracycline swish and swallow suspensions (250 mg/5 ml q.i.d) also offer some relief.

Major Aphthae

Major aphthae (periadenitis mucosa necrotica recurrens, Sutton's disease) is a disease of unknown cause affecting the oral mucosa; it is characterized by large (1 to 2 cm) single or multiple necrotic ulcerations of the lips, cheeks, tongue, soft and hard palates, and anterior tonsillar pillars. Apparently, the gingiva is rarely, if ever, involved. Ulceration also may occur on the pharyngeal and laryngeal walls. The condition is recurrent, with multiple episodes spaced over several years—in some cases, up to 15. After healing, the ulcer leaves a fibrous retractile scar. Pain and systemic manifestations are present during the acute state of the disease.

Females are slightly more frequently affected than males. The onset can take place at any age but is more common around puberty.

Treatment is generally ineffective, but some relief is provided by the use of 5 per cent Xylocaine ointment. Topically applied 0.05 per cent triamcinolone acetonide or fluocinonide ointment, four to five times per day, is also helpful.

Herpes Zoster

Herpes zoster is a recurrent neurotrophic manifestation of reactivated chickenpox virus. Presumably, the virus persists in ganglion cells, becoming reactivated when immunity has decreased through injuries such as local trauma, stress, neoplasia, or massive new infection with chickenpox-zoster virus.

After an incubation period of 4 to 20 days, the disorder appears with a neuralgic prodromal phase. Within two to three days, grouped vesicles form in the area innervated by the involved nerve. When the face is affected, as in zoster ophthalmicus or zoster oticus (Ramsay Hunt syndrome), the pain is especially severe, and general prodromal symptoms such as fever and nausea are marked. With the appearance of the vesicles, rarely before, a painful regional lymphadenitis develops. Herpes zoster occurs more commonly in males than in females and principally affects individuals over 45 years of age.

In herpes zoster of the cranial nerves, several types can be distinguished: (1) trigeminal type (attack of the gasserian ganglion with involvement of one or more branches), (2) zoster oticus (attack on the geniculate ganglion), (3) zoster of the glossopharyngeal nerve, (4) zoster of the vagus nerve, and other segmental types. Ophthalmic zoster is especially dangerous, since the conjunctiva and cornea are often involved, and iritis, glaucoma, and even panophthalmitis may occur.

On the oral mucosa, the lesions are more diffuse. The unilocular zoster vesicle is especially short-lived. It rapidly changes into a painful aphtha surrounded by a red halo. When the second trigeminal division is involved, unilateral vesicles appear on the palate, uvula, maxillary gingiva, and upper buccal and labial mucosa. Involvement of the lower lip, mandibular gingiva, and oral floor is seen in third division zoster.

Postzoster neuralgias are extremely painful for months or even years, especially in elderly persons. A combination of anesthesia or hypesthesia of the affected segment, often with very severe neuralgia, is especially distressing. In addition, herpes zoster may simulate lancinating trigeminal neuralgia.

In the immunocompromised patient, intravenous acyclovir or vidarabine affords help. However, in the immunocompetent patient, the disorder will run its course and help is largely supportive.

Pemphigus

A bullous disease of autoimmune etiology, pemphigus can be subdivided into many clinical types, all of which are histologically characterized by intraepithelial vesicles or bullae. Immunofluorescent studies have demonstrated autoantibodies to the intercellular cement substance of the stratified squamous epithelium of the oral mucosa and skin of patients with pemphigus. The most severe type, pemphigus vulgaris, often resulted in rapid death prior to the use of corticosteroids. It occurs almost exclusively in middle-aged and elderly persons and has no sex predilection. Lesions start in the mouth in 50 per cent of the patients, and there is oral involvement at some stage in the disease in all patients. The pharynx, larynx, and nasal, anal, and vaginal mucosae are also involved. Vesicles and bullae tend to arise on relatively normal-appearing skin and may be precipitated by pressure or friction (Nikolsky's sign). They are ordinarily tense and round but do not last long on a mucosal surface. They rupture, leaving peripheral epithelial tags.

Areas involved by pemphigus, especially the larynx, can heal with cicatricial formation.

Microscopically, the vesicle is usually suprabasilar and contains acantholytic cells as well as variable numbers of nonspecific inflammatory cells, among which there is a moderate number of eosinophils.

Various immunosuppressive agents, alone or in combination, are successful (prednisone, methotrexate, cyclophosphamide, azathioprine). A soft diet and topical Xylocaine can be used until control is achieved.

Mucous Membrane Pemphigoid

This disorder, also known as cicatricial pemphigoid, is a chronic vesiculobullous disease of autoimmune etiology. It involves primarily oral and ocular mucous membranes. It is characterized by bullae or erosions, or both, the ocular lesions tending to heal with scarring, which, if unattended, may lead to blindness.

The oral lesions are present in 90 to 100 per cent of the patients. They occur most commonly during the seventh decade. There may be some female predilection. The oral lesions frequently present as a desquamative gingivitis. Minor trauma wipes away the epithelium, leaving a raw hemorrhagic surface. The vesicles that occur on the buccal mucosa, tongue, or soft palate are more stable than those of pemphigus, the split taking place at the basal lamina. In contrast to pemphigus, there is no acantholysis and frequently there is a moderate, chronic, inflammatory infiltrate in the subepithelial connective tissue. Immunofluorescent studies show linear deposition of complement and immunoglobulins in the basement membrane zone.

Ocular lesions appear late in the disease process. There is redness, swelling, burning, tearing, and photophobia. The patient often complains of a foreign body sensation. Fibrous adhesions develop between the palpebral and bulbar conjunctivae. Scarring produces trichiasis, entropion, and corneal damage with resultant blindness.

As in the case of pemphigus, various immunosuppressive agents such as prednisone or azathioprine may be employed.

Erythema Multiforme (Fig. 15–18)

Erythema multiforme is an acute, recurrent, self-limited eruption of skin and mucous membranes. The disorder is probably a hypersensitivity reaction. It is characterized by various clinical types of lesions, including bullae, vesicles, papules, macules, and wheals. When vesicles and bullae predominate, the disease is known as erythema multiforme bullosum. The mucous membranes (oral, ocular, vulvovaginal, and urethral), as well as joints, may be involved in more severe disease. In some patients, the lesions are

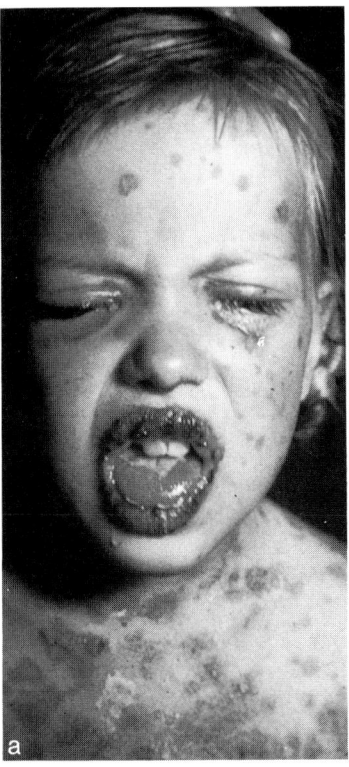

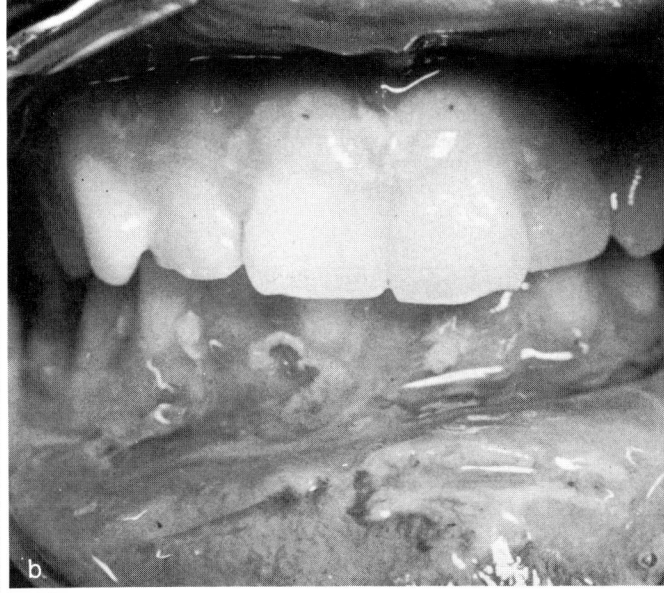

FIGURE 15–18. Erythema multiforme. *A*, Note generalized involvement of skin, a well as lips, tongue, and other areas. *B*, Oral mucosa is extremely fragile and looks scalded.

restricted to the mucous membranes. Stevens-Johnson syndrome is a severe form of bullous erythema multiforme characterized by a toxic, acute, febrile course. Precipitating factors include viral disorders, especially herpes simplex and *Mycoplasma* infections, and many drugs but especially long-acting sulfonamides. In our experience a short tapering course of systemic corticosteroids with an initial dose of 40 to 60 mg/day is helpful.

White Lesions of the Oral Mucosa

A change in color of the normally reddish oral mucosa to white constitutes one of the most frequently encountered oral abnormalities. The term *leukoplakia* has been used so differently by so many that it has come to signify only a "white patch" that does not rub away.

Increased retention and production of keratin by mucosal stratified squamous epithelium constitute the most frequent cause of white patches of the oral cavity. This is termed *hyperkeratosis* and may be associated with chronic mechanical irritation and other factors. Biopsies of oral white patches may demonstrate cytologic alterations of such a degree as to warrant consideration as "premalignant"; these changes include those of dyskeratosis—abnormal nuclear shapes and size and increased numbers of mitotic figures.

Lichen Planus (Fig. 15–19)

The oral lesions that are present in 30 to 40 per cent of the patients with cutaneous lichen planus appear on the buccal mucosa, tongue, gingiva, and lips. In approximately 25 per cent of the cases only oral lesions are present. They may precede the appearance of cutaneous lesions by several years.

The typical buccal and labial mucosal lesions present as a fine lacework of white reticular hyperkeratotic papules (Wickham's striae) and gray plaque-like or annular lesions on the dorsum of the tongue. On the buccal mucosa,

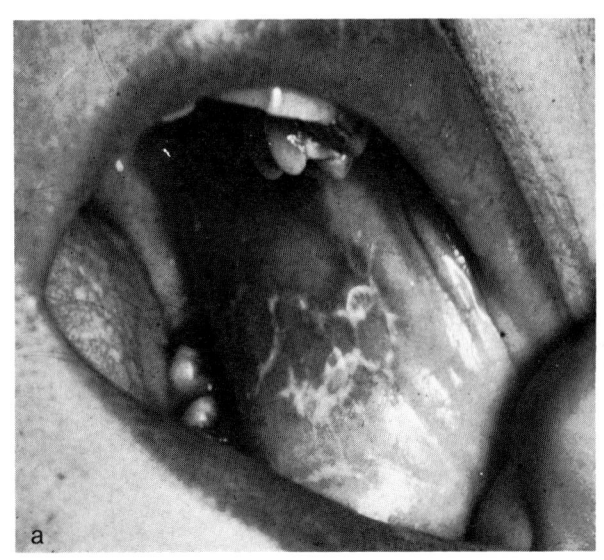

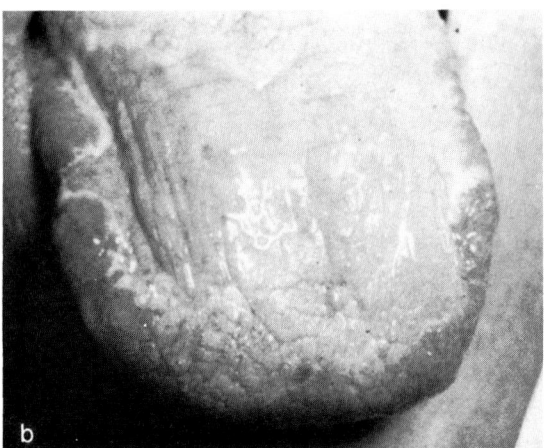

FIGURE 15–19. Lichen planus. *A*, Note the lace-like striae on the buccal mucosa. *B*, Whitish plaques on the dorsum of the tongue. Note striae on the lateral borders.

the lesions originate in the posterior area and spread anteriorly. Generally, they are asymptomatic, although a metallic taste or mild discomfort is common. Superficial erosions, bullous lesions, and deep, chronic, painful ulcerations occasionally occur.

Candidiasis (Fig. 15–20)

Candida albicans is universal and can be found in about 35 per cent of oral smears taken routinely from patients. Newborns may be infected by mothers with candidiasis of the vaginal tract. Neonatal monilial stomatitis usually becomes evident on the fifth to sixth postpartum day. *Candida albicans* has been identified in the mouths of up to 40 per cent of newborn infants.

The presence of *Candida albicans*, however, does not necessarily signify clinical candidiasis. To become virulent, the infection must be promoted by various factors such as age (infants, elderly persons), hormonal status (diabetes, pregnancy), and heredity. Moreover, local factors are important such as edentulousness, ill-fitting dentures, and in general, lowered body resistance due to such conditions as malabsorption, systemic malignancy, uremia, and various chronic infections. In recent years, the extensive therapeutic use of antibiotics has led to an increase in *Candida* infections of the mouth, respiratory and digestive tracts, and skin, especially in the anogenital area. Oral candidiasis may be diffuse or localized as angular cheilosis, superficial monilial stomatitis, denture stomatitis, and deep granulomatous candidiasis.

In *superficial monilial stomatitis,* the clinical picture ranges from mild erythema with fine, whitish deposits to diffuse, inflamed "white mouth." In infants, the first changes appear on the anterior dorsal third, edges, and ventral surfaces of the tongue and later in the oral vestibule. The lesions, resembling snow-white, curdled milk, can present as strips, plaques, and diffuse pseudomembranes and usually can be removed more easily than a

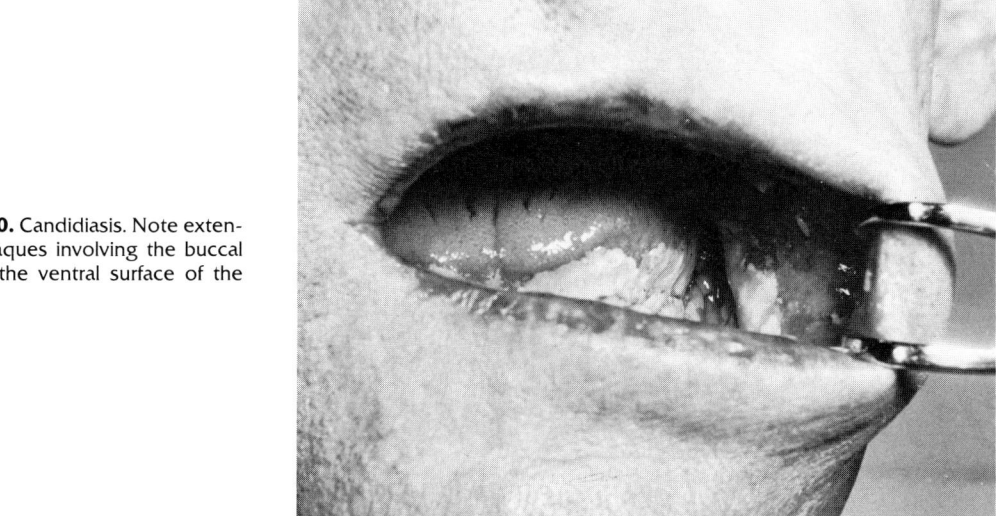

FIGURE 15–20. Candidiasis. Note extensive white plaques involving the buccal mucosa and the ventral surface of the tongue.

diphtheritic membrane. Generally, the easier the mechanical removal, the more superficial and less harmful the epithelial invasion. The white spots are composed of a dense matting of *Candida albicans* together with cell detritus, residual food particles, and bacteria. The surface of the lesions has a velvety appearance, whereas the adjacent mucous membrane appears dark red and moderately swollen.

In *denture stomatitis*, the patient complains of swelling, sensitivity, and pain of the oral mucous membrane at points of denture contact.

The treatment of oral candidal stomatitis consists of improved oral hygiene and nutritional status (especially serum iron), correction of the irritating factor, correction of the underlying disorder where possible, and the use of oral nystatin suspension, ointment, or tablets. Clotrimazole troches (10 mg q.i.d.) may also be used.

Halitosis

Halitosis (fetor oris), or bad breath, is a common complaint. Offensive mouth odor depends upon many factors such as decreased salivary flow rate resulting in mucosal dryness (due to antihistamines, Sjögren's syndrome, astringent mouthwashes, radiation sialoadenitis); poor oral hygiene (food remnants, unclean dentures); odoriferous foods (garlic, onion, fatty diet); periodontal disorders, especially if there is marked tissue destruction (periodontitis, necrotizing ulcerative gingivitis); necrotic soft tissue lesions; and heavy smoking.

Rarely a systemic cause can be implicated, such as the fetid odor of a disorder of the respiratory system, the acetone breath of uncontrolled diabetes mellitus, or the ammoniacal odor of uremia.

The efficacy of a mouthwash is only transient. The cause of the halitosis must be eliminated.

ORAL TUMORS

Odontogenic Tumors

The more common odontogenic tumors will be discussed in this section (Table 15–2).

TABLE 15–2. ODONTOGENIC TUMORS

Benign tumors
  Ameloblastoma
  Adenomatoid odontogenic tumor
  Calcifying epithelial odontogenic tumor
  Ameloblastic fibroma
  Odontomas
  Cementomas
  Myxoma
Malignant tumors
  Ameloblastic carcinoma (malignant ameloblastoma)
  Ameloblastic fibrosarcoma

From Gorlin RJ: *In* Anderson's Pathology (JM Kissane, ed): Vol 2. 8th ed. St Louis, The CV Mosby Co, 1985, p 1025.

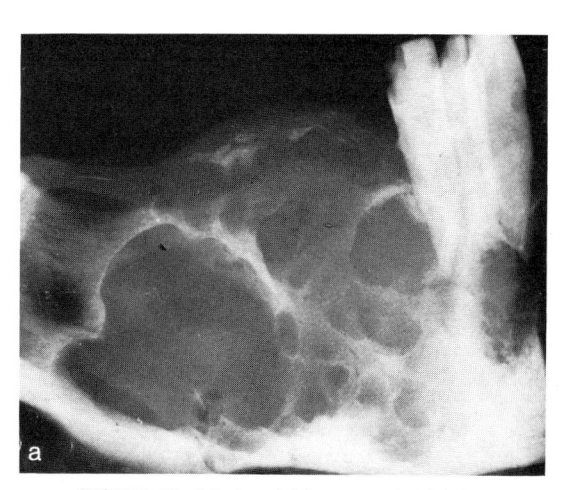

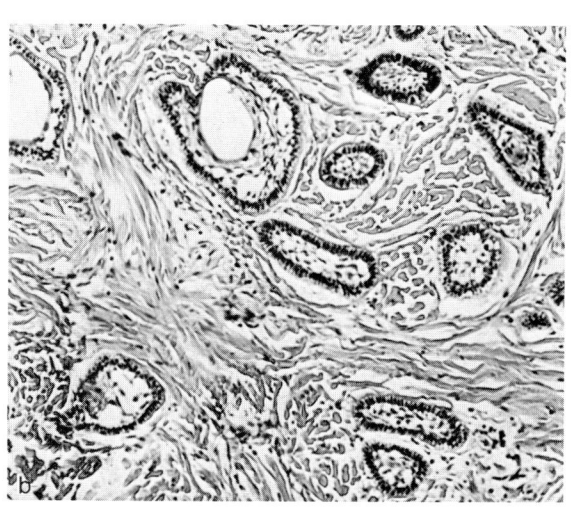

FIGURE 15–21. Ameloblastoma. *A,* Multilocular radiolucency of the mandible. *B,* Follicular ameloblastoma. Note that the pattern simulates that of tooth formation.

Ameloblastoma (Fig. 15–21)

Ameloblastoma has a relatively low incidence, comprising only about 1 per cent of the tumors and cysts of the jaws. Several origins have been suggested, including the epithelial lining of a dentigerous cyst, the remnants of the dental lamina of the enamel organ, and the basal layer of the oral mucous membrane.

The ameloblastoma most commonly occurs in the age group of 20 to 49 years, with the average age of initial diagnosis being about 39 years. Although at least one third of the tumors have a duration of two years or less prior to diagnosis, some have been present for more than 50 years.

The tumor arises in the mandible in more than 90 per cent of the cases, and 70 per cent of these have been in the molar-ramus area. About 10 to 15 per cent are associated with an unerupted tooth. In the maxilla, the canine and antral areas seem especially susceptible. Tumors encountered in this location may extend into the maxillary sinus, nose, orbit, or even the cranial base.

Because of the tumor's relative insensitivity to radiation therapy, surgical resection or even hemisection remains the treatment of choice. Rarely has the tumor metastasized.

Adenomatoid Odontogenic Tumor

Adenomatoid odontogenic tumor has been reported under a variety of names: adenoameloblastoma, ameloblastic adenomatoid tumor, and odontogenic adenomatoid tumor. This tumor is somewhat more common in females and usually occurs in the second decade of life. More than 90 per cent of affected individuals have been between ages 12 and 30. It arises somewhat more frequently in the maxilla and predominantly (over 90 per cent) in the anterior region of both jaws. In about three fourths of the patients, it is associated with an unerupted tooth, most often a canine and far less frequently a maxillary lateral incisor or mandibular first premolar.

Radiographically, it is most frequently radiolucent, resembling a dentigerous cyst or lateral periodontal cyst. The tumor expands the cortical plate but is not invasive and surgically "shells out" easily.

Calcifying Epithelial Odontogenic Tumor

The calcifying epithelial odontogenic tumor may be invasive and locally recurrent, behaving similarly to the ameloblastoma. As the tumor grows, it expands the surrounding bony structures and produces noticeable swelling. It occurs in the same age group (20 to 49 years) as the ameloblastoma. About 75 per cent of these tumors have arisen in the mandible, with the majority in the premolar-molar area. The radiographic appearance has usually been a combination of radiolucency and radiopacity, with numerous dense islands of various sizes scattered throughout.

Ameloblastic Fibroma

The vast majority of patients with this tumor have been between ages 5 and 20 years.

This tumor usually produces painless, asymptomatic, slow expansion of the cortical plates of the premolar-molar area of the maxilla or, far more frequently, the mandible. Radiographically, it is a smooth, outlined, cystlike lesion that cannot be differentiated from the unilocular ameloblastoma.

Ameloblastic Odontoma

Ameloblastic odontoma is characterized by the simultaneous occurrence of ameloblastoma and a complex or compound odontoma within the same tumor.

With few exceptions, the tumor is found in children, over 90 per cent of the patients being under age 15. It is more common in males and is found somewhat more frequently in the maxilla.

Growth is slow and often is associated with swelling of the alveolar process. Radiographs reveal areas of cystlike destruction.

Complex Odontoma

Complex odontoma differs from ameloblastic odontoma by the virtual absence of ameloblastic tissue. In normal tooth development, degeneration of the dental lamina occurs soon after hard tissue formation, and the complex odontoma corresponds to this more complete stage of induction. At least 70 per cent occur in the second and third molar area and are somewhat more common in the mandible. Usually they are asymptomatic and are found on routine dental radiographic examination. They appear as irregular radiopacities surrounded by a narrow radiolucent band.

Compound Odontoma (Fig. 15–22)

The compound odontoma differs from the complex odontoma in having a high degree of morphologic and histologic differentiation. However, the morphologic appearance may differ considerably from case to case, and it may be difficult to decide whether one is dealing with a complex or a compound odontoma. When the calcified structures exhibit sufficient anatomic similarity to normal teeth, although the teeth be small and deformed, the tumor is called compound.

At least 60 per cent of these tumors are diagnosed in the second and third decades. In contrast to the complex type, the vast majority of compound odontomas occur in the incisor-canine region of the upper jaw. The tumor is small and nonaggressive. It is usually diagnosed on routine dental x-ray examination.

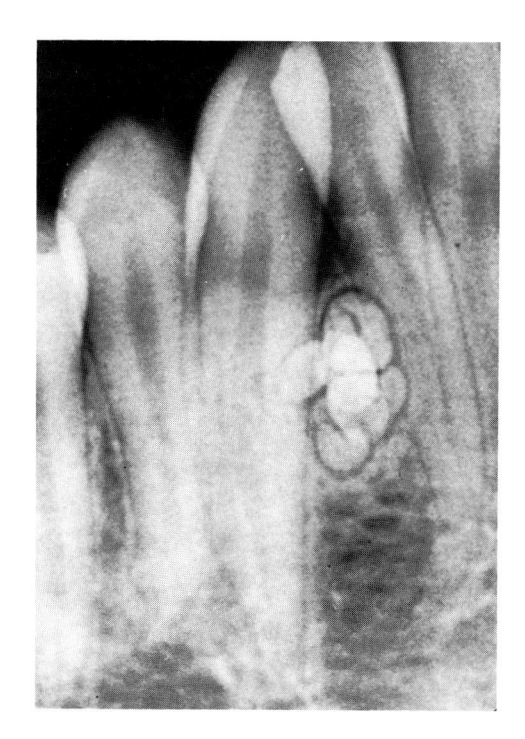

FIGURE 15–22. Compound odontoma. Several small teeth can be seen in the area between the lower lateral incisor and the canine tooth.

Myxoma

The myxoma (myxofibroma) of the jaw is a locally aggressive, nonmetastasizing tumor of odontogenic origin, probably arising from the connective tissue of the dental papilla.

Only rarely does the myxoma occur before the age of 10 years or after age 50. Approximately 60 per cent arise within the second and third decades. The tumor is slow-growing, and, on the average, it has been present for about five years prior to therapy.

Radiographically, differentiation from other jaw radiolucencies is difficult, if not impossible, and this lesion cannot easily be distinguished from fibrous dysplasia, central giant cell granuloma, or ameloblastoma. The tumor is not well defined but tends to be honeycombed, perforating the cortex of the jaw only if it reaches great size. In the mandible, it involves the ramus and body with equal frequency. Those tumors that arise in the maxilla may perforate and invade the antrum, filling it completely and producing exophthalmos. The antral walls are expanded but seldom are destroyed. The teeth are often displaced.

Cementoma

Cementoma most commonly involves the periapical regions of the mandibular anterior teeth. The frequency is roughly 2 to 3 per 1000 patients, with 70 to 90 per cent occurring in females.

The average age at which the lesion is discovered is about 40 years. Only rarely is it seen in persons under 25 years of age and almost never below the age of 20 years. It is more common in blacks than in whites.

The teeth involved are nearly always mandibular. The lesions are often multiple, and some individuals have as many as eight mandibular teeth involved. Because of a lack of symptoms, diagnosis is usually made during routine dental radiographic examination.

Nonodontogenic Tumors

Numerous types of benign and malignant neoplasms may occur in the oral regions. Two of the more fascinating benign tumors seen in infancy are the *melanotic neuroectodermal tumor* of neural crest origin and the *congenital epulis*, which is a granular cell myoblastoma.

Congenital Epulis

This benign tumor is present at birth; it is usually pedunculated and located on the maxillary or mandibular gingiva, generally in the anterior region. It is limited almost exclusively to females. Histologically, it is similar to a granular cell myoblastoma (schwannoma) but without associated pseudoepitheliomatous hyperplasia. Treatment consists of simple surgical excision.

Pigmented Neuroectodermal Tumor of Neural Crest Origin

This benign tumor usually occurs in the anterior maxillary gingiva of infants less than six months of age. It may grow rapidly and is usually deeply pigmented. Surgical excision is necessary. Even though it is benign, postsurgical recurrence has been noted in about 10 per cent of cases.

BONE DISORDERS AFFECTING THE JAWS

Only the more frequently occurring disorders will be reviewed here.

Fibrous Dysplasia (Fig. 15–23)

Fibrous dysplasia may involve only a single bone (monostotic) or several bones (polyostotic). The monostotic type is by far the more frequent and more often affects females in childhood or in early adolescence. In about 10 to 15 per cent of cases of monostotic fibrous dysplasia the skull or jaw is involved. Rarely, the polyostotic form may be associated with precocious puberty and café au lait pigmentation (McCune-Albright syndrome).

With polyostotic involvement, more often bilateral, the bones most frequently involved are the femur, tibia, fibula, and pelvic bones. Less often, the bones of the upper extremity are involved. In general, about 15 per cent of patients with the polyostotic form have jaw involvement. With severe polyostotic fibrous dysplasia, the skull or facial bones are almost always involved.

The process, which usually begins in childhood, tends to "burn out" during late adolescence, and surgical intervention is best delayed until that time. *In no case should radiation be employed, since it predisposes to malignant development.*

The maxilla is more frequently involved than the mandible, and the lesion is usually monostotic. The mass is hard and rounded, producing a painless, nontender facial asymmetry and, at times, exophthalmos or nasal obstruction.

Radiographically, the jaw lesion is dense, resembling ground glass with poor demarcation from normal bone. Microscopically, the lesion is composed of bone trabeculae in a fibrous connective tissue stroma.

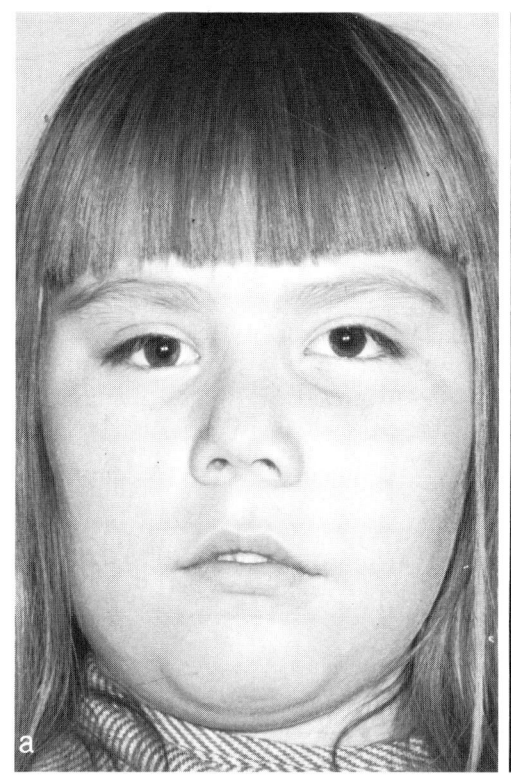

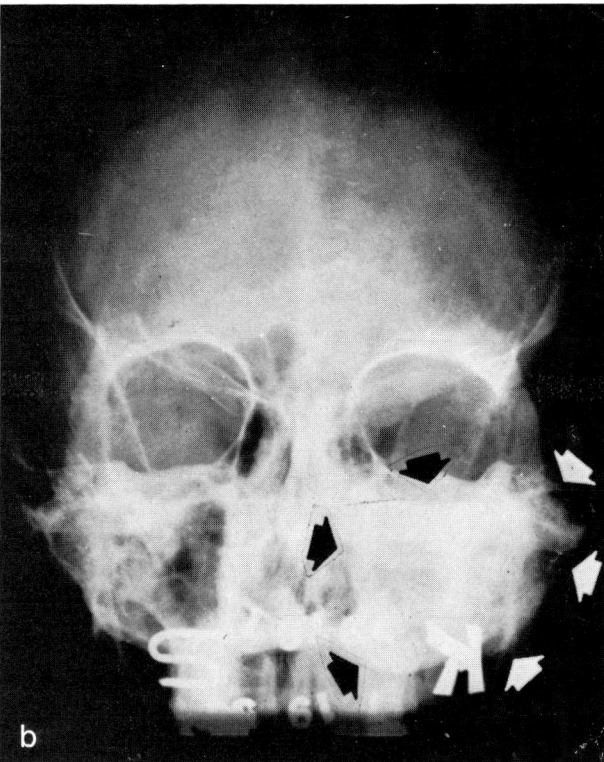

FIGURE 15-23. Fibrous dysplasia. A, Asymmetry of the face with swelling beneath the left eye. B, Ground glass appearance of the lesion in the patient shown in A.

Infantile Cortical Hyperostosis

This relatively rare disorder is probably inherited as an autosomal dominant trait. Typically, an affected child two to four months of age manifests bilateral, tender soft-tissue swelling over the mandibular rami. Other bones may be affected. Pain, fever, and irritability are common and may precede the swelling and bone involvement. Anemia, leukocytosis, and an elevated sedimentation rate are frequent findings. Radiographic examination shows thickening of the periosteum and new bone formation. The disorder is self-limiting, and surgical intervention is not warranted.

ACUTE TRAUMA OF DENTAL AND ORAL TISSUES

Hemorrhage

Oral hemorrhage usually results from acute trauma. Rarely, unusual bleeding may follow minor oral surgical procedures, such as tooth extraction. All wounds are managed by examination and debridement of necrotic tissue and foreign material. Primary closure or application of folded sterile gauze pressure dressings for 15 to 45 minutes is usually sufficient. The mouth should not be rinsed, since clots are easily dislodged from their moist environment. The application of warm, moistened tea bags or absorbable gelatin sponge cut to size and saturated with thrombin has also been used for persistent bleeding.

Tooth Fracture

If a tooth receives a severe, sharp blow, fracture often occurs. This fracture may be visible and involve the clinical crown of the tooth, or it may not be clinically demonstrable if it involves the invested or root portion. In either instance, dental consultation should be immediate. It should be emphasized that the physician should recommend that the child see the family dentist or pedodontist within the shortest time possible.

Fractures of the crowns of teeth are treated by covering surfaces with a protective, crown-shaped plastic or metallic cap. The cap is secured in position by a mixture, such as zinc oxide and eugenol, which minimizes pulp hyperemia and protects against irritation by thermal and chemical factors. If fracture of the tooth crown involves the pulp portion, treatment consists of pulp removal with sealing (ideally), pulpotomy (slightly less successful), or extraction.

Root fractures, although rare in primary teeth, are immobilized in situ by supportive wire ligation of affected and neighboring teeth.

It is worth emphasizing that early dentition performs a valuable space-maintaining function for the subsequent permanent dentition. Early loss of primary teeth adversely affects the development of a properly aligned permanent dentition.

Tooth Displacement or Loss: Replantation

Intrusion or forceful impaction of primary maxillary incisors is common during the first three years of life. The entire clinical crown may become embedded in bone and soft tissue. Primary attention should be given to treatment of the soft tissues. No attempt should be made to reposition the teeth after the accident. A dental radiogram should be made to detect fracture of the root or alveolar process. It is almost never possible to predict with accuracy whether injury has occurred to the underlying permanent successor. Intruded teeth usually re-erupt within one month after injury. Over half of the teeth will be retained; the rest undergo either pulpal necrosis or inflammatory resorption.

Displaced, but not intruded, permanent (not deciduous) teeth are repositioned. If the teeth are severely loosened, prognosis is poor, especially if the roots are completely formed, and the teeth are permanent.

Replantation of an avulsed permanent tooth is usually unsuccessful, since it will probably undergo subsequent resorption. However, replantation is still recommended, since the tooth is occasionally retained and will serve as a space maintainer. The tooth is gently cleansed, care being taken not to remove adherent periodontal ligament. The tooth is then placed in mild antiseptic solution, and the child is referred to a dentist for root canal filling of the tooth, replantation and splint construction for immobilization.

References

Gorlin RJ, Goldman HM: Thoma's Oral Pathology. 6th ed. St Louis, The CV Mosby Co, 1970.
Gorlin RJ, Cohen MM Jr, Levin S: Syndromes of the Head and Neck. 3rd ed. New York, Oxford University Press, 1989.
Shafer W, Hine M, Levy BM: Textbook of Oral Pathology. 4th ed. Philadelphia, WB Saunders Co, 1983.

16

DISORDERS OF THE SALIVARY GLANDS

by George L. Adams, M.D.

ANATOMY

The *parotid gland* is the largest of the major salivary glands and occupies the space just anterior to the mastoid process and external auditory meatus. Anteriorly, it lies lateral to the ascending ramus of the mandible and masseter muscle. Inferiorly, it abuts on the sternocleidomastoid muscle and covers the posterior belly of the digastric muscle. It is separated from the submandibular gland by the stylomandibular ligament. The deep portion of the parotid gland extends posteriorly and medial to the ascending ramus of the mandible and is known as the retromandibular extension. It is this portion of the gland which is in close contact with the parapharyngeal space.

The facial nerve artificially divides the parotid gland into superficial and deep portions.

The facial nerve leaves the skull through the stylomastoid foramen and passes anteriorly just lateral to the styloid process. The nerve then enters the substance of the parotid gland and divides into two major trunks, the cervicofacial and the temporofacial. The temporofacial division then separates into the temporal and zygomatic branches, while the cervicofacial gives off the cervical branches, marginal mandibular division, and buccal division, which passes anteriorly just below the parotid duct. Passage of the facial nerve through the substance of the parotid gland divides the gland, for clinical purposes, into a superficial lobe and that portion medial to the facial nerve known as the deep lobe. It is the deep lobe that lies in close contact with the ninth, tenth, eleventh, and twelfth cranial nerves and the division of the external carotid artery into the superficial temporal and internal maxillary arteries.

The deep lobe of the parotid is in close proximity to both the internal and external carotid arteries.

The parotid duct is approximately 6 cm long and arises from the anterior portion of the gland. It crosses the masseter muscle and turns sharply over the anterior border of the muscle to pierce the buccinator muscle. It then continues for a short distance in the submucosal tissues of the mouth and enters the oral cavity through a small papilla just opposite the crown of the second upper molar tooth.

The *submandibular (submaxillary) gland* lies beneath the horizontal ramus of the mandible and is enclosed by a thin layer of connective tissue. It lies entirely within the digastric triangle formed by the anterior and posterior bellies of the digastric muscle. Medially it is bordered by the styloglossus and hyoglossus muscles, and anteriorly it is limited by the mylohyoid muscle.

The more medial portion of the gland is closely associated with the floor of the mouth. The submandibular duct (Wharton's duct) is also 6 cm in length. It passes between the mylohyoid and hyoglossus muscles just medial to the sublingual gland and enters the mouth just lateral to the lingular frenulum.

The paired *sublingual glands* lie just beneath the anterior floor of the mouth and are actually large collections of minor salivary glands. Secreted saliva enters the floor of the mouth through multiple short ducts.

The sublingual and submandibular glands are mixed glands in that they contain both serous and mucous glandular elements. The parotid gland contains almost entirely serous elements. In the resting state the submandibular gland produces approximately two thirds of the saliva, and the parotid glands supply approximately one third of the saliva.

Salivary response to stimulation is dependent upon neural reflexes carried along the parasympathetic nervous system. The parasympathetic supply of the parotid gland begins in the inferior salivatory nucleus. The fibers leave the brain through the glossopharyngeal nerve and pass through the middle ear, crossing the promontory in Jacobson's nerve. In the tympanic plexus, they enter the lesser petrosal nerve and thereby reach the otic ganglion. Postganglionic fibers from the otic ganglion reach the parotid gland through the auricular temporal division of the fifth nerve. The parasympathetic supply of the submandibular gland arises in the superior salivatory nucleus. The fibers enter the nervus intermedius (nerve of Wrisberg) and follow the facial nerve into its vertical portion in the mastoid. The fibers then leave the seventh nerve in the chorda tympani, pass through the middle ear, and join the lingual nerve. The fibers follow the lingual nerve to a small ganglion closely associated with the submandibular gland. Postganglionic fibers leave the submandibular ganglion to pass to the substance of the gland. Because sectioning of the chorda tympani nerve and Jacobson's nerve does not always reduce salivary secretion, other pathways of parasympathetic nerve supply to the glands must exist. It is suggested that these pathways involve the hypoglossal and glossopharyngeal nerves. The sympathetic nerve supply to the major salivary glands is from the superior cervical ganglion by way of the arterial plexus. Sympathetic stimulation of the major salivary glands is reported to cause an increased flow followed by a compensatory decrease in flow. Since there are no muscle elements within the glands themselves, it is believed that this increase in flow may be due to contraction of the myoepithelial, or basket, cells associated with the striated ducts.

Jacobson's nerve, a division of the ninth cranial nerve, passes across the promontory of the middle ear.

INFLAMMATORY DISORDERS

Acute Parotitis

The most common form of acute parotid swelling is *mumps*. Without a history of exposure, the diagnosis may not be easy. The white blood cell count may be low, and there may be a relative lymphocytosis. Serum amylase may be elevated. The mumps vaccine should reduce the incidence of this disorder and its possible complications of orchitis, oophoritis, pancreatitis, sensorineural hearing loss, and encephalitis. Another form of parotid swelling which occurs in children is *recurrent sialadenitis*. This disorder may occur at any time from the age of one month through late childhood and is charac-

Mumps can cause sensorineural hearing loss.

terized by inflammation of one or both glands. Pus can be expressed from Stensen's duct, and pneumococci have been present on culture. Sialographic studies will reveal dilatation of the peripheral ducts.

Acute suppurative parotitis is characterized by a sudden onset of pain, redness, and swelling of the parotid region. It may occur postoperatively and usually is seen in debilitated or elderly persons who may be partially dehydrated. Poor oral hygiene may also be associated with this entity, and it is probable that there is a retrograde infection from the oral cavity to the parotid gland. Almost always the responsible organism is coagulase-positive *Staphylococcus aureus.* Because of the urgency of the situation, immediate treatment with intravenous antibiotics is necessary. Cultures are prepared from the purulent secretions expressed from the parotid duct, but until culture results are available, treatment with a penicillinase-resistant antibiotic is initiated. Correction of the dehydration is instituted, warm packs and analgesics are given for symptomatic relief, and proper oral hygiene is provided. Generally the inflammation shows evidence of subsidence over the next 48 hours. If there is evidence of progression of the infection, in spite of adequate medical management, surgical drainage may be necessary. An incision similar to that utilized for parotidectomy is made, and the skin and subcutaneous tissue are elevated from the capsule of the gland. Several incisions through the capsule of the gland are then made parallel to the major divisions of the facial nerve in order to drain all loculated areas of pus. Drains are inserted in the wound, and it is approximated but not closed. Radiation therapy in the range of 400 to 600 rads total dosage at the rate of 200 rads per day has been utilized to diminish the parotid secretions and thereby reduce the inflammation. This additional treatment is most helpful when initiated within the first 48 hours of the inflammation.

Because a parotid abscess is often loculated, a series of incisions into the glandular tissue parallel to the pathways of the facial nerve may be required.

Acute Submandibular Gland Sialadenitis

Suppurative sialadenitis is less common in the submandibular gland unless there is an obstructive component secondary to either a salivary calculus or trauma to the gland or its duct. Whenever there is suppuration involving the submandibular space, dental evaluation is also necessary. The acute infection is managed by obtaining a culture of the purulent secretions expressed from Wharton's duct. Appropriate antibiotics are utilized, and heat is applied to the submandibular area for relief of discomfort.

Excision of the submandibular gland in the presence of acute inflammation is difficult.

Chronic Sialadenitis

Chronic sialadenitis is a general term applied to long-standing, frequently recurring episodes of glandular swelling and discomfort of the major salivary glands. The etiology of such chronic inflammation can be in the gland parenchyma or in the ductal system, such as a stone. The terms given to describe these disorders reflect either their underlying cause, radiographic appearance demonstrated by sialography, which is injection of a dye into the major salivary duct, or pathologic appearance.

Chronic sialadenitis of the *parotid gland,* associated with recurrent calculi, mucous plugs, or strictures, is known as sialodochiectasis (Fig. 16–1). Chronic nonobstructive sialodochiectasis or sialectasis may involve one or all of the major salivary glands. The parotid gland is most frequently involved, and

FIGURE 16-1. *A*, Right parotid area mass, not obviously in parotid gland. *B*, Ultrasonogram demonstrating cystic appearance of mass. *C*, Axial CT scan with intravenous contrast shows a large mass in the parotid region. *D*, Sialogram demonstrates chronic sialadenitis and sialodochitis (destruction and inflammation of parotid ducts). *E*, CT scan combined with sialogram shows that the mass has displaced the parotid gland laterally and actually lies deeper in the neck.

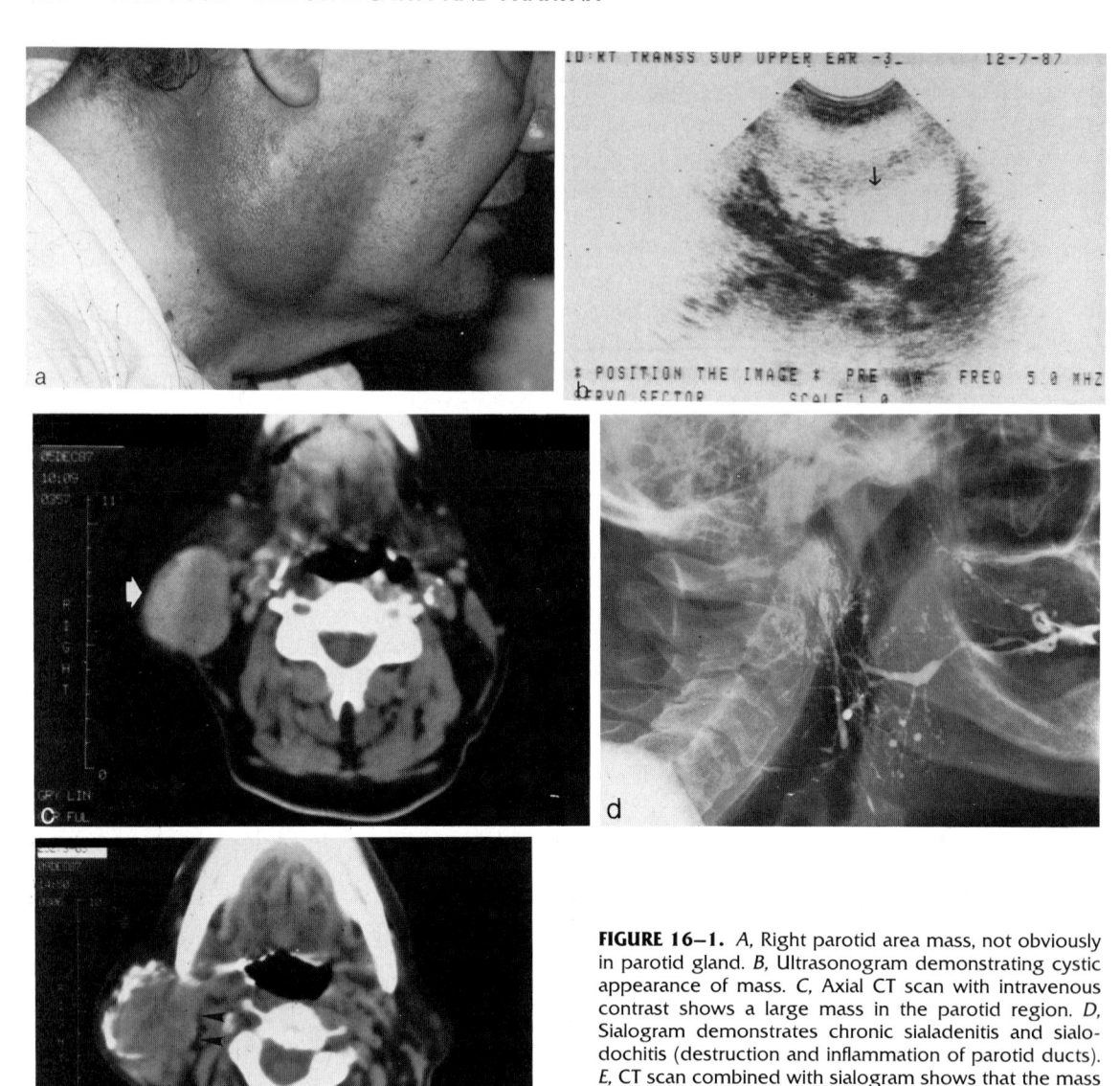

the symptoms include recurrent swelling and pain over the parotid region. A very viscous salivary secretion can be expressed from the duct by applying pressure over the gland. Calculi are not present. Sialography performed in the quiescent phase shows a characteristic picture with degenerative changes in the tubular ducts suggestive of the bronchogram findings seen in bronchiectasis. Symptoms and pathologic characteristics may vary from mild initial changes to severe chronic changes, by which time the gland has become firm and enlarged as a result of numerous repeated infections.

In certain situations when there are repeated episodes and the cause of obstruction of the salivary gland is not evident, dilatation of the duct is performed. After application of a local anesthetic, such as 4 per cent topical cocaine or lidocaine (Xylocaine), lacrimal duct probes of increasing size are introduced into the duct throught the papillae. The stricture in the duct may be found and can be dilated. Occasionally there will be a sudden flow of saliva from the gland when the obstruction is released. The procedure can then be followed by a sialogram, introducing a small polyethylene tube into the dilated duct orifice. A sialogram may help to further elicit the cause of the recurrent obstruction.

When there is advanced chronic sialadenitis that no longer responds to medical management, it may become necessary to perform a parotidectomy. Parotidectomy under such circumstances may be difficult, and the possibility of injury to the facial nerve is increased. Because of these risks, other procedures have been developed in an effort to avoid parotidectomy. These methods include ligation of the parotid duct (which is expected to cause atrophy of the gland) and sectioning of Jacobson's nerve on the promontory of the middle ear through an endaural approach, thereby interrupting the parasympathetic supply to the parotid gland.

Salivary gland calculi (sialolithiasis) occur far more commonly in the submandibular gland than in the parotid gland. Ninety per cent of submandibular gland stones are radiopaque, while in the parotid gland, only 10 per cent are identifiable on a scout film. There may be either a single large stone or multiple small pieces of gravel. Symptoms include the sudden onset of swelling and pain over the submandibular region, usually shortly after a meal. Fever occurs when infection develops behind the obstruction. Treatment in the acute phase may require surgical removal of the salivary calculus from the duct as it passes along the floor of the mouth. Occasionally the stone may be milked out of the duct until it appears at the lingual papillae adjacent to the frenulum. At other times, following administration of a local anesthetic, an incision is made directly onto the stone for its removal. Initially it may be necessary to obtain a culture, treat with antibiotics, and wait until the acute phase subsides before any manipulation of the duct can be attempted.

Recurrent sialadenitis of the *submandibular gland* is more frequently treated by surgical resection of the gland, and this is a less hazardous procedure than parotidectomy under similar circumstances. Here, care is taken to preserve the marginal mandibular division of the facial nerve, the hypoglossal nerve, and the lingual nerve, all of which lie in close proximity to the enlarged, chronically infected gland.

Surgical treatment of chronic parotitis may include tympanic neurectomy, parotid duct ligation, and parotidectomy.

Surgical treatment of chronic submandibular gland sialadenitis requires submandibular gland resection including the duct.

SYSTEMIC DISEASE

The parotid glands are the salivary glands most often involved in systemic illnesses. The following are notable examples of systemic disease involving salivary glands.

Sarcoidosis involving the parotid glands is referred to as Heerfordt's syndrome, or uveoparotid fever. The gland becomes diffusely swollen with slight tenderness. Facial nerve paralysis can occur. The term uveoparotid fever is used because of the possible coexistence of uveitis. Other systemic manifestations of sarcoidosis such as hypercalcemia, enlarged liver and spleen, enlarged cervical nodes, and enlarged hilar nodes as demonstrated by chest radiographs may be present. Definitive diagnosis is made by biopsy. The only treatment available at the present time consists of administration of systemic steroids.

Benign lymphoepithelial disease of the salivary glands is a specific type of chronic punctate parotitis. It occurs almost exclusively in women and is believed to represent an autoimmune disease process. It is often associated with rheumatoid disorders. Clinically it presents with recurrent episodes of noncalculous chronic parotitis. The sialogram presents an almost pathognomonic picture of the punctate parotitis, or little dots of contrast material distributed through the parenchyma of the gland. The pathologic appearance is that of dilated ducts with lymphocyte infiltration and eventual acinar atrophy. With the progressive destruction of the glandular substance, oral dryness develops.

Sjögren's syndrome includes the chronic parotitis associated with at least two or three additional entities. Patients must have xerophthalmia or xerostomia or an associated rheumatoid disorder, most often rheumatoid arthritis. While the disease process involves primarily the parotid gland, the minor salivary glands also are involved. Thus a lip biopsy may demonstrate the same pathologic findings in the minor salivary glands as are seen in the parotid. These pathologic findings are similar to those seen in biliary cirrhosis and graft-versus-host disease. Treatment is almost always nonsurgical unless the chronic parotitis cannot be resolved medically, or there is a suspicion of an additional parotid neoplasm. Sjögren's disease is associated with a 44 times higher incidence of developing lymphoma than in the general population. The associated lymphoma is in extraparotid nodal sites, however.

> There is a significant increased rate of lymphoma development in patients with Sjögren's syndrome.

Other causes of salivary gland enlargement include such systemic disorders as diabetes mellitus. Enlargement has been associated with certain drugs, particularly iodine compounds. Enlargement of the parotid gland should be distinguished from benign hypertrophy of the masseter muscle.

SIALORRHEA

Sialorrhea, or drooling, occurs in certain advanced neurologic disorders such as cerebral palsy, demyelinating disorders, and Parkinson's disease. It is also seen after certain major operations for head and neck cancer. There is not an increase in the actual amount of saliva formed, but there is an inability of the patient to handle the saliva that builds up in the anterior mouth and eventually flows over the lip. Nonsurgical treatment once consisted of the use of anticholinergic drugs, such as atropine, or radiation therapy in an effort to decrease the amount of saliva formed. Because of the side effects, these methods are not commonly employed. Surgical procedures have been designed to divert the flow of the saliva so that it enters the pharynx posterior to the anterior tonsillar pillar. This includes rerouting the parotid and submandibular ducts through a submucosal tunnel to the region posterior to the tonsillar pillar. In severe cases the submandibular glands are actually excised. Reports of successful control of sialorrhea by tympanic neurectomy combined with chorda tympani resection have been described. This procedure decreases the amount of saliva formed without producing any harmful side effects or causing an excessively dry mouth. Its major disadvantage is that it has not proven to have long-term effectiveness, and frequently within two years the excess saliva recurs. Prior to performing any of these surgical procedures, it should be determined that the patient has no disability in swallowing but only in handling secretions in the anterior mouth.

> The most effective surgical procedure to control drooling is bilateral submandibular gland resection and parotid duct ligations.

16—DISORDERS OF THE SALIVARY GLANDS

TABLE 16–1. INDICATIONS FOR SIALOGRAPHY

Indications
- Chronic nonobstructive sialectasis
- Chronic obstructive diseases
- Trauma
- Extraglandular masses
- Tumors (sialography and CT scan)

Contraindications
- Presence of acute inflammation or suppuration
- Allergy to contrast material

RADIOLOGICAL ASSESSMENT OF THE MAJOR SALIVARY GLANDS

Radiosialographic Scanning

This technique depends on the increased concentration of iodine in saliva compared to plasma. Radioactive technetium-99, like iodine, is secreted by the intralobular ductal epithelium of major salivary glands. Both the parotid and submandibular gland can be demonstrated using this nuclear medicine technique. A normal gland appears symmetric and smooth, but a tumor mass will show an area of decreased uptake, or in the case of Warthin's tumor, an area of increased concentration. Since it was later established that increased uptake was not limited to Warthin's tumor, but could occur in pleomorphic adenoma and oncocytoma, the technique has become less helpful.

Sialography

This technique requires injection of water- or oil-soluble contrast material directly into the submandibular or parotid duct. After application of a topical

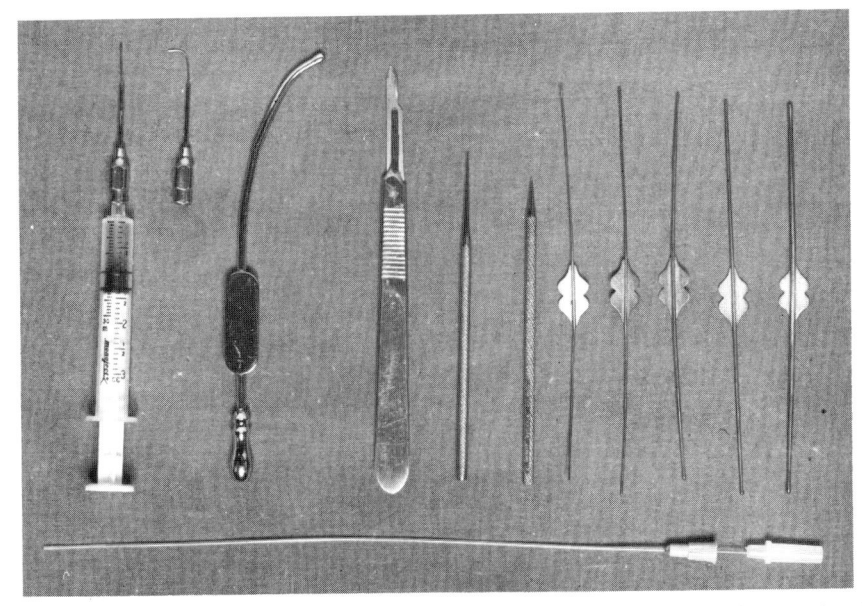

FIGURE 16–2. Instruments used for dilatation of Stensen's duct or Wharton's duct consist of the set of lacrimal duct dilators, a catheter for insertion into the duct, and a syringe for instilling contrast medium.

anesthetic to the area of the duct, pressure is gently applied to the gland, and the very fine orifice of the duct is identified by the saliva flow. The duct orifice is dilated with lacrimal probes (Fig. 16–2 and 16–3). An 18-gauge catheter, similar to the type used for administering intravenous fluids, or polyethylene tubing is gently inserted about 2 cm into the duct. The catheter is secured to the corner of the mouth. The technique is similar for both the parotid gland and submandibular gland. Cannulating the submandibular gland duct, however, may require more patience than dilation of the parotid duct. A scout x-ray film is obtained to make certain that there are no radiopaque substances, such as stones, in the gland. Between 1.5 and 2 ml

Always obtain a scout film before injection of contrast.

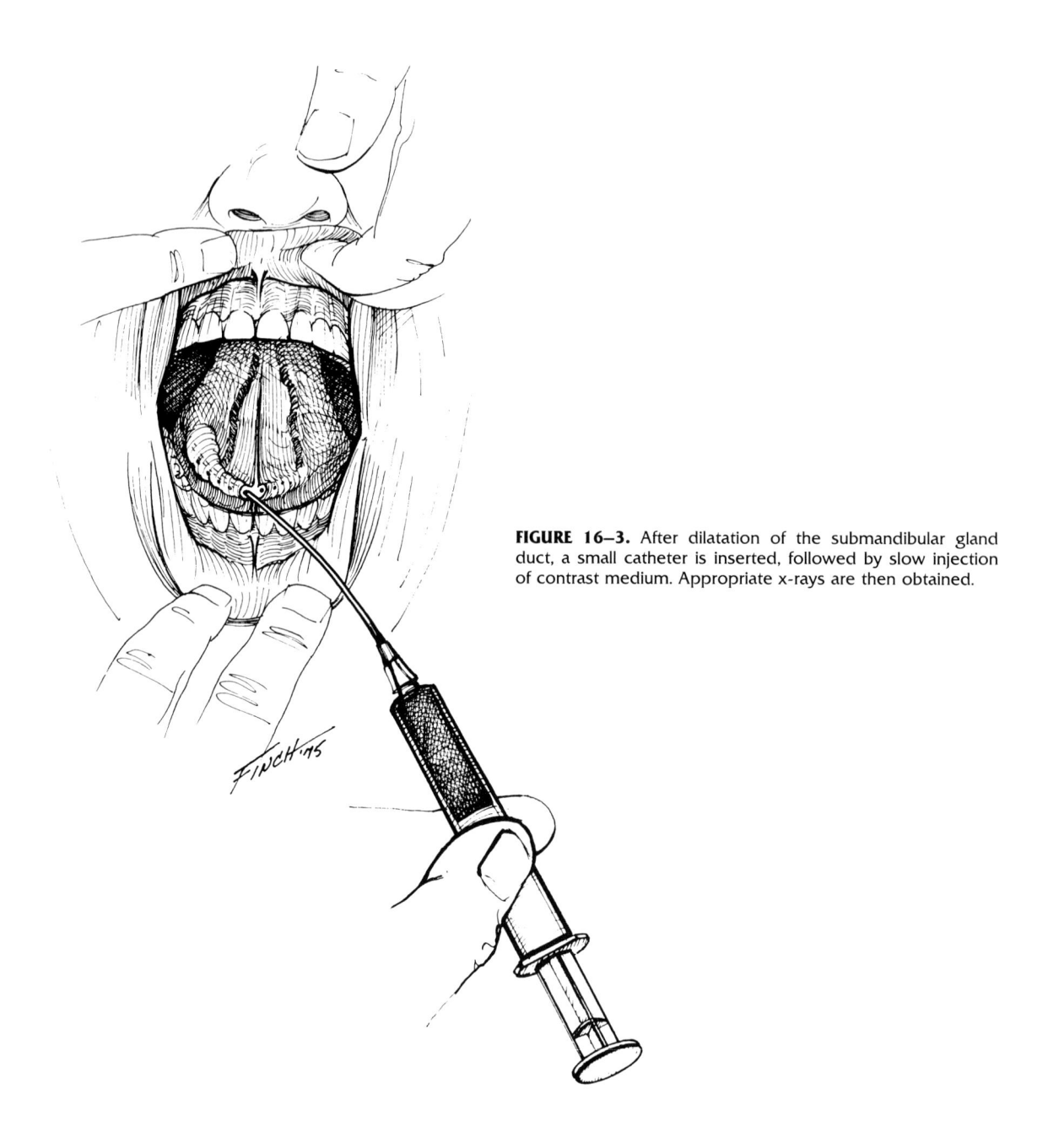

FIGURE 16–3. After dilatation of the submandibular gland duct, a small catheter is inserted, followed by slow injection of contrast medium. Appropriate x-rays are then obtained.

of contrast medium is injected gently through the catheter into the gland until the patient feels pressure but never beyond the point when the patient complains of pain. Appropriate lateral, oblique lateral, oblique, and anteroposterior films are obtained. When the catheter is removed, the patient may be given a small amount of lemon juice. In 5 to 10 minutes a repeat film is taken. Normally all contrast medium should have been expressed within that time. Persistence of contrast medium within the gland 24 hours after this test is definitely abnormal.

There are advantages and disadvantages to water-soluble and to lipid-soluble contrast materials. Currently, Pantopaque and Lipiodol are the most popular contrast materials.

Sialography is most useful in chronic disorders of the parotid gland such as recurrent sialadenitis, Sjögren's syndrome, or ductal obstruction such as stricture. It is of no value in differentiating a benign from a malignant mass. It is contraindicated in the presence of a recent, acute inflammation of the gland (Fig. 16–4).

Never inject contrast during an acute exacerbation of inflammation.

Computed Tomography

This is the single most useful radiologic diagnostic test of salivary gland masses. It requires the intravenous injection of a contrast material, first as a bolus and then with a continuous drip. Initially, this technique was combined with standard sialography, but with newer, high-resolution scanners this is seldom necessary. The parotid gland will appear less dense than surrounding structures and can be delineated from the masseter muscle. The most common tumor mass, pleomorphic adenoma, may appear as a well-defined, slightly enhancing mass. By this technique, it can be determined if the mass extends into the deep lobe or parapharyngeal space. Since the CT scan is not useful in differentiating benign from malignant lesions, biopsy remains imperative. It is helpful, however, to have a preoperative assessment of the size and location of any unusual mass or large mass, especially when it is not certain if the mass actually began within the substance of the parotid gland or is encroaching upon the parotid from adjacent areas.

MRI scanning will most likely replace the need for CT scan combined with sialography in most incidences.

BENIGN TUMORS OF THE SALIVARY GLANDS

In Children

The most common benign gland tumor of children is the *parotid gland hemangioma*. The skin overlying the mass may have a bluish discoloration, and there may be fluctuation in the size of the mass when the child cries. This tumor will show a gradual increase in size during the first four to six months of life but should begin to show evidence of resolution by age two. Similar to the hemangioma is the lymphangioma, which also arises in the parotid gland region. Pleomorphic adenoma is the third most common tumor, and the most common solid tumor, found in children. Other benign tumors include neurofibroma and lipoma. Salivary gland tumors in children most frequently involve the parotid gland, while the submandibular and minor salivary gland areas are uncommon sites.

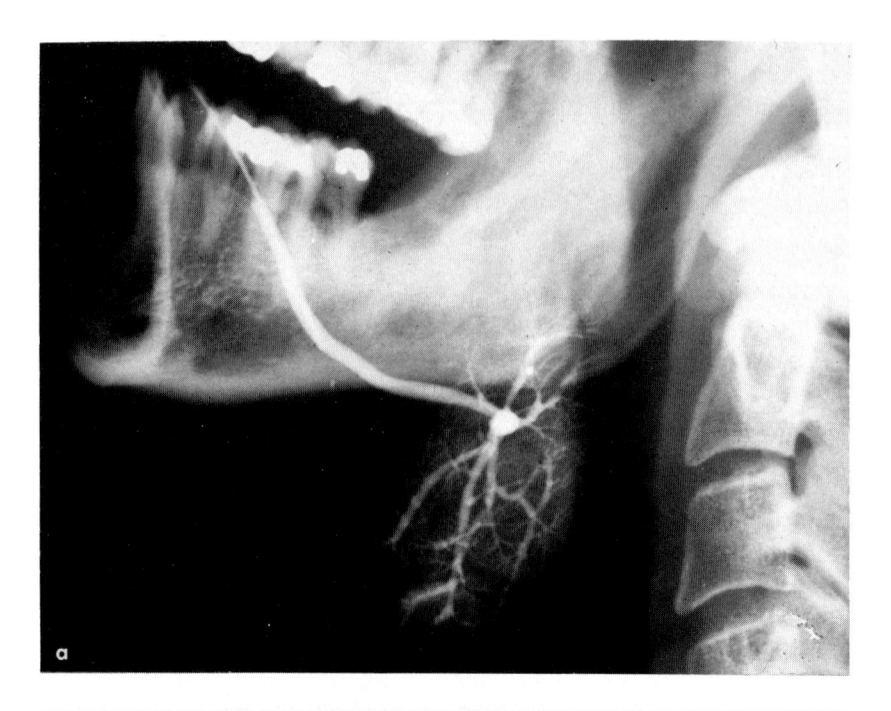

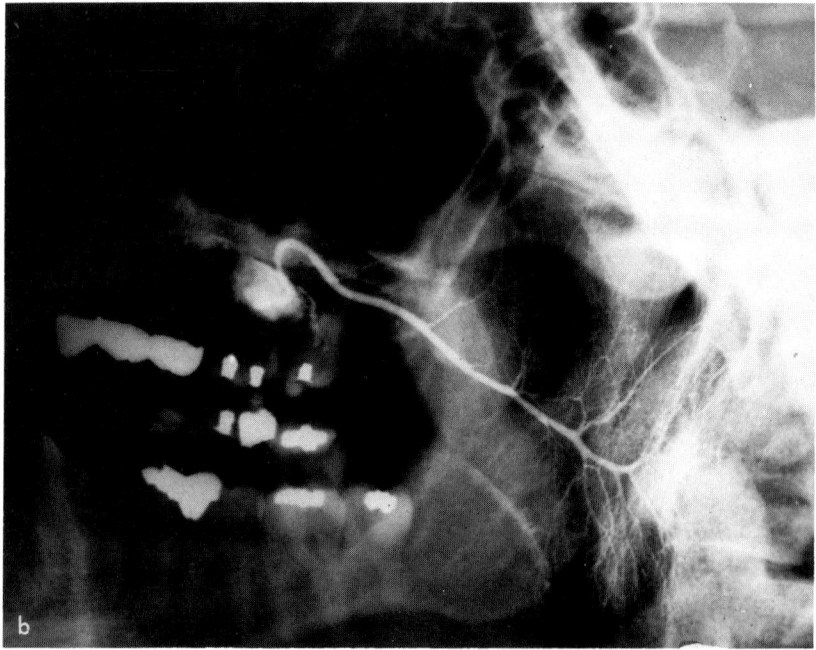

FIGURE 16–4. *A*, Normal submandibular duct (Wharton's duct) and gland. *B*, Normal parotid duct (Stensen's duct) and gland.

In Adults

The *pleomorphic adenoma (benign mixed tumor)* accounts for 75 per cent of parotid gland tumors, both benign and malignant, in the adult. It is most common in the parotid region, where it appears as a painless swelling of long duration in the preauricular area or the region of the tail of the parotid gland. There should be no pain or evidence of facial nerve weakness. In the parotid area, although classified as benign, the tumor may continue to increase in size and become locally destructive. Complete surgical resection is the only treatment. Care should be taken to prevent injury to the facial nerve, and the nerve is preserved even when immediately adjacent to the tumor. The tumor may develop primarily in the deep lobe and extend into the retromandibular region. In these circumstances the facial nerve is carefully preserved and gently retracted so that the tumor can be removed from its deep location extending into the parapharyngeal space.

Occasionally a deep lobe pleomorphic adenoma may present primarily intraorally. It can be recognized by the deviation of the soft palate and anterior tonsillar pillar toward the midline by a mass lateral to the tonsillar area. Resection should be performed through the neck rather than intraorally.

When removing parotid tumors, the entire superficial lobe, or that portion of the gland lateral to the facial nerve, is removed en bloc for biopsy purposes, dissecting out and preserving the facial nerve. Pathologic examination of the frozen section may not reveal the true nature of the tumor, and more radical surgery may be required when permanent section results are received. "Shelling out" a pleomorphic adenoma in the superficial lobe of the parotid gland is not recommended because of the high likelihood of recurrence. At the time of surgery the tumor mass appears encapsulated, but pathologic examination will show extracapsular extension. The incidence of recurrence when the entire tumor with a sufficient cuff of normal parotid gland is resected is less than 8 per cent. Should a pleomorphic adenoma recur, there is a high likelihood of injury to at least one of the divisions of the facial nerve when the tumor is re-resected. Although this tumor is considered benign, there have been cases of multiple recurrences with relentless growth in which the tumor expands to involve the region of the external canal and may actually extend into the oral cavity and parapharyngeal space. Recurrent tumors may undergo malignant degeneration, but the incidence of this is less than 6 per cent. Irradiation therapy to a tumor that has recurred and has become unresectable provides significant palliation.

Pleomorphic adenoma is also the most common tumor of the submandibular gland. Total surgical resection of the submandibular gland should provide an adequate margin for removal of this tumor. Pleomorphic tumor is also the most common benign tumor of the minor salivary glands. It occurs most frequently on the palate near the midline at the junction of the hard and soft palates. This location is also the most common for malignant salivary gland tumors of the palate. A wide local resection of the tumor in this location should be adequate.

Papillary adenocystoma lymphomatosum (Warthin's tumor) is another relatively common benign salivary gland tumor. It is most common in 50- to 60-year-old males. It is also the most common tumor to occur bilaterally. Treatment consists of surgical resection with facial nerve preservation. The tumor is encapsulated, and recurrence is unlikely.

Benign tumors of the parotid gland outnumber malignant tumors 4:1. There is no method short of excision to be certain a lesion is benign. Skinny needle biopsy is of benefit if positive but does not obviate the need for surgery. Even diagnosis by frozen section at surgery can be difficult.

Warthin's tumor is the most common tumor to occur bilaterally.

Other benign salivary gland tumors include the oxyphil adenoma (acidophilic cell), serous cell adenoma, and oncocytoma. Treatment is similar to that for pleomorphic adenoma.

The *parapharyngeal space* may be the primary site of origin for benign tumors. Most commonly these are salivary gland tumors that may have arisen from the deep lobe of the parotid gland and extended into the parapharyngeal space. Tumors of neurogenic origin such as schwannomas may originate in this area from the vagus nerve or cervical sympathetic chain. These tumors present as a smooth mass pressing the lateral pharyngeal wall medially. These tumors should be approached through the neck rather than intraorally because of the presence of major vessels and important cranial nerves in this space. A preliminary arteriogram not only may demonstrate the effect of the tumor on the location of the internal carotid artery but also may be useful in detecting a chemodectoma or neurogenic tumor within this space.

The most common tumor of the parapharyngeal space is a pleomorphic adenoma. The second most common is a malignant adenocystic carcinoma. The largest group of other tumors are of neurogenic origin, such as schwannomas and neuromas. Any tumor of the parapharyngeal space should be treated via an external, transcervical approach. This allows better control of the major vessels in the area. It also prevents seeding of the tumor, which can occur through a transoral approach. Because of the extensive postoperative edema that can occur, tracheostomy is often required.

MALIGNANT TUMORS OF THE SALIVARY GLANDS

Malignant Salivary Gland Tumors in Children

Malignant parotid tumors in children are fortunately rare. The most common tumor in children is mucoepidermoid carcinoma, usually of the low-grade type. The survival statistics for children are definitely better than for adults with the same pathologic appearance. However, the high-grade form of this malignancy is known to metastasize and cause death. In select situations, even after adequate resection, if there is evidence of metastatic disease, postoperative radiation therapy is advised. Careful consideration is always given to irradiating a child in view of the future potential complications, but it is still considered necessary in certain select situations, such as when evidence of neural or vascular invasion or metastatic disease is present. Adenocarcinoma is the second most common childhood parotid malignancy.

TABLE 16–2. DIFFERENTIATING MASSES IN THE SALIVARY GLANDS

Benign	Increasing Likelihood of Malignancy →	Malignant
Parotid	Submandibular	Minor salivary gland
Younger age		Older
Female		Male
Facial nerve function intact	Paresis	Paralysis
Cystic	Firm	Rock hard
Long duration (>2 yr)	Rapid growth	Recent onset (<1 yr)
Asymptomatic	Discomfort	Pain
No adenopathy		Cervical adenopathy

While much rarer than mucoepidermoid carcinoma, the undifferentiated type of this malignancy has a poor overall survival rate. Acinic cell cancer and adenocystic carcinoma initially have an almost benign course, with long-term survival, only to demonstrate ultimate recurrence at the primary site or evidence of distal or pulmonary metastases. Treatment remains adequate, complete, regional resection.

Malignant Salivary Gland Tumors in Adults

The possibility that a mass in the salivary gland is malignant increases with age. A frequently quoted rule of thumb applied to persons over 40 years of age is that 25 per cent of parotid tumors, 50 per cent of submandibular tumors, and one half to two thirds of all tumors of the minor salivary glands are malignant.

Further, major salivary gland tumors have been divided into those with high-, intermediate-, and low-grade malignant potential. *Mucoepidermoid carcinoma, squamous cell carcinoma,* and *undifferentiated adenocarcinoma* comprise the high-grade malignant tumors. *Adenocystic carcinoma (cylindroma)* is a specific salivary gland tumor that could easily be included in tumors with high-grade malignant potential. It differs from the preceding tumors by its prolonged course characterized by frequent local recurrence, and recurrences up to 15 years later. Patients with adenocystic carcinoma have a high five-year survival rate; the overall ten-year survival rate is less than 20 per cent. Carcinoma arising in a pleomorphic adenoma must be included in this group. Treatment of these highly malignant tumors involves radical surgical resection of the primary tumor including, when necessary, adjacent vital structures such as the mandible, the maxilla, and even a portion of the temporal bone. In order to completely excise these malignant tumors, divisions of the facial nerve adjacent to the tumor have to be excised. When feasible, and when there is a sufficient distal segment, it is worthwhile to utilize a nerve graft to restore nerve continuity. When there is already evidence of facial nerve paralysis the prognosis is poor, and no effort is made to preserve facial nerve continuity.

Adenocystic carcinoma has a predilection for neural invasion.

Malignant tumors of intermediate and low grade include *mucoepidermoid carcinoma* and *acinic cell carcinoma.* When these tumors occur in the parotid

TABLE 16–3. MALIGNANT TUMORS OF THE SALIVARY GLANDS

Children (under age 20)
    Mucoepidermoid carcinoma (low grade)
    Adenocarcinoma
    Acinic cell cancer
    Adenocystic carcinoma
Adults
    Mucoepidermoid carcinoma
      low grade
      high grade
    Adenocystic carcinoma
    Acinic cell cancer
    Adenocarcinoma
      mucus-producing
      undifferentiated
    Carcinoma arising in a pleomorphic
      adenoma
    Clear cell carcinoma
    Squamous cell carcinoma

TABLE 16–4. TNM CLASSIFICATION OF SALIVARY GLAND TUMORS

Primary Tumor (T)
T1 Tumor 2.0 cm or less in greatest diameter without significant local extension*
T2 Tumor more than 2.0 cm but not more than 4.0 cm in greatest diameter without significant local extension
T3 Tumor more than 4.0 cm but not more than 6.0 cm in greatest diameter without significant local extension
T4a Tumor over 6.0 cm in greatest diameter without significant local extension
T4b Tumor of any size with significant local extension*

*Significant local extension is defined as evidence of tumor involvement of skin, soft tissues, bone, or the lingual or facial nerves.
From Beahrs OH, Myers MH (eds): Manual for Staging of Cancer. 2nd ed. Philadelphia, JB Lippincott Co, 1983, p 50.

Acinic cell carcinoma is the most common malignant parotid tumor to occur bilaterally. It occurs almost exclusively in the parotid gland.

gland, a total parotidectomy is performed and the facial nerve preserved if its preservation does not compromise the total resection of the malignancy. A direct invasion of the nerve precludes preservation of that division of the nerve. Frozen section must be performed to rule out neural invasion, as this invasion is always cephalad. When possible, a nerve graft is performed at the time of the surgical resection. Tumors in the submandibular gland are treated by a total resection of the gland and adjacent tissues and a radical or modified radical neck dissection.

One of the greatest difficulties in dealing with tumors of the major salivary glands is determination of the tumor type on frozen section. When there is some doubt as to the interpretation it is preferable to wait until permanent sections are prepared and evaluated before proceeding with one of the radical operative procedures. Difficulty can be encountered in determining the type of mucoepidermoid carcinoma or in differentiating between benign and malignant mixed tumors or between adenocystic carcinoma and pleomorphic adenoma.

Radical neck dissection is not routinely part of the initial resection for parotid malignancies but is required when palpable cervical metastases are present or when there is a recurrence of a malignant tumor in the parotid region. Radical neck dissection is then combined with the extended radical parotid resection. When it is established at the time of surgery that one is dealing with a malignant parotid tumor, the preferred procedure is total parotidectomy with removal of surrounding, adjacent soft tissues. The facial nerve is preserved when it does not compromise the resection of the tumor. Facial nerve grafting is performed when feasible, particularly if the trunk has to be resected. If possible, the division to the eye is preserved, as this causes the largest number of postoperative problems. The upper digastric nodes and those nodes in the region of the parotid gland are removed at the time of the initial operative procedure. If these nodes show evidence of malignancy, either a complete radical neck dissection or postoperative radiation therapy is advised.

High-grade mucoepidermoid carcinoma and squamous cell carcinoma are the tumors most likely to develop cervical metastases. There is a 40 per cent incidence of occult metastases for squamous cell carcinoma and 16 per cent for high-grade mucoepidermoid carcinoma. Adenocystic carcinoma, adenocarcinoma, and acinic cell carcinoma can metastasize directly to the neck but are more likely to spread there by direct extension. These tumors are also more likely to develop hematogenous metastases to the lung. For these tumors resection of the parotid and subdigastric nodes is performed. If there is evidence of metastases at that time, a complete neck dissection can be performed. As facial nerve paralysis is a sign of poor prognosis, it is also an indication of a greater likelihood of cervical metastatic disease and can therefore be considered an indication to perform a radical neck dissection.

Currently, postoperative radiation therapy is advised for most malignant parotid tumors. Comparing current studies with historical controls, the data are highly suggestive that the addition of radiation therapy reduces the local recurrence rate. It should be recognized that radiation therapy is not a substitute for adequate surgical resection and does not decrease the recurrence rate when tumor margins are positive. Prognosis for adults with malignant parotid tumors depends on the stage and size of the tumor at presentation, presence or absence of facial nerve paralysis, and evidence of cervical metastatic disease. Additionally, the specific pathologic type of tumor is important in determining survival and the extensiveness of the operative procedure required. It is interesting that an initial complaint of pain has been shown in several studies to be a poor prognostic sign.

Malignant tumors of the submandibular gland are equal in frequency to benign tumors. The most common malignant lesion is adenocystic carcinoma. Surgery includes a wide regional resection and radical neck dissection. Postoperative radiation therapy is advised. Because of earlier extension and metastases, tumors of similar pathologic appearance have a poorer prognosis when they occur in the submandibular or minor salivary glands than in the parotid gland.

References

Batsakis JG: The pathology of head and neck tumors: The lymphoepithelial lesion of Sjögren's syndrome. Head Neck Surg 5:150–163, 1982.
Bernstein L, Nelson R: Surgical anatomy of the extraparotid: Distribution of the facial nerve. Arch Otol 110:177–183, 1984.
Gates GA: Radiosialographic aspects of salivary gland disorders. Laryngoscope 82:115–130, 1972.
Goode RL, Smith RA: The surgical management of sialorrhea. Laryngoscope 80:1078–1089, 1970.
Hemenway W: Chronic punctate parotitis. Laryngoscope 81:485–509, 1971.
Johns M: Parotid cancer: A rational basis for treatment. Head Neck Surg 3:132–141, 1980.
Swartz JD, Saluk PH, Lansman A, et al: High resolution computerized tomography, part 2: The salivary glands and oral cavity. Head Neck Surg 7:150–161, 1984.

Parotid Tumors

Conley JJ: Problems with reoperation of the parotid gland and facial nerve. Otolaryngol Head Neck Surg 99:480–488, 1988.
Guillamondegui OM, et al: Aggressive surgery in the treatment for parotid cancer: The role of adjunctive postoperative radiotherapy. AJR 123(1):49–54, 1975.
Matsuba HM, et al: High-grade malignancies of the parotid gland: Effective use of planned combined surgery and irradiation. Laryngoscope 95:1059–1063, 1985.
Spiro RH, Armstrong J, Harrison L, et al: Carcinoma of major salivary glands. Arch Otolaryngol 115:316–321, 1989.

Radiological Assessment

Blatt IM, Rubin P, French AJ, et al: Secretory sialography in diseases of the major salivary glands. Ann Otol Rhinol Laryngol 65:295–317, 1956.
Byrne MN, Spector JG, Garvin CF, Gado MH: Preoperative assessment of parotid masses: A comparative evaluation of radiologic techniques to histopathologic diagnosis. Laryngoscope 90:284–292, 1989.
O'Hara AE: Sialography: Past, present and future. CRC Crit Rev Clin Radiol, Vol 4, 1973.

17

DISEASES OF THE NASOPHARYNX AND OROPHARYNX

by George L. Adams, M.D.

For clinical purposes, the pharynx is divided into three areas: nasopharynx, oropharynx, and hypopharynx.

For clinical purposes the pharynx can be divided into three major regions: the nasopharynx, the oropharynx, and the laryngopharynx, or hypopharynx. The upper third, or nasopharynx, is the respiratory portion of the pharynx and is immobile except for the lower soft palate. The middle portion of the pharynx, termed the oropharynx, extends from the inferior border of the soft palate to the lingual surface of the epiglottis. It includes the palatine tonsils with their pillars and the lingual tonsils located on the base of the tongue. The lower portion of the pharynx, known as the hypopharynx or laryngopharynx, represents the region of the separation of the upper airway from the upper digestive pathway.

Anatomy of the Nasopharynx

The relatively small nasopharyngeal space contains or is in close relationship to a number of structures that have clinical importance.

1. On the posterior wall extending toward the vault is the adenoid tissue.
2. There is lymphoid tissue on the lateral pharyngeal wall and in the recessus pharyngeus, known as Rosenmüller's fossa.
3. Torus tubarius—this reflection of pharyngeal mucosa over the rounded protrusions of the cartilaginous portion of the eustachian tubes projects as a thumblike intrusion into the lateral wall of the nasopharynx just above the attachment of the soft palate.
4. The posterior choanae of the nasal cavity.
5. The cranial foramina, which are in close proximity and can be involved by extension of nasopharyngeal disease, include the jugular foramina through which pass the glossopharyngeal, vagal, and spinal accessory cranial nerves.
6. Important vascular structures in the immediate proximity include the inferior petrosal sinus, the internal jugular vein, the meningeal branches from the occipital and ascending pharyngeal arteries, and the hypoglossal foramen, through which passes the hypoglossal nerve.
7. The petrous portion of the temporal bone and foramen lacerum is in proximity to the lateral portion of the roof of the nasopharynx.
8. The ostium of the sphenoid sinuses.

FIGURE 17–1. Nasopharynx as viewed through a nasopharyngeal mirror inserted into the throat through the mouth. Inset shows the amount of the nasopharynx seen with the mirror at each position. By moving the mirror, the entire nasopharynx can be examined, and information on all parts of nasopharynx, shown in the larger figure, can be obtained.

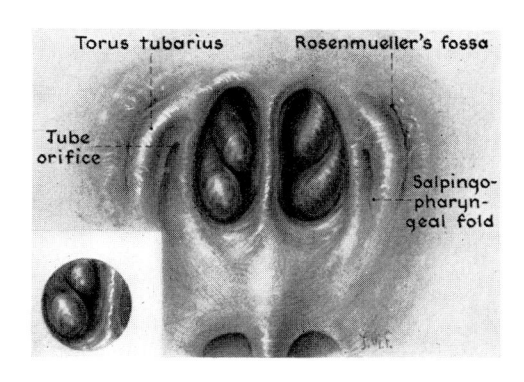

The nasopharynx can be examined in one of three ways. With the patient breathing through the mouth and with gentle downward pressure on the middle one third of the tongue with tongue blades, a mirror is introduced into the oropharynx. This examination differs from the laryngeal examination because of the small size of the mirror used and because the mirror must be rotated slightly from side to side to see the entire nasopharynx. Reflection in an upward direction permits visualization of the torus tubari on each side, the posterior choanae of the nasal cavity (Fig. 17–1), the posterior ends of the inferior turbinates, and the vault and posterior wall of the nasopharynx. Often patients require a topical anesthetic to decrease the "gag reflex" which prevents adequate visualization. Gagging does not justify inadequate visualization of the nasopharynx in any patient suspected of having a problem related to this area. If topical anesthesia alone does not permit adequate examination, it is possible to pass a small catheter through the nasal cavity, grasp it in the oropharynx, and direct it out through the mouth. This permits retraction of the soft palate (Fig. 17–2). Of course, anesthesia to both the nasal cavity and oropharynx is required.

An even better technique to visualize the nasopharynx is to pass a flexible nasopharyngoscope or a straight nonflexible nasopharyngoscope (Fig. 17–3) directly through the nose into the nasopharynx. This provides not only the best visualization but also magnification.

In cases in which it is strongly suspected that there is an underlying abnormality in the nasopharynx, general anesthesia in the operating room with bilateral retraction of the soft palate provides an opportunity to palpate the structures mentioned and obtain biopsies.

A flexible nasopharyngoscope passed through the nasal cavity provides the best visualization of the area.

FIGURE 17–2. Adenoid mass as seen at operation and drawn directly from life. A retractor is shown pulling the soft palate and uvula upward to expose the lower portion of the adenoid vegetations. Note the sharp inferior margin of the adenoid mass.

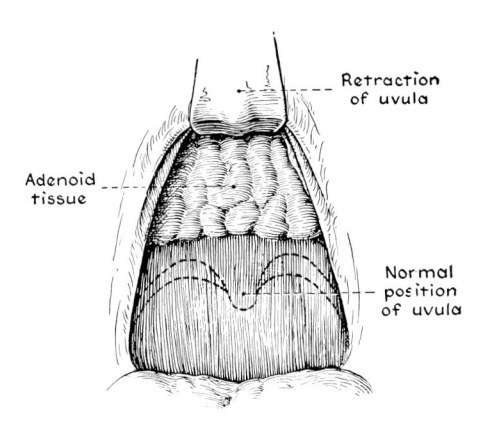

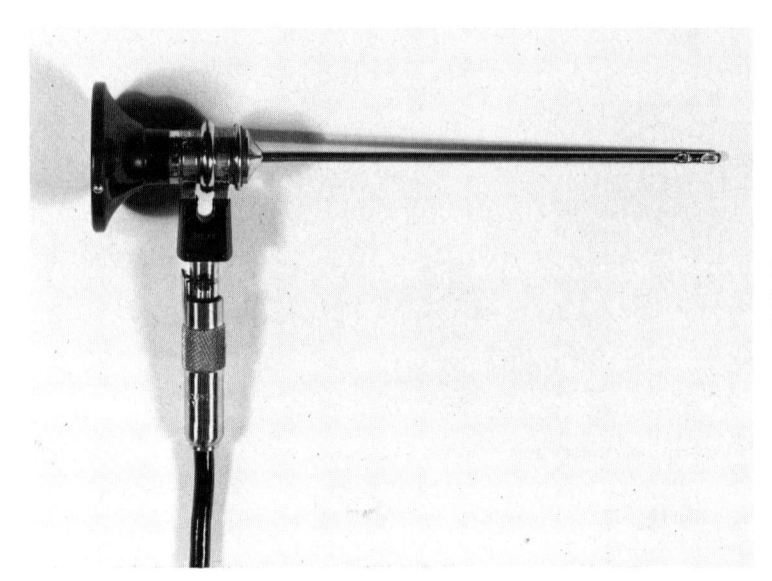

FIGURE 17-3. The nasopharyngoscope permits direct visualization of the nasopharynx and torus tubarius.

Radiographic and CT examination of the nasopharynx is helpful, but because of edema, normal asymmetry, or persistent adenoids, direct examination is still required.

Anatomy of the Oropharynx

The oropharynx includes a circumferential ring of lymphoid tissue referred to as Waldeyer's ring. The first component, or adenoid tissue, has been discussed as it relates to the nasopharynx. The other parts of the ring include the lymphoid tissue and the palatine or the faucial tonsils, the lingual tonsils, and the lymphoid follicles on the posterior pharyngeal wall. These all have the same basic structure: a lymphoid mass supported by a framework of connective tissue retinaculum. The adenoid (pharyngeal tonsil) has its lymphoid structures arranged in folds; the palatine tonsil has its lymphoid arrangement around cryptlike formations. The complex system of crypts in the palatine tonsil probably accounts for the fact that it becomes diseased more frequently than any of the other components of the ring. These crypts are more tortuous in the upper pole of the tonsil, become plugged with food particles, mucus, desquamated epithelial cells, leukocytes, and bacteria, and are an excellent place for the growth of pathogenic bacteria. During an acute inflammation, the crypts may fill with a coagulum that produces a characteristic follicular appearance on the surface of the tonsil.

The lingual tonsils have small crypts that are not particularly tortuous or branched as compared with the palatine tonsil. The same is true of the adenoids, and there is less marked crypt or crevice formation in other lymphoid collections in Rosenmüller's fossa and on the pharyngeal wall.

Anatomy of the Hypopharynx

The epiglottis serves as the divider between the oropharynx and the hypopharynx. The hypopharynx, which includes the pyriform sinuses, posterior pharyngeal wall, and postcricoid cartilage, is funnel-shaped. Food and liquids are directed downward into the esophagus. As the tongue thrusts the food into the hypopharynx, the cricopharyngeal muscle relaxes to permit passage of the food bolus.

The hypopharynx is discussed further in Chapters 19 and 20. It is mentioned here because inflammatory processes and abscesses involving the oropharynx can extend to include the hypopharynx.

DISORDERS OF THE NASOPHARYNX

Congenital Choanal Atresia

Some theorize that choanal atresia results from the embryologic failure of the bucconasal membrane to rupture prior to birth. This results in the persistence of a bony plate (90 per cent) or membrane (10 per cent) obstructing the posterior nares. A unilateral obstruction may not be symptomatic at birth but later will cause chronic unilateral nasal drainage in childhood. Bilateral choanal atresia presents an emergency situation at birth. The newborn depends totally on the nasal airway for breathing. Unless the infant cries, the nasal obstruction will produce pallor and cyanosis. The diagnosis should be suspected immediately and an attempt made to pass a small catheter transnasally to determine whether there is obstruction.

Bilateral choanal atresia presents as an airway emergency at birth. Newborns are obligate nasal breathers.

Inability to pass a soft catheter through the nose into the pharynx is diagnostic.

Emergency treatment consists of inserting a plastic oral airway into the infant's mouth. Another alternative is to tape a rubber baby bottle nipple (McGovern nipple) with a large opening on the tip into position in the infant's mouth. This has the advantage of permitting both breathing and feeding. Blindly perforating the bony plate or membrane is prohibited because of the narrow nasopharynx. When the infant's condition is stable, a transnasal airway can be established. Under general anesthesia and using the operating microscope, mucosal flaps are elevated and the bony plate is carefully curetted away. Silastic tubing is inserted for four weeks to maintain the opening while the area heals.

A transpalatal approach to the atresia plate provides more definitive correction. It is preferred by many surgeons, particularly when the atresia is unilateral or if the transnasal opening created shortly after birth has later closed. The infant soon learns to breathe through the mouth, and the transpalatal approach can be delayed until the child reaches at least one year of age. The direct access provided by this approach allows for resection of a portion of the palatine bone and vomer. Preservation of the palatine vessels permits closure of the incision on the palate with excellent healing. Unilateral choanal atresia is corrected at an older age.

The atresia plate can be approached surgically by (1) transnasal, (2) transeptal, (3) transpalatal approaches.

Nasopharyngeal Bursitis

Naopharyngeal bursitis, or Thornwaldt's disease, is a form of postnasal discharge that is produced by mucoid drainage from a pocket in the uppermost part of the posterior pharyngeal wall. The pocket is called the pharyngeal bursa. This is an unusual cause of postnasal drainage, and it is corrected by excision (Fig. 17–4).

Tumors of the Nasopharynx

A mass in the nasopharynx is frequently silent until it reaches sufficient size to interfere with surrounding structures. Symptoms may include posterior

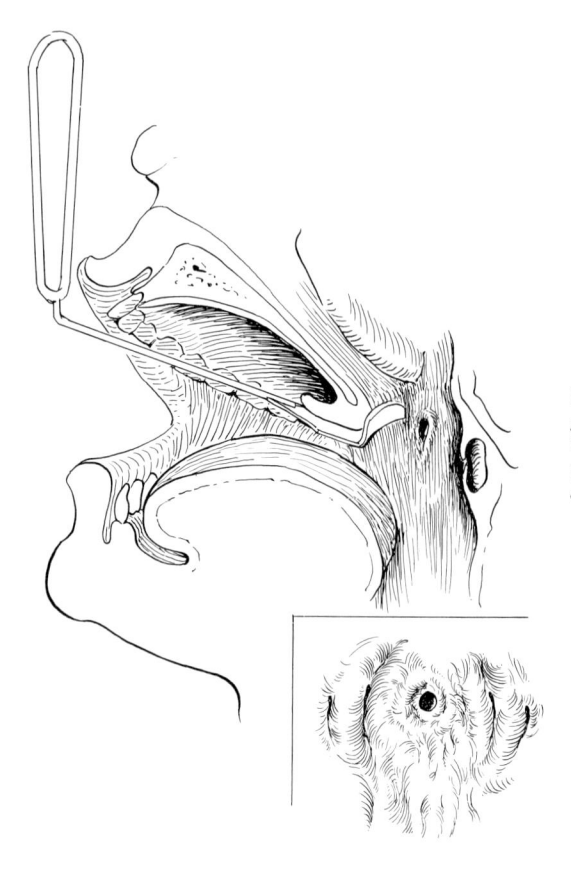

FIGURE 17–4. Diagrammatic representation of a nasopharyngeal bursa exposed by retraction of the soft palate. The inset indicates the site of the opening, which is rather high on the pharyngeal wall. Inflammation of this cystlike formation is known as Tornwaldt's disease or nasopharyngeal bursitis.

epistaxis, postnasal discharge, nasal obstruction, and hearing loss. Paralysis of cranial nerves III, VI, IX, X, and XI may occur but is usually a late sign. Serous otitis media develops because of eustachian tube obstruction. In every adult who develops a unilateral serous otitis media, a nasopharyngeal mass should be suspected and the nasopharynx examined.

Juvenile Nasopharyngeal Angiofibroma

Nasal obstruction and epistaxis in an adolescent boy suggest juvenile nasopharyngeal angiofibroma.

This uncommon tumor occurs almost exclusively in adolescent boys. Initial symptoms are epistaxis and nasal obstruction. Although histologically benign, these vascular tumors can invade the surrounding vital structures with eventual invasion of the base of the skull. Treatment modalities have included radiation, surgery, and hormonal therapy. Currently the preferred treatment, when feasible, is surgical resection. While radiation may be effective in certain cases, it is preferable to use radiation for residual disease or when surgery is not possible. There is always concern about irradiating a benign tumor in a young individual. Evaluation includes CT scanning and arteriography to determine the major vascular source of the tumor (Fig. 17–5). These highly vascular tumors obtain their blood supply from the ascending pharyngeal artery or internal maxillary artery. When the tumor transcends into the anterior or middle cranial fossa, an additional major blood supply may come from a branch of the internal carotid artery. It is essential to identify this vascular supply prior to surgical manipulation. Preoperative embolization to decrease vascularity and aid surgery has been used successfully but carries with it significant risk. CT scanning helps to determine the

CT scan may reveal the tumor to be larger than suggested by the arteriogram.

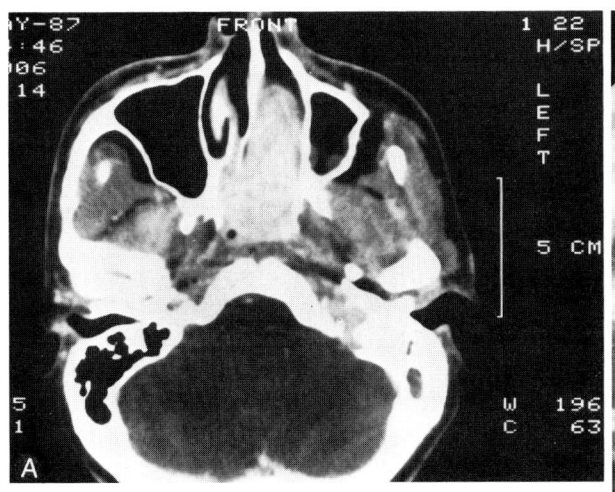

FIGURE 17–5. *A*, CT scan with contrast shows a large mass filling the posterior aspect of the nasal cavity and nasopharynx with extension to the left side in the region of the nasopharynx. *B*, The carotid arteriogram demonstrates the high vascularity of this juvenile nasopharyngeoangiofibroma. The internal maxillary artery is the main feeding vessel.

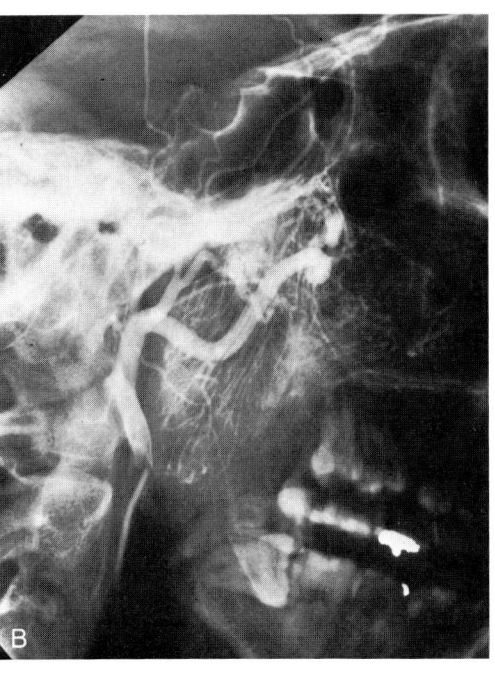

full extent of such tumors, as they rarely remain limited to the nasopharynx, but extend into the pterygomaxillary fossa, skull base, or sinuses. The diagnosis is so apparent by the very vascular appearance of the tumor and the history of epistaxis in an adolescent male that a preoperative biopsy is not obtained, for it may lead to uncontrollable hemorrhage. The arteriogram is sufficient to make the diagnosis.

Diagnosis is made by history, exam, CT, and arteriogram. A biopsy is not necessary and is hazardous.

Malignant Tumors

Management of malignant tumors is discusssed in Chapter 23. It is important only to mention the presenting symptoms of unilateral serous otitis media, cranial nerve paralysis (particularly the sixth nerve), and nasal obstruction. The most common presenting sign of nasopharyngeal carcinoma is a posterior high cervical lymph node. Nasopharyngeal cancers are not associated with smoking and can occur in young individuals. A particularly high incidence in Chinese has been noted. Research is being conducted on the association of the Epstein-Barr virus and nasopharyngeal carcinoma. Individuals with nasopharyngeal carcinoma have an elevated EB viral titer, and elevation of the titer after initial treatment often heralds recurrence.

A high posterior cervical lymph node suggests a nasopharyngeal source.

There is an association between Ebstein-Barr virus and nasopharyngeal carcinoma.

Adenoid Hypertrophy

The adenoids are an accumulation of lymphoid tissue along the posterior wall of the nasopharynx above the level of the soft palate. They normally hypertrophy during childhood, reaching their greatest size in the preschool and early school-age years. Spontaneous resolution is expected, so that by age 18 to 20 adenoid tissue will not usually be apparent on indirect nasopharyngeal examination. The adenoids often transiently enlarge with URI's, and spontaneous regression obviates the need for aggressive treatment. Adenoid tissue is seldom mentioned unless it interferes with normal function of one of the surrounding important structures. Hypertrophied adenoids have been related to eustachian tube obstruction and resultant serous otitis media as well as recurrent and repeated episodes of acute otitis media. The obstruction can interfere with nasal breathing. This may lead to a difference in voice quality. Adenoid hypertrophy may lead to some changes in dental structure and malocclusion.

Finally, and most importantly, adenoid hypertrophy can interfere with the normal respiratory process. In fact, children under age two with hypertrophied adenoids may have such interference with normal breathing that they may develop cor pulmonale or sleep apnea–type syndromes. This is discussed in more detail later in this chapter. Such children often have loud, sonorous breathing. Parents and physicians suspicious of the possibility of adenoid hypertrophy should request further evaluation of nasopharyngeal obstruction. Long periods of apnea suggest airway obstruction and sleep apnea. More elaborate testing can be performed in the hospital setting, including the sleep EEG and special sleep somnography studies. With a highly suggestive history, soft tissue lateral radiograph (Fig. 17–6) confirming the nasopharyngeal obstruction, and tape recording of the sleep, these more sophisticated studies may not be necessary. A more impressive form of upper airway obstruction related to adenoid hypertrophy can result in cor

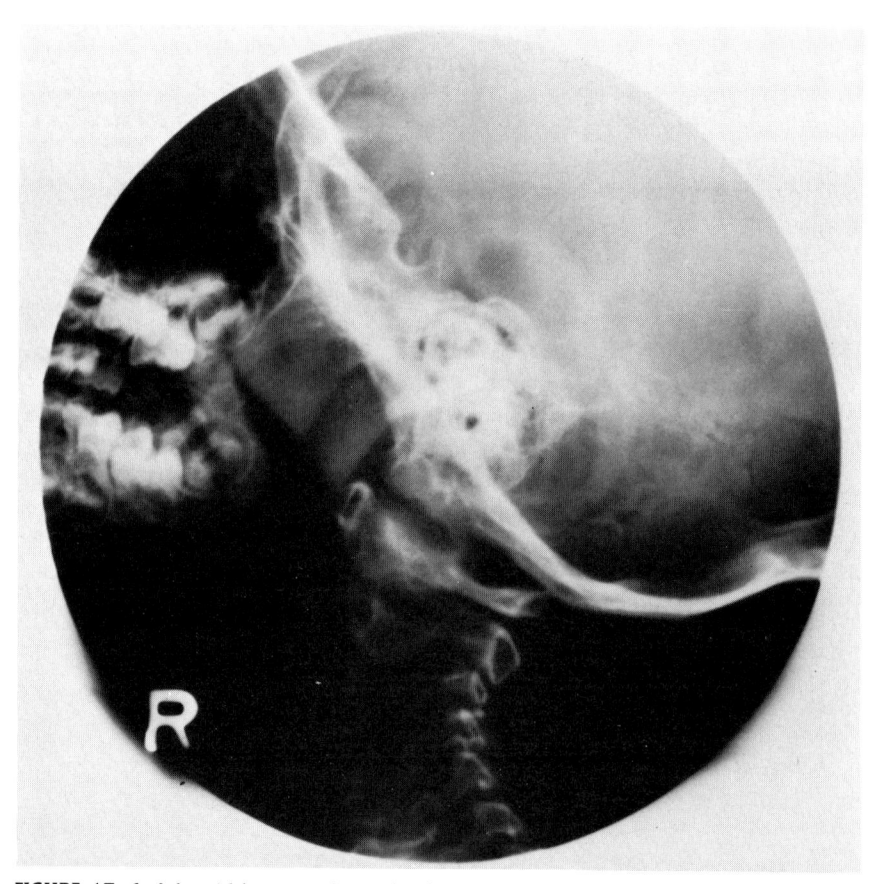

FIGURE 17–6. Adenoid hypertrophy in this four-year-old child obstructs the nasopharynx. The child presented with hyponasality to his voice, sleep disorders, and bilateral serous otitis media.

pulmonale. This form of right heart failure is refractory to management with diuretics but responds rapidly to adenoidectomy.

Indications for Adenoidectomy. Indications for adenoidectomy are based on one or more of the following conditions:

1. Chronic upper airway obstruction with resultant sleep disturbances, cor pulmonale, or sleep apnea syndrome
2. Chronic purulent nasopharyngitis despite adequate medical management
3. Chronic adenoiditis or adenoid hypertrophy associated with production and persistence of middle ear effusions (serous otitis media or mucoid otitis media)
4. Recurrent acute suppurative otitis media that has not responded to medical management with prophylactic antibiotics
5. Certain cases of chronic suppurative otitis media in children with associated adenoid hypertrophy
6. Suspicion of a nasopharyngeal malignancy (biopsy only)

The most common and preferred treatment for chronic serous otitis media that is refractory to medical management with antibiotics and other forms of conservative treatment is the insertion of ventilation tubes through the tympanic membrane. In children this is the most direct approach to alleviate the fluid accumulation and improve hearing. However, the tubes may remain in place only 6 to 12 months and the underlying problem is not always corrected. It is appropriate to look at the opposite end of the eustachian tube to determine whether the enlarged adenoids play a direct or indirect role in obstruction of this portion of the tube. Studies by Bluestone and others demonstrate that removal of enlarged adenoids can, in at least 50 per cent of cases, be effective in alleviating repeated episodes of otitis media and perhaps the need for ventilation tube insertion. These studies have not been effective in determining which group of patients would most benefit from adenoidectomy.

Adenoidectomy is beneficial in some individuals with recurrent serous otitis media.

Adenoidectomy for speech problems should be undertaken with great care. Speech pathologists should be consulted beforehand, for if a short palate, submucous cleft, or velopharyngeal insufficiency should result from the adenoidectomy, the voice may become hypernasal. In these situations full radiologic evaluation as well as a flexible nasopharyngoscopic exam is necessary.

Adenoidectomy should be avoided in cases of incipient velopharyngeal insufficiency, which might be created by removal of the adenoids in a patient with a very short soft palate or submucous cleft of the short or hard palate. It should certainly be avoided in patients with an obvious cleft palate. There may, however, be unusual cases in which a limited adenoidectomy is indicated for a patient with airway obstruction and a submucous cleft. In this case the parents must be warned of the possibility of further deterioration of voice quality if such an operative procedure is performed. There is no evidence to suggest that adenoidectomy will reverse dental changes that have already occurred, but removal can help prevent recurrence of malocclusion after orthodontia.

A bifid uvula serves as a "flag" to warn of possible submucous palatal cleft.

Because the adenoid tissue is not encompassed by a capsule like the tonsils, complete removal of all adenoid tissue is nearly impossible and recurrent hypertrophy or infection is possible.

DISEASES OF THE OROPHARYNX

The throat is considered to be the portal of entry of organisms that cause many diseases, and in some cases the organisms enter the body through this portal without causing any noticeable local symptoms. Oropharyngeal diseases can be divided into those that cause acute sore throat and those associated with chronic sore throat.

Diseases Associated with Acute Sore Throat

The following table lists the acute throat infections that originate in the nasopharynx or oropharynx:

DISEASE	FREQUENCY
Acute pharyngitis without membrane formation	Very common at all ages
Acute tonsillitis	Very common in children
Lingual tonsillitis	Moderately common in adults
Peritonsillar abscess	More common at ages 13–20
Acute pharyngitis with membrane formation or ulceration:	
Vincent's (Plaut's) angina	Common in young adults
Diphtheria	Uncommon
Pharyngitis associated with hematologic disorders:	
Infectious mononucleosis	Common
Acute leukemia	Uncommon

Acute Pharyngitis

Acute viral and bacterial pharyngitis are very common disorders. Numerous attempts have been made at classifications of an acute inflammation involving the pharyngeal wall. It probably is most logical to group a number of these infections under the relatively simple title of "acute pharyngitis." This includes acute pharyngitis occurring in the ordinary head cold, as a result of acute infectious disorders such as the exanthemas or influenza, and from the uncommon miscellaneous causes, such as herpetic manifestations and thrush (Fig. 17–7).

Etiology and Pathology. The cause of acute pharyngitis may vary from an organism producing a simple exudative or catarrhal change to one that produces edema and even ulceration. The organisms found include various streptococci, pneumococci, and the influenza bacillus, among others. In the

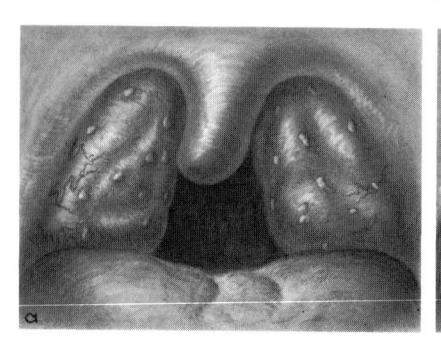

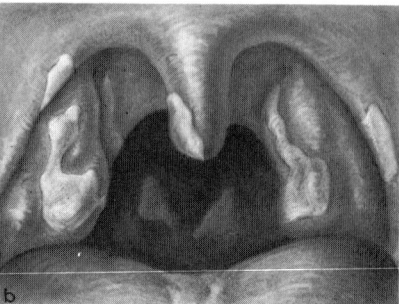

FIGURE 17–7. *A,* Acute follicular tonsillitis. *B,* Membranous involvement of the tonsils and pharynx.

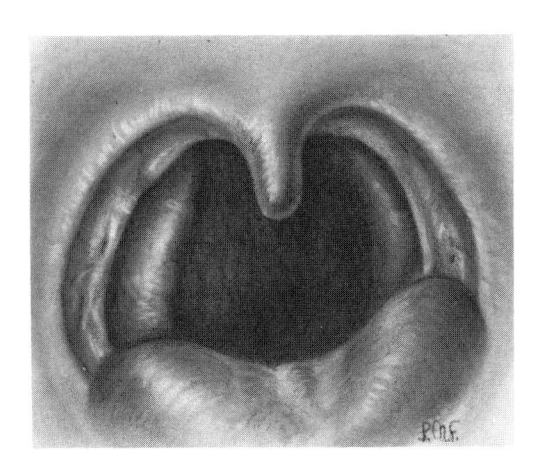

FIGURE 17-8. Chronic pharyngitis characterized by marked hypertrophy of lateral pharyngeal bands. This is also referred to as a "lateral pharyngitis."

early stages, there is hyperemia, then edema and increased secretion. The exudate is at first serous but becomes thicker or mucoid, and then tends to become dry and may adhere to the pharyngeal wall. With the hyperemia, the blood vessels of the pharyngeal wall become dilated. Small white, yellow, or gray plugs form in the follicles or lymphoid tissue. In the absence of tonsils, attention is usually focused on the pharynx, and it is observed that lymphoid follicles or plaques on the posterior pharyngeal wall, or localized more laterally, are inflamed and swollen. This lateral wall involvement, when isolated, has been referred to as "lateral pharyngitis" (Fig. 17-8). It is possible, of course, even in the presence of tonsils, for only the pharynx to be involved.

In recent years, with progress in the identification of viruses, reports of clinical problems related to a viral causative agent have become numerous. It is important to be aware of the probability of a viral etiology in acute pharyngitis associated with adenopathy in the absence of follicular pharyngitis membrane formation. Vesicle formation on the mucous membrane, as in herpes, strongly suggests a viral etiology.

A number of viruses have been identified in adenoid tissue during epidemics of acute pharyngitis (Table 17-1).

Symptoms and Signs. At the onset, the patient often complains of a dryness or "scratchiness" of the throat. Malaise and headache are common. There is usually slight elevation of temperature. The exudate in the pharynx invariably thickens. It may be dislodged with some difficulty, with a rasping, hawking effort and cough. A certain amount of hoarseness is present if the inflammatory process involves the larynx. In some cases, there may be dysphagia chiefly as the result of pain, referred pain to the ear, cervical adenopathy, and tenderness. The pharyngeal wall is reddened and may have a dry, glazed appearance and a coating of mucoid secretion. The lymphoid tissue usually appears red and swollen.

TABLE 17-1. CAUSES OF VIRAL PHARYNGITIS

Adenovirus	Respiratory syncytial virus
Epstein-Barr virus	Influenza virus (A and B)
Herpes simplex	Enteroviruses
Parainfluenza virus (types 1-4)	

Diagnosis. The diagnosis is usually made without difficulty, particularly in the presence of the symptoms and signs just described. Throat culture is helpful in determining the organism.

Treatment. The use of antimicrobials has changed the routine treatment of acute bacterial pharyngitis in recent years. As a result, the course of the disease has been shortened and the incidence of complications has decreased. An antibiotic should be given in therapeutic doses.

The use of warm throat irrigations, supportive care in the matter of an adequate fluid intake, a light diet, and aspirin when indicated may still be important in hastening the recovery, in spite of the fact that improvement follows the administration of an antibiotic.

Acute Tonsillitis

Etiology. Acute suppurative bacterial tonsillitis is most often caused by beta-hemolytic Streptococcus Group A, although pneumococci, staphylococci, and *Haemophilus influenzae* as well as viral pathogens can be involved. Occasionally nonhemolytic streptococci or *Streptococcus viridans* are cultured, usually in less severe cases. Nonhemolytic streptococci and *Streptococcus viridans* may be cultured from the throats of healthy persons, particularly in the winter months, and during epidemics of acute respiratory infections, hemolytic streptococci can be found in the throats of apparently healthy persons.

Pathology. There is a general inflammation and swelling of the tonsil tissue with an accumulation of leukocytes, dead epithelial cells, and pathologenic bacteria in the crypts. It is probable that differences in the strains or the virulence of the organisms may account for the following variations of pathologic phases:

1. A simple inflammation of the tonsil area
2. Formation of exudate
3. Cellulitis of the tonsil and its surrounding area
4. Formation of a peritonsillar abscess
5. Tissue necrosis

Symptoms. The patient complains of a sore throat and various degrees of dysphagia and, in the severe cases, refuses to take fluid or food by mouth. The patient may appear to be acutely ill and certainly experiences general malaise. The temperature is usually high, sometimes reaching 104°F. The breath is fetid. There may be otalgia in the form of referred pain. Occasionally otitis media is a complication of the inflammation in the throat. There is often tender cervical adenopathy.

The tonsils become enlarged and inflamed. They are usually spotted and sometimes covered with an exudate. This exudate may be grayish or yellow. It may become confluent and form a membrane, and in some cases an evident localized tissue necrosis occurs.

Treatment. In general, the patient with an acute tonsillitis and fever should have bed rest, an adequate fluid intake, and a light diet. Local applications, such as throat paints, are considered to have relatively little value. Oral analgesics are effective in controlling the discomfort.

GARGLES. The effectiveness of gargles has been questioned. It is true that the act of gargling does not bring much of the solution in contact with the pharyngeal wall, since in most instances it does not go beyond the fauces.

However, clinical experience indicates that gargling performed with a certain routine adds to the patient's comfort and probably influences to some extent the course of the disease.

Unless specifically instructed otherwise, the patient will probably feel that the treatment is finished when one glassful of lukewarm gargling solution has been used. This is inadequate. The patient should be instructed to use three glassfuls of the gargling solution each time. The first glassful should be warm as the patient can comfortably stand it. The second and the third glassfuls can be even warmer. It is advisable to specifically instruct the patient to use the gargling solution every two hours. It is practical to provide a list of the times for each treatment so that the patient can cross off each treatment as it is completed. This will ensure to a great extent that the instructions are carried out properly.

It is probable that the heat of the gargling solution is more effective than its medicinal content.

The following solutions, as well as available "over-the-counter" preparations, are useful:

1. Isotonic saline solution (½ teaspoon table salt in 8 ounces warm water).
2. Sodium perborate powder (1 teaspoon powder in 8 ounces warm water). This is especially useful in "Vincent's infections" or "trench mouth."

ANTIBIOTICS. Antibiotic therapy associated with appropriate cultures and sensitivities, when indicated, is the treatment of choice for acute bacterial pharyngitis. Penicillin is still the drug of choice, unless the organism is resistant or the patient is sensitive. In that case, erythromycin or a specific antibiotic that is effective against the organism should be used. Treatment should be continued for a full clinical course—between five and ten days. If group A beta-hemolytic streptococci are cultured, it is important to maintain adequate antibiotic therapy for ten days to reduce the possibility of nonsuppurative complications such as rheumatic heart disease and nephritis. A single intramuscular injection of 1.2 million units of benzathine penicillin is also effective and is preferred when there is doubt that the patient will complete the full course of antibiotic therapy by mouth.

Certain patients maintain a positive culture after adequate treatment with penicillin. The mechanism for this is most likely production of β-lactamase by coexisting organisms such as *Branhamella catarrhalis,* which is often present in mixed oral flora. A trial of clindamycin is advised to eradicate these resistant organisms.

B. catarrhalis present in the tonsil is capable of producing β-lactamase. This may explain persistent positive cultures after appropriate treatment.

Lingual Tonsillitis

The lingual tonsils do not have the complex crypt arrangement of the faucial tonsils, nor are they as large. For these reasons, lingual tonsil infections are much less common. Rarely are the lingual tonsils acutely inflamed along with the faucial tonsils. Lingual tonsillitis is more common in tonsillectomized patients and in adults.

The etiology and pathology are much the same as those of an acute inflammation of the faucial tonsils. The symptoms usually are soreness on swallowing, a sense of a lump in the throat, malaise, slight fever, and in some cases cervical adenopathy with tenderness. Inspection of the lingual tonsils with the aid of a laryngeal mirror and reflected light reveals a reddened, swollen lingual mass with whitish spots dotting the surface of the tonsil, similar to those seen in an acute tonsillitis involving the faucial tonsils.

Culture followed by appropriate antibiotic therapy is required. Lingual tonsillectomy by CO_2 laser has been performed in instances when medical management has not been effective.

Membranous Pharyngitis

Membranous pharyngitis has been described by some as a clinical entity, but membrane formation accompanies several forms of acute pharyngitis which are distinct entities but which resemble one another clinically. These diseases are Vincent's infection, diphtheria, the throat involvement accompanying certain blood disturbances, and the pseudomembranous character of a variety of throat disorders.

Vincent's (or Plaut's) Angina. This infection of the pharynx and mouth is often referred to as "Vincent's infection" or "trench mouth." It is caused by fusiform bacilli and spirochetes normally present in the oral cavity. It is more often encountered in a limited form without systemic reaction than in the more severe form, and it may be associated with other throat inflammations.

This form of membranous pharyngitis is commonly seen in young adults. Besides sore throat there are generally a low-grade fever, tender cervical adenopathy, and foul breath. Diagnosis is confirmed by the presence of numerous fusiform bacteria seen with Fontana stain. Treatment consists of supportive measures, sodium perborate or hydrogen peroxide mouthwash, and specific penicillin therapy.

Diphtheria. While the overall incidence of diphtheria is steadily declining in the United States, there is still an associated 10 per cent mortality rate. The pharynx remains the most common site for this infection. The disease occurs more frequently in unimmunized or inadequately immunized individuals. Individuals who are adequately immunized have a protective level of antitoxin for ten years or more. The most common initial complaint is a sore throat. In addition, patients may complain of nausea, vomiting, and dysphagia. The status of immunization has no effect on the presenting complaint. Examination reveals a characteristic membrane present over the tonsillar area with spread to adjacent structures. The membrane appears dirty and dark green and may even obstruct the view of the tonsils. Bleeding occurs with elevation of the membrane which is unlike other causes of membranous pharyngitis. The diagnosis is usually made earlier and treatment initiated sooner when it is known that an epidemic of diphtheria is present. There is often a delay in diagnosis of sporadic cases and in small epidemics.

The causative organisms are toxigenic strains of *Corynebacterium diphtheriae*. Smears of the nasopharynx and tonsil are obtained and placed in transport medium to be later cultured on MacConkey agar or Loeffler medium. Suspicious strains are then tested for toxigenicity.

Treatment of the disease consists of two phases: (1) use of a specific antitoxin and (2) elimination of the organism from the oropharynx. Before the antitoxin is administered, the patient should be tested for sensitivity to the serum. Patients should receive 40,000 to 80,000 units of antitoxin diluted in normal saline and administered slowly intravenously. Antibiotic therapy in the form of penicillin or erythromycin is initiated to eliminate the carrier state. Repeat culture should be performed to make certain the patient is not harboring the organism in the pharynx. Persistence of the organism requires long-term treatment with erythromycin.

Complications from diphtheria are common, and the patient who develops an airway obstruction may require tracheostomy. Cardiac failure and muscle paralysis may occur, and the inflammatory process may spread to the ears, causing an otitis media, or to the lungs, causing pneumonia.

Pharyngeal Manifestations of Blood Disorders

INFECTIOUS MONONUCLEOSIS. Infectious mononucleosis ("mono," "kissing disease") is an acute infectious disease characterized by fever, malaise, somnolence, lymph node enlargement (particularly in the posterior cervical region), and a peripheral smear revealing lymphocytosis with appearance of abnormal lymphocytes. The etiologic agent is thought to be a virus, most probably either Epstein-Barr (EB) virus or cytomegalovirus. Some physicians prefer to specifically divide the mononucleosis-type syndrome according to the suspected viral agent. The clinical pictures, however, are similar. Initially symptoms include a sore throat similar to that of acute pharyngitis or tonsillitis, fever, chills, and malaise. The patient complains of feeling tired. The lymphoid tissue of the pharynx becomes enlarged and often ulcerates. Often this tissue in the nasopharynx becomes so enlarged that it blocks the postnasal space, obstructing the nose and eustachian tubes. Splenomegaly occurs in 30 per cent of patients. Jaundice may develop in 5 per cent of patients. Approximately 40 per cent of patients develop a macular rash. The incidence of this rash, which is diffuse and of short duration, appears to be increased in patients receiving ampicillin. An exanthem can occur on the palate, also having a short duration of usually less than 48 hours and commonly occurring at the junction of the hard and soft palates.

Mononucleosis presents with persistent sore throat, fever, malaise, and tiredness.

Laboratory tests include a complete blood count and smear with examination for atypical lymphocytes. Initially there may be an elevated white blood cell count with neutrophils predominating, but this is later followed by a lymphocytic leukocytosis. A "Mono-spot" slide test is positive, and when the heterophil antibody test is performed the titer exceeds 1:60.

Initial "Mono spot" test early in the disorder can be negative.

Treatment of the patient with infectious mononucleosis is primarily symptomatic. Throat culture should be obtained because of the possibility of a coexisting beta-hemolytic streptococcal pharyngitis. When severe obstructive disease is present, steroids in the form of prednisone are administered in an effort to reduce the ancillary inflammatory process. The patient's activities should be substantially reduced during the acute phase, with a gradual return to normal activities.

A chronic or persistent form of mononucleosis caused by EB viral infection has been described.

Severe but unusual complications include a ruptured spleen, Guillain-Barré ascending paralysis, and cranial nerve paralyses.

Biopsy of a cervical lymph node during an acute episode of infectious mononucleosis can lead to an erroneous diagnosis of lymphoma.

ACUTE LEUKEMIA. The first manifestations of an acute leukemia may be oral lesions. These findings may include enlarged tonsils with ulcerative lesions, petechiae within the oral cavity, and bleeding associated with these areas. Gingival ulceration may occur. A low-grade fever and cervical adenopathy may be present. Positive diagnosis requires bone marrow aspiration and peripheral blood examination.

Peritonsillar Cellulitis and Abscess (Quinsy)

Etiology. Occasionally, infections of the tonsil proceed to a diffuse cellulitis of the tonsillar area extending onto the soft palate. A continuation of this process leads to a peritonsillar abscess. This may occur rapidly, with an early onset of tonsillitis, or late in the course of an acute tonsillitis. It can develop in spite of administration of penicillin. It is usually unilateral and is more common in older children and young adults.

Symptoms. In a moderately severe case, there is usually marked dysphagia, pain referred to the ear on the involved side, increased salivation, and, particularly, trismus. The swelling interferes with articulation and, if marked, speech is difficult. The fever hovers around 100°F, although occasionally it may be higher. A thorough inspection of the swollen area may be difficult because of the patient's inability to open the mouth. The examination causes the patient considerable discomfort. The diagnosis is seldom in doubt when the examiner sees the extensive peritonsillar swelling, pushing the uvula across the midline, with edema of the soft palate and bulging of these tissues toward the midline. The tonsil itself may appear normal as it is pushed medially, and the swelling develops lateral to the tonsil. Palpation, when possible, can help distinguish an abscess from cellulitis.

Pathology. A suppurative infiltration of the peritonsillar tissue occurs most often in the supratonsillar fossa (70 per cent). It causes edema of the soft palate on the involved side and displacement of the uvula across the midline. The swelling extends to adjacent soft tissues, causing painful swallowing and trismus.

Bacteriology. Throat cultures are taken but are often not helpful in identifying the responsible organism. The patient has invariably been treated with previous antibiotic therapy. Culture of the actual abscess drainage may reveal primarily *Streptococcus pyogenes* and, much less commonly, *Staphylococcus aureus* (Table 17–2). Sprinkle and others have identified a high incidence of anaerobic bacteria, which impart the foul odor to the drainage. Those organisms commonly found in the oral cavity include members of the Bacteroidaceae family.

Treatment. When an abscess forms it requires surgical drainage (Fig. 17–9), either by needle aspiration technique or by the incision and drainage technique. Difficulty can arise in determining whether one is dealing with an acute cellulitis or an actual abscess formation has occurred. When in doubt, a 17-gauge needle can be inserted (after application of spray anesthesia) into three locations most likely to yield aspiration of pus. When pus is encountered, this method may be sufficient for drainage when followed with antibiotics. If a large amount of pus is found and it is not adequately drained by this method, further incision and drainage can be performed. When no pus is found, it is more likely that one is still dealing with a cellulitis rather than a frank abscess. Those who object to this technique point to the fact that 30 per cent of abscesses are in the inferior aspects of the tonsillar fossa and are not reached by the needle technique.

The incision and drainage technique requires local anesthesia. First the

Peritonsillar abscess: fever, sore throat, trismus, cervical adenopathy.

Trismus: muscle spasm and pain which make it difficult to open the jaw.

Throat cultures may be negative in presence of an abscess.

Regardless of method preferred, all peritonsillar abscesses are drained.

TABLE 17–2. LIKELY PATHOGENS WITH A SELECTION OF ANTIMICROBIALS IN PATIENTS WITH A PERITONSILLAR ABSCESS

ETIOLOGY	ANTIBIOTIC
Streptococcus	Penicillin
Bacteroides	Cephalosporin
Haemophilus	Clindamycin
Fusobacterium	
Staphylococcus aureus	
Peptococcus	

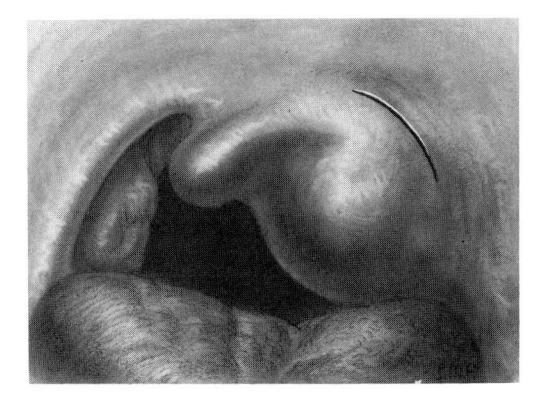

FIGURE 17-9. Appearance of a large, left peritonsillar abscess with a drainage site indicated. Incision should be through the mucosa only, with blunt dissection utilized in the deeper tissues.

pharynx is sprayed with a topical anesthesia. Then 2 cc's of Xylocaine with Adrenalin 1/100,000 are injected. A No. 12 tonsil blade or a No. 11 with tape to prevent deep penetration is used to make an incision through the mucosa and submucosa near the superior pole of the tonsillar fossa. A blunt hemostat is inserted through this incision and gently spread. Tonsil suction should be immediately available to collect the pus that is released. In older children and adults with severe trismus, surgical drainage for peritonsillar abscess may be performed after the application of 4 per cent cocaine solution to the site of the incision and to the area of the sphenopalatine ganglion in the nasal fossa. This sometimes alleviates the pain and trismus. Younger children require a general anesthetic. Advocates of immediate tonsillectomy (quinsy tonsillectomy) feel that this is a safe procedure that supplies complete drainage of the abscess when the tonsil is removed. It alleviates the need for a planned tonsillectomy six weeks later, at which time there is frequently scarring and fibrosis present and the tonsillar capsule is less easily identified. Indications for immediate tonsillectomy are listed in Table 17–3.

In addition to surgical drainage, whether by needle aspiration or by incision, the patient is treated with antibiotics and warm saline irrigations (Fig. 17–10). Even though cultures may show no growth because of previous antibiotic administration, antibiotics are administered which are effective against *Streptococcus*, *Staphylococcus*, and oral anaerobes. In individuals with repeated peritonsillar abscess or a history of repeated episodes of pharyngitis, a tonsillectomy is performed either immediately or as interval tonsillectomy six weeks later.

Atrophic Pharyngitis

A condition that is just the opposite of hypertrophic pharyngitis may occur. Varying degrees of atrophy of the mucosal elements of the pharynx are frequently encountered. In the mild cases, the mucosa appears thin and glistening or glazed, with an absence of all but a few of the lymphoid collections that are seen in an average pharynx. On careful inspection, one

TABLE 17–3. INDICATIONS FOR IMMEDIATE TONSILLECTOMY FOR PERITONSILLAR ABSCESS

Upper airway obstruction
Sepsis with cervical adenitis or deep neck abscess
History of previous peritonsillar abscess
History of recurrent exudative pharyngitis

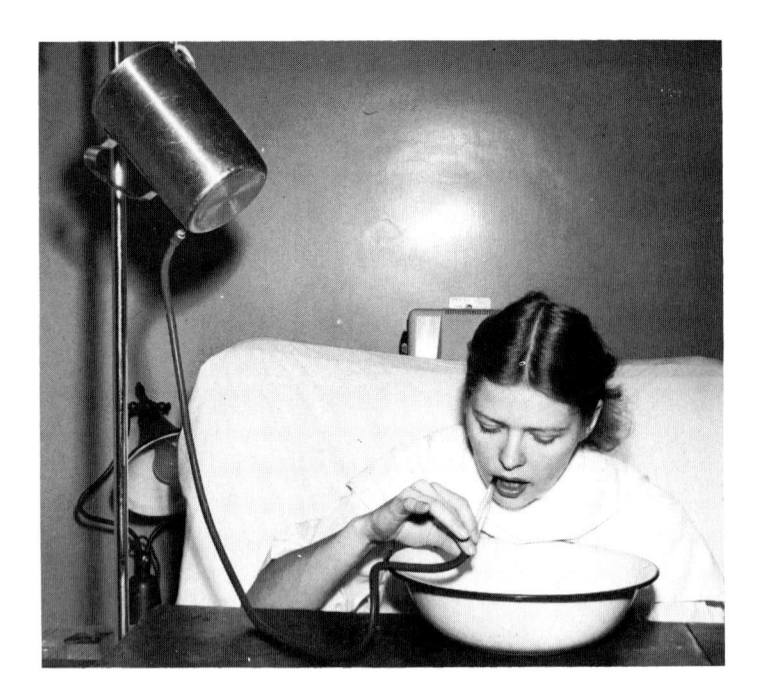

Figure 17–10. Warm saline throat irrigation provides symptomatic relief from the pain of pharyngitis or peritonsillar abscess.

can usually see that the blanket of mucus, which is normally transparent, seems thicker and semitransparent. It may be raised off the surface in spots.

In the advanced form of atrophic pharyngitis, the dryness is striking, the mucous coating is gluelike in its consistency, and at times an actual crust is seen. When this secretion is removed, the underlying mucous membrane has a dry, furrowed appearance. This advanced stage of atrophic pharyngitis has been termed "pharyngitis sicca" and is usually associated with an atrophic rhinitis, or "rhinitis sicca."

Etiology. The cause of atrophic pharyngitis is not definitely known. It has been claimed that it is caused by the air not being sufficiently warmed and humidified by the nasal mucosa, as would occur in chronic mouth breathing and in the instances of atrophic rhinitis in which the air-conditioning role of the nose is not functioning. There are apparently, however, trophic changes in the mucosa which result in a hyposecretion of mucus and which are influenced by some factor that is not understood.

Symptoms. The main symptom of atrophic pharyngitis is a sense of dryness and thickness in the upper pharynx. The patient's attempt to dislodge the adherent secretion consists of frequent attempts to clear the throat, usually by "hawking." Varying degrees of soreness are not uncommon. Hoarseness of a mild degree may accompany this disorder, owing to an extension of the process to the larynx and the irritation from frequent attempts to clear or cough out the sticky secretion. In some instances there is fetor.

Treatment. When an atrophic rhinitis is concurrently present, it should also receive therapeutic attention. Local application of Mandl's paint to the pharynx is beneficial. The purpose of this medication is to stimulate secretion. Potassium iodide may be given internally for the same effect. An average dose is 10 drops of a saturated solution three times daily with meals. A combination of the local application of a throat paint and the internal administration of the iodide is desirable. The breathing of warm moist air, such as can be accomplished by placing a hot, moist turkish towel across the nose and mouth, helps to moisten the inspissated secretion. Twenty to 30 minutes of this once or twice a day is desirable. Attention should also be given to matters of general health.

Pharyngitis Associated with Tobacco

Smoking has been implicated as a very common offender in the production of a dry, troublesome throat. These patients may begin by having symptoms of mild soreness and may eventually have difficulty with marked pharyngitis sicca. The throat of a heavy smoker is easily recognized by the dry, shiny, and hyperemic pharyngeal mucosa. Complete avoidance of smoking is needed to treat this chronic problem.

Chronic Tonsillitis

Diagnosis. Chronic tonsillitis is undoubtedly the most common of all recurring throat diseases. The clinical picture varies, and diagnosis depends largely upon inspection. In general, there are two rather widely differing pictures that seem to fit into the category of chronic tonsillitis. In one type the tonsil is enlarged, with evident hypertrophy and scarring (Fig. 17–11). The crypts seem partially stenosed, but an exudate, often purulent, can be expressed from them. In some cases one or two crypts are enlarged, and a considerable amount of "cheesy" or "putty-like" material can be expressed from them. A chronic infection, usually low-grade, is obvious. The other common clinical picture is that of the small tonsil, usually recessed and often referred to as "buried," in which the margins are hyperemic, and a small amount of thin, purulent secretion can often be expressed from the crypts.

The size of the tonsils in chronic tonsillitis does not necessarily correlate with severity of the problem.

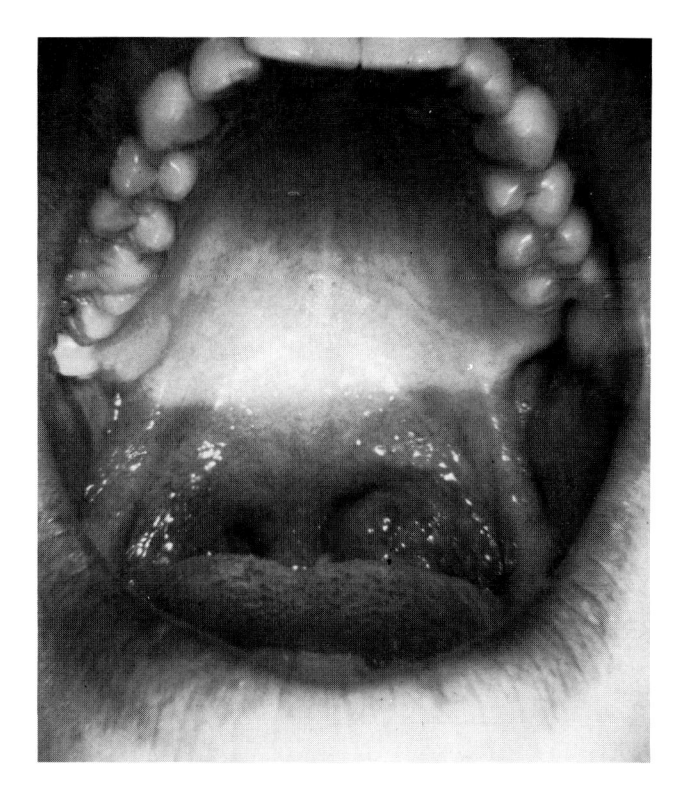

FIGURE 17–11. Chronic tonsillitis with a unilaterally enlarged obstructing left tonsil. In cases of unilateral tonsillar hypertrophy the possibility of underlying lymphoma must be considered.

Cultures from tonsils with chronic disease usually show several organisms of relatively low virulence and, in fact, rarely demonstrate beta-hemolytic streptococci.

Treatment. The one certain cure for chronic tonsillitis is surgical removal of the tonsils. This is reserved for those cases in which medical or more conservative management has failed to alleviate the symptoms. Medical management includes prolonged courses of penicillin, daily throat irrigations, and efforts to cleanse the tonsillar crypts with a dental or oral irrigating device. The size of tonsil tissue does not correlate with chronic or recurrent infection.

TONSILLECTOMY

Tonsillectomy constitutes one of the oldest surgical procedures still in existence. In 1867, Wise stated that Asiatic Indians were skilled in tonsillectomy in 1000 B.C. The frequency of the operative procedure has been drastically reduced since the advent of antibiotics. In addition, a better understanding of the indications for this operative procedure has reduced its frequency, from an estimated 1.5 million tonsillectomies in the United States in 1970, to an incidence of 350,000 to 400,000 per year in 1985. Because tonsil surgery is not free from morbidity and even mortality, it is prudent to recognize that this procedure, like every other operation, optimally should be performed by those skilled in the techniques.

Current Issues Regarding Tonsillectomy

Tonsillectomy with or without adenoidectomy has been performed frequently in an effort to control recurrent pharyngeal disease, upper airway obstruction, and chronic otitis media. With the advent of antibiotics and a better understanding of the immunologic function of the pharyngeal lymphoid tissue, it has become necessary to carefully reconsider indications for these procedures.

Mawson and Roydhouse performed the first classic prospective studies on the value of tonsillectomy and/or adenoidectomy in children.

In an effort to determine the benefits of adenotonsillectomy and to better select candidates requiring the operative procedure, prospective studies have been conducted. In recent years the best-known controlled studies are those of McKee in England in 1963, Mawson in England in 1967, and Roydhouse in New Zealand in 1970. These investigators compared children in various age groups with control groups with respect to episodes of tonsillitis, upper respiratory infections, and other associated infections. These studies demonstrated that preschool children with a significant history of pharyngeal disease received the greatest benefit from the operative procedure, and the benefit was most evident for one to two years immediately after the surgery. Thereafter, the beneficial effects between the two groups became less significant. The difficulty in interpreting these studies results from the fact that complete randomization could not be achieved, and patients who were strongly believed to require the procedure were removed from the control group and placed in the operative group. In addition, an exact definition of what constitutes adenotonsillitis that can be agreed upon by all physicians is still not available. Currently in the United States, adenotonsillectomy is frequently done not only for episodes of recurrent pharyngitis but also for episodes of middle ear disease. In particular, adenoidectomy is performed most frequently for the control of chronic or recurrent episodes of otitis media.

A prospective study was initiated in Pittsburgh, Pennsylvania, in 1973 under the direction of Drs. Bluestone and Paradise in an effort to answer the numerous questions that have arisen concerning the efficacy of tonsillectomy and adenoidectomy. To enter their study the patient had to have had a significant history of recurrent, documented tonsillitis, including seven episodes during the preceding year or pharyngitis associated with fever or positive culture for *Streptococcus* pharyngitis. Patients could also be entered if they had had at least five episodes per year for the preceding two years. It was essential that documentation of the frequency and severity of episodes was available. This study showed that children with this extent of disease did benefit from the operative procedure. However, the benefits were less apparent after the operative and control groups reached age ten. Again in this study, as in others, a certain number of children had to be removed from the control group and placed in the operative group because of the severity of their symptoms. The study raises the question of whether children with less severe disease would show the same benefit from the operative procedure, and the answer to this has yet to be established. This valuable study is still active and is pursuing answers to the numerous questions that arise regarding the efficacy of tonsillectomy and/or adenoidectomy.

In the past few years discussion has arisen concerning the role of the tonsils in the development of the immunologic system in children. Prior to the development of poliovirus vaccine, it was recognized that the incidence of bulbar paralysis during poliomyelitis epidemics was greater in recently tonsillectomized children. However, the overall incidence of poliomyelitis was equal in control and previously tonsillectomized individuals. More recently, sophisticated studies have demonstrated the presence of all major groups of antibody-producing immunoglobulins within the tonsils. In particular, these immunoglobulins include IgG, IgA (secretory type), IgM, and more recently IgE and IgD. The clinical significance of the presence of these antibodies is still not established, but the location of the pharyngeal lymph tissue places it in the anatomic position of the first line of defense against microorganisms. The significance of the tonsil in development of immunologic competence is probably greatest during the early years of life. Children with repeated episodes of pharyngitis and otitis media may have slightly decreased ability to develop certain immunoglobulins (IgA).

In 1971, Vianna pointed out a possible relationship between tonsillectomy and Hodgkin's disease because of the decrease in this lymphoid tissue barrier. Subsequent studies by Johnson and Johnson showed no correlation between the incidence of tonsillectomy and Hodgkin's disease. In addition, Freeman and colleagues showed that there is no correlation between tonsillectomy and the incidence of acute leukemia in childhood.

Indications

While there may be a variance in opinion on the exact indications for tonsillectomy in children, there is less disagreement on the indications for this procedure in adults. Tonsillectomy is commonly performed in young adults who have suffered repeated episodes of documented tonsillitis, peritonsillar cellulitis, or peritonsillar abscess. Chronic tonsillitis can result in extensive loss of time from work.

Children seldom suffer from chronic tonsillitis or peritonsillar abscess. Most commonly, they develop recurrent episodes of acute tonsillitis and associated hypertrophy. Such episodes may be of viral or bacterial origin. Discussion may then develop regarding at what point or after how many episodes surgical intervention is required.

The current commonly accepted guidelines are presented in this section.

Absolute Indications. Indications for tonsillectomy that have remained nearly absolute include the following:

1. Development of cor pulmonale by chronic airway obstruction
2. Tonsil or adenoid hypertrophy with sleep apnea syndrome
3. Hypertrophy to the extent of causing dysphagia with associated weight loss
4. Excisional biopsy for suspected malignancy (lymphoma)
5. Recurrent peritonsillar abscess or abscess extending into adjacent tissue spaces

Relative Indications. All other indications for tonsillectomy are considered relative. The most common such indication is recurrent episodes of documented group A beta-hemolytic streptococcal infection. The standard throat culture may not necessarily demonstrate the organism responsible for the current episode of pharyngitis. Culture of the tonsil surface does not always reflect flora in the depths of the tonsil. Likewise, culture alone cannot always be relied upon in the decision to treat with antibiotics. Sprinkle points out that while the majority of "sore throats" are caused by a viral infection, *Streptococcus pyogenes* was the responsible bacterial agent in 40 per cent of patients with recurrent exudative tonsillitis. Streptococci groups B and C, adenoviruses, EB virus, and even herpesviruses are also capable of producing an exudative tonsillitis. He believes that certain cases of recurrent adenotonsillitis may result from harboring such a virus in its dormant state within tonsillar tissue. At present, tonsillectomy may be the only way to establish a more normal oral flora in certain patients with recurrent adenotonsillitis.

The final decision to perform tonsillectomy will depend upon the judgment of the physicians who care for the patient. They should remain cognizant of the fact that this is a major operative procedure that even today is not free of serious complications.

Currently, in addition to the absolute indications, the most widely accepted indications for tonsillectomy in children include the following:

1. Documented recurrent bouts of tonsillitis (despite adequate medical management)
2. Tonsillitis associated with persistent and pathogenic streptococcal cultures (carrier stare)
3. Tonsil hyperplasia with functional obstruction (e.g., deglutition)
4. Hyperplasia and obstruction remaining six months after infectious mononucleosis (usually young adults)
5. Rheumatic fever history with heart damage associated with chronic recurrent tonsillitis and poor antibiotic control
6. Persistent chronic tonsil inflammation that does not respond to medical management (usually young adults)
7. Tonsil and adenoid hypertrophy associated with orofacial or dental abnormalities that narrow the upper airway

8. Recurrent or chronic tonsillitis associated with persistent cervical adenopathy

If there is recurrent streptococcal infection, there may be a carrier at home, and family culture and treatment may interrupt the cycle of recurrent infection.

Professional judgment and experience in evaluating the merits of these indications for a given patient are, of course, equally important. Just as there are indications for surgery, there are certain nonindications and contraindications that must be mentioned, since it has been fashionable to perform this type of surgery for these problems.

Contraindications. Nonindications and contraindications for tonsillectomy include the following:

1. Repeated upper respiratory infections
2. Systemic or chronic infection
3. Fevers of unknown origin
4. Enlarged tonsils without obstructive symptoms
5. Allergic rhinitis
6. Asthma
7. Blood dyscrasia
8. General inability or failure to thrive
9. Poor muscular tone
10. Sinusitis

Tonsillectomy can be performed in individuals who have a cleft palate deformity. However, there should be extenuating circumstances to indicate this operative procedure, and the patient must be informed of the possible effect on voice quality of the operative procedure.

Surgical Procedure

Preparation of the Patient

When the decision has been reached that tonsillectomy is to be performed, it must be realized that this may be the young patient's first surgical procedure. A complete history and physical examination should be performed with particular attention to existence of any familial or inherited disorders and specifically any bleeding tendency. In addition, a history of any relative who may have had difficulty with general anesthesia should be sought in an effort to exclude the remote possibility of malignant hyperthermia. The most commonly preferred screening tests for bleeding disorders include partial thromboplastin time, prothrombin time, and platelet count. The patient should not take any aspirin for two weeks before surgery. The history remains the most valuable guideline for the possibility of a bleeding tendency. Complete blood count and urinalysis are always required prior to a general anesthetic. Chest radiograph and electrocardiogram are recommended in adults over age 40. There should be documentation on the chart of the need and indication for the surgical procedure.

A history of a bleeding problem is more accurate than any single preoperative screening test.

The physician should explain to the patient in terms the young child can understand exactly what surgical procedure will be performed and that it is being done in an effort to help the patient and to prevent repeated episodes of infection or to improve hearing. It should be made clear that there may be discomfort in the immediate postoperative period but that the physicians, nurses, and parents will be available to help during this time. The family should then be asked to reinforce this and answer the child's questions honestly. A preoperative visit to the hospital may help to eliminate any fears the child may have. Instructions to the family on postoperative care in diet, activity, return to school, expected symptoms such as ear pain during the first postoperative week, and the possibility of delayed bleeding should be explained. Postoperative activities are individualized to the child's response and desires. No absolute limit to activity is necessary. In addition, if ventilating tubes were inserted at the time of the adenoidectomy and tonsillectomy, care and prevention of water in the ear canal should be explained.

Adults tend to have more postoperative discomfort than children. Persistent pharyngeal discomfort can be anticipated for seven to ten days. Adults should be made aware of this and of the possibility of delayed bleeding seven to eleven days after the operative procedure.

Technical Considerations

There is no substitute for proper training for the performance of these procedures.

Important anatomical relationships must be appreciated by the surgeon (Figure 17–12A) who performs tonsillectomy.

Surgical Anatomy

1. The structure of the two pillars—the palatoglossus muscle (anterior pillar) and the palatopharyngeus muscle (posterior pillar)
2. The lateral boundary of the tonsillar fossa—the superior constrictor muscle
3. The relationships of the plicae, particularly the plica triangularis
4. The blood supply, which is derived from five arteries—the dorsalis linguae from the lingual artery; the ascending palatine and the tonsillar, both from the external maxillary; the ascending pharyngeal from the external carotid; and the descending palatine from the internal maxillary.

Anomalous blood vessels in this area may offer certain difficulties in tonsil surgery.

The main lymphatic drainage from the palatine tonsils leaves the fibrous trabeculae of the tonsil to pass through the capsule to the superior constrictor muscle of the pharynx. Several trunks form at this site, pierce the buccopharyngeal fascia, and enter glands of the deep cervical chain from which drainage reaches the thoracic duct and then enters the general circulation. There has been no proof that there are effective afferent lymphatic vessels from the tonsils.

Such things as endotracheal anesthesia, nonexplosive anesthetics, intravenous fluids, and suction cautery for hemostasis have aided the surgeon technically. Local anesthesia for adults is safe and quite acceptable to the patient (Figures 17–12B, 17–13, and 17–14).

Postoperative Bleeding. Postoperative bleeding is categorized into immediate and delayed. Immediate persistent postoperative bleeding is generally handled by reanesthetizing the patient and controlling by ligature or suction electrocautery. Later bleeding of significance may be handled in

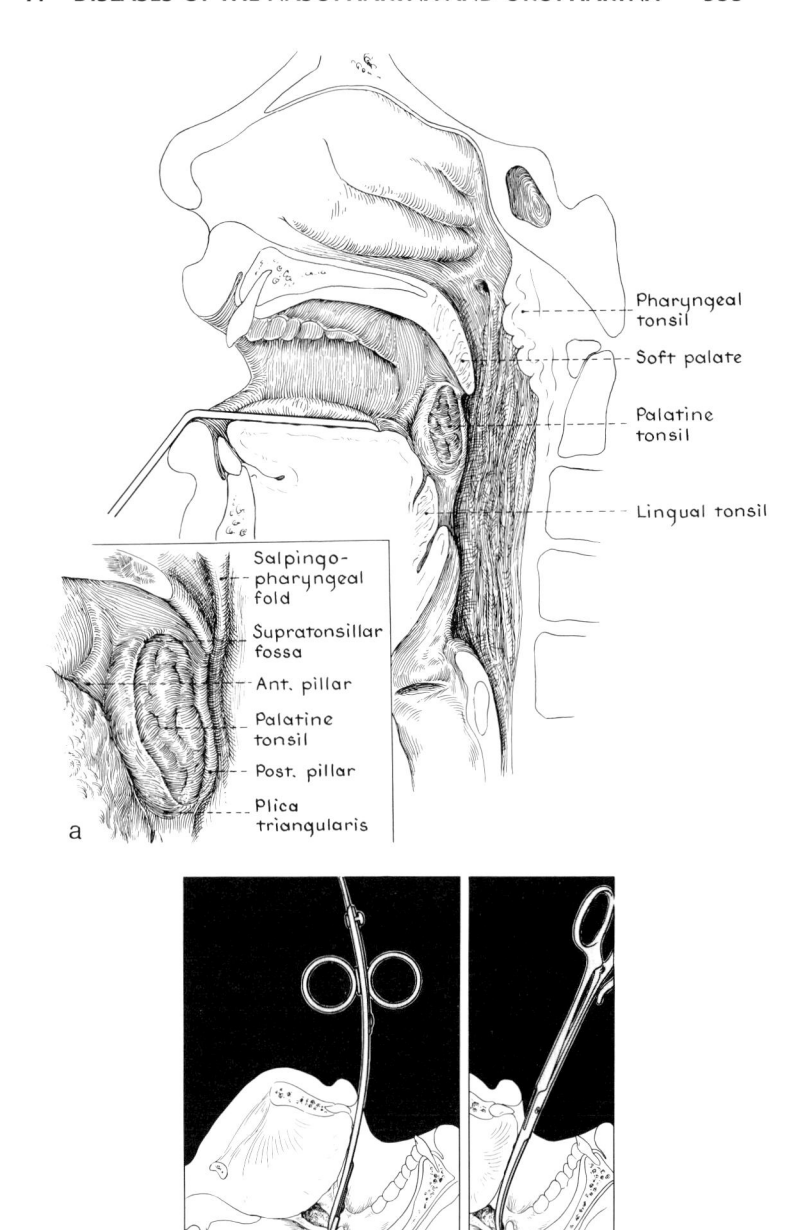

FIGURE 17-12. *A,* The relationships of the structures included in the oropharynx. The details of the structures surrounding the tonsils. (Redrawn from Hirsch.). *B,* The principle of adenoidectomy with LaForce adenotome requires insertion of the opened adenotome in the midline followed by additional insertion of the adenotome in lateral positions on either side of the midline. The advantage of this instrument is that it is less traumatic than the curet, the depth of incision is better controlled, and the adenoid removed is safely caught in the basket of the adenotome. After the adenoid is removed, or during phases of its removal, there is value in holding a sponge in the nasopharynx to control the bleeding so that the site of removal can be repeatedly inspected to ensure thorough removal of the adenoid mass and to visualize bleeding points on which to apply a hemostat. This technique is suitable only for the removal of an ordinary hypertrophic adenoid.

an outpatient situation, particularly if the youngster or adult is cooperative. This may occur up to the tenth postoperative day. Removal of the clot in the tonsillar fossa associated with silver nitrate cautery and pressure is generally all that is needed to control delayed postoperative bleeding. On occasion, because of uncooperativeness of the patient or profuse bleeding, it may be necessary to reanesthetize the patient in order to adequately control the bleeding.

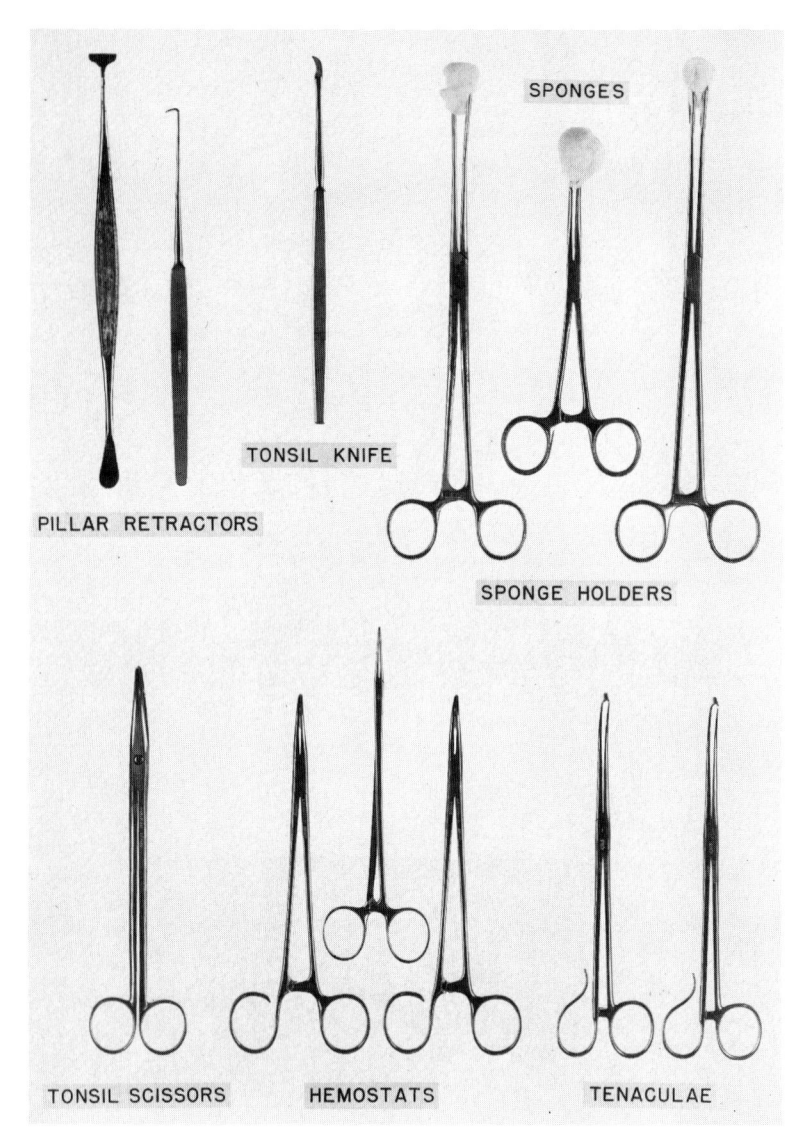

FIGURE 17–13. Instruments commonly used for tonsillectomy and adenoidectomy under general anesthesia.

Tonsillectomy can be performed as an outpatient operative procedure in many patients. However, some patients have persistent nausea and dysphagia and can develop dehydration if discharged prematurely. The decision as to the appropriateness of early discharge should remain with the surgeon. Patients undergoing tonsillectomy may require an overnight stay if oral intake is inadequate, they do not live close to a medical facility, or there is concern about bleeding.

DEEP NECK INFECTIONS

Deep neck infections develop in potential pharyngeal spaces. The source of infection may be of dental, pharyngeal, or traumatic origin, in which there is perforation of the protecting mucous membranes of the oral or pharyngeal cavity (Fig. 17–15).

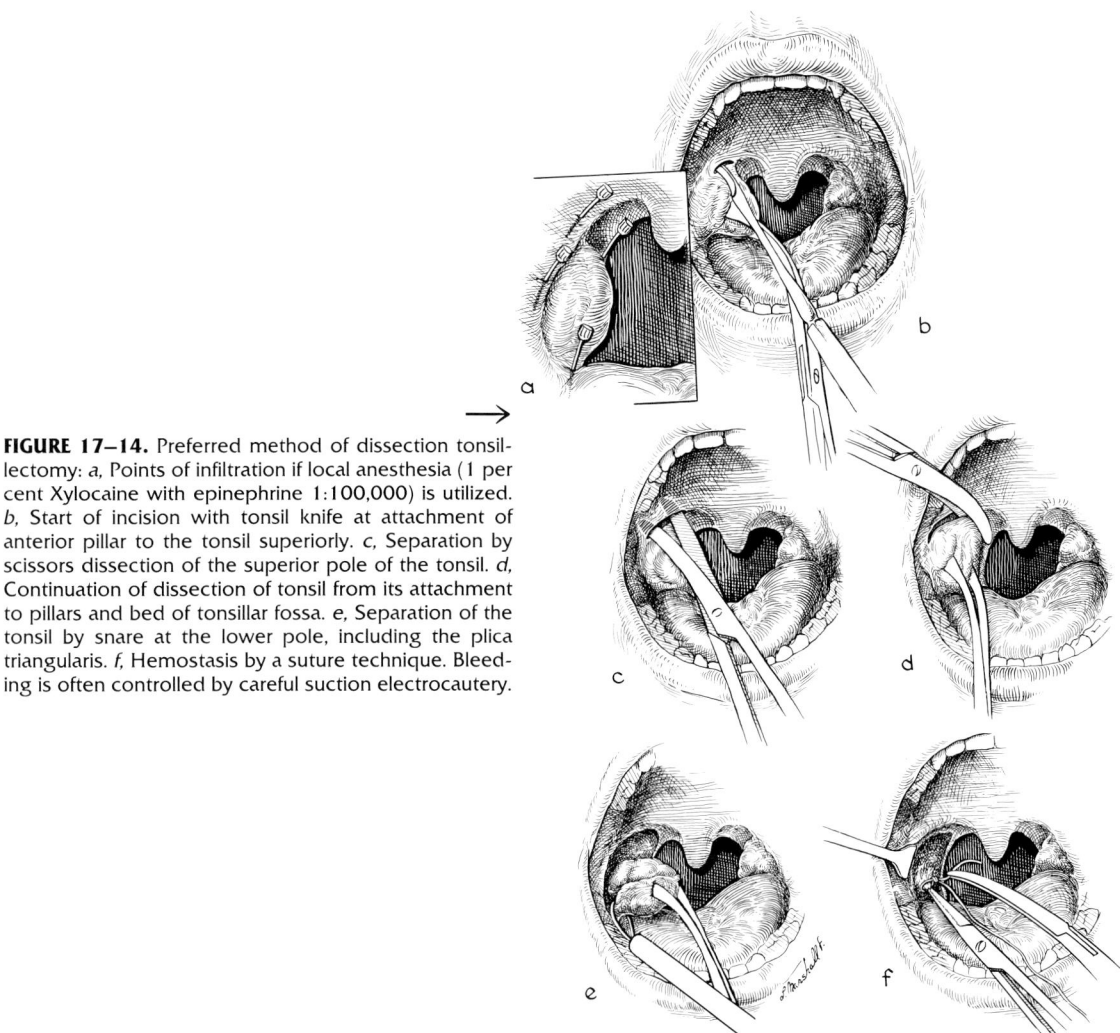

FIGURE 17–14. Preferred method of dissection tonsillectomy: *a*, Points of infiltration if local anesthesia (1 per cent Xylocaine with epinephrine 1:100,000) is utilized. *b*, Start of incision with tonsil knife at attachment of anterior pillar to the tonsil superiorly. *c*, Separation by scissors dissection of the superior pole of the tonsil. *d*, Continuation of dissection of tonsil from its attachment to pillars and bed of tonsillar fossa. *e*, Separation of the tonsil by snare at the lower pole, including the plica triangularis. *f*, Hemostasis by a suture technique. Bleeding is often controlled by careful suction electrocautery.

FIGURE 17–15. Potential deep neck spaces.

Pharyngomaxillary (Parapharyngeal) Space Infection

Pharyngeal space infection: dental, oral cavity, tonsils, parotid gland, traumatic, mastoid.

This potential space is funnel-shaped, with its base located at the base of the skull on each side close to the jugular foramen and its apex at the great horn of the hyoid bone. The inner boundary is the ascending ramus of the mandible and its attached medial pterygoid muscle and the posterior portion of the parotid gland. The dorsal boundary consists of the prevertebral muscles. Each fossa is divided into two unequal compartments by the styloid process and its attached muscles. The anterior (prestyloid) compartment is the larger. It may become involved in a suppurative process as a result of infected tonsils, some forms of mastoiditis or petrositis, dental caries, and surgery. The smaller posterior compartment contains the internal carotid artery, jugular vein, vagus, and sympathetic nerves. Only a thin layer of fascia separates this compartment from the retropharyngeal space.

Infection can spread rapidly from one potential space to another.

The fascial spaces of the neck have been previously described (Chapter 14). Pharyngeal infections can extend into the potential spaces surrounded by these fascial planes. Because patients have generally been treated with an antibiotic, the classic development of a fascial space deep neck infection is less common today (Fig. 17–16). The physician should initially determine which space is most likely involved as well as the probable causative organism.

When infection extends from the pharynx into this space, the patient will develop marked trismus. While the lateral pharyngeal wall may be pushed medially, as in a peritonsillar abscess, this infection should always be drained through a cervical incision. The neck becomes swollen near the angle of the mandible. CT scan aids in delineating the abscess.

A transverse incision, two fingerbreadths below the mandible, gives access to the anterior border of the sternocleidomastoid muscle (Fig. 17–17). The submaxillary gland is identified as well as the posterior belly of the digastric

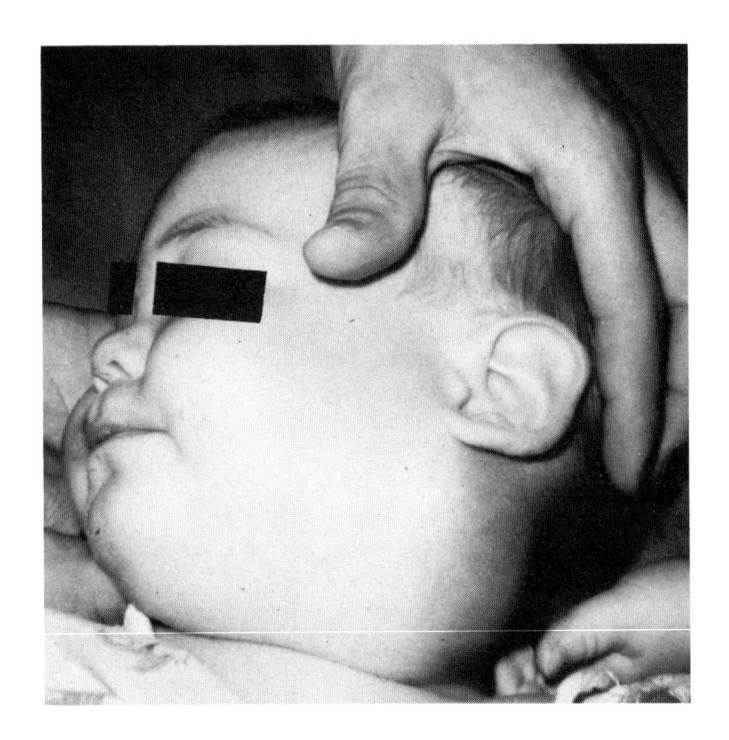

FIGURE 17–16. Parapharyngeal space abscess in an infant which will require drainage through a cervical incision.

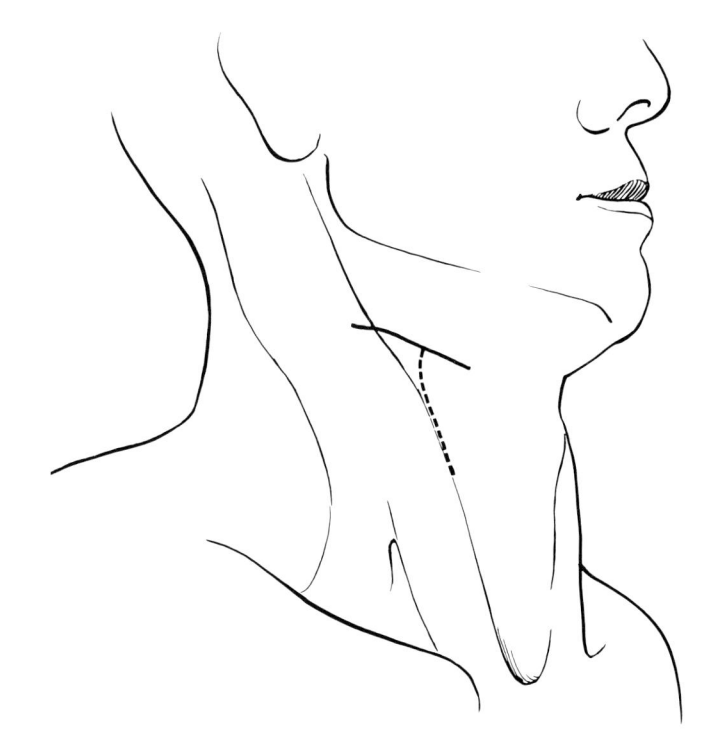

FIGURE 17–17. A transverse incision two to three fingerbreadths below the level of the mandible is made anterior to the anterior margin of the sternocleidomastoid muscle. The T extension as described by Mosher is often unnecessary. This extension is useful for identification of the carotid artery.

muscle. Blunt dissection toward the styloid process opens this space. After pus is collected for both culture and Gram's stain, drains are inserted into the abscess. The skin is approximated loosely.

The most serious complications of a pharyngomaxillary space infection involve the surrounding vasculature. Septic thrombophlebitis of the jugular vein can occur. There can be sudden massive hemorrhage from erosion of the internal carotid artery. An initial small hemorrhage (sentinel bleed) suggests this complication. Identification of the internal carotid arteries is mandatory when this complication is suspected and plans are made for drainage of the abscess. Thus, if hemorrhage occurs when the abscess is drained, immediate ligation of the internal carotid artery or common carotid artery can be performed.

Ludwig's Angina

Ludwig's angina is a cellulitis or phlegmonous inflammation of the superior compartment of the suprahyoid space. This potential space exists between the muscles attaching the tongue to the hyoid bone and the mylohyoid muscle. Inflammation of this space causes extreme firmness in the tissue of the floor of the mouth and forces the tongue upward and posteriorly and thus can potentially obstruct the airway. Ludwig's angina develops most frequently as a result of infection of dental origin, but it may develop from suppurative cervical lymph nodes in the submaxillary space. Treatment consists of surgical incision through the midline, thus interrupting the tightness that has formed in the floor of the mouth. Since this is a cellulitis, actual pus is seldom obtained. Before the incision and drainage are undertaken, preparations should be made for a possible tracheostomy because of inability to intubate the patient, as the tongue obstructs the view of the larynx and cannot be compressed by the laryngoscope (Fig. 17–18).

Free pus is not encountered when a Ludwig's infection is drained. Tissue edema is released by decompressing the submaxillary space.

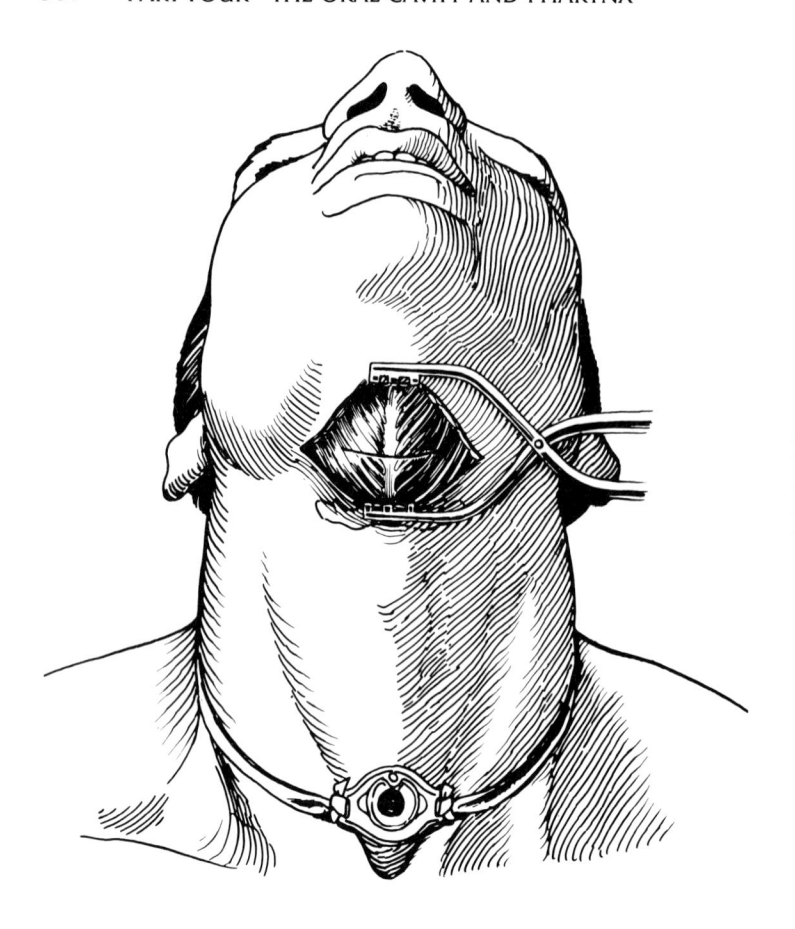

FIGURE 17–18. When there is no possibility of safe intubation, a preoperative tracheostomy is performed prior to incision of the geniohyoid muscle for release of tension in the region of the floor of the mouth.

Masticator Abscess

This potential space is in close proximity to the pharyngomaxillary space. This space includes the internal pterygoid muscle, masseter muscle, and ramus of the mandible. While infections in the adjacent pharyngomaxillary space are primarily the result of infection in the pharynx, the masticator space is most frequently involved secondary to infection of dental origin. Swelling and tenderness occur over the ramus of the mandible as well as firmness developing along the lateral floor of the mouth. It is not possible to depress the tongue because of the swelling and edema in the floor of the mouth. Infections in this space should be treated initially and vigorously with appropriate antibiotics. If the infection fails to resolve after a week of intensive antibiotic therapy, surgical drainage is required. A transverse cervical incision is made two fingerbreadths below the mandible and carried down to the mandibular periosteum. Blunt dissection is then used to drain the abscess. It may also be necessary to make a separate incision intraorally, thus draining the infection into the mouth.

Retropharyngeal Abscess

Etiology. This disease occurs primarily in infants or small children under the age of two. In older children or adults it is almost always secondary to spread from a parapharyngeal space abscess or traumatic interruption of the posterior pharyngeal wall lining by trauma from a foreign object or during instrumentation or intubation. In children there is an accumulation of pus between the posterior pharyngeal wall and prevertebral fascia which results from a suppuration and breaking down of lymph nodes in the retropharyngeal tissue. These nodes are immediately anterior to the second cervical vertebra and are no longer present in older children.

Symptoms. The disease should be suspected in an infant or young child when unexplained fever follows an upper respiratory infection and there is a loss of appetite, change in speech, and difficulty swallowing. Stridor occurs when the abscess becomes larger or edema extends downward to involve the larynx. Adults present with dysphagia, pain on swallowing, and symptoms suggesting airway obstruction. In adults, as the abscess increases there is pain and swelling in the neck, as the parapharyngeal spaces are usually simultaneously involved.

General anesthesia is administered provided that intubation is feasible and will not cause rupture of the abscess. In small infants it has been possible to drain the abscess under local anesthesia as an emergency procedure, but safe intubation by an experienced anesthesiologist is preferable.

Safe intubation is required to avoid rupture of the abscess.

Diagnosis. In the small infant the swelling of the pharyngeal wall may not be readily detected by inspection or palpation. In these cases, a lateral soft tissue radiograph of the neck may reveal a marked increase in the soft tissue shadow between the pharyngeal airway and the bodies of the cervical vertebrae. The larynx and trachea are demonstrated in a forward position. If there is question about the radiograph, it can be confirmed by a barium-swallow radiograph.

Treatment. Because of early administration of antibiotics, the true abscess stage may never develop, but there is extensive retropharyngeal adenitis, which will respond to appropriate intravenous antibiotics. When a diagnosis of an actual abscess is confirmed, the abscess should be drained. The airway must be protected. The head is lowered so that escaping pus will not be aspirated, and a small, pointed scalpel blade is used to make a short vertical incision at the point of greatest swelling (Fig. 17–19). As a safety factor, the knife may be guided by an index finger placed on the abscess. If pus does not escape, a small closed hemostat may be inserted into the wound, gently pushed to a deeper level, and spread.

FIGURE 17–19. Incision and drainage of retropharyngeal space abscess.

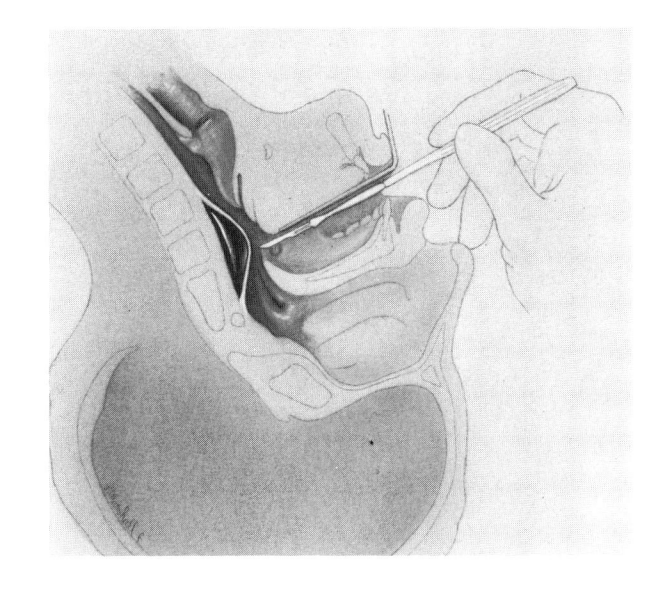

Cultures are obtained for aerobic and anaerobic organisms as well as tuberculosis. A stat Gram's stain is also obtained. Antibiotic treatment should include *Staphylococcus, Streptococcus,* and common oral anaerobes, including penicillin-resistant strains of *Bacteroides (B. fragilis).*

More recently young infants have presented with an identical clinical picture suggestive of a retropharyngeal space abscess. Soft tissue radiographs confirm the edema present in the retropharyngeal space. A lateral cervical approach has been used in older infants. The findings have been soft or necrotic, massively enlarged and edematous lymph nodes. The tissue is sent for pathologic evaluation to rule out leukemia and lymphoma as well as for culture. The airway is improved as the tissue edema subsides, and a tracheostomy is often avoided. This clinical picture most likely reflects a change in the classic presentation due to the early intervention with antibiotic therapy in patients with suspected retropharyngeal space abscess.

Complications. Asphyxia due to aspiration of septic debris and hemorrhage are the feared complications of a retropharyngeal abscess. Asphyxia has occurred when a mouth gag has been inserted for examination and drainage or from sudden rupture of a large abscess, flooding the larynx with pus. When hemorrhage occurs, the bleeding is usually profuse and may possibly require ligation of the internal carotid artery on the involved side for control.

Infection in this space can extend into the mediastinum with resultant mediastinitis.

OBSTRUCTIVE SLEEP APNEA*

During the past ten years the effects of long-term upper airway obstruction with development of sleep apnea syndrome or the cardiopulmonary syndrome have received significant attention. The severity of these long-term effects had not been previously appreciated. Sleep apnea and associated snoring are no longer considered psychosocial problems. Their interrelationships with significant cardiac and pulmonary problems have been recognized.

Obstruction can occur anywhere from the nasal cavity to the supraglottic larynx, or anyplace where the tissues are pliable rather than fixed.

The cardiopulmonary syndrome results from the efforts of the heart and lungs to compensate for long-term chronic obstruction (Table 17–4). Other findings associated with this syndrome include systemic hypertension (in 30 to 50 per cent of individuals), polycythemia, and cardiac arrhythmias (bradycardia and ventricular tachycardia).

Clinical Presentation:

Obstructive sleep-disordered breathing primarily affects adult males (95 per cent) and occurs in perhaps 1 to 3 per cent of the adult population. The clinical syndrome is associated with snoring in all individuals, and the

*Conrad Iber, M.D., and Robert Maisel, M.D., contributed to the section on Obstructive Sleep Apnea.

TABLE 17–4. PROGRESSIVE COMPLICATIONS OF LONG-TERM UPPER AIRWAY OBSTRUCTION

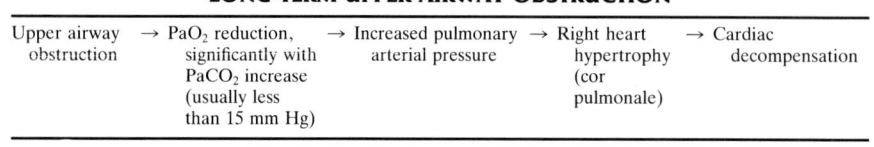

Upper airway obstruction	→	PaO_2 reduction, significantly with $PaCO_2$ increase (usually less than 15 mm Hg)	→	Increased pulmonary arterial pressure	→	Right heart hypertrophy (cor pulmonale)	→	Cardiac decompensation

accompanying sleep fragmentation causes excessive daytime sleepiness in 80 per cent. Since excessive daytime sleepiness may be caused by other clinical disorders (narcolepsy, sleep restriction, depression, idiopathic hypersomnolence syndrome), and since snoring occurs in 50 per cent of the adult male population, it is not surprising that the history of snoring and daytime sleepiness alone are not pathognomonic of sleep apnea. Hypertension, enuresis, nocturnal headaches, and daytime personality disturbances are less common. Clinically evident right heart failure occurs in less than 10 per cent and is due to pulmonary hypertension from chronic hypoxia and respiratory acidosis. Right heart failure is more common in patients with associated obstructive lung disease and daytime hypoxia. Cardiac dysrhythmias may occur only during sleep apnea events and include vagally mediated bradycardia and asystoles as well as ventricular dysrhythmias. Children typically have noisy nocturnal respiration and daytime nasal discharge and are less likely to have daytime sleepiness than adults. In severe cases, children may present with reversible underdevelopment and heart failure.

Mechanisms

Obesity and increasing age are associated with an increased risk of sleep-disordered breathing. Although prospective studies of adults with sleep apnea demonstrate reduced pharyngeal size and increased compliance with evidence of mild retrognathia, most adults do not have clinically evident disease of the upper airway. Narrowing of any portion of the supraglottic airway can contribute to pharyngeal collapse during sleep. Nasal obstruction due to septal deviation, massive adenoidal hypertrophy, or other anatomic or functional problems may produce sleep apnea. Most of the common aerodigestive pathway (pharynx) is composed of soft tissues capable of collapse and airway narrowing. Continuous muscle tone is required to maintain patency at the level of the nasopharynx, tongue base, and supraglottis. Sleeping in the supine position and relaxation of muscle tone, which accompanies sleep, can create obstruction. Although loss of phasic pharyngeal dilator activity was initially implicated in obstructive sleep apnea, recent studies show phasic inspiratory activation of upper airway muscles more commonly in patients than in normal subjects. Presumably the obstructive sleep apnea patient requires greater upper airway muscle activation than normal to maintain airway patency.

Coexisting anatomic obstruction of the upper airway combined with functional relaxation of the muscle tone and the sphincters increase the likelihood of pharyngeal collapse. Individuals with good daytime muscle tone may demonstrate disturbances during sleep and frank obstructive sleep apnea, with no apparent findings during waking hours. Obstruction may result from redundant tissue in the superior hypopharynx, base of tongue, or oropharyngeal areas. At night during both REM (rapid eye movement) and non-REM sleep, there is loss of muscle tone, and obstructive apnea will develop with continued inspiratory diaphragmatic and intercostal muscle contraction.

Provocative factors in adults include anatomic derangements (lymphomatous involvement of the nasopharynx, allergic rhinitis, and acquired retrognathia) as well as causes of pharyngeal collapse (alcohol, benzodiazepines, androgens, hypothyroidism). Correction of congestive heart failure may result in significant improvement or resolution of sleep apnea in some patients with biventricular failure. The provocative factors may precipitate obstructive episodes during sleep in susceptible individuals and should be corrected before considering surgical management of disease.

Obstructive hypopneas are more common than apneas in children and are more typically a result of identifiable anatomic abnormalities such as tonsillar and adenoidal enlargement, choanal atresia, mucopolysaccharidoses, or micrognathia.

Obstructive sleep-disordered breathing includes the related conditions of obstructive apnea and hypopnea. Obstructive apnea (cessation of airflow for greater than 10 seconds) or hypopnea (transient reduction in tidal volume) are due to occlusion or narrowing of the hypopharynx during sleep. Patients with the obstructive sleep apnea syndrome average 60 to 80 obstructive events per hour and may spend more than 50 per cent of their sleep time apneic. Each apneic event is terminated by arousal; thus sleep fragmentation and daytime sleepiness are a necessary complication of sleep apnea. The frequency of arousals correlates with daytime sleepiness. The severity of oxygen desaturation is usually worse in REM sleep and is related to the duration of the apnea as well as to the severity of the associated obesity and obstructive lung disease. Patients may have severe sleep disruption and daytime sleepiness without significant oxygen desaturation.

Apnea: cessation of airflow for > 10 secs.

Diagnosis

For a patient suspected of having obstructive sleep apnea, a careful interview is held preferably in the presence of another household member. Many patients deny or do not realize the symptoms are a result of the disease. Apnea causes arousal from sleep with disruption of the normal sleep cycle and subsequent symptoms of sleep deprivation—most notably daytime somnolence. These patients, or more usually their families, complain about significant or even heroic snoring. This may be so bad that a spouse has to move out of the room or work and travel partners are unable to stay in the same hotel room with the patient. Patients complain of morning headaches and impotence; families report that in severe cases the patient does not participate in family activities or decisions. Many of the patients are able to function in the workplace but immediately come home, eat dinner, and fall asleep. They may partake of meals with the family but may not participate in any other activities. Despite what appears to be an excess of sleep, these people are chronically sleep deprived from the recurrent awakenings associated with sleep-disordered breathing.

Daytime somnolence often is associated with sleep apnea.

Physical examination of the head and neck may be quite normal, although the physician should always look for obstructive lesions in the nose, nasopharynx, oropharynx, and hypopharynx. Specific lesions sought in the examination include nasal-septal deformity, nasal polyps, hypertrophic turbinates, and adenoid hypertrophy. In some apnea patients, the uvula is edematous and wrinkled, looking much like an earthworm. The soft palate may appear long, although no relationship of these anatomic landmarks to the degree of sleep apnea has been confirmed. Many patients are obese, some by 50 to 100 per cent over normal body weight.

Obstructive sleep apnea is a disease that causes two significant problems. The fragmentation of sleep disturbs the psychosocial activities of the patient, disenchants the family, and destroys emotional relationships. And because of excessive daytime sleepiness, the patient may be a hazard in the workplace

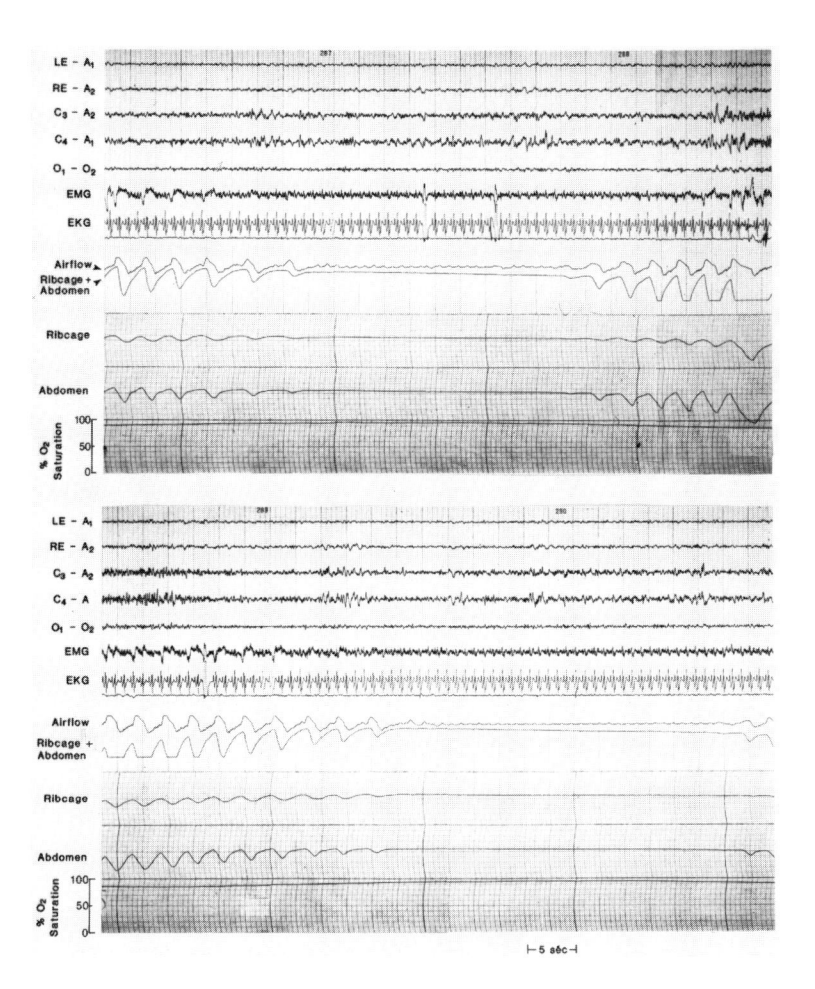

FIGURE 17-20. Obstructive sleep apnea. Cessation of airflow with continued respiratory attempts evident as paradoxical rib cage and abdominal movements lasting two minutes and associated with severe progressive oxygen desaturation terminated by arousal from REM sleep. (Seventy-two seconds of the continuous obstruction were removed to facilitate display.)

and while operating machinery, including automobiles. Cardiac complications including dysrhythmias and right heart failure may also be clinically apparent.

The diagnosis of obstructive sleep apnea is confirmed by overnight sleep and respiratory monitoring such as with nocturnal polysomnography (Fig. 17-20). The frequency of airway obstruction and associated sleep disruption is tabulated before and after therapeutic intervention. The frequency of apneas per hour (apnea index), apneas and hypopneas per hour (apnea-hypopnea index), and arousals per hour (arousal index) are objective measures of apnea and arousal frequencies. The frequency and grade of cardiac dysrhythmias and the severity of oxygen desaturation can best be determined during this testing. Home monitoring, such as oximetry and continuous EKG recording, is insufficiently reliable and specific for sleep apnea and is more useful for determining response to therapy or defining worsening of disease.

Treatment

Treatments of sleep apnea include bypassing the upper airway (tracheostomy), correcting identifiable anatomic abnormalities (uvulopalatopharyngoplasty, genioplasty, nasal septoplasty, tonsillectomy, adenoidectomy, mandibular or midface advancement), using devices to maintain airway patency (continuous positive airway pressure or CPAP), tongue retaining devices, jaw positioning devices, and weight loss. Tracheostomy cures obstructive sleep apnea in virtually all cases as long as the tracheostomy tube is patent and is positioned properly. It bypasses the site of obstruction and allows the patient and those living with him or her a complete, restful night. However, it is often not socially acceptable because of the open neck wound and can be difficult to manage chronically for obese patients because of the need for local wound care. Tracheostomy tube size may be difficult to match to the patient's stoma. Perhaps 30 per cent of patients will experience minor complications of infection and obstructing granulation tissue in the first few months after surgery as well as the need for humidification during the winter months. Many of these problems have been reduced in frequency and intensity by using new tracheostomy techniques, which include developing skin-lined flaps as well as combining that procedure with a submental lipectomy in the obese patients (Fig. 17–21). Tracheostomies planned around the Montgomery straight cannula tracheostomy tube also offer distinct advantages for patient tolerance compared with routine tracheostomy (see Chapter 25).

The flaccidity of the muscular structures and redundancy of tissues noted in the oral pharynx and hypopharynx in patients with obstructive sleep apnea suggest the value of uvulopalatopharyngoplasty (UPPP) (Fig. 17–22). This operation was first described by Fujita and consists of excision of excess oral pharyngeal tissue and tonsillectomy (if it had not been previously performed). The excess soft palate, particularly the posterior pillar of the tonsillar fossa, is carefully excised during this operation. Pharyngoplasty results in significant improvements in nocturnal oxygen saturation and arousals from obstructive events. Responders to pharyngoplasty have objective improvements in daytime sleepiness. The published literature harbors large discrepancies in

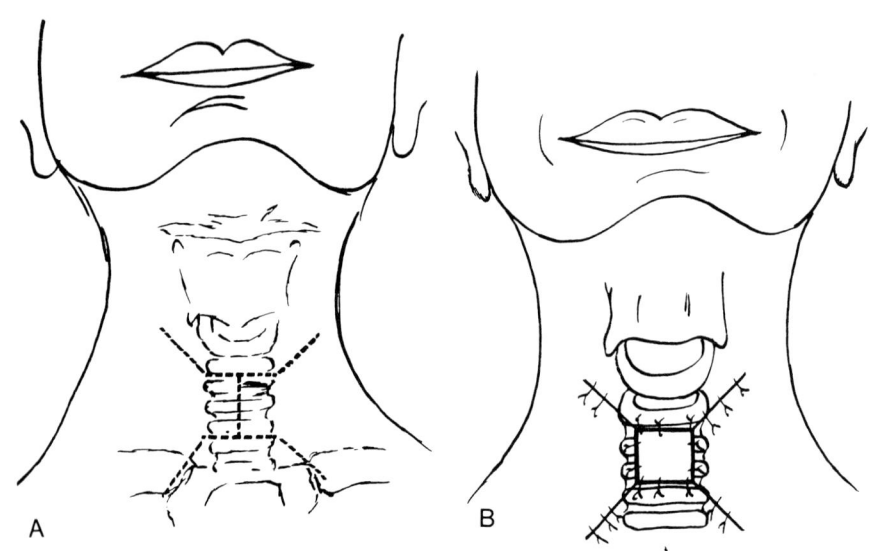

FIGURE 17–21. *A*, Anterior cervical skin incisions. *B*, Stoma after tracheocutaneous flap approximation. (From Sahni R, Blakley B, Maisel RH: Flap tracheostomy in sleep apnea patients. Laryngoscope 95:221–223, 1985.)

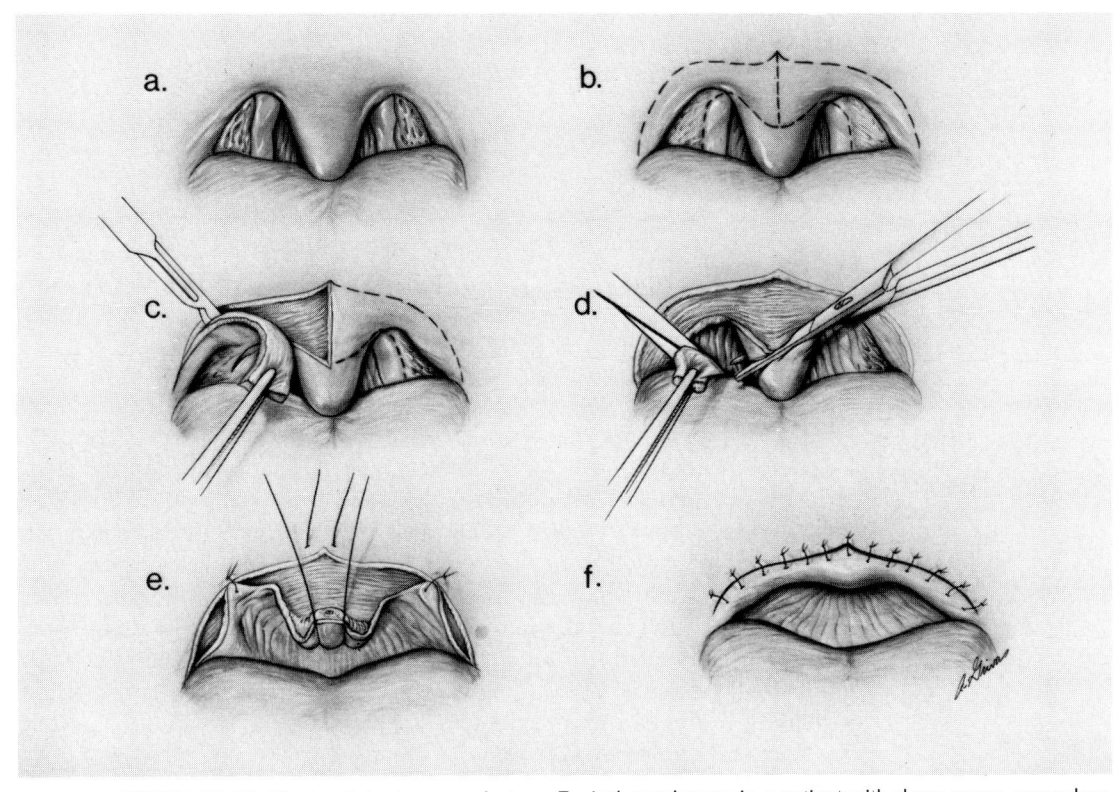

FIGURE 17–22. Uvulopalatopharyngoplasty. *a*, Typical oropharynx in a patient with sleep apnea secondary to oropharyngeal obstruction. Note elongated, engorged uvula, and thick, redundant folds of tissue. The tonsils are removed initially if this has not previously been done. *b* and *c*, Mucosal flaps based inferiorly, extending to the midline, are elevated. *d*, Excessive redundant submucosal tissue is excised and the uvula is partially amputated. *e*, Midline sutures are placed and reapproximated to the soft palate. *f*, Completion of procedure. (Adapted from Fujita.)

the response rates and predictors of response to pharyngoplasty. These discrepancies are due in large measure to differences in patient selection and definitions of response. If "response" is defined as a reduction of apneas and hypopneas to less than 20 per hour, only 30 to 40 per cent of patients are "responders." As yet, there is no consensus regarding the role of the physical examination, weight reduction, use of cephalometrics, or acoustic reflectance measurements in predicting response to pharyngoplasty. The response to other upper airway surgical procedures in sleep apnea remains largely anecdotal. Patients with moderate or severe apnea will often have a tracheostomy in conjunction with a UPPP. A repeat sleep study to demonstrate improvement to a more satisfactory level allows removal of the tracheostomy in about one-third of these patients.

TABLE 17–5. MEDICAL MANAGEMENT OF SLEEP APNEA

Avoidance of CNS depressants, especially alcohol
Appropriate use of medications
    a. Protriptyline (tricyclic antidepressant) reduces period of time in REM sleep
    b. Acetazolamide stimulates ventilation and reduces oxygen desaturation
    c. Thyroid supplement corrects hypothyroidism when present
Weight loss
Continuous low oxygen (1.5 L/min): Beneficial and deleterious effects have been reported
Airway maintenance: Intubation, tongue retainers
Continuous positive airway pressure (CPAP)

TABLE 17–6. OPTIONS FOR SURGICAL CORRECTION OF UPPER AIRWAY OBSTRUCTION IN SLEEP APNEA

	SITES OF OBSTRUCTION	TREATMENT
Nose	Nasal septal deflection	Septoplasty
	Enlarged inferior nasal turbinate	Submucous resection or cautery of turbinate
Nasopharynx	Adenoid hypertrophy, small slitlike configuration	Adenoidectomy
Oropharynx	Redundant tonsillar folds, prominent uvula, floppy soft palate	Uvulopalatopharyngoplasty (UPPP)
	Tonsil hypertrophy, enlarged lingual tonsil	Tonsillectomy Limited laser tonsillectomy
Hypopharynx	Collapse of pharyngeal constrictors, retrodisplacement of tongue	Tracheostomy, hyoid or mandibular advancement

Therapy with respiratory stimulants (progesterone, almitrine) or with other drugs (protriptyline, nicotine, strychnine) results in marginal improvement and is often complicated by intolerable side effects. In some cases where excessive daytime sleepiness and cardiac dysrhythmias are not paramount, oxygen alone may be sufficient to correct right heart failure. Although placing some patients with mild sleep-disordered breathing in a semireclining or lateral decubitus position results in marked improvement, this is often difficult to accomplish at home. Gastric weight reduction surgery usually results in dramatic improvement of sleep-disordered breathing in the morbidly obese, reduces health risks for other medical complications of obesity, and has perhaps a 10-fold increased likelihood of achieving weight reduction compared with dietary methods. In the moderately overweight, weight reduction of 10 to 20 lb may result in significant improvement in the frequency of sleep-disordered breathing (Table 17–5).

Continuous positive airway pressure by nasal mask (nCPAP) is now the most commonly prescribed treatment for sleep apnea in certified sleep disorders centers and has resulted in a dramatic reduction in the use of tracheostomy. nCPAP provides pneumatic stenting of the upper airway during sleep and corrects sleep apnea in over 80 per cent of patients who are able to tolerate the mask. Intolerance to the equipment results in significant attrition after initiation of nCPAP at home. Periodic follow-up by a nurse-specialist clinic may result in more successful long-term use. The tongue-retaining device results in marginal improvement in sleep-disordered breathing. The experience with other devices is anecdotal. A list of possible surgical options and their indications is given in Table 17–6.

References

Bartlett JG, Gorbach SL: Anaerobic infections of the head and neck. Otol Clin North Am 9(3):655–675, 1976.

Bierman CW, Furukawa CT: Medical management of serous otitis in children. Pediatrics 61(5):768–774, 1978.

Blakley BW, Maisel RH, Mahowald M, Ettinger M: Sleep parameters after surgery for obstructive sleep apnea. Otolaryngol Head Neck Surg 95:23–28, 1986.

Bluestone CD: Eustachian tube function and allergy in otitis media. Pediatrics 61(1):753–760, 1978.

Bluestone CD, Beery QC: Adenoidectomy in relationship to otitis media. Ann Otol Rhinol Laryngol 85(Suppl):280, 1976.

Christiansen TA, Duvall AJ, Rosenberg Z, Carley RB: Juvenile nasopharyngeal angiofibroma. Trans Am Acad Ophthalmol Otolaryngol 78:140, 1974.

DeDio RM, Tom LWC, McGowan KL, et al: Microbiology of the tonsils and adenoids in a pediatric population. Arch Otolaryngol Head Neck Surg 114:763–765, 1988.
Donovan R, Southill JE: Immunological studies in children undergoing tonsillectomy. Clin Exp Immunol 14:347–357, 1973.
Fairbanks DNF: Snoring: Surgical vs. nonsurgical management. Laryngoscope 94:1188–1192, 1984.
Feinstein AR, Levitt M: The role of tonsils in predisposing to streptococcal infections and recurrence of rheumatic fever. N Engl J Med 282:285, 1970.
Freeman AJ, et al: Previous tonsillectomy and the incidence of acute leukemia of childhood. Lancet 1:1128, 1971.
Fujita S, Conway W, Zorick F, Roth T: Surgical correction of anatomic abnormalities in obstructive sleep apnea syndrome: Uvulopalatopharyngoplasty. Otolaryngol Head Neck Surg 89:923–934, 1981.
Guilleminault C, Simmons FB, Motta J, et al: Obstructive sleep apnea syndrome and tracheostomy. Arch Intern Med 141:985–988, 1981.
Herzon FS: Permucosal needle drainage of peritonsillar abscess: A five year experience. Arch Otolaryngol 110(5):104–105, 1984.
Holt GR, Tinsley PP Jr: Peritonsillar abscesses in children. Laryngoscope 91:1226–1230, 1981.
Iber C, Davies S, Chapman R, Mahowald M: A possible mechanism for mixed apnea in obstructive sleep apnea. Chest, 89:800–805, 1986.
Johnson AK, Johnson RE: Tonsillectomy history in Hodgkin's disease. N Engl J Med 287:1122–1125, 1972.
Kornblut AD: The tonsils and adenoids. Otol Clin North Am 20:2, 1987.
Levitt GW: Cervical fascia and deep neck infections. Otol Clin North Am 9(3):703–716, 1976.
Manford RS, Orey HW, Brooks GF, Feldman RA: Diphtheria deaths in the United States. JAMA 229:1890, 1974.
Mawson GR, Adlington P, Evans M: A controlled study evaluation of adenotonsillectomy in children. J Laryngol Otol 81:777–790, 1967.
McCurdy JA Jr: Peritonsillar abscess: A comparison of treatment by immediate tonsillectomy and interval tonsillectomy. Arch Otolaryngol 103:414–415, 1977.
McKee WJE: A controlled study of the effects of "tonsillectomy and adenoidectomy." Br J Prev Soc Med 17:49–69, 1963.
Miller AH: Relationship of surgery of the nose and throat to poliomyelitis. JAMA 150:532–534, 1952.
Olsen KD, Kern EB, Westbrook PR: Sleep and breathing disturbance secondary to nasal obstruction. Otolaryngol Head Neck Surg 89:804–810, 1981.
Olsen KD, Suh KW, Staats BA: Surgically correctable causes of sleep apnea syndrome. Otolaryngol Head Neck Surg 89:726–731, 1981.
Orr WC: Sleep-related breathing disorders: An update. Chest 84:475–480, 1983.
Orr WC, Martin RJ: Obstructive sleep apnea associated with tonsillar hypertrophy in adults. Arch Intern Med 141:990–992, 1981.
Orr WC, Moran WB: Diagnosis and management of obstructive sleep apnea: A multidisciplinary approach. Arch Otolaryngol 111:583–588, 1985.
Paradise JL, Bluestone CD, Bachman RZ, et al: Efficacy of tonsillectomy for recurrent throat infection in severely affected children. N Engl J Med 310(11):674–683, 1984.
Roydhouse N: A controlled study of adenotonsillectomy. Arch Otol 92:611–623, 1970.
Sprinkle PM, Veltri RW: The tonsil adenoid dilemma: Medical or surgical treatment? Otolaryngol Clin North Am 7(3):909–925, 1974.
Sullivan CE, Issa FG, Berthon-Jones M, et al: Home treatment of obstructive sleep apnea with continuous positive airway pressure applied through a nose mask. Respir Physiol 20:49–54, 1984.
Templer JW, Holinger LD, Wood RP II, et al: Immediate tonsillectomy for the treatment of peritonsillar abscess. Am J Surg 134:596–598, 1977.
Vianna NJ, Greenwald P, Daview JNP: Tonsillectomy and Hodgkin's disease: "The lymphoid tissue barrier." Lancet 1:431, 1971.
Workshop on tonsillectomy and adenoidectomy. Ann Otol Rhinol Laryngol 84(Suppl 19), 1975, Chapters I, II, and III.

18

INFECTIONS IN THE IMMUNOCOMPROMISED HOST

by Norman T. Berlinger, M.D., Ph.D.

Our knowledge of the operation of the immune system has advanced remarkably in the last 20 years. Consequently, congenital and acquired immune deficiency diseases are being diagnosed with increasing frequency. Therapeutic manipulations of the immune system in the forms of bone marrow transplantation, solid organ transplantation, and high-dose cytotoxic chemotherapy are becoming commonplace and even preferred forms of treatment. As a result, otolaryngologists are now encountering increasing numbers of immunocompromised patients with head and neck infections that present diagnostic and therapeutic challenges.

BONE MARROW TRANSPLANTATION

Bone marrow transplantation was once considered a desperate or heroic form of therapy. However, improvements in conditioning regimens, in medical and surgical support strategies to reduce the risk of fatal infections, and in methods to treat and prevent graft-versus-host disease (GVHD) have allowed marrow transplantation to emerge as a potentially curative form of therapy. The largest number of bone marrow transplants has been performed for hematologic malignancies such as acute leukemia, chronic myelogenous leukemia, Hodgkin's disease, and non-Hodgkin's lymphoma. Transplants have also been performed for nonmalignant diseases such as thalassemia major, aplastic anemia, congenital immunodeficiency diseases, and inborn errors of metabolism such as the mucopolysaccharidoses.

Irradiation and chemotherapy break down mucosal barriers to infection.

Two major factors contribute to the inordinate incidence of infection among bone marrow transplant recipients. One is the breakdown of mucosal barriers due to cytotoxic agents and total body irradiation. Proper functioning of the mucosal cilia facilitates microbe clearance. The mucous membrane secretions contain soluble factors such as IgA, lactoferrin, lysozyme, and alpha-antitrypsin, all of which have some antimicrobial activity. The second is, of course, the immune deficiency associated with the transplantation process itself.

Immunologic Abnormalities with Bone Marrow Transplantation

Soon after transplantation, the circulating white cell count drops to levels of less than 50/cu mm and usually remains at that level for two to three weeks. Furthermore, the absolute neutrophil count may remain below 500/cu mm for up to four or five weeks. It is during this neutropenic period of profound immunosuppression that the marrow recipient is inordinately susceptible to serious or fatal infections, often with unusual or unfamiliar organisms. Even after recovery of normal or nearly normal numbers of circulating neutrophils, neutrophil chemotaxis or intracellular killing of organisms may remain abnormal.

Nonspecific immune mechanisms such as antibody-dependent cell-mediated cytotoxicity and natural killing similarly recover rapidly with marrow engraftment. Serum immunoglobulin levels can return to normal within several months after engraftment. However, maturation of the humoral immune system may be prolonged so that the production of antibody to some antigens may be poor despite the ability to produce sufficient immunoglobulin.

T cell and B cell levels may return to normal soon after engraftment, but T cell subpopulations may remain abnormal for prolonged periods of time.

The occurrence of infection early during the course of marrow transplantation is directly related to the duration of the neutropenic period. The occurrence of infection after engraftment is related to the rapidity of maturation of the immune system and to the development of GVHD, which itself is immunosuppressive and often must be treated with immunosuppressive drugs.

Early Infections

Confounding the prompt and accurate diagnosis of infectious complications during this period of profound neutropenia is the fact that the usual signs and symptoms of inflammation are not likely to be evident. The clinical presentation of localized infection in neutropenic patients is often subtle. Localized infections may elude diagnosis and be discovered only at autopsy. In neutropenic patients, erythema and pain seem to be the only reliable indicators of localized infection. The other classic signs of localized infections, such as exudates, local warmth, edema and swelling, regional adenopathy, cough, sputum production, sputum purulence, and radiographic air-fluid levels, are all less prevalent. The degree of subtlety of these latter signs is directly proportional to the degree of patient neutropenia, with a major reduction of these signs and symptoms occurring with an absolute neutrophil count of 0 to 100/cu mm.

Signs and symptoms of inflammation are less obvious with immunosuppression.

Otitis Media

This is a relatively infrequent problem. Again, pain and erythema are the only reliable clinical signs. Pain is sometimes misleading in patients who have a concurrent oral or pharyngeal mucositis, which may cause referred pain in the ear. Tympanic membrane retraction is minimal, and frank effusion is seldom seen at the time of either otoscopy or myringotomy.

When otitis media is suspected in the presence of an otherwise unexplained fever, the patient ought to undergo bilateral tympanocentesis with saline lavage and aspiration of the middle ear clefts to obtain a Gram's stain, a KOH preparation, and cultures for aerobes, anaerobes, and fungi. A solution of 90 per cent phenol can be applied to the myringotomy site for hemostasis in these thrombocytopenic patients, as has been recommended for tympanostomy tube placement in children with hemophilia A. Tympanostomy tubes should usually be inserted to allow aeration of the middle ear cleft and to prevent the need for a myringotomy later in the course of the transplantation process.

Otomycosis

A fungal infection of the external auditory canal in an immunologically normal patient is called an otomycosis and usually represents a harmless saprophytic growth that often resolves without treatment. In the bone marrow recipient, however, fungal infection of the external auditory canal can persist and spread to involve the middle ear and mastoid. The fungi invade the vasculature of the infected part of the ear and cause tissue destruction by infarction and secondary necrosis. The facial nerve can be involved directly by fungal invasion or indirectly by infarction to yield a facial nerve paralysis. *Aspergillus* species seem to be the most common pathogenic organisms, although infections with *Scopulariopsis* and *Coccidioides* have occurred.

The usual presentation of a complicated otomycosis in a bone marrow recipient is a dry, gangrenous involvement of the external auditory canal. Some granulation tissue may be present, and there is often anesthesia of the uninvolved portions of the ear canal. Middle ear or mastoid involvement should be suspected in the presence of a tympanic membrane perforation. In the presence of an intact tympanic membrane, hearing loss, facial nerve paresis, or pain out of proportion to the physical findings should similarly raise the suspicion of middle ear or mastoid involvement.

Prompt and aggressive surgical debridement of the external auditory canal should be performed. When indicated, middle ear exploration or a mastoidotomy should be performed to obtain mucosal specimens for fungal cultures and fungal stains. When mastoid involvement is proved, a radical or modified radical mastoidectomy should be performed to allow aeration and inspection of the entire mastoid cavity. Systemic antifungal agents and granulocyte infusions are the usual medical adjuncts, as for any fungal infection in a bone marrow recipient.

Sinusitis

Mucosal thickening is the usual presentation of maxillary sinusitis in the immunocompromised host.

The majority of cases are bacterial in origin, and the causative bacteria usually are the ones encountered in a routine practice. The presentation of sinusitis is almost always the radiographic detection of maxillary sinus mucosal thickening in a patient with an unexplained fever. Air-fluid levels are rarely seen. The clinical examination is usually unremarkable. If the fever persists, surgical intervention is the treatment of choice when the patient is expected to remain profoundly neutropenic for at least several more days. surgical intervention in the form of nasoantral windows allows representative cultures, prompt and effective treatment of the sinusitis, and a biopsy of diseased mucosa for detection of any possible invasive fungal elements. Thus, sinus lavage or aspiration is an insufficient treatment.

Aspergillus is the most common fungus causing sinusitis.

Fungal sinusitis is relatively infrequent but not rare. It is the most lethal sinus infection, with the mortality rate for fulminant necrotizing aspergillosis being estimated as high as 80 per cent. *Fusarium* species are less common pathogens but also cause a fulminant form of infection. *Penicillium* and *Alternaria* are relatively uncommon fungal pathogens. These latter organisms tend to cause indolent and less aggressive disease, although they invade local blood vessels also.

Early diagnosis of fungal sinusitis requires a high index of suspicion and a careful clinical examination. Early ethmoid sinusitis often presents as a black necrotic patch of mucosa, which may be only several millimeters in diameter, on the anterior end of the middle turbinate or as a slight erythema at the medial canthal area. Early maxillary sinusitis presents as erythema or tenderness over the cheek. In a neutropenic patient, fungal sinusitis can demonstrate a unilateral opacified antrum, and this is usually not the case with a bacterial pathogen.

Since *Aspergillus* and *Fusarium* species seem to be the most common fungal pathogens, surgery is the treatment of choice to interrupt a potentially fulminant infection that can rapidly spread to the orbit, facial soft tissues, and central nervous system. The surgical treatment should be identical to that for mucormycosis of the paranasal sinuses. The surgical treatment is justified even though the specific fungus may not have been identified or speciated at the time of surgery. A delay of even several days can allow rapid local spread, aerosol dissemination to the lungs, and hematogenous spread to distant organs.

Once engraftment occurs, adequate numbers of circulating neutrophils halt local progression and dissemination so that the disease may become indolent. Reactivation can occur later on in the sinuses previously affected if the patient subsequently develops severe GVHD, requires immunosuppressive agents, or again becomes severely neutropenic.

Rhinitis

Bacterial and fungal infections can occur on the nasal septum. It appears that only the fungal infections assume any clinical importance, since, as in fungal sinusitis, local tissue destruction can occur. The infection can spread distally to the soft tissues of the face (Fig. 18–1) or can spread proximally to the cribriform plate. The fungal infection of the septum can be detected as a dry, dark or black patch of anesthetic mucosa, most commonly occurring at the area of Kiesselbach's plexus. A wide septectomy is usually indicated.

Laryngitis

Upper airway problems are usually due to the extension of infectious problems in the mouth and nasopharynx. With the breakdown of mucosal barriers, oral infections with *Candida* or herpes simplex virus are common. Obstructive laryngitis can be caused by these organisms as well as by *Aspergillus*. The respiratory obstruction is seldom due to airway edema, but rather to marked mucosal ulceration resulting in the formation of obstructing crusts, pseudomembranes, or casts caused by bleeding, serous exudation, or the sloughing of necrotic tissue (Fig. 18–2). The performance of an urgent tracheostomy can be especially treacherous, since the obstructing crusts can extend well below the site of the tracheostomy. In such a situation, surgical entry into the trachea can precipitate total acute airway obstruction, which

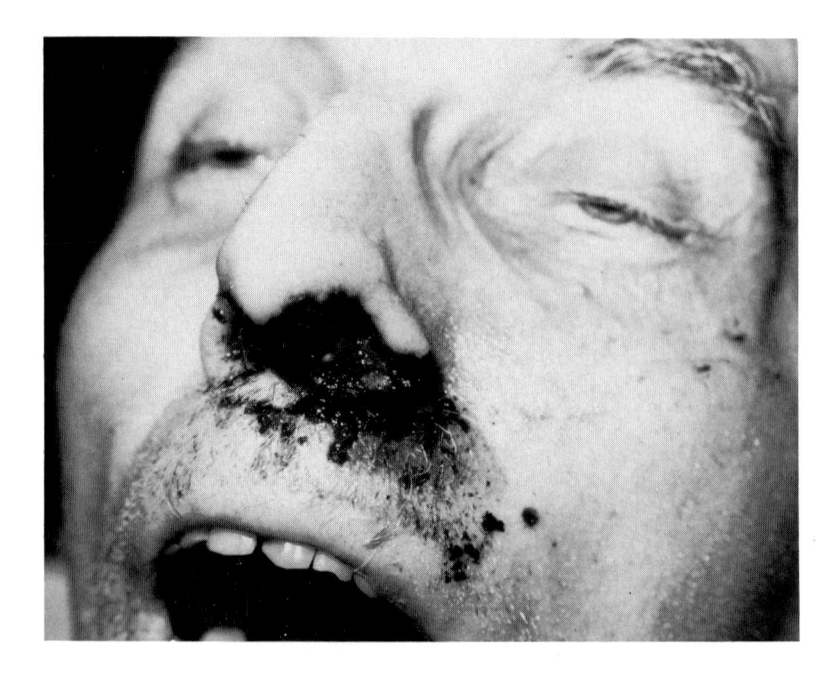

FIGURE 18–1. An *Aspergillus* infection of the nasal septum had quickly progressed externally to cause gangrenous erosions of the nasal columella, rim, ala, and lip.

may not be promptly relieved by the passage of a bronchoscope. To try to avoid this problem, it is wise to obtain a CT scan or MRI scan of the major airways prior to the tracheostomy, if time allows, to assess all the areas of large airway obstruction.

Esophagitis

This is most frequently caused by *Candida* species and often results from the swallowing of *Candida*-contaminated saliva. Some patients are asymptomatic, whereas others complain of dysphagia or burning retrosternal pain.

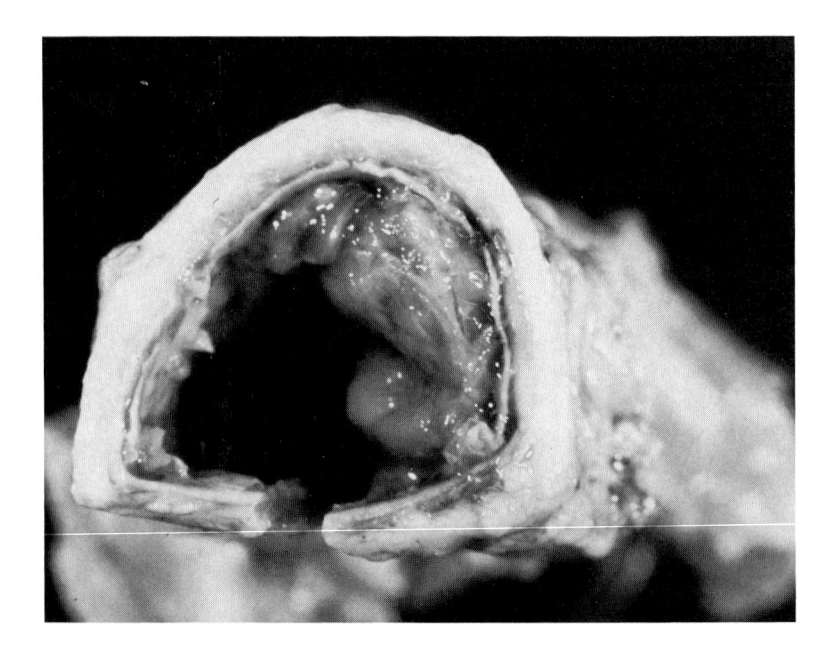

FIGURE 18–2. Cross-section of the trachea. A large *Aspergillus* mycetoma occludes half of the cross-sectional area of the trachea. In this patient, many such lesions were found at other sites in the trachea and bronchi.

The radiographic appearance of candidal esophagitis can be characteristic. A ragged esophageal mucosa with deep ulcerations and pseudopolypoid formation is said to be typical or even pathognomonic. Nevertheless, the immunocompromised patient may not be able to manifest a typical inflammatory reaction to *Candida,* and the barium swallow may therefore not be reliable. Esophagoscopy is the preferred form of diagnosis when a mucosal biopsy is obtained both for culture and for light microscopy. Cytology instead of a biopsy may yield false-negative results. The decision to perform an esophageal biopsy in a thrombocytopenic patient may be difficult and should be individualized for each case. Nevertheless, definitive diagnosis is very important, since candidal esophagitis is associated with esophageal perforation or candidal sepsis.

Esophagoscopy and biopsy are required for the definitive diagnosis of candidal esophagitis.

Esophagitis may also be due to herpes simplex virus and presents with the same symptoms as does candidal esophagitis. It appears to be due to the swallowing of saliva contaminated with virus particles. An extensive patchy ulceration can occur in the esophagus. At times, the lesions may not be recognizable as typical herpetic ulcers. Cytology is often an inadequate way to diagnose this disease, and both culture and biopsy may be necessary. Definitive diagnosis is necessary, since viremic herpes simplex infections can occur in the bone marrow recipient with dissemination of the virus particles to the lungs, liver, and brain.

Cervical Cellulitis

Inflammatory swellings of the neck can occur by means of direct extension of oral bacteria into fascial spaces or of retrograde infection of Stensen's duct or Wharton's duct. Diffuse edema and erythema can occur, but there is usually no fluctuance, since neutropenia does not allow the production of copious pus. These infections are treated with a regimen of antibiotics such as tobramycin, ticarcillin, and vancomycin. Resolution almost always occurs spontaneously as engraftment begins. Surgery is seldom, if ever, necessary.

INFECTIONS AFTER MARROW RECOVERY

This period is arbitrarily considered to be the time between marrow engraftment and approximately day 100 after transplantation. Most infections after initial marrow recovery are due to latent opportunistic organisms that undergo reactivation. These organisms tend most commonly to be DNA viruses. Orofacial herpes simplex viral infections are common and can be especially troublesome in a small but significant percentage of patients with widespread involvement of the lingual, buccal, and gingival mucosa. Oral and intravenous acyclovir has been effective in the treatment and prophylaxis of these infections.

Varicella-zoster virus infections are also common and can present in a trigeminal distribution with the complications of blindness or local scarring of the skin. Ramsay Hunt syndrome has been reported. Hand-foot-and-mouth disease, most commonly due to coxsackievirus A16, has also been observed.

LATE INFECTIONS

Otitis media and sinusitis are common late infections.

Infections six months or more after bone marrow transplantation are relatively unusual. They tend to occur most frequently in patients with GVHD. In a recent study, the most frequent infections involved the head and neck region. Otitis media occurs in about 7 per cent of patients and sinusitis in about 11 per cent. These infections usually are due to gram-positive cocci and only seldom to fungi. It has been speculated that the high incidence of sinus infections is due in part to a sicca-like syndrome induced in the upper airway mucosa by chronic GVHD. Oral candidiasis occurs in about 9 per cent of patients and may be related to the use of corticosteroids for chronic GVHD. Chronic GVHD may occur in up to 40 per cent of bone marrow transplant recipients. Its onset varies from 70 to 400 days after transplantation and resembles several naturally occurring autoimmune diseases such as scleroderma, Sjögren's syndrome, and systemic lupus erythematosus.

ACQUIRED IMMUNODEFICIENCY SYNDROME

AIDS is a devastating disease caused by an RNA retrovirus, the human immunodeficiency virus (HIV). The virus preferentially infects helper T lymphocytes and causes their lysis. The protean manifestations can be attributed to the resulting deficiency of this crucial component of the immune system. Approximately 40 per cent of adults with AIDS eventually come to the attention of the otolaryngologist for head and neck manifestations of the disease, including Kaposi's sarcoma. Of these, about one third present with head and neck infections.

Mouth, Larynx, and Esophagus

Cervical adenopathy is a nearly constant finding in patients with AIDS.

The most common infection so far appears to be oral candidiasis. This can occur at the onset of the disease before definitive diagnosis. Therefore, any adult patient with oral candidiasis should undergo a thorough social history, especially in a geographic area with a high incidence of AIDS. Furthermore, the physical examination should emphasize the detection of cervical lymphadenopathy (a nearly constant finding in AIDS), weight loss, and evidence of other opportunistic infections.

A small but significant percentage of AIDS patients eventually demonstrate extension of the candidiasis to the larynx or to the esophagus. Candidal laryngitis causes the usual symptoms but also can progress to a process that obstructs the upper airway. Candidal esophagitis has been associated with a 50 per cent mortality rate secondary to candidal sepsis in these patients.

Sinusitis

Sinusitis is usually due to bacteria, and the pathogens tend to be the ones encountered in a routine practice such as *Haemophilus influenzae, Streptococcus pneumoniae,* and *Staphylococcus aureus.* These infections are appropriately treated with an antral lavage and antibiotics chosen according to sensitivity testing. More unusual organisms such as *Klebsiella* and *Gardnerella* usually require a Caldwell-Luc procedure to eradicate diseased mucosa and provide adequate drainage. In one series, *Pseudallescheria boydii,* a ubiquitous soil fungus, and *Aspergillus* species were the most common fungal pathogens. Therapeutic lavage is not appropriate therapy in these cases, and consideration should be given to a nasal antral window or, preferably, to a Caldwell-Luc procedure.

Children

In HIV-infected children, recurrent otitis media and chronic sinusitis can be presenting illnesses before the onset of opportunistic infections or the definitive diagnosis of AIDS. For children with these types of infections, it is recommended that a careful history be taken for blood transfusions and to assess whether the parents are at risk for AIDS.

SOLID ORGAN TRANSPLANT RECIPIENTS

Infection is the leading cause of death among allograft recipients. This is especially significant among kidney transplant recipients, since azotemia and hyperglycemia are associated with a higher incidence of infection.

During the first month after organ transplantation, infections tend to be caused by nonopportunistic organisms. Head and neck infections tend to be only slightly more frequent than in a normal population. Opportunistic infections seem to occur in patients undergoing intensive or prolonged immunosuppression and in those undergoing repeated courses of antirejection therapy. This is especially true during the second through sixth month after transplantation. It is during this period that the allograft recipient may experience numerous rejection episodes and be subjected to intensive immunosuppressive therapy.

Sinusitis tends to be the most frequent head and neck infection, with most episodes due to bacterial pathogens. *Pseudomonas* has been notable among these patients and can cause a necrotizing type of infection. This must be treated aggressively and with the instillation of irrigation catheters into the maxillary sinuses and nose for frequent daily saline lavages of infected areas. Fungal sinusitis with *Aspergillus, Alternaria,* and Phycomycetes has also been reported. Candidal pharyngitis and esophagitis occur rather frequently.

Pseudomonas sinusitis requires aggressive therapy.

INFECTIONS IN THE CANCER PATIENT

Infections are a major source of morbidity in the patient with cancer and often are the major cause of death. Cancer patients are susceptible to infectious complications due to altered host defense mechanisms, which may be deficient secondary to the malignancy itself or to its treatment.

Immunologic Milieu

A number of immune functions can be adversely affected by cancer therapy.

Granulopoiesis, of course, can be inhibited by cytotoxic agents and granulocyte reserves can be exhausted, with granulocytopenia occurring in about one week. Neutrophil chemotaxis and phagocytosis can be inhibited by corticosteroids. Certain chemotherapeutic agents and craniofacial irradiation can impair the intracellular killing of organisms by neutrophils. The macrophage is not as sensitive to chemotherapy and can provide residual phagocytic capacities during periods of neutropenia.

Numerous T cell functions can be impaired in cancer patients, even in the absence of cytotoxic therapy. Decreased lymphocyte responses to mitogens and antigens, the appearance of monocytes that nonspecifically suppress T cell blastogenesis, and cutaneous anergy are frequent.

The humoral immune system can be severely affected by chemotherapy. Impaired antibody production, inadequate agglutination and lysis of bacteria, and deficient opsonization all can occur.

Malnutrition contributes to the breakdown of mucosal barriers.

Malnutrition is a frequent occurrence in the cancer patient and can be responsible for other deficiencies in the immune system such as diminished macrophage mobilization, impaired phagocytosis, and certain lymphocyte deficiencies. Malnutrition also contributes to the breakdown of mucosal barriers to microorganisms.

Infections

Sinusitis is frequent in the cancer patient undergoing chemotherapy. When the symptoms appear chronic, the possibility of anaerobic bacteria must be entertained and appropriate cultures obtained and antibiotics chosen. It appears that anaerobic pathogens can be isolated in at least 50 per cent of the cases of chronic maxillary sinusitis. Fungal sinusitis is common in the cancer patient also. The incidence of *Aspergillus* infection seems to be increasing, and one cancer treatment center has reported that 20 per cent of adults with acute leukemia developed *Aspergillus* sinusitis during a five-year period (Fig. 18–3).

Esophagitis is most commonly caused by *Candida,* but herpes simplex virus and bacteria can also be etiologic agents.

In general, the greater the degree of neutropenia, the more likely the infectious complications will resemble those in the bone marrow transplant recipient, both in the types of etiologic organisms and in the subtlety of clinical presentation.

CONGENITAL IMMUNODEFICIENCY DISEASES

The most common recurrent head and neck infections in children with congenital immunodeficiency diseases are rhinitis, sinusitis, tonsillitis, and suppurative otitis media. The majority of these children who present to the otolaryngologist already have a known and proven diagnosis of the immunodeficiency disease.

Nevertheless, a small but significant number present with the basic immunologic abnormality undiagnosed. To aid in the identification of patients who deserve an immunologic evaluation, careful attention should be paid to certain factors in the history and physical examination. These include a family history suggestive of immune deficiencies, a history of other recurrent infectious processes such as skin infections or recurrent pneumonias

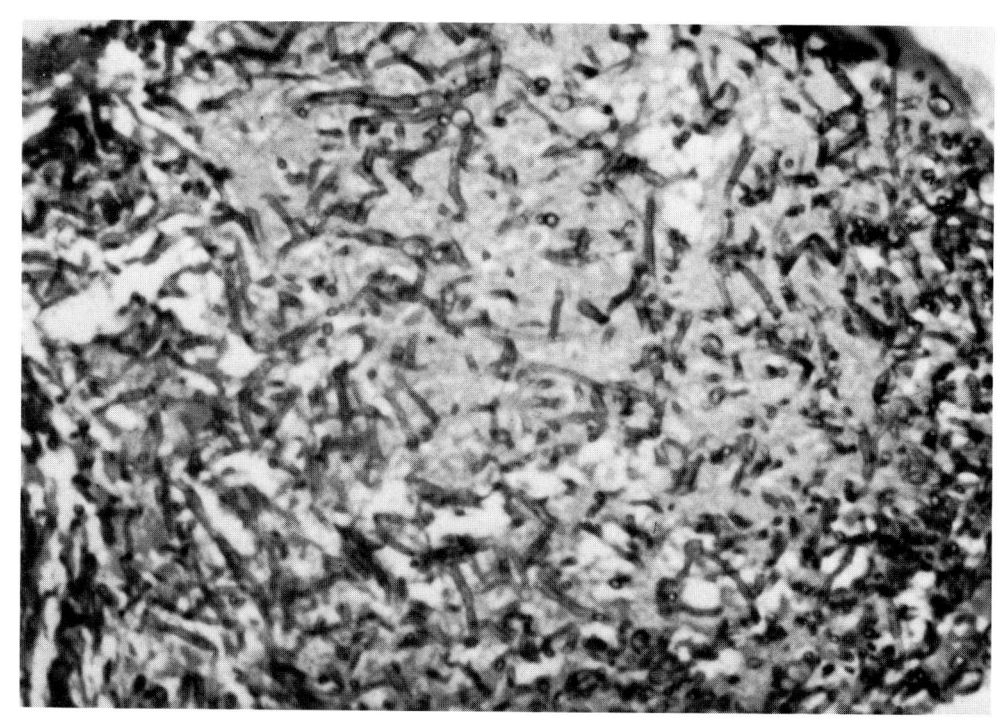

FIGURE 18–3. Giemsa silver stain demonstrating *Aspergillus* organisms in the mastoid cavity of a patient with acute leukemia.

with unusual organisms such as *Pneumocystis carinii* or *Nocardia,* recurrent infections with the same organism, chronic diarrhea, a family history of fetal wastage or infant deaths, failure to thrive, and hepatosplenomegaly.

If immunodeficiency is suspected, a screening immunologic evaluation should be performed. This should include a complete blood count and differential, quantitative circulating immunoglobulins, erythrocyte sedimentation rate, and skin tests for delayed hypersensitivity to *Candida, Trichophyton,* and tetanus toxoid. If an immunodeficiency is still suspected in a child with normal immunoglobulin levels, a total hemolytic complement assay should be obtained, especially if documented recurrent infections are due to *S. pneumoniae* or meningococci. Also, IgG subclasses should be measured, since a recent report has documented deficiencies of IgG2 and IgG3 in children with recurrent sinus and pulmonary infections. The IgG antibody response to many bacterial capsular polysaccharide antigens, including those of *H. influenzae,* resides chiefly within the IgG2 subclass. Children with these subclass deficiencies should receive either antibiotic prophylaxis for their infections or gamma globulin replacement.

IgG subclass deficiencies can lead to sinusitis or otitis media in children.

References

Berkow RL, Wisman SJ, Provisor AJ, et al: Invasive aspergillosis of paranasal tissues in children with malignancies. J Pediatr 103:49–53, 1983.
Berlinger NT: Sinusitis in immunodeficient and immunosuppressed patients. Laryngoscope 95:29–33, 1985.
Harris JP, South MS: Immunodeficiency diseases: Head and neck manifestations. Head Neck Surg 5:114–124, 1983.

Marcusen DC, Sooy CD: Otolaryngologic and head and neck manifestations of acquired immunodeficiency syndrome (AIDS). Laryngoscope 95:401–405, 1985.

McGill TJ, Simpson G, Healy GB: Fulminant aspergillosis of the nose and paranasal sinuses: A new clinical entity. Laryngoscope 90:748–754, 1980.

Shannon KM, Ammann AJ: Acquired immune deficiency syndrome in children. J Pediatr 106:332–342, 1985.

Wong KK, Hirsch MS: Herpes virus infections in patients with neoplastic disease: Diagnosis and therapy. Am J Med 76:464–478, 1984.

PART FIVE

THE LARYNX

19

ANATOMY AND PHYSIOLOGY OF THE LARYNX

by James I. Cohen, M.D., Ph.D.

Embryology

The pharynx, larynx, trachea, and lungs are derivatives of the embryonal foregut, which appears at about 18 days after conception. Soon thereafter, the median pharyngeal groove arises, containing the first indications of the respiratory system and the anlage of the larynx. The laryngotracheal sulcus or groove then becomes apparent at around 21 days of embryonic life (Fig. 19–1). Caudal expansion of this groove represents the pulmonary primordium. It deepens and becomes saclike and then bilobed at 27 to 28 days. The most proximal portions of this enlarging tube will become the larynx. The arytenoid swellings and the epithelial lamina are recognizable by 33 days, and the cartilages and muscles, including vocal folds for the most part, develop during the subsequent three to four weeks.

Only the cartilage of the epiglottis does not appear until midfetal life. Since the development of the larynx is closely linked to the development of the branchial arches of the embryo, many of the laryngeal structures are derivatives of the branchial apparatus.

FIGURE 19–1. Development of the human larynx. *A*, Four weeks; *B*, five weeks; *C*, six weeks; *D*, seven weeks; *E*, ten weeks; *F*, infant larynx at birth. Roman numerals refer to visceral arch derivatives. (From Bluestone CD, Stool SE (eds): Pediatric Otolaryngology. Philadelphia, WB Saunders Co, 1983, p 1136.)

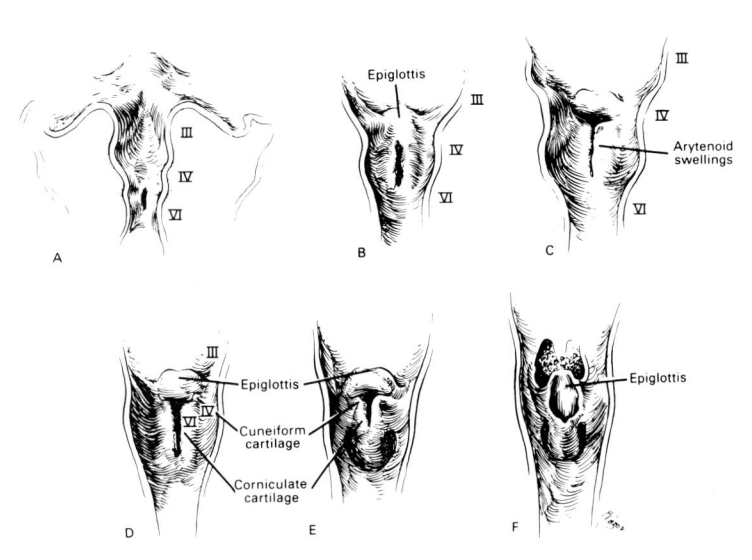

Incomplete closure of the cricoid cartilage results in a laryngotracheal esophageal cleft.

Defective development may result in a variety of abnormalities that can be diagnosed by direct examination of the larynx. The larynx itself may be small, or there may be a variable degree of webbing between the true vocal cords. Rarely, the posterior arm of the T of the laryngotracheal sulcus may persist, leaving an opened laryngeal cleft between the esophagus and trachea. Laryngomalacia, an abnormal degree of flaccidity in the laryngeal framework which allows it to collapse during respiration, is the most common congenital laryngeal abnormality seen as a cause for stridor in the newborn. It is almost always a benign self-limiting condition that will resolve with growth and development. Developmental disorders of the larynx are discussed in Chapter 20; disorders of the esophagus and tracheobronchial tree are discussed in Chapter 24.

ANATOMY OF THE LARYNX

Supporting Structures

The laryngeal skeletal structure is composed of one bone and several paired and unpaired cartilages (Fig. 19–2). Superiorly is the hyoid bone, the U-shaped structure that can be palpated both anteriorly on the neck and transorally in the lateral pharyngeal wall. Extending from each side of the central portion, or body, of the hyoid bone is a posteriorly directed long process and a small, superiorly oriented short process. Attached to the superior surface of the body and to both processes are tendons and muscles from the tongue, mandible, and skull. During swallowing, contraction of these muscles elevates the larynx. However, when the larynx is stabilized, these muscles open the mouth and contribute to tongue motion. Inferior to the hyoid bone, and suspended by the thyrohyoid ligament, are the two alae, or wings, of the thyroid (shield) cartilage. The alae join in the midline at an angle that is more acute in the male, producing the visible "Adam's apple." On the posterior border of each ala are the superior and inferior cornua. The inferior cornu articulates with the cricoid cartilage, allowing a small amount of gliding and rocking between the thyroid and cricoid cartilages.

The cricoid cartilage, also easily palpable subcutaneously, is attached to the thyroid cartilage by the cricothyroid ligament. Unlike all other supporting

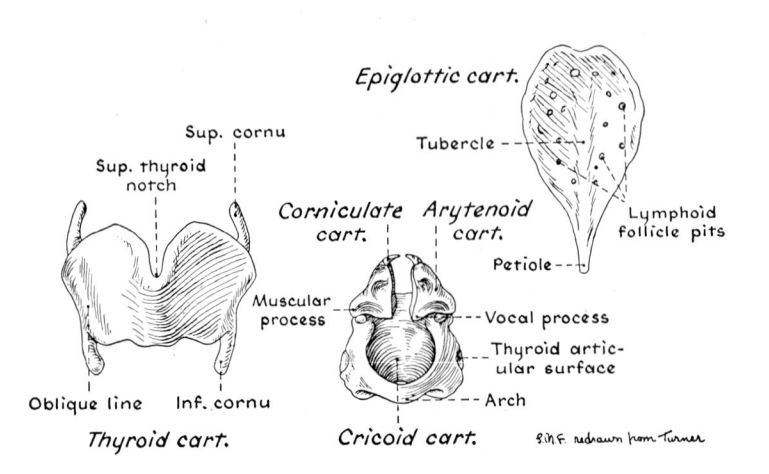

FIGURE 19–2. The cartilages of the larynx. (Redrawn from Turner.)

structures of the airway, the cricoid cartilage is a complete circle, unable to expand. The posterior surface, or lamina, of the cricoid is quite wide, giving this cartilage the appearance of a signet ring. Prolonged endotracheal intubation is often damaging to the mucosal lining within the ring and may lead to acquired subglottic stenosis. Inferiorly, the first tracheal cartilage attaches to the cricoid by an intercartilaginous ligament.

Because the cricoid cartilage cannot expand, prolonged intubation results in subglottic stenosis.

On the superior surface of the lamina sit the paired arytenoid cartilages, each shaped like a three-sided pyramid. The bases of the pyramids articulate with the cricoid at the cricoarytenoid joints, allowing medial to lateral sliding and rotation. Each arytenoid cartilage has two processes, an anterior vocal process and a lateral muscular process. Extending anteriorly from each vocal process and inserting into the thyroid cartilage in the midline is a vocal ligament. The vocal process makes up the posterior two fifths of the vocal cord, while the vocal ligament forms the remaining membranous, or vibratory, portion of the cord. The free edge and superior surface of the vocal cord make up the glottis. The larynx above this is the supraglottis and that below it is the subglottis. There are two small paired cartilages in the larynx which have no function. The corniculate cartilages are located in the tissue over the arytenoids. Lateral to these, within the aryepiglottic folds, are the cuneiform cartilages.

The epiglottic cartilage is a single midline structure shaped like a ping-pong paddle. The handle, or petiolis, is attached by a short ligament to the thyroid cartilage just above the vocal cords, while the racquet portion extends upward behind the body of the hyoid into the lumen of the pharynx, separating the base of the tongue from the larynx. In most adults, the epiglottis is mildly concave posteriorly. However, in children and some adults, it is markedly curved and is called an omega, or juvenile, epiglottis. The epiglottis functions as a keel, forcing swallowed food to the side of the laryngeal airway.

The epiglottis is more Ω (omega) shaped in the infant.

Additional support is given to the larynx by elastic tissue. Superiorly on each side is the quadrangular membrane, which extends from the lateral border of the epiglottis back to the lateral border of the arytenoid cartilage. This membrane is therefore the dividing wall between the larynx and the piriform sinus, and its superior border is called the aryepiglottic fold. The other paired elastic tissue of importance is the conus elasticus. It is much stronger than the quadrangular membrane and extends upward and medially from the arch of the cricoid cartilage to join the vocal ligament on each side. The conus elasticus thus lies beneath the mucosa on the undersurface of the true vocal cords.

Laryngeal Musculature

The laryngeal muscles may be divided into two groups (Fig. 19–3). The extrinsic muscles act mainly on the larynx as a whole, whereas the intrinsic muscles cause movements between the various laryngeal structures themselves. The extrinsic muscles may be categorized by function. The depressors, or strap muscles (omohyoid, sternothyroid, sternohyoid), originate inferiorly. The elevators (mylohyoid, geniohyoid, genioglossus, hyoglossus, digastric, stylohyoid) extend from the hyoid bone to the mandible, tongue, and styloid process of the skull. The thyrohyoid, although considered a strap muscle, functions mainly as an elevator. Attached to the hyoid bone and posterior

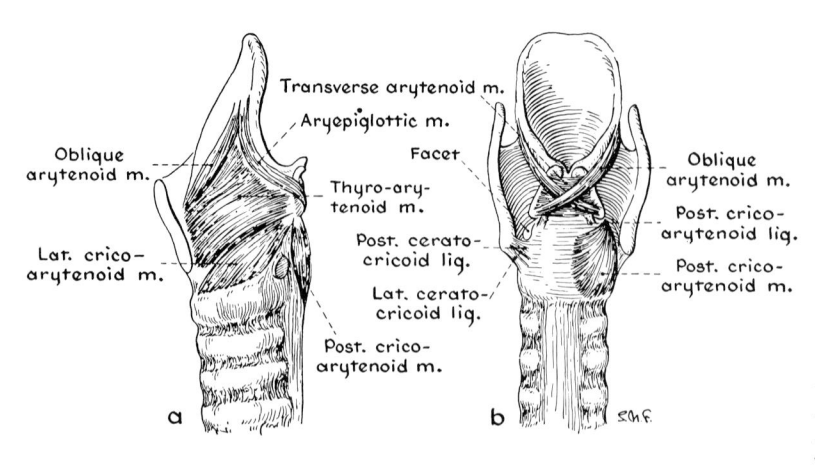

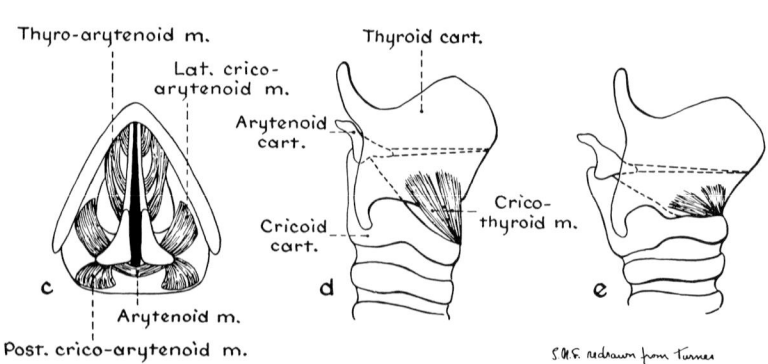

FIGURE 19–3. The appearance of the larynx and attached trachea after removal of all but the muscular and ligamentous structure. *a*, Side view; *b*, posterior view; *c*, a diagrammatic representation of the arrangement of the intrinsic muscles; *d* and *e*, position, attachments, and action of the cricothyroid muscle. (Redrawn from Turner.)

edge of the thyroid cartilage alae are the middle and inferior constrictors, which encircle the pharynx posteriorly and function during swallowing. The lowermost fibers of the inferior constrictor arise from the cricoid to form the strong cricopharyngeus, which serves as the upper esophageal sphincter.

The anatomy of the intrinsic laryngeal musculature is best understood by relating it to function. Extending between the two arytenoids are the transverse and oblique fibers of the interarytenoid (or arytenoid) muscle. When it contracts, the arytenoid cartilages glide toward the midline, adducting the cords. The posterior cricoarytenoid muscle extends from the posterior surface of the cricoid lamina to insert on the muscular process of the arytenoid; it rotates the arytenoid outward, abducting the vocal cord. Its main antagonist, the lateral cricoarytenoid, takes origin on the lateral cricoid arch; it inserts also on the muscular process and rotates the arytenoid medially, causing adduction. Making up the bulk of the vocal cords are the barely separable vocalis and thyroarytenoid muscles, which contribute to cord tension. In older individuals, the vocalis and thyroarytenoid muscles may lose some tone; the cords appear bowed outward, and the voice becomes weak and hoarse. The other major laryngeal muscles are the paired cricothyroids, fan-shaped muscles that originate anteriorly from the cricoid arch and insert on the broad lateral surface of the thyroid alae. Contraction of this muscle pulls the thyroid cartilage forward, stretching and tensing the cords. This also tends to passively rotate the arytenoid medially, so the cricothyroid is also considered an adductor. In summary, then, there are

The cricothyroid muscle tenses the vocal cords.

one abductor, three adductors, and three tensors, all of which are listed as follows:

ABDUCTORS	ADDUCTORS	TENSORS
Posterior cricoarytenoid	Interarytenoid	Cricothyroid (external)
	Lateral cricoarytenoid	Vocalis (internal)
	Cricothyroid	Thyroarytenoid (internal)

Innervation, Blood Supply, and Lymphatic Drainage

Two pairs of nerves supply the larynx with both sensory and motor innervation. These two superior laryngeal nerves and two inferior, or recurrent, laryngeal nerves are all branches of the vagal nerves. The superior laryngeal nerve leaves the vagal trunk just below the nodose ganglion, curves anteriorly and medially beneath the internal and external carotid arteries, and divides into an internal sensory branch and an external motor branch. The internal branch pierces the thyrohyoid membrane to provide the sensory innervation for the vallecula, epiglottis, piriform sinus, and all the internal laryngeal mucosa superior to the free margin of the true cords. Each external branch is the motor supply for just one muscle, the cricothyroid. Inferiorly, the recurrent nerve ascends in a groove between the trachea and esophagus, enters the larynx just behind the cricothyroid articulation, and provides the motor supply to all the intrinsic laryngeal muscles except the cricothyroid. The recurrent nerve also provides sensation to the undersurface of the true cords (the subglottic region) and the superior trachea. The differing courses of the right and left recurrent nerves are illustrated in Figure 19–4, which also shows the higher neural pathways involved in laryngeal innervation.

The superior laryngeal nerve is primarily sensory. It supplies motor function to only one muscle—the cricothyroid.

FIGURE 19–4. A pen sketch by Dr. Chevalier Jackson "schematically illustrating in a simplified way the fundamentals of innervation of the larynx. For clearness, intervening central structures have been omitted. The laryngeal nerves originated in the nuclei ambigui of which there are two, one on each side of the medulla. Here are activated the autonomic functions of respiration and reflex laryngeal movements. For volitional movements the nuclei ambigui are activated and dominated by impulses, 'orders' received from the cortical executive centers. These bilateral executive centers in turn receive their 'orders,' as to words, from the unilateral language (or word) area located on the left side of the brain (in right handed individuals), represented diagrammatically as distributing its impulses bilaterally. To avoid impairing simplicity, only efferent pathways are indicated in this scheme. It must be understood that all these pathways have their complementary afferent pathways." (From Jackson C, Jackson CL (eds): Diseases of the Nose, Throat, and Ear. 2nd ed. Philadelphia, WB Saunders Co, 1959.)

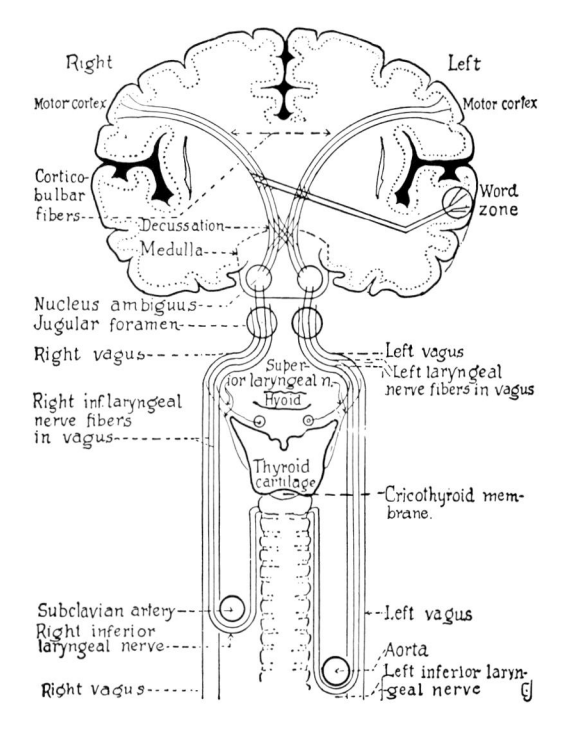

The superior laryngeal nerve, superior laryngeal artery, and vein enter the larynx laterally between the hyoid bone and thyroid cartilage.

Because of the longer course of the left inferior nerve and its relationship to the aorta, it is more vulnerable to injury than the right.

The arterial supply and venous drainage of the larynx closely parallel the nerve supply. The superior laryngeal artery and vein are branches of the superior thyroid artery and vein, and they join the internal branch of the superior laryngeal nerve to form the superior neurovascular pedicle. The inferior laryngeal artery and vein arise from the inferior thyroid vessels and enter the larynx alongside the recurrent laryngeal nerve.

Knowledge of the lymphatic drainage of the larynx is important in cancer therapy. There are two separate drainage systems, superior and inferior, with the dividing line being the true vocal cord. The cords themselves have a poor lymphatic supply. Superiorly, the flow accompanies the superior neurovascular pedicle to join the upper lymph nodes of the deep cervical chain at the level of the hyoid bone. The subglottic drainage is more diverse, going to the pretracheal nodes (one in particular is just anterior to the cricoid and is called the Delphian node), the lower deep cervical nodes, the supraclavicular nodes, and even the superior mediastinal nodes.

Internal Laryngeal Structure

For the most part, the larynx is lined by columnar ciliated mucosa known as respiratory epithelium. However, those parts of the larynx which are exposed to the most airflow, such as the lingual surface of the epiglottis, the superior surface of the aryepiglottic folds, and the superior surface and free edge of the true cords, are covered with the hardier stratified squamous epithelium. Mucus-secreting glands are numerous in the respiratory epithelium.

The first structure noted on mirror examination is the epiglottis (Fig. 19–5). Three mucosal bands (one median and two lateral glossoepiglottic folds) extend from the epiglottis to the tongue. Between the median and each lateral band is a small pocket, the vallecula. Below the free margin of the epiglottis the arytenoids can be seen, appearing as two small mounds connected by the thin interarytenoid muscle. Extending anterolaterally from each arytenoid to the lateral free edges of the epiglottis are the aryepiglottic

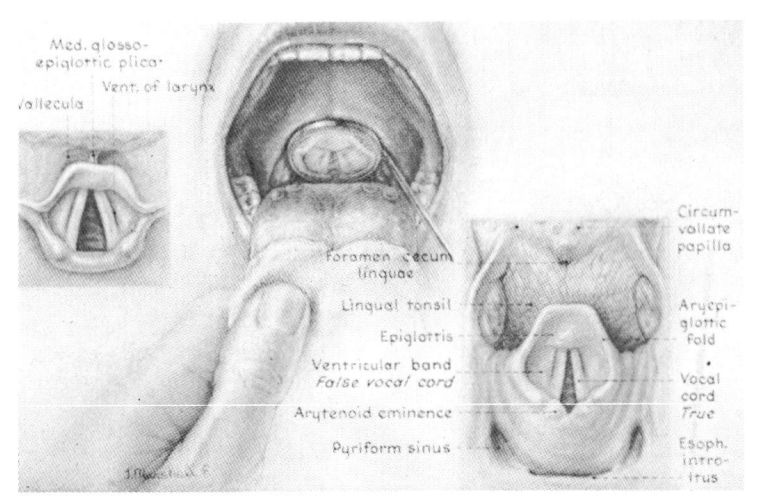

FIGURE 19–5. The important structures to visualize in an examination of the laryngopharynx are the valleculae, the epiglottis, the aryepiglottic folds, the ventricular bands ("false" cords), the vocal cords ("true" cords), the openings of the ventricles of the larynx, the anterior commissure, the arytenoid eminences, the piriform sinuses, and the posterior pharyngeal wall down to the esophageal introitus.

folds, which are the mucosa-covered quadrangular membranes. Lateral to each aryepiglottic fold is the piriform sinus, or recess. These are, as seen from above, triangle-shaped pouches in which there is no posterior wall. The medial wall is the quadrangular cartilage above and the arytenoid with its attached lateral musculature below, and the lateral wall is the internal surface of the thyroid ala. Posteriorly, the piriform sinus is continuous with the hypopharynx. The piriform sinuses and pharynx converge inferiorly into the esophageal introitus, which is encompassed by the strong cricopharyngeal muscle.

Within the larynx itself, two pairs of horizontal bands arise from the arytenoids and insert into the center of the thyroid cartilage anteriorly. The superior bands are the false cords, or ventricular bands, and are lateral to the true cords. The false cords are found by the inferior free margin of the quadrangular membrane. The edge of the true (vocal) cords is the superior margin of the conus elasticus. The vocalis and thyroarytenoid muscles make up the bulk of this cord. Because the superior surface of the vocal cord is flat, the mucosa reflects light and appears white on indirect laryngoscopy. Separating the true and false cords are the laryngeal ventricles. At its anterior end, the ventricle extends superiorly as a small diverticulum known as the laryngeal saccule, which harbors the mucous glands thought to lubricate the cords. An enlargement of this saccule is known clinically as a laryngocele.

Light reflection from the surface of the vocal cord makes it appear white.

Surrounding Structures

Anteriorly, the isthmus of the thyroid gland covers the first few tracheal rings, while the thyroid lobes rest on the lateral tracheal wall and may even extend up onto the thyroid alae. The isthmus must be elevated, and occasionally incised, when placing a tracheostomy through the third tracheal cartilaginous ring. The strap muscles cover the larynx and thyroid gland except in the midline, where the median raphe places the laryngeal structures in a subcutaneous position. The cricothyroid membrane is easily palpable and, in an emergency, can be rapidly incised to establish an airway. Not infrequently, the innominate artery passes anteriorly to the cervical trachea, necessitating careful palpation during any tracheostomy procedure. Lateral and posterior to the larynx are the carotid sheaths, each containing the carotid artery, jugular vein, and vagus nerve.

The thyroid isthmus is elevated or incised during tracheostomy.

PHYSIOLOGY OF THE LARYNX

Although the larynx is usually thought of as an organ for the production of voice, it serves three major functions—protection of the airway, respiration, and phonation. In fact, phylogenetically, the larynx first developed as a sphincter to protect the respiratory tract, and the development of voice is a relatively recent event.

Protection of the airway during the act of swallowing comes about through a variety of separate mechanisms. The laryngeal inlet itself is closed by the sphincteric action of the slips of the thyroarytenoid muscle in the aryepiglottic folds and false cords in addition to the adduction of the true vocal cords and arytenoids brought about by the other intrinsic muscles of the larynx.

The major function of the larynx is to protect the airway.

Laryngeal functions: protect the airway, cough, speech, Valsalva maneuver (as in lifting), central intrathoracic pressure.

Elevation of the larynx under the base of tongue further protects the larynx as it serves to push the epiglottis and aryepiglottic folds down over the inlet. These structures then divert food laterally away from the laryngeal inlet into the pyriform sinuses and through the esophageal introitus. Simultaneous relaxation of the cricopharyngeal muscle promotes the passage of food into the esophagus rather than the larynx. In addition, respiration is inhibited during swallowing owing to a reflex mediated by receptors present in the mucosa of the supraglottic area. This prevents inhalation of food or saliva.

In animals such as the deer the epiglottis extends superiorly to contact the nasal surface of the soft palate. This configuration allows simultaneous breathing while eating so that the animal can still smell and thus protect itself while grazing. Similarly, in infants, the higher position of the larynx allows contact of the epiglottis with the posterior surface of the soft palate. They are thus able to breathe while nursing without passage of food into the airway.

During respiration, the intrathoracic pressure is controlled by varying the degree of closure of the true vocal cords. This modulation of pressure assists the cardiac system inasmuch as it affects pulmonary and cardiac filling and emptying. In addition, the intrinsic design of the true and false vocal cords allows the larynx to serve as a pressure valve that, when closed (Fig. 19–6), allows the build-up of intrathoracic pressure necessary for straining acts such as lifting or defecation. Sudden release of this pressure produces a cough, which is useful in maintaining the expansion of the terminal alveoli of the lungs and clearing any secretions or food particles that end up in the laryngeal inlet despite all the other protective mechanisms mentioned above.

Voice production, however, is perhaps the most complex and certainly the best studied of the laryngeal functions. The advent of fiberoptic viewing systems and stroboscopes that can be coordinated with voice frequency has helped a great deal in understanding this phenomenon. It is currently thought that the adducted true vocal cords serve as a passive reed that vibrates as a result of the air forced up between them by contraction of the expiratory muscles. The fundamental tone that is produced can be modified in a number of ways. The intrinsic muscles of the larynx (and the cricothyroid) play a major role in the adjustment of pitch by changing the shape and mass of the free edges of the true vocal cords and the tension in the cords themselves.

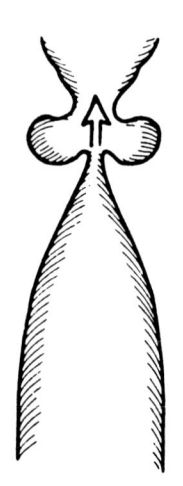

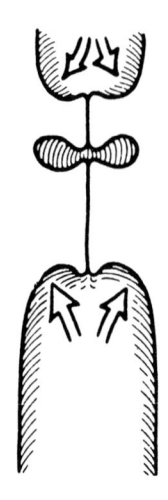

FIGURE 19–6. With the cords in tight apposition, rising supraglottic and subglottic pressure tend to force the vocal cords more tightly together, thus sealing the glottis. (from Tucker HM: Surgery for Phonatory Disorders. New York, Churchill Livingstone, 1981, p 9; by permission.)

The extralaryngeal muscles may also play a role. Also, because of the lower position of the larynx in humans, a large portion of the pharynx is available, in addition to the nasal cavity and paranasal sinuses, for modulation of the tone produced by the larynx. All of this is monitored by a feedback mechanism consisting of the human ear and a system within the larynx itself which is poorly understood. By contrast, the loudness of the voice is essentially proportional only to the pressure in the subglottic airstream that is setting the true vocal cords in motion. Whispering, on the other hand, is believed to be due to escape of air through the posterior commissure between the abducted arytenoids without vibration of the true vocal cords themselves.

Any disease that affects the action of the intrinsic and extrinsic muscles of the larynx (nerve paralysis, trauma, surgery) or the mass of the true vocal cords (i.e., vocal cord polyps or carcinoma) affects laryngeal function, and disorders of either swallowing (i.e., aspiration) or voice will result. Such disease processes will be discussed in detail in subsequent chapters.

References

Crelin ES: Development of the upper respiratory system. CIBA Clinical Symposia, Vol 29, No 4, 1977.
Fink RB, Demarest RJ: Laryngeal Biomechanics. Cambridge, MA, Harvard University Press, 1978.
Hollinshead HW: Anatomy for Surgeons, Vol 1: The Head and Neck. New York, Harper and Row, 1968.
Kirchner JA: Physiology of the larynx. *In* Paparella MM, Shumrik DA (eds): Otolaryngology. Philadelphia, WB Saunders Co, 1980, pp 377–388.
O'Rahilly R, Tucker JA: The early development of the larynx in staged human embryos. Ann Otol Rhinol Laryngol 82 (Suppl 7):1–27, 1973.
Tucker HM: Monographs in Clinical Otolaryngology—Surgery for Phonatory Disorders, Vol 3. New York, Churchill Livingstone, 1981, pp 6–11.
Van Alyea OE: The Embryology of the Ear, Nose, and Throat. Rochester, MN, American Academy of Ophthalmology and Otolaryngology, 1944.
Wyke BD, Kirchner JA: Laryn-Neurology. *In* Hinchcliffe R, Harrison D (eds): Scientific Foundations of Otolaryngology. Chicago, Year Book Medical Publishers, 1976, pp 546–573.

20

BENIGN LARYNGEAL DISORDERS

by John D. Banovetz, M.D.

PATIENT COMPLAINTS

The history of a patient with a laryngeal disease usually includes the symptoms of hoarseness, pain, cough, stridor, or dysphagia. Hemoptysis is an unusual symptom. In many instances of laryngeal disease, the early symptoms are very slight and do not alarm the patient. This is particularly true for lesions in the base of the tongue, the piriform sinus, or the epiglottis. Hoarseness is an early symptom of glottic lesions but a late symptom for tumors that originate in areas away from the glottic aperture. Any patient who has been hoarse for more than three weeks should have visual examination of the larynx. Pain, particularly pain referred to the ear, is often the first symptom of laryngeal disease from the base of the tongue, the epiglottis, or the piriform sinus. Cough resulting from laryngeal irritation may also be an early symptom of serious laryngeal disease. Dyspnea and stridor are usually late and serious symptoms. They demand immediate visualization. Any child who has had two or more episodes of croup should be examined for a possible laryngeal lesion. It should be kept in mind that wheezing does not necessarily indicate asthma. Unresponsive asthmatics should have the upper air passages examined. Any change in swallowing ability, particularly dysphagia related to solid foods, should always be evaluated radiologically and perhaps endoscopically.

SPECIFIC METHODS OF DIAGNOSIS

The key to laryngeal examination is visualization. Fortunately this can often be accomplished by indirect (mirror) laryngoscopy or by a flexible fiberoptic instrument (Fig. 20–1). When this is impossible, direct examination with a local or general anesthetic can be done. Auscultation of the larynx, listening directly over the larynx with the stethoscope, is also of value in determining the volume of air the patient moves with each respiration. This maneuver is particularly useful for differentiating laryngeal stridor from bronchial stridor. The larynx itself and the neck should be carefully palpated. During palpation the examiner feels each neck structure carefully as though performing a surgical dissection. Each neck structure is examined for size, texture, and mobility. Lateral soft tissue radiographs often show the size of the airway and can be invaluable in detecting tumors of the trachea or

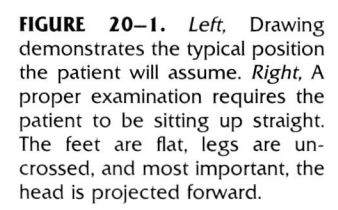

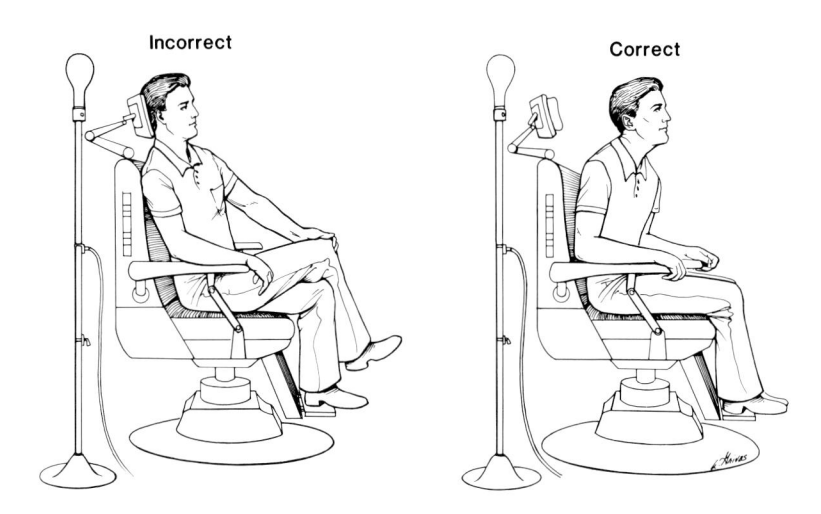

FIGURE 20–1. *Left*, Drawing demonstrates the typical position the patient will assume. *Right*, A proper examination requires the patient to be sitting up straight. The feet are flat, legs are uncrossed, and most important, the head is projected forward.

larynx. A chest film may also help localize stridor to upper or lower airway. Computed tomography and magnetic resonance imaging are valuable in evaluating masses because they accurately visualize laryngeal spaces and detect changes in laryngeal cartilages not visible by other means. Esophagograms, particularly those done with videoradiography, are also useful. Voice recordings can also be diagnostic of the type of vocal disorder and can be used to compare pre- and postoperative status.

CONGENITAL ANOMALIES

The normal infant larynx is situated higher in the neck than that of the adult. The infant larynx is softer, less rigid, and more compressible by airway pressures. In the infant, the larynx is at the level of C2 to C4, whereas in the adult it lies anterior to C4 to C6. The size of the newborn larynx is approximately 7 mm in the anteroposterior length and opens approximately 4 mm in a lateral direction. The symptoms that arise from disease here concern respiratory obstruction, dysphagia, the quality of cry or noise produced, and a failure to thrive. Airway obstruction may in itself lead to a failure to thrive, which may be more obvious than the airway obstruction.

The infant larynx is located more superiorly in the neck.

Laryngomalacia

There is no underlying pathologic or progressive disorder in laryngomalacia. Rather, it is an exaggeration of the soft, flabby state that is normal for newborns. As the infant inhales, the soft larynx falls together, narrowing the inlet, and stridor results. Swallowing is unaffected. The cry should be normal. The weight gain and development of these infants are usually normal. Stridor is the major symptom, and it may be constant or may occur only with excitement. With the stridor may come retraction of the sternum and chest; laryngomalacia has been named as a cause of pectus excavatum. Usually infants are several weeks old when laryngomalacia begins, in contrast to the respiratory distress syndrome of the newborn. On direct examination the physician can see the larynx fall together with inhalation. The subglottic

Laryngomalacia is usually not apparent until a few weeks of age.

area is normal, and the stridor ceases if the larynx is held open with a laryngoscope. The prognosis is good for this most common laryngeal anomaly, as the cartilages gain rigidity. Most infants cease to have the stridor by the twelfth to fifteenth month. Twenty per cent of infants with laryngomalacia have an additional cause of airway obstruction.

Laryngomalacia can be associated with a second upper airway abnormality.

Tracheomalacia is a similar disorder of the trachea due to lack of rigidity of the tracheal cartilages. Tracheomalacia and compression of the airway by an anomalous great vessel are similar conditions and must be differentiated. This can usually be done endoscopically. Arteriograms may be necessary to effectively study the great vessels. Esophagograms also help delineate vascular abnormalities, especially anomalous vascular rings.

Congenital Subglottic Stenosis

Congenital subglottic stenosis is defined as a subglottic diameter less than 4 mm. A normal newborn larynx should permit passage of a 3.5-mm bronchoscope. Some neonates present with stridor shortly after birth, whereas other infants have recurrent episodes of laryngotracheitis. Diagnosis is made endoscopically. Mild cases may require only observation, but most cases require tracheotomy. Growth tends to resolve the relative stenosis, but laser excision or reconstructive surgery may be necessary. More than one congenital anomaly can exist in a child's airway.

Webs

Congenital webs may be glottic (75 per cent), subglottic (12 per cent), or supraglottic (12 per cent). Usually both the airway and the cry or voice are affected, with the symptoms beginning at birth. Webs must first be diagnosed by endoscopic visualization. Then treatment, consisting of laser or surgical excision, repeated dilatation, or tracheotomy and the use of laryngeal inserts, can be accomplished. The long-term prognosis for congenital laryngeal webs is favorable.

Congenital Cysts

Newborns who have congenital cysts usually have airway obstruction or simply do not grow. The episodes of airway obstruction can be confusing and may be thought to be due to a seizure disorder. Usually the voice and swallowing are normal. The cyst may arise from the base of the tongue, the aryepiglottic folds, or the false cords. Whenever possible, these cysts should be excised, preferably endoscopically. If this is not possible, then aspiration or marsupialization may be done. In an exceptional patient tracheotomy and external surgery are necessary.

Hemangioma

Hemangioma of the subglottic area of the larynx is considered here because it is a tumor that occurs primarily in infants under six months of age. Half of the patients with laryngeal hemangiomas have an external hemangioma on the head or neck. Stridor plus a visible hemangioma strongly suggests this diagnosis. These tumors are not true neoplasms but rather vascular abnormalities, and they do tend to regress, usually by the age of 12 months. The symptoms of the hemangiomas are not those of bleeding but of airway obstruction. The voice and swallowing are usually normal. The hemangioma is very close to the vocal cords above the site of a tracheotomy and is truly subglottic. A lateral radiograph shows a mass in the airway. Endoscopically there is a smooth, compressible mass, often on the posterior or lateral wall. Treatment has often been tracheotomy and allowing time for regression. Laser excision is currently being used. Low-dose irradiation has also been employed but is now avoided because of concern about late thyroid carcinoma.

Laryngocele

Laryngocele is a special type of congenital cyst that develops as a residual from a small appendix or saccus of the laryngeal ventricle. Like a thyroglossal duct, it may present at any age, but its origin is congenital. As the cyst begins, it first causes a bulging of the false vocal cord on that side. With enlargement, the cyst dissects along the superior laryngeal nerve and vessels to present as a mass in the neck. Since this cyst may communicate with the airway, a radiograph may show an air-fluid level. These cysts do not necessarily contain air but may be solid, containing only fluid. As they enlarge, they encroach on the airway and may cause stridor and airway obstruction. The diagnosis can be suggested by aspirating the mass with a large needle. The only effective treatment for laryngocele is dissection of the cyst, using an external approach. Usually this is accompanied by a temporary tracheostomy.

Laryngotracheoesophageal Cleft

This rare congenital abnormality is a result of a failure of fusion of the dorsal portions of the cricoid cartilages. There is an associated failure of closure of the tracheoesophageal septum, thus creating a groove in the region of the cricoid cartilage that resembles in many respects the more common H-type tracheoesophageal fistula. The infant may have cyanosis, respiratory distress, and recurrent episodes of pneumonia. In addition, there may be associated changes in the cry as well as inspiratory stridor. Direct laryngoscopy reveals the larynx to be normal. Cineradiography may be a useful study to help determine the position of the fistula. Endoscopic examination is also useful, but the physician must be searching specifically for this rare abnormality, or the fistula site may not be recognized.

Clefts may not be apparent on routine direct laryngoscopy.

Neurogenic Disorders in the Newborn

Infants can develop vocal cord paralysis from birth canal trauma. Congenital disorders involving the central nervous system or chest such as a meningocele or mediastinal mass also cause vocal cord paralysis. Increased intracranial pressure from any cause, especially in children, may result in vocal cord dysfunction. Infants with unilateral vocal cord paralysis may show varying symptoms. In many the cord is lateral enough to give a breathy poor cry but no respiratory distress. Other infants may have the cord median

Unilateral vocal cord paralysis is more common on the left.

enough so as to limit respiratory exchange. Stridor, especially with crying or activity, results. Infants with bilateral vocal cord paralysis have a good cry but poor respiratory exchange and need prompt airway support. An endotracheal tube forced between the cords gives short-term relief, but tracheotomy is necessary eventually. Paralysis often recovers in 6 to 9 months but may take up to 14 months. The tracheotomy is left until the airway enlarges by growth, reinnervation, or a lateralization procedure.

Children with bilateral vocal cord paraylsis can have a normal cry.

LARYNGEAL TRAUMA

Contusions of the Larynx

Mild contusions of the larynx are manifested by internal hematomas and occasionally by dislocation of the arytenoid cartilage. Usually the trauma is caused by some blunt object striking an extended neck. The key to treatment of laryngeal injury is immediate diagnosis. Contusions can be observed while preparations for tracheotomy are kept in reserve, but they must be differentiated from the more severe cartilaginous fracture and from laryngotracheal avulsions by mirror or fiberoptic examination and lateral radiograph. Usually the patient with a contusion can cooperate sufficiently for the larynx to be visualized. The hematoma can usually be observed. Direct laryngoscopy usually reduces the dislocated arytenoid cartilage. The patient should not have subcutaneous emphysema with a contusion or hematoma.

Laryngeal Fracture

Sharp compression of the larynx, hyoid, and upper trachea between the cervical spine and the unyielding force of an automobile or motor bike can cause a fracture. Hyoid fractures usually do not cause airway obstruction, since the pharynx is very wide at this level. The greater cornu of the hyoid does not normally unite to the body until age 35. This fact must be known when radiographs of the hyoid are interpreted. Actual separation of the greater cornu from the body must occur before a fracture can be diagnosed here. The epiphyseal line is not a fracture line. Treatment of hyoid bone fractures can usually be expectant.

Signs of laryngeal fracture: hoarseness, stridor, hemoptysis, subcutaneous emphysema.

Fractures of the thyroid cartilage itself are common. These injuries are characterized by (1) a history of a blow to the neck, (2) hoarseness, (3) inspiratory or expiratory stridor (or both), (4) hemoptysis, and (5) subcutaneous emphysema. The most likely fracture runs in a vertical plane from the bottom of the thyroid notch to the lower border of the cartilage. Avulsion of the thyroid cartilage from the cricoid and trachea may also occur. Facial pain, aphonia, and subcutaneous emphysema are the most common symptoms. Airway obstruction may develop explosively. On palpation, the cervical area is usually flat and there is loss of the prominence of the thyroid cartilage and cricoid. These patients, if not unconscious, are nearly impossible to examine with a mirror because their pain and hematoma are too great. If fracture is suspected and the thyroid cartilage is not palpated, tracheostomy should be done. Intubation is hazardous in these patients, since it may be impossible to do without compromising the little remaining airway. Tracheostomy under local anesthesia is preferred in these injuries.

When laryngotracheal separation occurs, the trachea will retract into the lower neck. Emergency tracheostomy is required.

Laryngeal fractures often are accompanied by cervical spine injuries. A force sufficient to fracture the larynx often dislocates the cervical spine as well. Cervical spine films must be taken before treatment is begun. Injuries to the recurrent laryngeal nerves can often result from avulsion.

Cervical spine films and neurologic examination are required in anyone with a laryngeal fracture.

Gunshot wounds of the larynx are characterized by a loss of tissue and a greater likelihood of associated cervical spine, great vessel, or esophageal injury. Esophageal injury is evaluated by radiography with contrast swallow or by endoscopy. Injuries to the laryngeal cartilage should be repaired as soon as possible. Therefore, as soon as the central nervous system and cardiovascular system permit, repair should begin. If feasible, immediate open repair and reduction of the laryngeal cartilage should be undertaken. Such immediate surgery tends to prevent the development of hard fibrotic stenosis. Since torn cartilage without its blood supply is quite susceptible to absorption, repair should be done quickly.

Laryngeal and Subglottic Stenosis

Scar tissue narrowing the airway is a sequela of disease or injury, and its treatment is extremely difficult. Blunt or perforating trauma, high tracheotomy, caustic ingestion, a gunshot wound, and irritation from an endotracheal tube cuff are the more common causes of laryngeal stenosis. Usually patients who require long-term endotracheal intubation with cuffed tubes are desperately ill, and the laryngeal stenosis occurs as a result of the heroic therapy they receive. Because of its more resilient cartilage, the child's larynx is more forgiving in long-term intubation than are those of adults. CT scans can be used to delineate laryngeal and subglottic stenosis. Nevertheless, cuffed endotracheal tubes should be used for as short a time as possible with the cuff deflated intermittently. Low-pressure cuffs lessen but do not completely prevent stenosis. Cuffed tubes should be made of new, nonirritating plastic and should be free of sterilization gas contamination before being used. Treatment of chronic laryngeal stenosis is very complicated and must be individualized. Dilatation, excision, direct re-anastomosis, skin grafting over a mold, and partial or total laryngectomy are all used.

Intubation Granuloma

Rarely an endotracheal tube abrades the vocal process of the arytenoid cartilage, causing an intubation granuloma. This may occur any time an endotracheal tube is used; it is not a complication of laryngeal surgery only. A perichondritis develops, and the healing process produces a raised polypoid lesion in the posterior portion of the glottic chink (rima glottidis). The patients are usually not very hoarse, but they know the voice is changed. The airway is not obstructed because the lesion is in the wide posterior portion of the glottis. Occasionally a large granuloma or one that suddenly increases in size because of hemorrhage may cause obstruction. Often granulomas are bilateral. Their treatment consists of endoscopic surgical removal, often using the CO_2 laser.

ALLERGIC DISEASE OF THE LARYNX

Allergic reactions in which the loose areolar tissue about the glottis is the shock organ may cause a rapid airway obstruction. Obstructive edema may develop in only a few minutes after contact with an exciting antigen. Fortunately, such situations are rare, but when they occur heroic measures, including steroids and tracheostomy, are necessary.

INFECTIOUS DISEASE OF THE LARYNX

Croup

Croup is a rapidly developing infection of the larynx resulting in stridor and airway obstruction. Although it can develop at any age, even in adults, croup is most common in children under six years of age.

Both the laryngeal surface of the epiglottis and the area just below the vocal cords in the larynx contain loose areolar tissue that is prone to swell when inflamed. Hence, croup can be divided into acute supraglottitis (epiglottitis) and acute subglottic laryngitis. Although both can be rapid in onset and severe, acute epiglottitis tends to be more explosive, often terminating fatally in a few hours without treatment. Both disorders appear clinically the same—with restlessness, apprehension, stridor, retraction, and cyanosis—but there are some subtle differences. A child with epiglottitis tends to sit up with mouth open and chin forward, is not hoarse, tends not to have as croupy a cough, but is more likely to have dysphagia. Because it is painful to swallow, the child may drool. Dysphagia in epiglottitis may be a sign of impending collapse. It results from spread of inflammation into the adjacent esophageal inlet and means that the inflammatory process has swollen the epiglottis markedly.

Children with acute subglottic laryngitis are hoarse with a very croupy cough and usually want to lie down. Other characteristics that differentiate these two forms of croup are listed in Table 20–1.

Arterial blood gas studies are of little value in acute upper airway obstruction.

These children must be rapidly treated without long delay in the radiology or emergency department and must not be upset or agitated. A soft tissue lateral radiograph of the neck may show narrowing of the subglottic area or an enlarged epiglottis. A chest radiograph should be normal but is taken to rule out pneumonia, the presence of a foreign body, or asthma. Blood gas studies and the finding of leukocytosis are academically interesting, but in the rapidly changing child results are not obtained in time to aid in planning treatment. Depressing the tongue to see the epiglottis may force the swollen epiglottis into the larynx like a cork and should not be done unless one is equipped to pass a bronchoscope or endotracheal tube.*

Blood culture may isolate H. influenzae.

Treatment must begin quickly. Intravenous fluid therapy is started in order to prevent dehydration and drying of secretions. Cold, moist humidity, preferably with the smallest particulate size of water vapor, is necessary. Antibiotic therapy to actual *Haemophilus* or *Staphylococcus* is initiated while awaiting the culture results. Antibiotics should not be withheld because, clinically, it may be difficult to distinguish between the types of croup, and the course can be very rapid. While smears and cultures should be taken, their results arrive too late to be of value. Steroids are given in large doses to reduce inflammation. The patient must be carefully observed and consideration given to intubation or tracheostomy. The indication for airway

---

*For selection of tube size, see Table 25–1.

TABLE 20-1. CLINICAL FEATURES IN CROUP

SUPRAGLOTTITIS	LARYNGOTRACHEOBRONCHITIS (INFRAGLOTTITIS)	BACTERIAL TRACHEITIS	SPASMODIC CROUP
3-6 years	Under 3 years	8-15 years	1-5 years
Onset hours	Onset days	1-2 week period of respiratory infection with rapid deterioration	Rapid onset, usually evening
Voice clear	Hoarse	Barking cough	No associated infection
Dysphagia	None	Inspiratory stridor	Exposure to humidity or cold relieves
Drooling	None		May be noninflammatory edema of subglottic area
Sitting up	Recumbent	Recumbent	
Rarely recurs	May recur	Intubation needed to remove secretions or pseudomembranes	
Rapid course	Days to weeks		
Lateral radiograph shows supraglottic edema	Normal neck films	Tracheal radiographs show irregular margins	
Haemophilus influenzae most common; *Streptococcus* or viral etiology less common	Viral etiology	*Staphylococcus aureus* most typical; *Streptococcus* or *H. influenzae* less common	

support is deterioration in spite of humidity, antibiotics, and steroids. To evaluate the croup one must monitor pulse, respiratory rate, degree of restlessness and apprehension, the use of accessory muscles of respiration, the degree of cyanosis, the degree of retraction, and the overall fatigue of the patient. If the patient can sleep, airway support is not necessary. On the other hand, a respiratory rate over 40, a pulse rate greater than 160, and increasing restlessness and retraction indicate the need for support.

Acute epiglottitis can occur in 30- to 40-year-old adults.

Some authors recommend sedation for croup patients, but it is our belief that no sedation or narcotics should be given. The status of the patient should be watched at all times. Croup is one of the few disorders that require the physician to be in constant attendance at the bedside. Racemic epinephrine given by inhalation has been valuable, especially in laryngotracheobronchitis, and has reduced the need for airway support. Intubation or tracheotomy can be used to maintain the airway. If the child collapses, an Ambu respirator with positive pressure is used to force oxygen through the edematous airway. Nasal intubation can be accomplished and may remain for days. Children's larynges allow longer intubation than do adults'. When it must be done, tracheotomy should be performed in an orderly manner in an operating room over a tube. Most cases of croup resolve in 48 to 72 hours and the patient can be extubated. Chest radiography must be done after tracheotomy because, especially in children, the pleura rises into the neck. Its injury results in pneumothorax.

In selecting an antibiotic for H. influenzae *supraglottitis, recognize that 20 per cent of organisms are ampicillin resistant.*

Acute Laryngitis

Vocal abuse, toxic fume inhalation, and infection produce acute laryngitis. Usually the infection is not limited to the larynx but is a paninfection involving the sinus, ear, larynx, and bronchial tubes. The influenza virus, adenoviruses, and streptococci are the most common causative organisms. Diphtheria must always be suspected in laryngitis, particularly if there is any evidence of a membrane or lack of immunization history. Mirror examination usually shows a diffuse erythema of the larynx. Cultures of the throat should be taken. Treatment consists of voice rest, antibiotics, increased humidity, and cough suppressants. Medications whose side effect is to cause drying should be avoided in laryngeal treatment. Singers and voice professionals must be advised to let the inflammatory process subside before resuming their careers. Attempting to sing during the infection may result in hemorrhage in the larynx and the subsequent development of vocal cord nodules.

SYSTEMIC DISORDERS WITH LARYNGEAL MANIFESTATIONS

Rheumatoid Arthritis

Because the cricoarytenoid joint is a true joint, it may be involved by a rheumatoid process. Pain radiating to the ear, dysphagia, and hoarseness are symptoms of acute cricoarytenoid arthritis. On visualization the affected arytenoid is edematous, erythematous, and immobile. In order to differentiate a vocal cord paralysis from rheumatoid fixation the joint must be palpated directly. In vocal cord paralysis the joint should move passively, whereas it is fixed in an arthritis. In addition to systemic rheumatoid treatment, steroids may be injected directly in and about the cricoarytenoid joint.

Hypothyroidism

The larynx is involved early in hypothyroidism with the deposit of mucopolysaccharides submucosally; hoarseness may be an early symptom of hypothyroidism.

Infiltrative Disorders

The lesions of *sarcoid* and *amyloid* may infiltrate the larynx. If localized, they can be surgically removed. Only 1.5 per cent of patients with sarcoidosis have laryngeal involvement. The supraglottic larynx is primarily involved as the true cords are spared. Patients present with hoarseness and dysphagia. Endoscopic findings show diffuse edema without ulceration of the supraglottic larynx. Biopsy demonstrates noncaseating granulomas with giant cells. Treatment requires systemic steroids or direct intralesional injection of steroids. Obstructing lesions may require tracheostomy.

Histoplasmosis can cause simultaneous mucosal ulceration in the larynx and oral cavity. These nodular ulcerations may be the initial sign of the disease and are often confused with carcinoma or tuberculosis. Diagnosis depends upon identifying the fungus or detecting a serologic change.

Pemphigus vulgaris may affect the larynx primarily or may be associated with oral mucosal involvement. Typical blebs are not seen in the larynx, but the laryngeal surfaces are ulcerated or covered with a whitish membrane. If the associated findings and history suggest pemphigus, treatment should be begun.

Treatment of laryngeal pemphigus requires dapsone and steroids. Even then, cicatricial stenosis can result.

Chronic Granulomatous Infections

Tuberculosis of the larynx is rarely primary but almost always associated with pulmonary tuberculosis. Infected sputum bathes the larynx, causing ulceration and infiltration of the walls with tuberculous granuloma. As the disease progresses, edema, fibrosis, and perichondritis develop. Usually the posterior commissure is involved first. The diagnosis is based on the clinical findings of swelling or ulceration plus a positive tuberculosis smear. Usually a pulmonary lesion is also obvious. Laryngeal biopsies may show tuberculous granuloma. The treatment of laryngeal tuberculosis is not surgical but is based on antituberculosis drugs.

Tuberculosis more often involves the posterior aspect of the cords.

Syphilis in its secondary or tertiary state usually affects the larynx. A diffuse erythema may be a symptom of secondary lues. Tertiary gumma can invade and destroy the larynx.

Leprosy affects the nose and the larynx together. *Mycobacterium leprae* cannot be cultured but can be identified in smears in the lepromatous state of leprosy. Nasal secretions or sputum may be cultured in studies. The laryngeal picture is primarily one of infiltration and ulceration.

Mycotic infection of the larynx as a primary disease is rare. Usually oral pulmonary or cutaneous infection coexists with the laryngeal involvement. Candidiasis occurs in the immunosuppressed patient or after antibiotic or steroid therapy.

Androgen Therapy

The vocal signs of virilization occur in women treated with androgens. Androgens combined with estrogens are sometimes given to women, resulting in vocal masculinizing changes. As a rule, these changes are not reversible, even though the androgen therapy is discontinued. The decision to use androgens in women must be based on the disease process involved and not on the possible laryngeal complications.

CHRONIC NONSPECIFIC LARYNGITIS

Chronic nonspecific laryngitis includes a variety of conditions that are all characterized by hoarseness and are all examples of long-standing inflammatory changes in the laryngeal mucosa. Such patients may have repeated attacks of acute laryngitis, may be exposed to irritating dust or smoke, or may use their voices improperly in a neuromuscular sense. Cigarette smoking can produce laryngeal erythema and edema. Esophageal disorders such as Zenker's diverticulum or hiatus hernia may, through reflux, cause chronic laryngitis. Rarely, systemic disorders such as allergy, hypothyroidism, or Addison's disease are associated with vocal weakness and hoarseness. Anxiety and tension may also be factors in producing persistent nonspecific inflammatory changes.

The diagnosis of chronic nonspecific laryngitis is, in a sense, a "catch-all" diagnosis; in an individual patient there are often unknown factors that can produce such chronic inflammatory changes. On examination the vocal cords appear reddened or thickened. Vocal cord mobility should be unaffected, since the changes are primarily mucosal and submucosal.

Treatment of chronic laryngitis consists of removing the offending cause, correcting treatable related disorders, and re-educating vocal habits through speech therapy. Vocal sprays or syrups may be soothing but offer no real benefits. Antibiotics and short courses of steroids may lessen the inflammatory changes in a short-term episode but are not of value over the long period of rehabilitation. Elimination of drugs with "drying" side effects also helps the larynx.

BENIGN TUMORS OF THE LARYNX

Vocal Nodules

Vocal cord nodules that do not respond to conservative treatment are excised by microscopic laryngoscopy.

A variety of clinical synonyms exist for the vocal nodular polyp, including screamer's nodules, singer's nodes, or teacher's nodes. Benign nodules may be unilateral and result from prolonged or improper use of the vocal cords. Often when there is some coexisting inflammation, the vocal cords strike firmly together, causing formation of a polyp or nodule. The nodule may vary histologically from a soft, loosely edematous tumor to a firm, fibrous growth or a vascular lesion with many small vessels as its most outstanding feature. Some patients respond to vocal restraint and re-education, but many require endoscopic surgery.

Diffuse Vocal Cord Polyposis

Polypoid degeneration all along the length of the vocal cord is usually associated with prolonged vocal use, smoking, and persistent inflammation. Surgical removal must be done on one side at a time to prevent the development of synechiae in the anterior commissure. The surgery must be followed by cessation of smoking and vocal re-education. If it is not, recurrence of the thick polypoid tissue along the vocal cord is likely.

Contact Ulcer

The mechanical action of the vocal cords against each other is more likely to form vocal nodules in women and children, whereas in men it is more likely to form a contact ulcer. Men forcefully bring the arytenoid cartilages together, and the resulting irritation forms a granuloma called a contact ulcer. Characteristically the patient complains of pain and notices only a slight vocal change. Contact ulcers heal slowly, usually over two to three months. Speech therapy usually aids their resolution. Biopsy is of value to reduce some of the excessive granulation tissue and to give assurance to the patient that the granuloma is not malignant.

Juvenile Papilloma

Papilloma is the most common tumor of the larynx in children. The onset of the papilloma usually occurs in children between 18 months and 7 years of age, and involution often occurs at puberty. The duration of the disorder can extend over 10 years with many recurrent papillomas. Many children require multiple hospital admissions to maintain the voice and airway. Hoarseness and abnormal cry are the initial symptoms. Occasionally croup is suspected, but the papilloma is diagnosed when there is no response to therapy. Papillomas can enlarge to cause airway obstruction and present as an emergency requiring tracheostomy. Papillomas can be hormone-dependent, regressing with pregnancy and puberty. If they persist into adult life, they tend to be less aggressive and slower to recur. Papillomas are considered to have a viral etiology, although the virus has not yet been isolated.

With such a socially devastating disease, requiring dozens of hospital admissions in some patients, many treatments have been proposed. Irradiation has been discarded because of the late development of carcinoma. The most effective current therapy is precise surgical removal, often using a microscope with a CO_2 laser. In some cases a tracheotomy must be maintained for years. Repeated surgical excisions can lead to laryngeal scarring or webbing. Other therapies include tetracycline, steroids, smallpox vaccine, autologous vaccines, and alpha N_1 interferon. Fortunately, papillomas are not common. Malignant transformation in the absence of irradiation is rare and usually occurs in older patients with a history of smoking or long-standing papilloma.

Granular Cell Myoblastoma

These tumors tend to occur on the tongue and larynx. Hoarseness is the main symptom of this small tumor, and recurrence is unlikely after endoscopic removal. The mucosa over the granular cell myoblastoma may show pseudoepithelial hyperplasia, which can be confused with carcinoma.

Chondroma

Chondromas are slow-growing tumors of hyaline cartilage arising from the cricoid, thyroid, arytenoid, or epiglottic cartilages. Hoarseness related to restriction of the vocal cord and dyspnea due to airway obstruction are the main symptoms. Many of these tumors are calcified and can be suspected from radiographic examination. The treatment is surgical, with the origin and the extent of the tumor determining the surgical technique. Because these tumors are slow-growing, they can sometimes be partially removed, relieving the patient's symptoms without sacrificing the larynx.

Leukoplakia or Erythroplakia

Persistent irritation of the larynx, particularly by smoking, may lead to the development of whitish areas. Clinically the whitish area is termed leukoplakia. Paradoxically, areas with the histology and clinical significance may appear reddened (erythroplakia). Any area of the larynx may be involved, but usually the vocal cords are most affected. Commonly hoarseness is the patient's complaint. Biopsy of these areas shows hyperkeratosis, carcinoma in situ, or frank carcinoma. Hyperkeratosis is found in most biopsies. Its treatment requires total endoscopic removal and careful follow-up of the patient. Smoking must be curtailed. Hyperkeratosis may become invasive carcinoma over time but does not do so commonly. Most authors put the incidence at 15 per cent or less.

Surgery of Benign Laryngeal Tumors

Benign, small laryngeal tumors are usually removed endoscopically. Local anesthesia plus sedation or general anesthesia with an endotracheal tube can be used. The operating laryngoscope can be stabilized by suspension devices, and then an operating microscope is employed to give magnification. Laryngoscopy done with a binocular microscope allows very precise surgical technique. The carbon dioxide laser has added a new dimension to laryngeal surgery.

Attached to the binocular operating microscope, the CO_2 laser has permitted surgical resection of tumors of the larynx and trachea. The major advantage of the laser is the possibility of resection without bleeding and with minimal postoperative edema. In the past, these two factors restricted

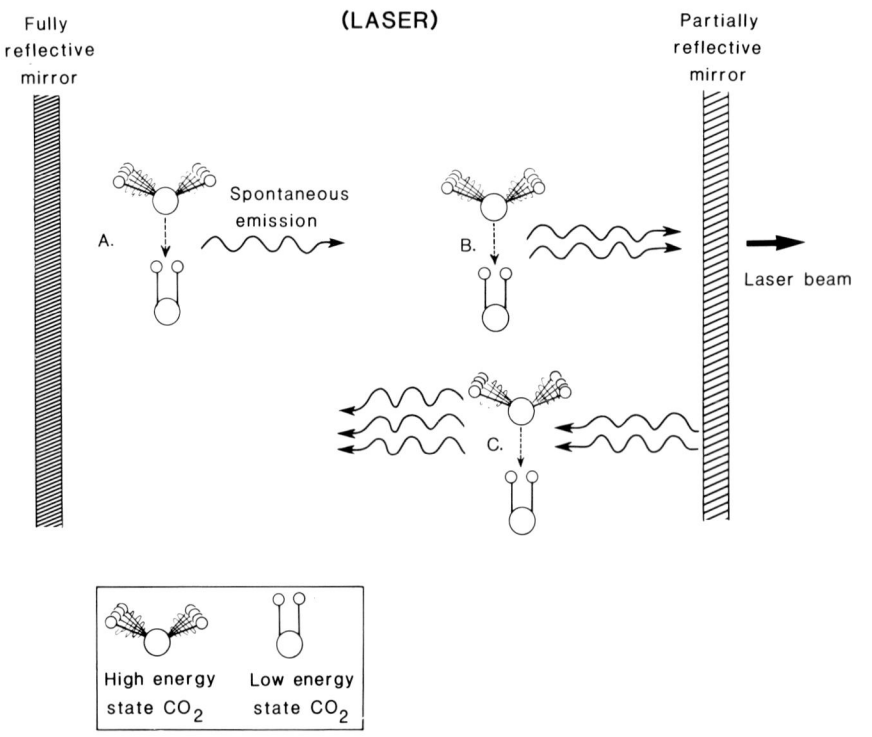

FIGURE 20–2. Generation of coherent light by means of (L)ight (A)mplification of (S)timulated (E)mission of (R)adiation (LASER). Laser medium molecules can be in one of two states: high energy or low energy. The laser pump puts molecules into the high energy state. One of the molecules ("A") *by chance* spontaneously emits in the direction of the axes of the two mirrors. The light generated by the spontaneous emission (at molecule "A") can stimulate other high energy molecules to emit additional light that is in phase and of the same frequency as the original light wave. "Stimulated light emissions" are much more likely to occur in the direction of the axes of the mirrors. The process proceeds as the stimulated light makes multiple reflections within the optical cavity. Only light traveling in the direction of the mirror axes is reflected multiple times and therefore significantly propagated. The energy pump restores the molecules that have emitted and dropped to a lower energy state back to the high energy state. (Illustration by Barry P. Kimberley, M.D., M.Sc., Medical Fellow, Department of Otolaryngology, University of Minnesota.)

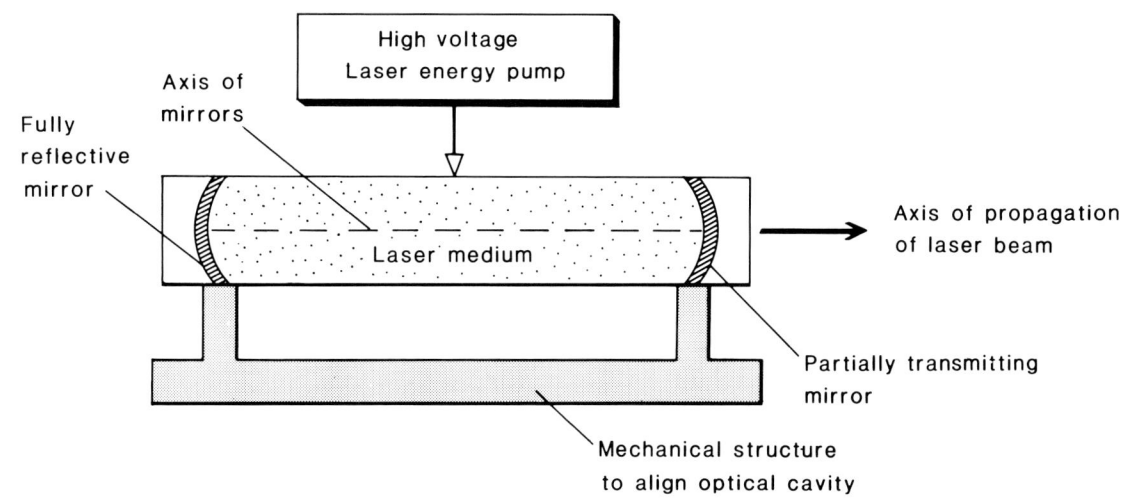

FIGURE 20-3. Laser components. Basic components of any laser are (1) a laser medium, i.e., CO_2, N_2, He in the case of a CO_2 laser; (2) a source of energy called a laser pump that causes a "population inversion" in the laser medium; (3) an optical cavity formed by the two mirrors and the space between them; and (4) a mechanical structure to align the axes of the two mirrors. (Illustration by Barry P. Kimberley, M.D., M.Sc., Medical Fellow, Department of Otolaryngology, University of Minnesota.)

the surgical procedures that could be done transorally. Thus the carbon dioxide laser has reduced the necessity for operative procedures on the larynx.

Figures 20-2 and 20-3 explain the mechanism of the laser, which is an acronym for "light amplification of stimulated emissions of radiation." Rather than allowing the light source to illuminate and propagate in multiple directions with multiple light frequencies, the radiation is made (1) coherent (that is, in phase), (2) collimated (parallel directions), and (3) monochromatic (one frequency only). This creates a high-power density at one focal spot. Whether a CO_2 (Table 20-2) or a YAG laser is used, the light generation in an active medium is the same. The operating room and the patient are protected from any stray laser beams. The surgeon, sitting at the head of the table and using the operating microscope, directs the beam onto the area of tissue that is to be removed for biopsy or vaporized. Currently the laser is frequently employed for the treatment of subglottic stenosis, subglottic hemangioma, and most particularly, for the removal of juvenile laryngeal papillomas.

Large benign laryngeal tumors require an external approach. Usually a

TABLE 20-2. CO_2 LASER

PHYSICAL PROPERTY	CLINICAL FEATURE
Light energy	Focused through microscope. Controls bleeding in small vessels (≤ 0.5 mm)
Power adjustable	Depth and size of vaporized area variable
Deactivated by cellular water	More power (energy) needed in dense tissue (bone)
Small zone of tissue reaction outside lasered area	Postoperative edema is minimal and healing is rapid. Less pain, and scarring may be lessened.
Tissue vaporized	Suction carries away debris.
Ignition of anesthesia	Not a problem with precautions
Deflected by mirrors	Not yet available in fiberoptics

tracheostomy is done to guarantee the airway. The larynx can be entered through the midline of the thyroid cartilage or laterally through the pharynx. The primary principle of benign tumor surgery is removal of only the tumor, preserving all normal tissue and hence normal laryngeal function. A midline laryngeal opening is not thought to affect later growth. After laryngeal surgery for benign disease, most patients are advised to rest their voices and gradually resume full use over two to three weeks. Cough suppressants are also used to control explosive coughing. Speech therapy may be essential to provide vocal re-education and lessen the chance of recurrence.

NEUROGENIC DISORDERS OF THE LARYNX

Vocal Cord Paralysis

Generally five positions of the vocal cord are recognized in describing the degree of opening of the larynx: median, paramedian, intermediate, slight abduction, and full abduction. If a paralysis is bilateral, these positions are designated by observing the size of the glottic chink (Table 20–3). If a paralysis is unilateral (Fig. 20–4), the observer must first estimate the true midline position and then relate the cordal position to that.

Any lesion along the course of the recurrent laryngeal nerves can cause laryngeal paralysis. Intracranial lesions usually have other associated symptoms and present as neurologic problems rather than as voice or articulation disorders. Lesions of the brain stem may seem to involve the voice primarily, but they also have other neurologic signs. Multiple sclerosis, brain stem tumors, and amyotrophic lateral sclerosis may have significant voice symptoms. A careful examination of all the cranial nerves plus cerebellar testing and examination for Horner's syndrome must be done.

Lesions of the base of the skull that will selectively catch one or more of the cranial nerves include tumors of the nasopharynx, aneurysms, and neurogenic tumors. Tumors arising in the lateral pharyngeal space, as well as from the deep lobe of the parotid, may also cause vocal cord paralysis. Thyroidectomy or other neck surgery can cause vocal cord paralysis. If recognized immediately after surgery, re-exploration of the nerves should be accomplished to look for surgical trauma. This should be done before fibrosis obliterates the surgical field, making nerve identification impossible. Neoplasms of the thyroid, esophagus, and lung are common causes of vocal cord paralysis. Mechanical pressure from dilated or abnormal cardiovascular structures, distended cysts, or rapidly increasing hilar adenopathy can cause vocal cord paralysis.

Even after thorough evaluation, a number of vocal cord paralyses will still be unexplained. These idiopathic paralyses are thought to be viral. If a

TABLE 20–3. VOCAL CORD POSITION, OPENING

POSITION	VOCAL CORD OPENING
Median	Both cords in midline
Paramedian	3–5 mm
Intermediate	7 mm
Slight abduction	14 mm
Full abduction	18–19 mm

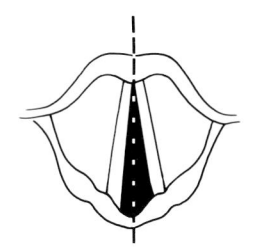

FIGURE 20–4. The left vocal cord is paralyzed and partially abducted (paramedian position). With phonation, the right cord comes to the midline, but the left cord remains unchanged.

Unilateral vocal cord paralysis (During normal breathing)

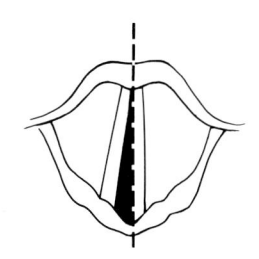

Unilateral vocal cord paralysis (Quiet)

paralysis is termed idiopathic, a careful long-term follow-up with repeated examination should be done. Occult carcinoma, particularly of the thyroid, can in its early stages appear to be idiopathic. A list of diagnostic procedures that might be done for evaluation of vocal cord paralysis includes chest radiography (both anteroposterior and lateral views), esophagram, CT scans, radioactive iodine thyroid scan, cervical spine radiography, skull radiography, white blood cell count (for leukemia), blood urea nitrogen, viral titers, and glucose tolerance test (diabetic neuropathy). Examination of the larynx must, of course, be done directly or by mirror examination. Palpation of the cricoarytenoid joint is done to differentiate inflammatory fixation from vocal cord paralysis. Such fixation may result from rheumatoid arthritis, laryngeal trauma, or an indwelling endotracheal tube.

Motor and sensory function of the larynx is from a superior and inferior nerve on each side. Table 20–4 describes the pathology, its effect, and the findings on examination. An isolated superior laryngeal paralysis is very subtle to diagnosis, but the other lesions are clinically obvious.

Unilateral vocal cord paralysis in children has an additional feature.

TABLE 20–4. LARYNGEAL PARALYSIS

	SUPERIOR LARYNGEAL PARALYSIS	UNILATERAL RECURRENT NERVE PARALYSIS	BILATERAL RECURRENT NERVE PARALYSIS	COMPLETE PARALYSIS
Pathology	Paralysis of cricothyroid muscle; sensory loss in half of larynx	Paralysis of all intrinsic muscles on that side	Paralysis of all intrinsic muscles	Vagus nerve lesion above the superior laryngeal nerve; may be unilateral or bilateral
Effect	Loss of pitch; aspiration	Hoarse; good airway except in small children; breathy voice; poor cough	Good voice; poor airway, especially on exertion	Similar to corresponding lesions of recurrent paralysis; more likely to aspirate
Examination	Anterior commissure looks tilted to side of lesion; arytenoid on that side tilts in	Cord in paramedian position; no lateral motion	Vocal cords do not move laterally; some patients adapt and exist with decreased exercise tolerance	Cord(s) are immobile but in intermediate position due to loss of adduction by cricothyroid muscle

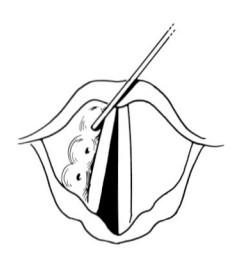

Injecting Teflon lateral to true vocal cord.

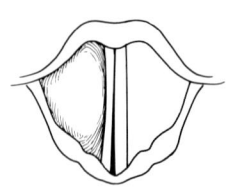

Cords now able to approximate in midline during phonation.

FIGURE 20–5. The left vocal cord is paralyzed and cannot reach the midline. The voice is breathy and hoarse. Injecting Teflon lateral to the cord under local anesthesia pushes the cord to the midline. Now during phonation the cords can approximate.

Because of the small size of the glottis, unilateral paralysis in a child may compromise the airway to result clinically in stridor. Many patients recover their vocal cord function either because the nerve recovers and again moves the cord or because the opposite vocal cord compensates by crossing the midline to once again firmly abut against the paralyzed cord. This is possible if the paralyzed cord is in a paramedian position. Before restorative procedures are done, 6 to 12 months should elapse to allow time for compensation. If these mechanisms do not occur, Teflon paste can be injected lateral to the true cord to increase its bulk and move it medially so that the normal moving cord can approximate, producing a pleasing voice (Fig. 20–5).

Bilateral vocal cord paralysis (Fig. 20–6) presents a different problem. Because both vocal cords are usually in a paramedian position, the voice is less affected, yet the glottic chink is not wide enough to permit any exertion. The patient may even be dyspneic at rest. Usually patients with bilateral cordal paralysis have vocal cords that are nearly together, and the majority of them require a tracheostomy to relieve their airway obstruction. Very rarely does a patient with a bilateral vocal cord paralysis have the cords widely separated. Such adducted cords do not result from neurogenic lesions but can result from laryngeal trauma. In this case the airway is satisfactory, but the voice is weak and breathy. More commonly in bilateral paralysis from neurologic lesions, the vocal cords are adducted, and the patient has a good voice with a very poor airway. These patients often require a tracheostomy. A valve in the tracheostomy tube allows air to be inhaled through the tube and then closes on expiration, diverting the air stream through the vocal cords to produce a voice. Many patients do not accept valve tubes, and a variety of surgical procedures are done to increase the airway while sparing the voice. These operations all involve compromise; they trade vocal

Normal (Quiet breathing)

Bilateral vocal cord paralysis

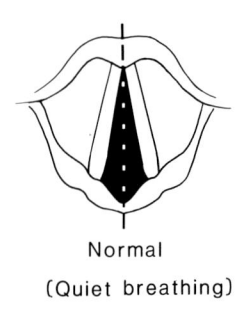

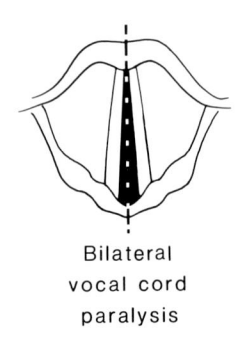

FIGURE 20–6. During normal inspiration the cords adduct as seen on the left. When there is bilateral vocal cord paralysis, the cords are just off the midline, allowing a slit-like airway. Tracheostomy or arytenoidectomy is generally required.

ability for airway patency and occasionally some degree of aspiration. In these surgical procedures the arytenoid cartilage is removed or turned laterally to increase airway size. Some patients may get excellent results and feel they have good voices as well as a good airway, but for most, the airway is adequate but the voice is husky and hoarse.

Idiopathic Laryngeal Aspiration

In addition to being a vocal organ, the larynx is also a valve separating the food and air passages. After trauma or surgery this valve function may be compromised, and the patient may aspirate foods or liquids. Usually thin liquids like water are the most difficult to swallow. Fortunately these symptoms are usually temporary, and the patient can regain nearly normal swallowing. In the uncommon disorder of idiopathic laryngeal aspiration, an otherwise healthy patient has a feeling of mucus or saliva going the wrong way. Then a paroxysm of coughing, choking, and laryngospasm follows. The patient and on-lookers are frightened. After the spasms relent, the patient is again asymptomatic. Repeated episodes may occur. Examination and laboratory testing show no abnormality. The disorder is self-limited and usually disappears. No medication seems to be of any value.

Brain stem disorders can produce aspiration both of ingested nourishment and of oral secretions. Treatment of these disorders is difficult and may include tracheostomy and gastrostomy, esophagostomy, or procedures designed to close the larynx at the level of the vocal cords.

Spastic Dysphonia

Spastic dysphonia is a strained, hoarse voice, often staccato-like, due to hyperadduction of the true and false cords. This "tension larynx" usually starts in young adults, who become very self-conscious and may change occupation to avoid speech. Psychotherapy, drugs, biofeedback, voice therapy, and hypnosis have been of limited success. Surgical section of the right recurrent laryngeal nerve has been the best therapy, although voices do not return to complete normalcy and some redevelop the dysphonia in time. The pathophysiology of the disorder is unknown.

Myasthenia Gravis

All ages can be affected by myasthenia, a disease that usually starts with bulbar involvement. Characteristically muscles weaken with use and recover after rest. Often the eye or facial muscles are involved, but speech and swallowing dysfunction may cause the patient to seek medical help. A diagnostic test can be done with Prostigmin, 15 mg orally (or 0.5 to 1.0 mg IM); improvement should occur within 30 minutes.

Amyotrophic Lateral Sclerosis

Typically patients are in their 50's or 60's. Bulbar symptoms of swallowing and speech dysfunction may be prominent, although tongue dysfunction with fasciculations is more common.

FUNCTIONAL DISORDERS OF THE LARYNX

Functional disorders with no obvious diagnostic abnormality form a special group of laryngeal disorders.

Psychogenic Aphonia

The patient may complain of a total inability to talk, but on examination the larynx looks and moves normally. Upon request the patient is able to cough normally, and this is the key to the psychogenic etiology. Often there is a history of emotional disturbance, particularly if the patient is questioned directly.

Dysphonia Plicae Ventricularis

Phonation with the false cords vibrating instead of the true vocal cords produces a husky voice. On visualization the larynx appears normal, but the false cords seem to overhang or cover the true cords. The diagnosis can be clinically suspected and proved by planigrams done during phonation. The false vocal cords meet and vibrate while the true cords remain apart.

Vocal Weakness

Many older patients complain of vocal weakness. Their voice lacks its usual tone and vigor. Frequently the voice breaks or drops in pitch. On examination the vocal cords appear slightly bowed. As the larynx ages, this bowing occurs normally to a variable degree. The vocal change then is an extension of a normal physiologic aging process.

When older patients are weakened after illness or surgery, their voices suffer because of their overall debility and improve as they gain muscle strength. Excessive emotional tension in the young also can produce a functional weakness with a cracking, breaking voice. A feeling of dryness or of a lump in the throat is often an accompanying symptom.

FOREIGN BODIES OF THE LARYNX

Any foreign body in the larynx is an immediate emergency. Often the patient was holding the object in the mouth between the teeth and accidentally inhaled. If the patient is not in respiratory distress, no attempt should be made to remove the object in an emergency room. Removal should be done in the operating room with anesthesia personnel available. Dislodging the foreign body may produce airway obstruction. In small children an upper esophageal foreign body can compress the airway by dilating the esophagus.

A special example of a laryngeal foreign body is the so-called café coronary. There is no cardiac involvement, but foreign material, usually meat, is lodged in the glottic opening. Suddenly the victim collapses after taking a large bite of food. An attempt can be made to dislodge the foreign body by squeezing the chest from behind. This bellows action may dispel the obstruction like a cork from a bottle. If not successful, a cricothyrotomy must be done rather than a tracheostomy. The usual tracheostomy site is low in the neck to enter the trachea. The thyroid gland overlies the trachea, and in a restaurant, entering the trachea can be both bloody and difficult. The cricothyroid membrane is subcutaneous between the thyroid and cricoid cartilages. There are no major vascular structures here and entry is much easier. After the airway is secure, the foreign body can be removed in a leisurely manner. If necessary, an orderly tracheostomy can be done later in a hospital setting. In an emergency with poor facilities, a cricothyrotomy is preferred over tracheostomy.

References

Bailey BJ, Biller HF: Surgery of the Larynx. Philadelphia, WB Saunders Co, 1985.
Cotton RT, Richardson MA: Congenital laryngeal anomalies. Otolaryngol Clin North Am 14:203–218, 1981.
DeSanto L, et al: Cysts of the larynx; classification. Laryngoscope 80:145–176, 1970.
Fried MP (ed): The larynx. Otolaryngol Clin North Am 17(1): February 1984.
Friedman ER, et al: Bacterial tracheitis—two-year experience. Laryngoscope 95:9–11, 1985.
Hodge KM, Ganzel TM: Diagnostic and therapeutic efficiency in croup and epiglottitis. Laryngoscope 97:621–625, 1987.
Linscott MS, Horton WC: Management of upper airway obstruction. Otolaryngol Clin North Am 12:351–373, 1979.
Nau TW, et al: Management of neonatal subglottic stenosis. Otolaryngol Clin North Am 20:153–162, 1986.
Simpson GT, Shapshay SM (eds): The use of lasers in otolaryngologic surgery. Otolaryngol Clin North Am 16(4): November 1983.
Tucker JA: Obstruction of the major pediatric airway. Otolaryngol Clin North Am 12:329–342, 1979.

21
SPEECH AND LANGUAGE DISORDERS

by Virginia Wigginton, M.A., C.C.C.,
   Meredith Gerdin, M.A., C.C.C., and
   Frank M. Lassman, Ph.D.

The development of speech and language is essential to most forms of human interaction. When there is a disruption in communicative ability, human development suffers. For this reason, the physician must understand speech and language development and factors that can alter its normal, orderly progression and must be aware of available services for treatment.

Definitions

Language is a system of symbols used for the understanding and expression of ideas and feelings. Attributes of language include not only vocabulary and grammar but also the abilities to remember, classify, order, and abstract.

In contrast, speech is one mode for conveying language. Among other modes are writing, gesturing, and signing. Attributes of speech include pitch, loudness, and quality of voice; vowels, consonants, diphthongs, and the blending of these into syllables, words, and phrases; and rate, intonation, and rhythm. "Language" and "speech" are distinguished here for purposes of clarity. This is not meant as an argument that they are dynamically separable. For example, there is a considerable amount of language information contained in intonation.

In defining speech and language disorders, there are three primary considerations: (1) Can the language and speech be understood with little or no difficulty? (2) Is the language usually appropriate to the substantive requirements of the communication? (3) Does the manner of communicating call attention to itself and divert attention from the message? When disorders of speech or language are judged to exist, there is usually a problem in one of these areas. With children, this possibility should follow a careful comparison of the child's performance against the general developmental description that follows.

NORMAL SPEECH AND LANGUAGE DEVELOPMENT

Prelinguistic Development

There are skills and knowledge learned in infancy which are necessary for the development of language and communication. These primary skills are in the areas of cognition and social interaction. Cognitively, the infant must learn to be aware of objects and events in his environment and to realize their uniqueness. It is this knowledge base that is the subject of early communications. Socially, the infant must learn that he can have a specific effect on caregivers by what he does, to be both an initiator and responder in interactions, to jointly attend to activities, and to interact with others for a variety of reasons. Many children with communication problems have had disturbances in the development of social and cognitive skills in infancy.

Communication problems in children may develop because of disturbed social and cognitive skills in infancy.

Linguistic Development

Language comprehension seems to precede language usage. Imitation may occur without comprehension, but functional language for communication purposes appears to require prior comprehension. Even though there are fairly predictable stages and ages for development, the range of normality is great.

Language comprehension precedes language usage.

Receptive language is that which the child hears and must interpret. The child progresses from simply alerting to a speaker to understanding meaning based on grammatical construction within the first five years of life.

Expressive language is that which the child expresses to others. Speech progresses from simple reflexive vocalization to complex sentences. Correspondingly, nonverbal communication progresses from unintentional behaviors to refined, conventional gestures.

General guidelines for both receptive and expressive language are listed in Table 21–1.

TABLE 21–1. DEVELOPMENT OF RECEPTIVE AND EXPRESSIVE LANGUAGE

AGE LEVEL	RECEPTIVE LANGUAGE	EXPRESSIVE LANGUAGE
0–6 months	Startles and turns to sound; understands tone of voice (e.g., angry vs. happy)	Cooing and babbling for pleasure; differential crying
6–12 months	Understands gestures; understands some words and phrases	Use of vocalization with inflection; may develop use of first word
12–18 months	Understands common short and simple sentences; points to some body parts; can identify familiar picture	Use of single words, using that word to mean several things; continues to use own jargon (syllables with intonation)
18–24 months	Understands a few prepositions and personal pronouns; listens to and understands simple stories; points to pictures when asked	Uses 2- and 3-word combinations; expresses negation by using "no"
2–3 years	Can follow 3-part directions; understands most adult sentences; understands concepts like "one" and "many"	3- and 4-word sentences; uses some pronouns and prepositions; about 50% intelligible
3–4 years	Can identify object when given function; understands more prepositions; understands information about more abstract events	Mostly intelligible; 4- to 6-word sentences with various sentence types (interrogative, imperative, negative)
4–5 years	Except for vocabulary limitations, understands most adult communication	90% of learning to talk completed; expression at a colloquial adult level

Physician's Screening

Commonly, parents become concerned enough to bring a child who is not talking or who uses only a few words to a physician at age 24 to 30 months. An alert physician, however, may recognize problems even earlier. Children not falling within accepted guidelines for language development should be referred for consultation with an audiologist and speech pathologist. Speech pathologists can determine whether behavior is outside acceptable limits and thereby minimize long-term effects.

SPEECH AND LANGUAGE DISORDERS IN CHILDREN

Three major considerations are important for the development of communication skills. Disruption of one or more can cause delayed or disordered development.

1. The child's physiologic status: Conditions that affect development include hearing loss, cleft palate, and CNS dysfunction, among others.
2. The child's environment: Conditions to consider include cultural factors, long-term hospitalization, and impoverished stimulation, ranging from disadvantage to deprivation.
3. The child's emotional status: Conditions to consider include ability to relate, disorders of thought processes, and behavioral problems.

Hearing Loss

Failure to develop speech or language requires evaluation for hearing impairment.

The quality of speech and language reflects the ability to hear and perceive. There is usually a direct relationship between speech/language abilities and the amount of residual hearing. Hearing loss, from the minimal to the profound, negatively affects speech and language development.

The effects of profound deafness tend to be obvious. Vocabulary, word order, and grammatical usage are faulty. Voice distortion, speech sound errors, and rhythm deviations are characteristic, making speech very difficult to understand.

The use of hearing aid amplification is important for reducing the effective hearing impairment, enabling the child to hear others as well as himself. The value of the hearing aid for maintaining speech skills is less obvious but should not be underestimated.

The hearing aid is but one aspect of the habilitation process. Children should not be expected to develop communication skills on the basis of amplification alone. Remediation is further discussed in Chapter 4, which deals with hearing impairment.

Age of onset is critical. Children who have normal hearing beyond age two years, even for a short while, are likely to have significantly better language/speech skills than those who are deaf at birth or very early in life.

Children with moderately severe hearing impairments usually have better speech and language than those with more profound losses. Attention is usually not drawn to the speech and language of those with mild hearing impairment. Yet children with mild, chronic hearing impairment are at risk for reduction in language skills. A hearing loss of 20 dB in young children (three years old and under) has been shown to affect language/speech

A hearing loss of 20 dB may affect speech.

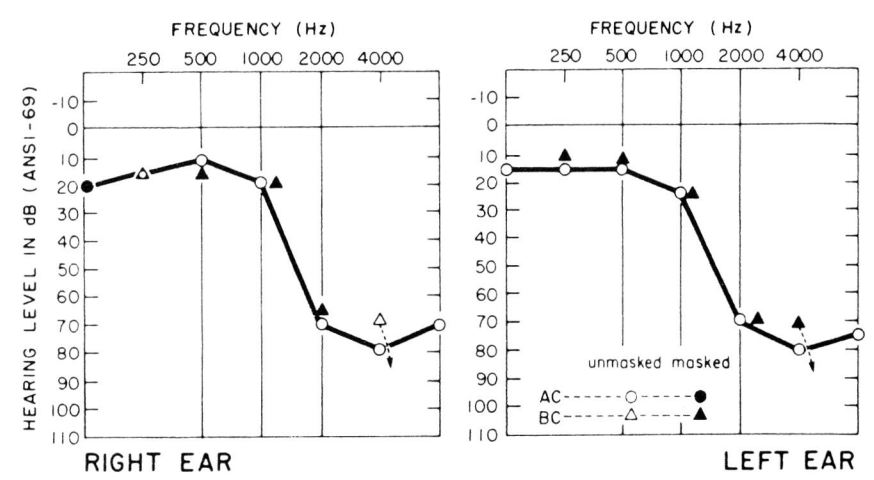

FIGURE 21–1. The audiogram (representing both ears) of the child with a hearing impairment for the higher frequencies. Because of better hearing sensitivity for low frequencies, the child often appears to have normal hearing to gross inspection. Speech/language delay may be ascribed to other factors such as assumed intellectual retardation.

learning. A mild intermittent hearing loss may cause additional problems involving attention and behavior, which in turn affect school learning.

Many children do poorly in speech production yet pass a gross screening test of hearing. Some of these are later found to have selective hearing impairment, often for the higher frequencies (Fig. 21–1). They appear to have normal hearing because they can perceive a portion but not all of the acoustical information, coupled with situation cues. They may respond correctly to their name, more predictable messages, and gross environmental sounds. Parents, teachers, and physicians falsely are led to believe that these children have normal hearing and that poor speech and school performance must be attributable to other factors such as attention, intellect, motivation, and emotional problems.

Because of the possibilities for erroneous conclusion, as described in the previous paragraph, it is advisable for the physician to consider the speech/language delay itself as the reason for a carefully conducted clinical examination of hearing, including pure tone threshold measures at frequencies 250 Hz (middle C) through 8000 Hz (five octaves above middle C).

Apparently one normally functioning ear is sufficient for normal language development. Very little hard data are available on this issue, but clinicians are not of the impression that the speech and language of unilaterally deafened (e.g., following mumps, virus) children are noticeably different from those of children with two normally functioning ears.

Voice Disorders

A common childhood voice disorder is hoarseness resulting from vocal abuse. Unchecked, the condition of the vocal folds can progress from mild irritation and edema to formation of nodules. Nodules respond to vocal rest and often to a change in pitch. Group as well as individual therapy has been successful in locating the causes of the abuse and helping the individual to take responsibility for vocal output. Behavior modification—e.g., counting uses of loud voice and timing total use of voice—has been effective.

Nasality following adenoidectomy is not uncommon, and most patients become normal in a few hours or days. Occasionally, nasality continues and the child is found to have palatal insufficiency or submucous cleft. In such cases, the adenoid tissue served to fill in the nasopharyngeal space. The necessity of preoperative recognition of a submucous cleft, velopharyngeal insufficiency, or congenitally short palate is discussed in Chapter 17.

Cleft Palate

The child born with a cleft lip/cleft palate faces years of restorative procedures and rehabilitation. Among the disciplines needed are pediatrics, prosthodontics, pedodontics, nutrition, education, audiology and speech pathology, otolaryngology, and maxillofacial surgery. Therefore, coordinated management is essential.

Cleft palate deformity is often associated with conductive hearing loss.

Vocal play helps the baby develop a perception of his oral structure and of the sounds he is producing. Cleft palate not only compromises oral sensation but also is frequently accompanied by hearing loss, impairing auditory feedback and environmental stimulation.

In cases of cleft palate, the speech product is excessively nasal. Problems related to nasal resonance are discussed later in the section on voice disorders of adults. Of equal significance are the articulation problems that accompany velopharyngeal insufficiency. That is, the precision of plosive (p-b-t-d-k-g), fricative (s-z-f-v-th-sh-zh), and affricate (ch-dzh) consonants is reduced through nasal escape. The child may grimace in an effort to occlude his nares to prevent the escape of air. In the case of repaired cleft lip, sounds likely to be affected are those requiring lip closure, rounding, and extension (p-b-m-oo-ee).

Regardless of whether surgery, prosthesis, or both affect structural repair, the child may still have inadequate velopharyngeal closure for speech. Assistance with precise, rapid articulation of speech is necessary. Speech outcome is one criterion for success of surgical/prosthetic management.

The cleft palate child is at risk for oral sensation deficits, feeding problems, social/emotional problems, developmental delay, and speech and language problems associated with hearing impairment.

Stuttering

Stuttering is a fluency disorder or an abnormality of speech rate or rhythm. All speakers experience normal dysfluency, such as pauses or word repetitions. When the dysfluencies call attention to themselves or the speaker struggles to avoid the dysfluency, the speaker is considered a stutterer. The stutterer may repeat words or sounds, prolong sounds, or "block," thus producing no sound at all. In addition, these speech behaviors may be accompanied by muscular tension and struggling. Secondary characteristics may include head jerks, eye blinks, and facial contortions.

The speech of many children with dysfluencies at ages 3 and 4 will improve spontaneously.

It is important to know that many children have exaggerated dysfluencies at around three to four years of age. These interruptions are not associated with any struggle or tension in speaking and usually disappear spontaneously. Parents may need reassurance about normal dysfluencies. They should avoid overreacting to the dysfluencies while responding positively to the sense of the child's communication. If marked dysfluencies continue, the child and his parents should be referred to a speech pathologist.

Approximately 1 per cent of the population consider themselves to be stutterers. Most begin to stutter before they enter school. There are a number of schools of thought regarding the cause and nature of stuttering, each with a preferred approach to therapy. Each method has been shown to be successful for some patients.

Behavioral/Emotional Disorders

Children with behavioral/emotional disorders often have associated language disorders, including mutism, disordered content of speech, comprehension deficits, poor communicative interaction, and atypical vocal characteristics. The specific type of language disorder, e.g., neologisms, pronoun reversals, echolalia, excessive talkativeness, is often useful in establishing a differential diagnosis. Children with the most severe disturbances, autistic disorder or schizophrenia, always exhibit extreme language disturbance.

There are some children whose emotional disturbance is thought to be a primary "cause" of the language problem. Emotional disturbance can also "result" from the inability to communicate. In either case, the communication problem warrants evaluation by a speech pathologist.

Cerebral Palsy

The child with cerebral palsy requires a specialized orientation of the speech pathologist and of the physician as well. Knowledge of body tone, sensation, posture, and reflexes is essential.

Before speech can be acquired, the child needs an oral musculature that can manage basic vegetative functions such as eating or swallowing. The optimum posture for breath support to produce voice should be established. The speech of the cerebral palsied child reflects his basic neurophysiologic condition. Voice quality, speech sound articulation, respiration rate, and rhythm are distorted by flaccidity, spasticity, rigidity, tremor, or athetosis.

The language of the physically disabled child is frequently affected by his experiential limitations. Moreover, because by definition cerebral palsy involves brain damage, the child may manifest many or all of the features associated with language disability or organic mental retardation. In the case of cerebral palsy related to Rh incompatibility and kernicterus, sensorineural hearing loss with the resultant speech and language difficulties may occur.

The ability to communicate is more crucial than the ability to speak. When a child has severe motor speech limitations, alternate or supplementary communication systems (e.g., word or symbol boards or computer-assisted communication) may be necessary.

Coordinated rehabilitation services including those of the physician and occupational and physical therapists, social worker, speech pathologist, and others are necessary.

Specific Language Disabilities

Children with specific learning disabilities have deficits in one or more of the processes basic to normal, efficient learning. Although there are other characteristics, most learning disabled children have some language disorder. As a group, learning disabled children have average intelligence. They may have problems forming verbal abstractions and performing the logical operations required to interpret the complex relationships expressed in language. Their oral language problems may lead to deficits in perceiving and interpreting as well as in formulating and producing spoken language. The difficulties may also be reflected in subject areas such as reading, spelling, writing, and other academic areas that require adequate language abilities.

While some language disabilities change over time, others persist throughout life. A child with language disorders requires special services. Remedial and compensatory education and therapy are available through schools, hospitals, and special clinics.

Mental Retardation

In contrast to children with specific language disorder or emotional disturbance, retarded children are retarded generally. They are delayed in socioemotional, intellectual, and perceptual-motor development as well as in language. The greater the severity of general retardation, the greater the language delay. The profoundly retarded child may not talk at all.

Articulation Disorders

The child who has defective speech articulation may have difficulty with the precision or sequencing of speech sounds. At any given age, certain articulation errors fall within normal developmental expectations (Table 21–2).

In the rare incidence that a tight lingual frenum affects speech, a simple "Z" plasty can be performed.

Parents are sometimes concerned that a child's speech problem is related to being "tongue-tied" when, in fact, a lingual frenum would need to be extremely restricted to account for an articulation disorder. Almost all children compensate for "tongue-tie," and, in many cases, the restriction lessens over time.

The most prevalent type of articulation disorder is called functional misarticulation. There are four types: substitution, omission, distortion, and addition. Functional articulation disorders (the largest single disorder category) are common among young school-aged children.

Two other types of articulation disorders are associated with physiological problems. Children with dysarthria have imprecise speech for reasons of paralysis, weakness, or lack of coordination of the speech mechanism. When the difficulty involves the selection, programming, or sequencing of sounds,

TABLE 21–2. ACQUISITION OF ENGLISH CONSONANTS

DEVELOPMENTAL AGE	SOUNDS MASTERED*
2	p, h, n, b, k, f
2½	m, g
3	w, d, y, v
3½	s
4	sh
4½	t, ng, ch, r, l, z, th

*By 50% of children in all positions of a word. Source: Olmsted D: Out of the Mouths of Babes. The Hague, Mouton, 1971.

it is called apraxia of speech. Dysarthria and apraxia can severely limit the child's ability to develop fluent speech.

SPEECH AND LANGUAGE DISORDERS IN ADULTS

Adult communication disorders can refer to any number of difficulties that lead to impaired or ineffective communication. The disorders most frequently encountered by otolaryngologists are voice disorders of laryngectomees. However, an adult may have other disorders affecting communication that can have implications for medical and therapeutic intervention.

Voice Disorders

Voice is an acoustical end-product of a smooth, balanced, dynamic, interrelated system involving respiration, phonation, and resonance. A subglottic pressure of air from the lungs, compressed by abdominal and thoracic musculature, is addressed against the vocal folds. Sound is produced by rapid opening and closing of the cords, set into vibration by a smooth combination of muscular tension and rapid air pressure changes. The pitch is largely determined by the frequency of cord vibration.

Sound produced at the glottis is amplified and is supplied with characteristic quality (resonance) as it moves through supraglottic passages, especially the pharynx. Disturbance of this system can result in voice disorder.

Voice problems have been estimated to occur in 1 per cent of all people in the United States. Reported incidence of voice disorders in school children ranges from 6 to 23.4 per cent.

Organic versus Functional Disorders

Voice problems may be functional, organic, or an interaction of both. Functional voice disorders result from improper use of an otherwise normal mechanism. Frequently, functional voice disorders occur with vocal abuse or personality disturbances. Emotional stress may produce musculoskeletal tension that can contribute to improper vocal use. Organic voice disorders result from pathophysiologic disease that alters laryngeal structure or function. Some disorders (e.g., papillomata, leukoplakia) require medical or surgical intervention. Most functional disorders and many organic problems (e.g., nodules, unilateral adductor paralysis) respond to symptomatic remediation.

Emotional stress can contribute to improper vocal use.

Vocal Parameters (Pitch, Loudness, Quality)

Most people speak at a habitual *pitch* level natural and appropriate for their physiology. Inappropriate pitch that is inconsistent with the person's appearance or his vocal physiology may or may not be socially acceptable. Pitch deviations can be responsible for laryngeal strain or insult and quality disorders.

The average speaker should have little difficulty modulating vocal intensity. Since *loudness* control depends upon auditory feedback, evaluation of the hearing of the patient who has difficulty should be considered. Although there may be an emotional basis for habitual excessive loudness, the relationship of excessive loudness to background noise is striking. At times, excessive loudness may be habituated and sustained in the absence of background noise.

Vocal *quality* can be subjectively described by numerous terms, two of which are "harshness" and "hoarseness," vocal attributes denoting roughness and rough-breathiness. They often accompany or follow periods of vocal abuse. Singers, teachers, and others who must vocalize in public for prolonged periods of time develop harsh or hoarse voices, especially when amplifying equipment is absent. Sports fans and others who shout are also likely to be in this category. The majority have only temporary difficulty allayed by a few hours of vocal rest, but a semichronic condition is not uncommon under these circumstances.

Adductor hyperfunction seems to be implicated in all vocal abuse. In many, vocalization is initiated with a hard glottal explosion called the "glottal attack." Over a period of time, irritation and edema of the vocal folds may develop. The hyperfunction unchecked, the edges of the folds are at risk for the development of nodule(s). As the nodule grows, vocal pitch may drop due to larger mass, the rough quality will increase, and breathiness may be noticed as air escapes around the nodule.

Adductor spastic dysphonia, which is characterized by a choked, strained, harsh voice, seems to be an extreme example of hyperfunction, although it is seemingly "resistant" to therapeutic techniques. The suspicion remains that spastic dysphonia has an important psychological component, but this has not often been verified by successful response to psychotherapy. It has also been considered a possible manifestation of regional neurologic disturbance. Fortunately, its incidence is low.

Long-term results of recurrent laryngeal nerve section for spastic dysphonia have not been as effective as immediate results. Injected botulinum toxin is currently being evaluated.

Surgical therapy by intentionally interrupting the recurrent laryngeal nerve has been of benefit in very carefully selected patients but is never preferred prior to thorough evaluation and attempted correction by more conservative means. Long-term results have not been as beneficial as initially predicted.

Breathiness seems to result from adductor hypofunction. The breathy quality betrays a short approximation phase and in the whisper, the cords do not touch at all. Breathiness is usually responsive to symptomatic treatment. In these disorders, thorough evaluation of vocal cord movement, preferably by magnified fiberoptic examination, is required.

"Hyponasality" and "hypernasality" are resonance problems involving the functioning of the oral, nasal, and pharyngeal cavities and their attachments. The nasopharyngeal sphincter demands a functioning soft palate in relation to a dynamic superior constrictor muscle on the posterior pharyngeal wall. The sphincter remains relatively closed through most speech sounds with the exception of "m," "n," and "ng." Consider the speed and ballistic precision required to include nasal consonant sounds without contaminating adjacent non-nasal sounds. Chronic failure to accomplish this is "assimilated nasality."

Many good speakers demonstrate some nasality. Persons with cleft palates have obvious difficulties. Chronic hypernasality should lead to further evaluation.

Hyponasality requires evaluation of the nasal cavity and the nasopharynx.

Hyponasality is the reduction or absence of nasality when it normally should occur. Thus, it affects only three speech sounds (m, n, and ng). "Something is in my nose" becomes "subthig is id by doze." And often that is the case. The phenomenon is associated with the congestion and edema of upper respiratory tract infection, but continued denasality requires examination for hypertrophic adenoids, a mass of some kind, or structural deformity.

Voice Therapy

Following medical examination, the speech and language pathologist can utilize several techniques that may help the voice patient achieve a more normal voice. The first step is to increase the patient's ability to monitor his own vocal production and to increase awareness of situations in which vocal abuse can occur. Other treatment goals may include (1) educating the patient regarding normal anatomy and physiology of the vocal mechanism; (2) eliminating faulty speaking habits; (3) reducing vocal abuse; (4) decreasing musculoskeletal tension; and (5) counseling.

Prior to surgical intervention, the patient should receive a trial period of voice therapy. Therapy for non–life-threatening disorders can often alleviate the need for surgery. Then the physician, with input from the speech and language pathologist, can determine the best course of action for the patient.

Post-surgical patients, if not referred to the speech and language pathologist prior to surgery, can benefit from therapeutic intervention to reduce trauma to the vocal folds. A brief period of voice rest, no more than a few days, may help patients recovering from vocal fold surgery. However, there is no evidence that voice rest is of benefit to patients in general, and it may be harmful to those with psychogenic disorders.

Alaryngeal Speech

A person who has undergone laryngectomy must make many adjustments afterward. One of the most difficult is that of learning to communicate again.

Mechanistic Effects of Laryngectomy

Removal of the larynx separates respiration from speech, eliminates the vibratory source for phonation as it has existed (the glottis), and leaves articulation relatively intact. The laryngectomized person breathes through the tracheal stoma. Instead of the same passage for pulmonary and phonatory air, the trachea serves only for pulmonary exchange. Usually, in cases of total laryngectomy, the esophagus remains intact as a connecting passage from the mouth and pharynx to the stomach. It is in the pharyngoesophageal region that a new vibratory source for voice production must be established. This region is identified as the pseudoglottis or neoglottis. The new voice is called "esophageal" or "alaryngeal." Approximately 60 to 75 per cent of all laryngectomees learn some form of esophageal speech, but not all become excellent or even adequate speakers. Another 15 per cent communicate only by means of artificial devices, and the remainder do not learn to communicate orally.

Methods for Achieving Esophageal Voice

There are essentially two methods for air intake to produce esophageal voice: injection and inhalation. Swallowing as a method of air intake is not encouraged because the act of swallowing does not allow for the rapid injection and expulsion of air required for speech.

During injection, air in the mouth or nose is compressed by movement of the lips or tongue and injected into the esophagus. This may be accomplished by consciously placing the lips together, or the tongue tip against the alveolar ridge, or the dorsum of the tongue against the hard palate, and pushing the

Alaryngeal speakers do not swallow air but use the tongue to inject air into the esophagus.

"ball of air" into the throat. Certain consonant sounds (e.g., p, t, and k) serve to drive air into the esophagus. This is called "consonant injection." The laryngectomee who is able to use consonant injection has a built-in "pumping action," so that in connected speech, he is continually "recharging."

During inhalation, the patient maintains a patent airway between the nose or lips and the esophagus. As he inhales through the stoma, there is increased negative pressure in the esophagus, creating a partial vacuum. If the pharyngoesophageal segment is relaxed, the higher pressure in the mouth and hypopharynx pushes air into the esophagus. The inhalation method has the advantage of being very natural, since pulmonary and phonatory air are in synchrony. It is quite possible for a laryngectomee to use a combination of methods.

Inhalation of air into the esophagus is possible if there is relaxation of the nasopharynx.

The Artificial Larynx

The artificial larynx is another means for producing voice for speech. There are several types of devices. A common device is one which is held in the hand, usually against the neck. Sound is transmitted through tissue and then articulated into words. A similar electronic device is one in which a tone generator held in the hand is connected to a plastic tube inserted into the mouth. This device is of particular value to the laryngectomee who cannot use an instrument on his neck because of extensive neck surgery or radiation. A third type of device is pneumatic; air is driven from the stoma to the mouth, using a vibrating reed as sound source (Fig. 21–2). The speech and language pathologist can assist the laryngectomee in selection and use of an appropriate artificial larynx.

In the past it was sometimes believed that the artificial device should be withheld from the laryngectomee, lest it serve as a "crutch" and thus reduce the motivation to learn esophageal voice. This has never been proved to be so. In fact, there is some evidence that patients using the artificial larynx will talk more, thus promoting the development of esophageal voice. In most centers today, the artificial larynx is demonstrated and sometimes lent

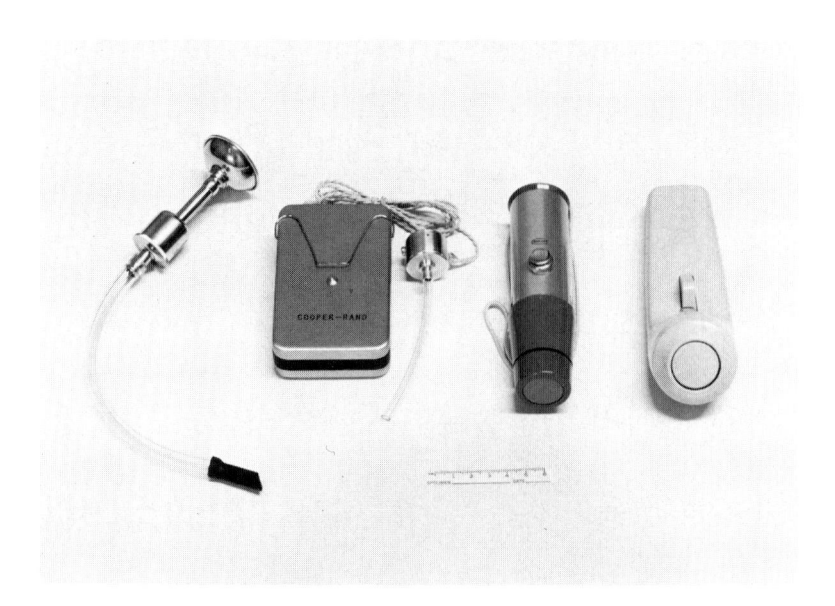

FIGURE 21–2. Some instruments for alaryngeal speech communication. From left to right, Tokyo Artificial Larynx, Cooper-Rand Artificial Larynx, Servox Speech Aid, and Western Electric #5 Electrolarynx.

to the patient at the first visit. Esophageal speech is presented as an ultimate objective, but the patient is also advised that not all laryngectomees are able to learn it. Some refuse the artificial larynx, which sounds less like the normal voice than does esophageal speech. Sometimes the patient will request it later. The decision should be the patient's. The artificial larynx may be particularly useful for telephoning while the patient is at the beginning stages of learning esophageal voice.

Tracheoesophageal Puncture and Voice Prosthesis

Dr. Mark Singer, an otolaryngologist, and Eric Blom, Ph.D., a speech and language pathologist, have reported and popularized a surgical procedure that allows a laryngectomee to speak on his own lung air. While the puncture can be made at the time of the laryngectomy, most surgeons prefer to wait for six months to allow the patient to try to learn esophageal speech and the stoma to be fully matured. The puncture is made through the posterior tracheal wall into the esophagus, and a one-way valve tube is inserted. The laryngectomee's exhaled air is shunted through the silicone prosthesis into the esophagus when the stoma is occluded, and fluent speech is possible (Fig. 21–3). Selection of a prosthetic low-pressure valve is now available. The valve is removed, cleaned daily, and reinserted. It has an average life span of three months. The speech and language pathologist works with the surgeon in patient selection, fitting the prosthesis, and educating the patient in use and care of the prosthesis and in troubleshooting techniques.

Course of Treatment

Rehabilitation should begin, whenever possible, before surgery. A presurgical visit to the patient by a speech pathologist and, when indicated, by a successful laryngectomized speaker informs him that help will be available. Some laryngectomized patients have reported after surgery that they were

A presurgical visit and discussion about rehabilitation is essential.

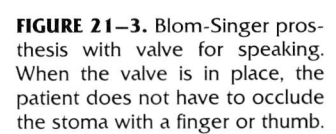

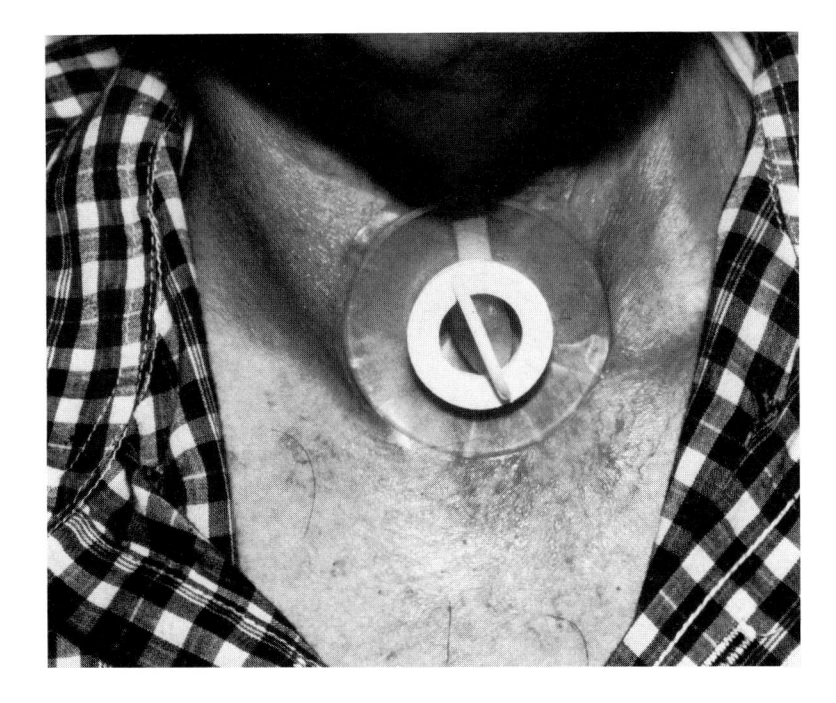

FIGURE 21–3. Blom-Singer prosthesis with valve for speaking. When the valve is in place, the patient does not have to occlude the stoma with a finger or thumb.

frightened or unimpressed by visiting esophageal speakers. Some were unaware that speech would be possible.

The presurgical visit provides an opportunity to assess communication skills and to determine whether faulty speech habits, unrelated to the loss of the larynx, need attention. Cognition and hearing can be appraised. The physician should be especially alert for selective hearing impairment that might compromise the discrimination of consonant sounds.

Instruction in the use of an artificial larynx is necessary in order to obtain the best speech product. Treatment goals include effective tube placement, accurate on/off timing, accurate articulation, correct phrasing and appropriate rate, and appropriate inflection and stress.

Patients are fed through a nasogastric tube for 7 to 10 days after a laryngectomy.

Esophageal speech instruction commonly begins as soon as the nasogastric tube has been removed and the surgeon indicates that there is little chance of a fistula. Some laryngectomees can produce a sound in the first few sessions, although the sound is not yet useful for communication purposes. The rehabilitation of functional communication skills takes months, sometimes years. Early esophageal speech instruction can help to prevent undesirable speech behaviors such as "duck voice," "klunking," and stomal blast.

Factors Related to Success and Failure

Some laryngectomees learn esophageal speech more readily than others, and some speakers are more proficient than others. Approximately 25 to 40 per cent do not master functional esophageal voice.

The relationship between speaking skill and various physical and psychological factors has been explored by many investigators. A number have concurred that type and extent of surgery or radiation have little effect on the ability to learn esophageal speech. Some motivated individuals who are unable to learn esophageal speech may be experiencing pharyngoesophageal spasm during attempted phonation. An esophageal insufflation test will reveal such spasms. In addition, a videofluoroscopic swallowing study may reveal an otherwise unrecognized problem such as a web, stricture, or spasm which precludes developing speech. In selected incidences, a myotomy of the constrictors may benefit these patients. In addition, hearing impairment, medical problems, cognitive impairment, and psychological characteristics have also been cited as reasons for failure to learn esophageal speech.

Group Support

Laryngectomees help each other, providing information and encouragement to the new patient. The patient should be made aware of the International Association of Laryngectomees, in care of the American Cancer Society, 90 Park Avenue, New York, New York 10016.

Other Communication Disorders

Aphasia is a language disorder resulting from a dominant hemisphere cerebrovascular accident, head trauma, or disease process. There are several types of aphasia, usually classified according to site of lesion. All aphasic persons exhibit deficits in comprehension, reading, verbal expression, and writing to a greater or lesser degree.

Occasionally, when the lesion producing the aphasia is anterior, the patient may have a concomitant motor speech disorder. *Apraxia of speech* is a disorder in the selection, programming, or sequencing of speech sounds and their combinations to form words. The most common characteristics of apraxic speech are sound substitutions, inconsistent and unpredictable errors, and groping behaviors indicating awareness of errors.

Dysarthria is a motor speech disorder due to abnormal tone, paralysis, weakness, or incoordination of the speech mechanism. Dysarthria can involve respiration, phonation, resonation, articulation, and prosody. Speech may sound slurred, uneven, distorted, or nasal. The general goal of speech therapy is to compensate for unintelligibility.

Patients with *right hemisphere deficits* may exhibit disturbances in attention, orientation, perception, pragmatic communication skills, memory, and integration. Speech and language may be intact, but the cognitively impaired patient may have much more difficulty in communicating appropriately than the aphasic patient.

The *head injured* patient may demonstrate any of the previous disorders, most notably aphasia, dysarthria, and cognitive deficits. During recovery, the head-injured patient usually goes through rather predictable stages of recovery.

ORAL DYSFUNCTION/DYSPHAGIA

Dysphagia, a deficit in the ability to swallow, can occur in both children and adults. Children with neurologic, behavioral, or structural deficits may have oral motor and/or swallowing problems such as weak or inefficient suck, poor oral intake, failure to thrive, choking, refusal to eat orally, and inability to handle foods of differing texture at appropriate developmental ages. Problems can be congenital or acquired. Children frequently develop oral aversion if not fed by mouth for extended periods of time (three weeks or longer). Following medical examination, speech and language pathologists evaluate the problem with a clinical feeding/swallowing assessment and/or a videofluoroscopic study to determine the reasons for the problem and to plan a therapeutic feeding program. Intervention can include oral stimulation or desensitization, oral motor training, or modification of position, equipment, or food consistencies.

In adults, anatomic or neuromuscular disorders may result in dysphagia. A patient may complain of difficulty chewing or swallowing, food "sticking" in the throat, coughing/choking while eating or drinking, and other symptoms. Following a thorough medical examination, the speech and language pathologist can perform a clinical swallowing evaluation to gain valuable information regarding history, oral function, and symptoms. If the speech and language pathologist suspects pharyngeal dysfunction, which may occur without observable clinical symptoms, a modified barium swallow should be performed in cooperation with the radiologist. In some medical facilities all tracheotomized and head and neck cancer patients are routinely evaluated by a swallowing team.

The modified barium swallow is a videofluoroscopic or cineradiographic procedure that allows the swallowing process to be viewed and stored on tape or film for further study. It involves giving the patient several textures (liquid, paste, solid) of contrast medium and viewing the swallowing process.

The clinician may change the patient's position or use special techniques to facilitate the swallow during the study. Information gained from the modified barium swallow, particularly the presence or absence of aspiration, is necessary for making decisions regarding oral feeding and treatment procedures.

SOURCES OF SPEECH PATHOLOGY SERVICES

A referral to a speech and language pathologist should be made if any of the previously discussed problems is observed by the physician or family. The speech pathologist is a health professional specialized by academic preparation, supervised practice, internship experience, national board examination, and certification to rehabilitate patients with speech, language, and swallowing disorders. The private practice of speech pathology tends to be concentrated in large cities, although these services are beginning to have broader distribution. Speech pathologists may also be attached to hospitals, speech and hearing centers, school systems, and departments of education and health. In some states, licensing boards maintain registries of certified speech pathologists. Many state speech and hearing associations have annual directories identifying their members. A national directory of speech pathologists can be obtained from the American Speech-Language-Hearing Association, 10801 Rockville Pike, Rockville, Maryland 20852.

References

Aronson AE: Clinical Voice Disorders. 2nd ed. New York, Thieme, Inc, 1985.
Gabbard SA: References for communication disorders related to otitis media. Semin Speech Lang Hear 3:351, 1982.
Hall P, Tomblin J: A follow-up study of children with articulation and language disorders. J Speech Hear Disord 43:227–241, 1978.
Logemann J: Evaluation and Treatment of Swallowing Disorders. San Diego, College Hill, Inc, 1983.
McClean J, Snyder-McClean L: A Transactional Approach to Early Language Training. Columbus, OH, Charles E. Merrill, 1978.
McClowry D, Guilford A, Richardson S: Infant Communication: Development, Assessment, and Intervention. New York, Grune and Stratton, Inc, 1982.
Milisen R: The incidence of speech disorders. *In* Travis L (ed): Handbook of Speech Pathology and Audiology. New York, Appleton-Century-Crofts, 1970.
Salmon S: Factors that may interfere with acquiring esophageal speech. *In* Keith R, Darby F: Laryngectomee Rehabilitation. 2nd ed. San Diego, College Hill Press, Inc, 1986.
Senturia B, Wilson F: Otorhinolaryngologic findings in children with voice deviations. Preliminary report. Ann Otolaryngol Rhinol Laryngol 22:1027–1042, 1968.
Shames G, Florance C: Disorders of Fluency. *In* Shames G, Wiig E (eds): Human Communication Disorders. Columbus, OH, Charles E. Merrill, 1982.
Silverman E, Zimmer C: Incidence of chronic hoarseness among school-aged children. J Speech Hear Disord 40:211–215, 1975.
Singer EM, Blom E: An endoscopic technique for restoration of voice after laryngectomy. Ann Otolaryngol Rhinol Laryngol 90:529–533, 1980.
Wiig E, Semel E: Language Assessment and Intervention for the Learning Disabled. 2nd ed. Columbus, OH, Charles E. Merrill, 1984.

PART SIX

NEOPLASMS OF THE HEAD AND NECK

22

BENIGN NECK MASSES

by James I. Cohen, M.D., Ph.D.

The neck is an exposed area of the body and therefore swellings in this area are easily recognized by the patient or detected during routine examination. In addition, congenital, inflammatory, and malignant cervical lesions are relatively common. Thus physicians are often confronted with the problem of a new lump in the neck. The purpose of this chapter is to develop a rational approach to the management of the most commonly encountered neck masses, excluding thyroid disease.

ANATOMIC CONSIDERATIONS

The anatomic boundaries of the neck are as follows: superiorly the lower border of the mandible, the mastoid tips, and the superior nuchal line; inferiorly the suprasternal notch, the clavicles, and a horizontal line through the spinous process of the seventh cervical vertebra (Fig. 22–1). For descriptive purposes, the neck is divided into two halves by the vertical midline, and each side is further divided into an anterior and posterior triangle by the sternocleidomastoid muscle. Most masses appear in the anterior cervical triangle.

The sternocleidomastoid muscle divides each side of the neck into two triangles.

The surface landmarks of the neck, which are normally palpable, include the mandible, the submandibular glands, the tail of the parotid glands, the hyoid bone, the larynx, the thyroid, the trachea, the sternocleidomastoid muscles, the clavicles, and the cervical vertebrae (Fig. 22–1). These structures are therefore used to further define a number of regions in the neck (Fig. 22–2), which are important in describing the position of a lump in the neck.

DIAGNOSTIC EVALUATION

The evaluation of any neck mass begins with a careful history. A logical series of questions can quickly narrow down the diagnostic possibilities and streamline subsequent investigations and management (Table 22–1). These questions and their significance are listed below:

1. What is the age of the patient? Congenital lesions are far more common in younger individuals, whereas malignant lesions are more likely in the elderly.

   The older the patient, the more likely the neck mass is malignant.

2. Is the mass growing rapidly? In the absence of signs of infection, malignant lesions (lymphoma, metastatic cancer) are far more likely to experience rapid growth than benign ones.

430 PART SIX—NEOPLASMS OF THE HEAD AND NECK

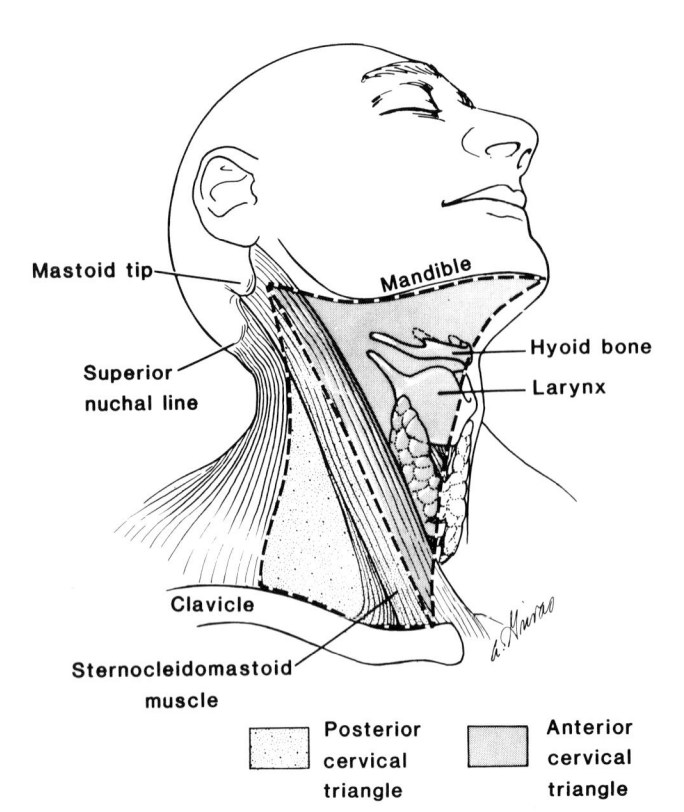

FIGURE 22–1. Surface anatomy and anatomic boundaries of the neck. The normally palpable structures in the neck are shown.

3. Is there evidence of infection or inflammation? While any neck mass can become infected, those masses that appear inflamed or infected are far more likely to be benign.
4. Where in the neck is the mass located? The position of the mass should be carefully described in the following terms: Is it midline or lateral?

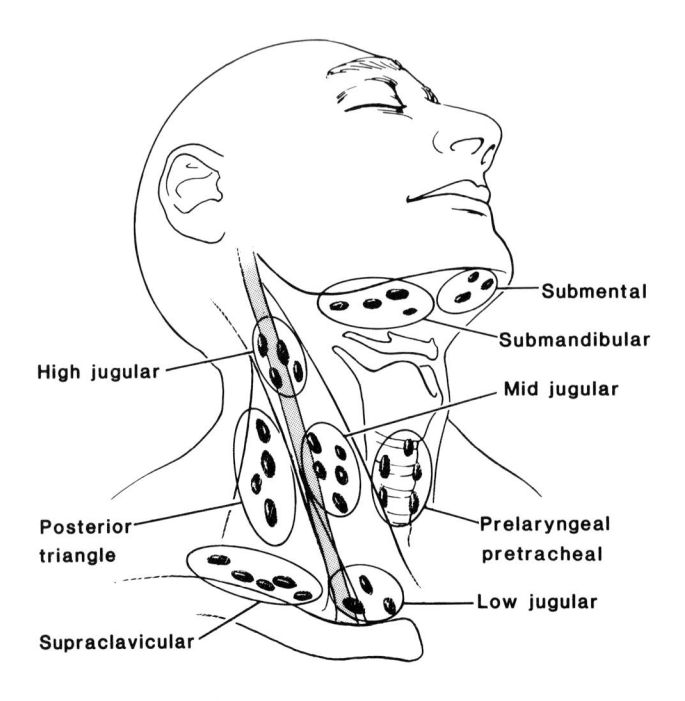

FIGURE 22–2. Anatomic regions of the neck. The neck is divided into a number of regions that are useful in describing the location of a neck mass.

TABLE 22–1. DIAGNOSIS OF A NECK MASS: PERTINENT QUESTIONS

1. What is the age of the patient?
2. Is the mass growing rapidly?
3. Is there evidence of infection or inflammation?
4. Where in the neck is the mass located?
5. Is the mass cystic or solid?
6. Is there evidence of infection or malignancy elsewhere in the head and neck?

If it is lateral, is it in the anterior or posterior triangle (Fig. 22–2)? In addition, the relation of the mass to any of the normally palpable structures and regions of the neck defined above (Figs. 22–1 and 22–2) should be stated. Midline masses are more likely to be related to the thyroid, whereas supraclavicular masses are far more likely to contain metastatic disease.

5. Is the mass cystic or solid? Cystic masses are more often congenital lesions such as branchial cleft cysts and thyroglossal duct cysts.
6. Is there any evidence of a source of infection or malignancy elsewhere in the head and neck?

Whenever a cystic or infected mass is drained, a portion of the cyst wall must be sent for pathological examination.

History and physical examination alone may answer all of these questions and establish a diagnosis, but often more information and tests are required. However, to avoid unnecessary investigations, each test should be designed (in advance) to answer a specific question and the answer would be important to the subsequent management of the mass.

Diagnostic tests for neck masses can be classified into two broad categories: (1) those that supply information about the physical characteristics or position of the mass (indirect tests) and (2) those that seek a histologic diagnosis (direct tests) (Table 22–2). Ultrasonography, CT scans, MRI scans, and angiography are examples of indirect tests. Ultrasound distinguishes solid from cystic lesions and should be used in the rare situation in which only this information is required. Angiography alone is useful to evaluate the vascularity, the specific blood supply of a mass, or the status of the carotid artery but gives little information about the physical characteristics of the mass itself. Alternatively, CT and/or MRI scans can provide information about both the physical characteristics and the vascularity of the mass and in addition define its relationship to adjacent structures (Fig. 22–3). Hence, they are the most useful of the indirect tests and are ordered most commonly.

Direct tests involve histologic examination of tissue from the mass. This tissue can be obtained in one of three different ways: (1) fine needle aspiration, (2) needle biopsy (Fig. 22–4), or (3) "open" biopsy. A fine needle aspiration involves the insertion of a small needle (23 to 25 gauge)

Fine needle aspiration (F.N.A.) is the preferred method of diagnosing a neck mass when immediate excision is not indicated.

TABLE 22–2. DIAGNOSTIC TESTS FOR NECK MASSES

Indirect Tests	Direct Tests
Ultrasound	Fine needle aspiration
CT scans	Needle biopsy
MRI scans	Open biopsy
Angiography	
Thyroid scan	

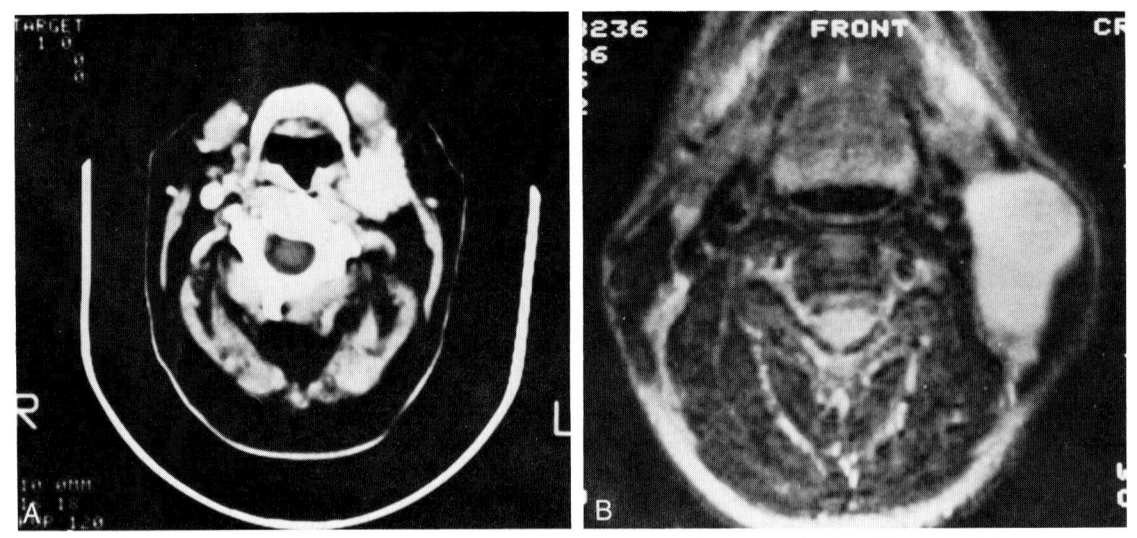

FIGURE 22–3. *A*, CT scan of a neck mass. A large mass is seen adjacent to the hyoid bone and deep to the sternocleidomastoid muscle. *B*, MRI scan of a neck mass. A large mass is seen deep to the sternocleidomastoid muscle. The carotid artery and internal jugular vein are seen deep to the mass.

Interpretation of a fine needle aspirate requires experience.

attached to a syringe into the mass to obtain sufficient cells for cytologic examination (Fig. 22–4). This procedure is generally well tolerated by patients and is both safe and accurate in experienced hands. Hence it is the preferred method at present. By contrast, large-bore needle biopsy methods (which obtain a "core" of tissue) (Fig. 22–4) and operative "open" biopsy techniques are more invasive and have a higher risk of "seeding" the malignancy and complicating future management.

By appropriate work-up most neck masses can be classified into one of the categories listed in Table 22–3. These will each be discussed separately below.

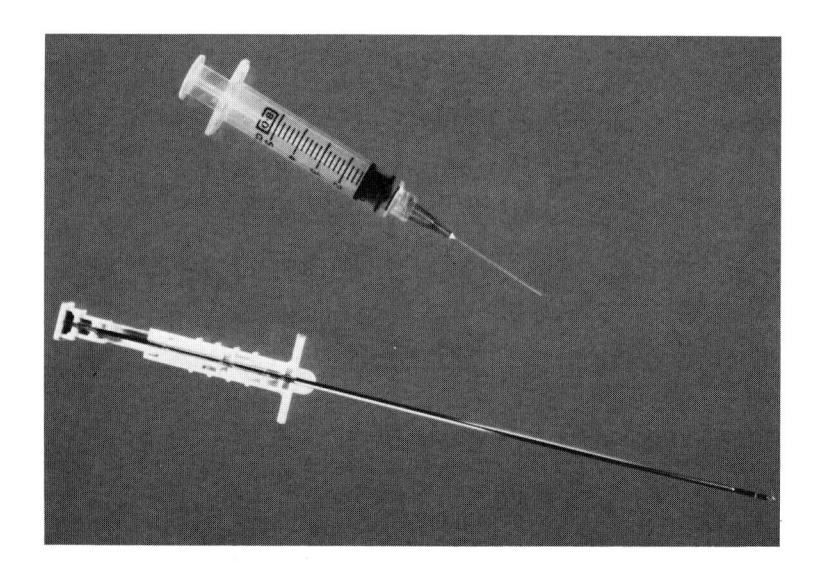

FIGURE 22–4. Needle biopsy techniques. The upper needle (25 gauge) attached to a syringe is used for fine needle aspiration of neck masses. The larger needle is used for "core" needle biopsies of neck masses.

TABLE 22–3. CLASSIFICATION OF NECK MASSES

Congenital Cystic Masses
  Thyroglossal duct cyst
  Branchial cleft cyst
  Cystic hygroma
Solid Masses
  Lymph node masses
    Infectious disease
    Lymphoma
    Metastatic disease
  Tumors of the neurovascular structures
    of the neck
    Neurogenic tumors
    Carotid body tumors
  Thyroid masses

CONGENITAL CYSTIC MASSES OF THE NECK

Branchial Cleft Cysts

Branchial cleft cysts are vestigial remnants of the fetal branchial apparatus from which all neck structures are derived. Early in development there are five branchial arches and four grooves (between them) present in the embryo (Fig. 22–5A). The rapid growth of the first and second arches and the epipericardial ridge (the future sternocleidomastoid muscle—Fig. 22–5B) submerges the third and fourth branchial arches and the second, third, and fourth branchial clefts into a large cavity known as the cervical sinus of His. Hence, most branchial cleft cysts (those that develop from the second, third, and fourth arches) usually present as a bulge or sinus tract opening along

Tracts from first branchial cleft cysts drain near the external auditory canal. The tract lies close to the facial nerve.

FIGURE 22–5. *A,* Development of the branchial arch apparatus. Early in development, there are five branchial arches and their associated clefts visible on the external surface of the embryo. *B,* Development of the branchial arch apparatus. As the embryo matures, the epipericardial ridge submerges the arches caudal to the second arch, thereby forming the cervical sinus of His.

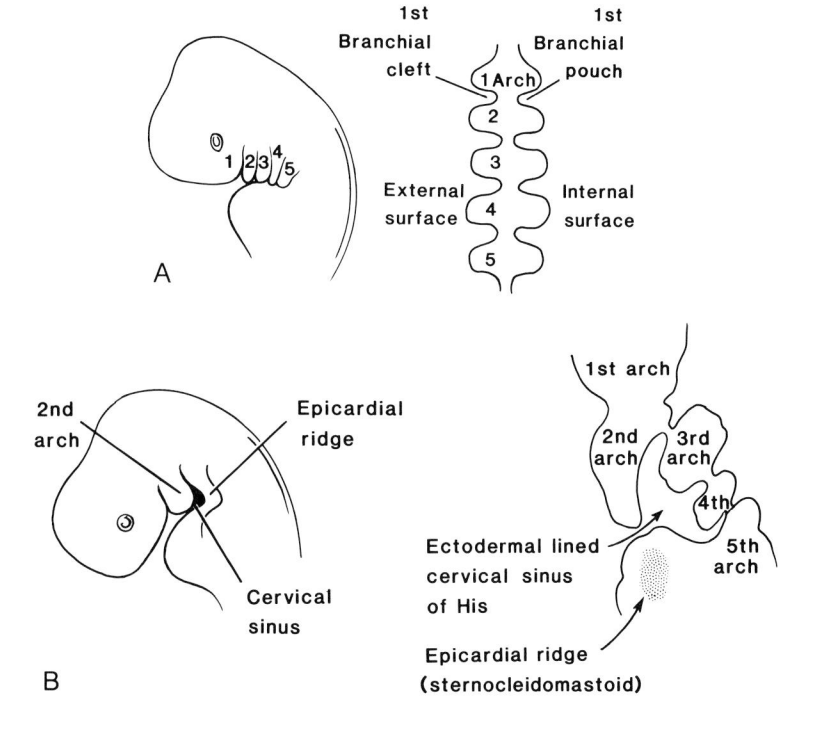

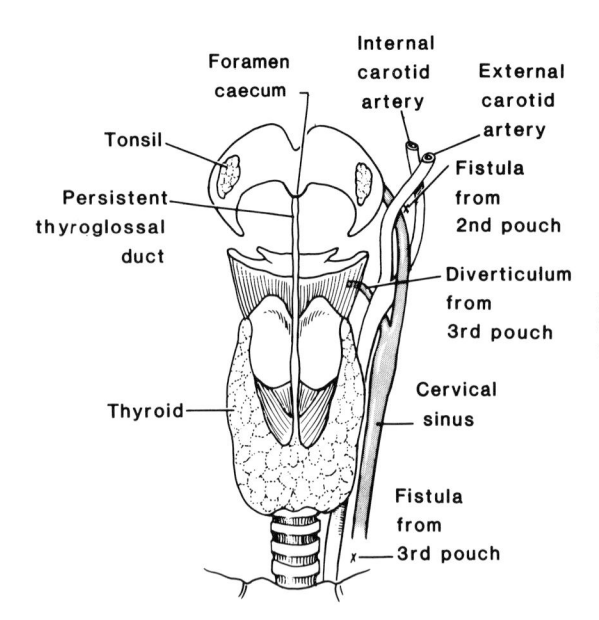

FIGURE 22–6. Branchial arch and thyroglossal duct vestiges. Cystic swellings may appear anywhere along the course of the development of these structures.

the anterior border of the sternocleidomastoid muscle. The internal tract or opening of such a cyst is situated at the embryologic derivative of the corresponding pharyngeal groove, i.e., the tonsil (second arch) or pyriform sinus (third and fourth arches). The position of the cyst tract is also determined by the embryologic relationship of its arch to the derivatives of the arches cephalad and caudal to it.

A branchial cleft cyst usually presents between the ages of 20 and 30 as a smooth, painless, slowly enlarging mass in the lateral neck. Infection of the cyst may be the reason for the first symptoms. Treatment consists of complete surgical removal of the cyst and tract. If infection or inflammation is present, this should be treated and allowed to settle prior to removal. Second branchial cleft cysts are by far the most common type. The tract of these cysts passes between the internal and external carotid arteries, above the hypoglossal nerve, and enters the pharynx in the tonsillar fossa (Fig. 22–6).

Thyroglossal Duct Cysts

A midline cyst that elevates with swallowing is most likely a thyroglossal duct cyst.

The thyroid gland is first seen as a ventral midline diverticulum of the floor of the pharynx just caudal to the junction of the first and second branchial arches at the site known as the foramen cecum. The developing thyroid migrates caudally along a tract that passes ventral to the body of the hyoid, then curves underneath it and downward to the level of the cricoid cartilage (Fig. 22–7). Thyroglossal duct cysts are vestigial remnants of this tract. Hence, they are usually midline cysts (Fig. 22–8) found anywhere between the base of the tongue and superior border of the thyroid gland.

Resection of the midportion of the hyoid bone reduces the recurrence rate of thyroglossal duct cysts.

Papillary carcinoma has been reported within thyroglossal duct cysts.

The treatment of a thyroglossal duct cyst consists of complete excision of both the cyst and the entire thyroglossal duct tract up to the foramen cecum at the base of the tongue. The intimate association of the tract with hyoid bone mandates simultaneous removal of the central portion of the hyoid to ensure complete removal of the tract (Sistrunk procedure). Failure to do this is the most common cause of recurrence. It is preferable to treat infected cysts with antibiotics until the inflammation subsides before excision.

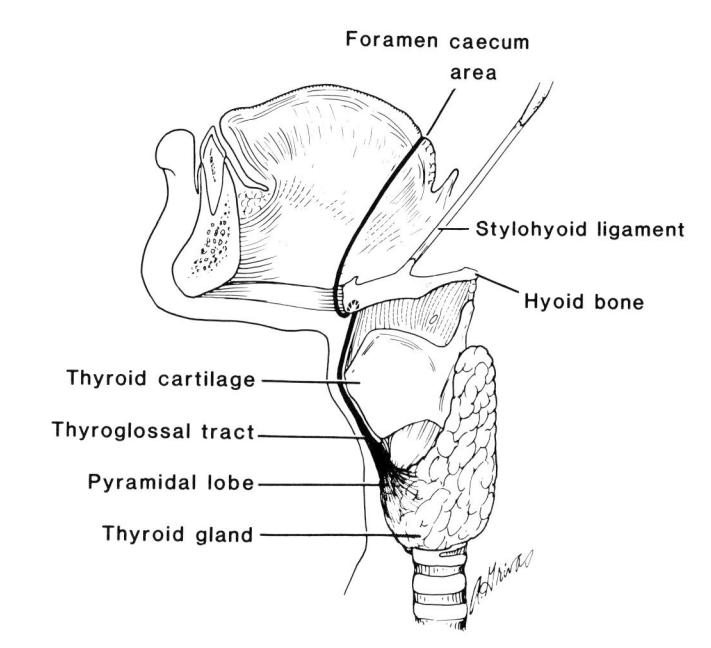

FIGURE 22–7. Course of the thyroglossal duct tract. The thyroglossal duct tract is intimately associated with the body of the hyoid bone. Therefore, this structure must be removed to ensure complete removal of the tract.

Cystic Hygroma

A cystic hygroma is a lymphangioma that arises from vestigial lymph channels in the neck. It may present as a relatively simple thin-walled cyst in the floor of the mouth or may involve all the tissues from the floor of the

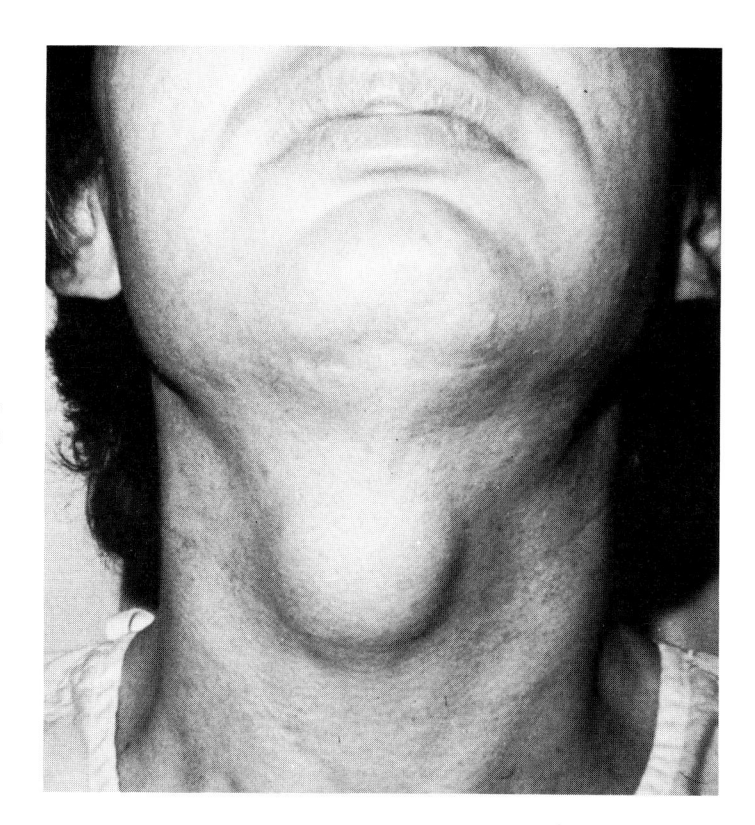

FIGURE 22–8. Typical appearance of a thyroglossal duct cyst. These cysts usually present as midline structures in the region of the hyoid bone.

436 PART SIX—NEOPLASMS OF THE HEAD AND NECK

mouth down to the mediastinum. However, approximately 80 per cent of the time there is only a painless cyst in the posterior cervical triangle or in the supraclavicular area. The majority of these tumors are present by the age of two. Sudden increases in size occasionally occur as a result of upper respiratory infections, infection of the mass itself, or hemorrhage into the tissues. If the mass becomes sufficiently large, it can cause compression of the trachea or difficulty in swallowing.

Treatment usually consists of complete surgical excision. However, because spontaneous regression has been known to occur, in the absence of pressure symptoms (obstruction of the airway or interference with swallowing) or gross deformity, these lesions should be treated expectantly at first. If regression fails to occur, then surgery should be undertaken. Excision can be difficult because of the numerous satellite extensions that often surround the main mass and because of the association of the tumor with vital structures such as the cranial nerves. Preservation of these nerves is recommended, and this often necessitates dissection through the mass itself. Hence, recurrences are common and staged procedures for complete excision are often necessary.

Complete surgical excision of a cystic hygroma can be difficult because of the numerous extensions of the cyst.

EVALUATION OF CERVICAL LYMPH NODES

Enlarged lymph nodes are by far the most common type of neck masses encountered. The cervical lymphatic system consists of interconnected groups or "chains" of nodes which parallel the major neurovascular structures in the head and neck (Fig. 22–9). The skin and mucosal surfaces of the head and neck all have specific and predictable nodes associated with them. Thus, the location of an enlarged lymph node is an important clue to the position of the primary disease.

There are general guidelines that may be helpful in the assessment of a

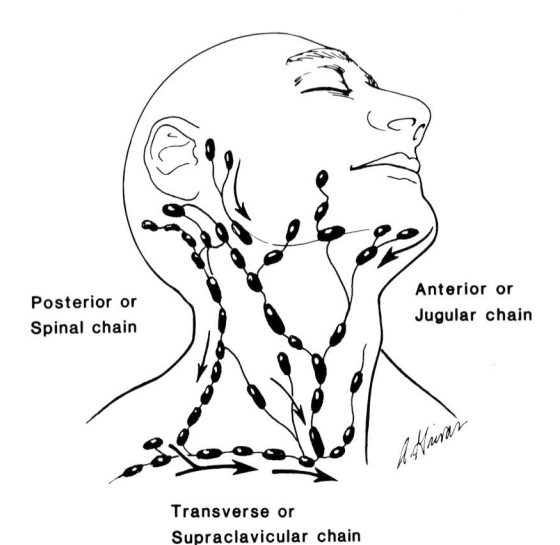

FIGURE 22–9. The cervical lymphatics. The lymph nodes of the neck are connected in a systematic and orderly fashion. The flow of lymph is believed to be unidirectional (arrows).

neck node. Tender neck nodes are more likely to be infectious in origin, whereas painless nodes are more likely to contain metastatic disease. Multiple regions of enlarged lymph nodes usually represent systemic disease such as lymphomas, tuberculosis, or infectious mononucleosis, whereas solitary nodes are more often metastatic. Low neck nodes are more likely to contain metastatic disease from a source other than the head and neck, whereas upper cervical nodes are more likely secondary to a head and neck source.

Open biopsy is the last step in the work-up of a neck mass. Prior to biopsy, direct examination of the nasopharynx, larynx, hypopharynx, and esophagus under anesthesia should be performed to rule out small lesions that are difficult to see with the patient awake. Only when all of these examinations fail to reveal a source of disease should an open biopsy be considered. Where possible, node biopsies should be excisional without violation of the mass itself. Vital structures must be preserved until a definitive diagnosis of cancer has been established. Skin incisions should be oriented in such a manner that they can be extended for the performance of a neck dissection, should it prove necessary.

> Consider an enlarging cervical lymph node in an individual over 60 years of age as malignant until proven otherwise.

> When a lymph node is excised for diagnosis, the incision should be planned for possible later incorporation for a radical neck dissection.

Nodal Enlargement Associated with Acute Infections

Many types of infectious diseases can cause lymph node enlargement, but most often the source is an acute infection of the mouth or pharynx. In this situation, the enlarged nodes are usually just posterior and inferior to the angle of the mandible. The patient usually has signs of acute infection such as fever or malaise and the localizing symptom of a sore mouth or throat. Treatment should be directed toward the primary disease.

Chronic Infections

Chronic infections that involve cervical lymph nodes include tuberculosis, fungal disease, syphilis, sarcoidosis, cat scratch fever, and AIDS (acquired immunodeficiency syndrome). Owing to their chronicity, these lymph node infections are easily confused with neoplasms, especially the lymphomas. While biopsy is occasionally necessary for diagnosis, skin tests and serologic study are often more useful. Treatment of all of these conditions is primarily medical, with surgery reserved for residual sinus tracts or other complications.

Malignant Lymphoma

Cervical adenopathy is one of the most common presenting symptoms in patients with Hodgkin's and non-Hodgkin's lymphoma. The nodes themselves tend to be softer, smoother, more elastic, and more mobile than nodes with metastatic carcinoma. Rapid growth is not unusual, particularly with non-Hodgkin's lymphoma. Extranodal sites, particularly Waldeyer's ring, are often involved in non-Hodgkin's lymphoma, and enlargement in this area may provide a clue to the diagnosis of this disease. Complete diagnosis requires an excisional biopsy of an intact lymph node. Fine needle aspiration alone is not enough. Treatment involves the use of radiation therapy and/or chemotherapy depending upon the pathologic type and clinical stage of the disease.

> Lymphoma can present as rapid growth of any area of Waldeyer's ring.

METASTATIC DISEASE

Metastatic malignancy should always be suspected when a firm, nontender enlarging mass is encountered in an older individual. In the great majority of cases the primary malignancy is located above the clavicle. This is particularly true for masses in the upper two thirds of the neck.

Metastatic Squamous Cell Carcinoma

The most common cancer that metastasizes to the cervical lymph nodes is squamous cell cancer from the skin of the face, scalp, lips, tongue, oral mucosa, nasopharynx, paranasal sinuses, oropharynx, hypopharynx, or larynx. A complete examination of these areas reveals the primary lesion in the majority of cases. If it can be discovered prior to biopsy of the metastatic site, then appropriate treatment can be planned to encompass both the primary and metastatic disease. By contrast, hurried neck biopsy without this search for a primary may contaminate the neck with cancer cells and complicate or delay treatment of the primary. Such factors can diminish the chances of cure.

When a thorough search for the source of the primary malignancy is made, and none is found, the metastatic cervical node is referred to as an "unknown primary" or "occult primary." The primary site is most likely in the base of the tongue, nasopharynx, or hypopharynx. A biopsy of these sites at the time of endoscopy, even when no primary tumor is apparent, is called a "directed biopsy."

The location of the node can be helpful in the diagnosis. For example, isolated supraclavicular nodes with squamous cell cancer in them usually represent metastatic disease from the lung. By contrast, squamous cell cancer in posterior triangle nodes is usually metastatic disease from the nasopharynx. Occasionally, however, despite the extensive search, no primary source of a metastatic squamous cell carcinoma of a cervical lymph node is found. In this situation, a neck dissection that encompasses the involved nodes should be done. Adjunctive postoperative radiation therapy should then be given to the neck and upper aerodigestive tract in most cases.

Metastatic Adenocarcinoma

Adenocarcinoma in a cervical node most frequently represents metastatic disease from the thyroid gland, salivary glands, or gastrointestinal tract. Thus, this situation also requires a thorough search for the primary tumor through endoscopic and radiologic study of the bronchopulmonary, gastrointestinal, and genitourinary tracts, salivary glands, and thyroid. In women, breast and pelvic tumors must also be considered.

Carotid Body Tumors

Carotid body tumors are one of a group of tumors known as chemodectomas which are derived from the chemoreceptive tissue of the head and neck. This specific tumor presents as a firm, round, slowly growing mass at the carotid bifurcation. The diagnosis can be made by CT scan and/or arteriography, which will demonstrate a characteristic highly vascular mass at the carotid bifurcation (Fig. 22–10). Biopsy should thus be avoided. These tumors are seldom malignant but should be removed in younger, healthier individuals to avoid subsequent growth and pressure symptoms from the mass. By contrast, in the absence of symptoms, the risks of bleeding at operation (due to this tumor's intimate association with the internal and external carotid arteries) and the tendency for slow growth allow expectant treatment in older or debilitated individuals.

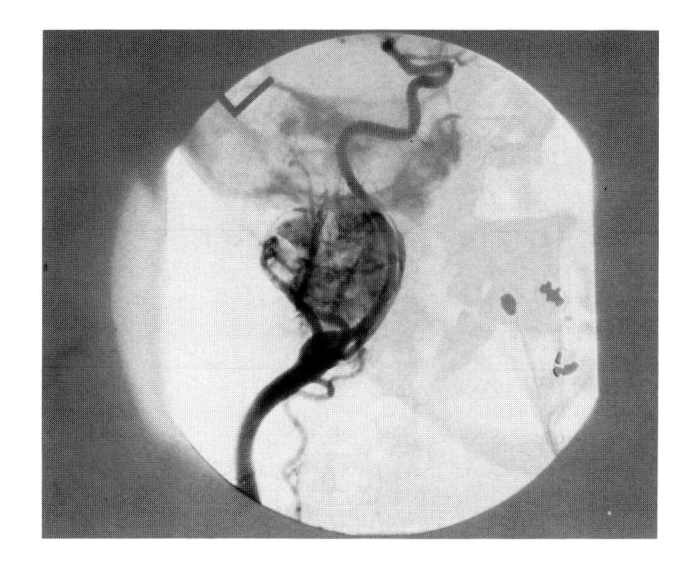

FIGURE 22–10. Typical angiographic appearance of a carotid body tumor. The vascular blush seen here at the carotid bifurcation at the time of angiography is characteristic of a carotid body tumor.

Neurogenic Tumors

The large number of nerves in the head and neck make the area susceptible to tumors of neurogenic origin. Neurilemmomas (schwannomas) and neurofibromas, which are the most common types seen, are quite similar. Both arise from the neurilemmal (Schwann) cell of myelinated nerves and both usually present as painless, slowly growing masses in the lateral neck. Differentiation between these two types of tumor can be accomplished only by histologic examination. Owing to their potential for malignant degeneration and their slow but progressive growth, surgical resection is indicated. This, however, may involve resection of the involved nerve(s), particularly with neurofibromas, which tend to be more invasive and less encapsulated than neurilemmomas.

Paralysis of the involved nerve usually results when a neuroma is excised.

THYROID MASSES

Thyroid disease is a relatively common cause of a lump in the neck. Although the diagnostic approach to the thyroid is similar to that of other neck masses, there are enough unique features to warrant a separate discussion here. The specific features of each type of thyroid disease and the controversies surrounding the management of the various malignant thyroid conditions will not be discussed.

Diagnostic Approach

Unless there is a concern that thyroid cancer may be present, thyroid swellings are often treated by medical therapy rather than surgery. Hence, it becomes extremely important when considering any thyroid mass to identify those thyroid lumps that might contain malignancy. This discussion will focus on this issue.

For any individual with a thyroid swelling, clues to the presence of malignancy are initially sought in the history and physical examination. The history should specifically ask about prior radiation exposure. Even though thyroid cancer is relatively uncommon in the general population (1 per cent of all cancers), it is more common in a subset of patients who were treated with radiation therapy for benign disease such as acne, tonsillar and adenoid hypertrophy, and thymic enlargement, as was the practice in some areas in the past. Hence, these people require frequent thyroid examinations, even in the absence of any signs or symptoms, and thyroid surgery is probably indicated for any detectable thyroid abnormality.

A normal thyroid gland can be difficult to palpate. Thus, easily palpable masses in the midline compartment of the neck (between the sternocleidomastoid muscles and overlying the larynx and upper trachea) generally represent thyroid abnormalities, particularly if they move up and down with swallowing. Firm, discrete nodules are more likely to contain malignancy than diffuse or cystic swellings. Abnormalities of vocal cord function or the presence of palpable lymph nodes also suggest malignancy.

Thyroid function tests (T3, T4, and TSH) and a thyroid scan are done in almost all patients with a detectable thyroid abnormality. In the latter test, the patient is given a radioactive substance (I-131, I-123, Tc-99m) which is then taken up and concentrated by the thyroid gland so that it can be imaged. The scan can help determine if the function of the gland is normal (Fig. 22–11) or increased either diffusely or locally. If a discrete nodule is present, the scan can help determine whether it is functional ("hot" and not likely malignant) (Fig. 22–12A) or nonfunctional ("cold"—a higher incidence of malignancy) (Fig. 22–12B).

Fine needle aspiration plays an important role in the diagnosis of thyroid masses.

Ultrasound and CT scans can also be helpful in determining the character (cystic or solid), number (single or multiple), and location of thyroid masses but should be used only if this information will not be made available through other more routine tests such as thyroid scans or fine needle aspiration.

Diffuse Thyroid Disease

Diffuse thyroid enlargement may be due to nodular goiter, thyroiditis (inflammatory lesions of the thyroid), acute hyperthyroidism, Graves' dis-

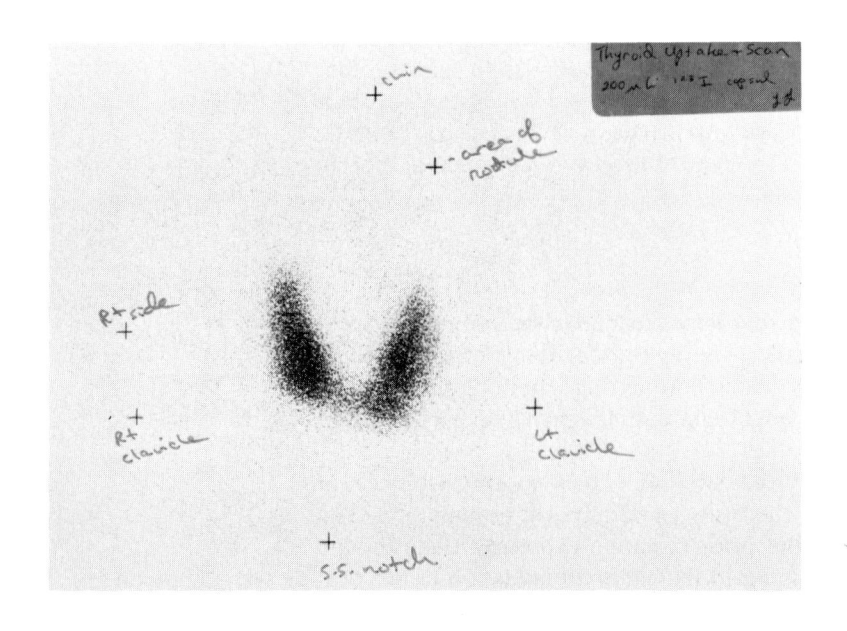

FIGURE 22–11. A normal thyroid scan. The two lobes of the thyroid and isthmus are well seen.

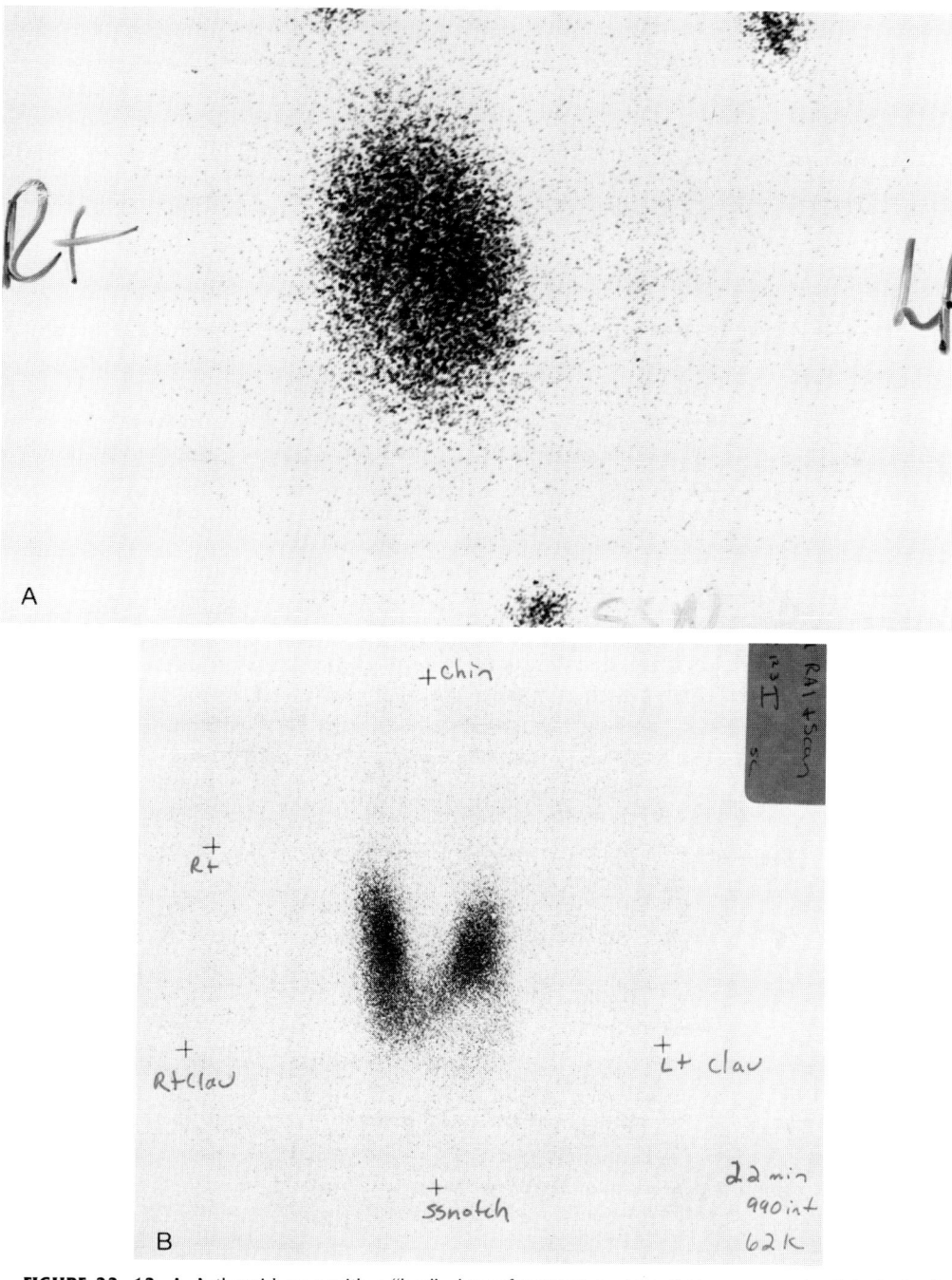

FIGURE 22-12. *A,* A thyroid scan with a "hot"—hyperfunctioning—area that corresponds clinically to the position of a palpable thyroid nodule. *B,* A thyroid scan with a "cold" thyroid nodule. There is decreased uptake seen in the left inferior pole of the thyroid which corresponds clinically with the position of the palpable nodule in the thyroid.

ease, or advanced carcinoma. Routine thyroid function tests, history and physical examination, and thyroid scans can usually help distinguish between these types of disease. For example, tenderness or signs and symptoms of infection are important diagnostic clues to the presence of thyroiditis. By contrast, a positive test for antithyroglobulin antibodies suggests the diagnosis of autoimmune thyroiditis. Fine needle aspiration (see below) may also be useful.

Treatment of most of the above conditions is medical and involves symptomatic measures for pain and suppression of normal thyroid function by the administration of exogenous thyroid hormone. Surgery is indicated only if a malignancy is suspected or if medical therapy fails and the enlarged gland is causing pressure symptoms or cosmetic problems.

Thyroid Nodules

If physical examination and thyroid scans suggest a discrete thyroid nodule, then the diagnostic approach is somewhat different from that used for diffuse disease. Most nodules are benign. However, those that are truly solitary, firm or hard, growing rapidly, or nonfunctional ("cold") on scan are more likely to be malignant. Similarly, if a nodule appears in either a young male, a pregnant female, or an individual with a history of irradiation or family history of thyroid cancer, the chances of malignancy are higher.

Fine needle aspiration of thyroid nodules properly done or interpreted has proven helpful in determining the presence or absence of malignancy within a thyroid nodule. An aspiration that is positive or suspicious for the presence of malignancy suggests the need for surgery, whereas those nodules that are histologically benign and disappear with aspiration can often be treated with thyroid suppression and observation.

Hyperfunctioning ("hot") nodules and those in which the suspicion of malignancy is extremely low can be treated with a trial of thyroid hormone replacement therapy to see whether this will make the mass disappear. However, if this is ineffective or signs of malignancy appear, then surgery is necessary.

Surgery for thyroid nodules involves an excisional biopsy consisting of total lobectomy and not enucleation alone. More extensive surgery is performed if the frozen section of the resected specimen reveals carcinoma.

References

Allard RHB: The thyroglossal duct cyst. Head Neck Surg 5:134–146, 1982.
Bonnadonna G, Molinari R, Banfi A: Hodgkin's and non-Hodgkin's lymphoma presenting in the head and neck. *In* Suen JY, Myers EN (eds): Cancer of the Head and Neck. New York, Churchill Livingston, 1981, pp 699–717.
Bumstead RM: Thyroid disease: A guide for head and neck surgeons. Ann Otol Rhinol Laryngol 89(Suppl):72, 1980.
Chandler JR, Mitchell B: Branchial cleft cysts, sinuses and fistulas. Otolaryngol Clin North Am 14:175–186, 1981.
Hamaker RC, Singer MI, DeRossi RV, Shockley WW: Role of needle biopsy in thyroid nodules. Arch Otolaryngol 109:225–228, 1983.
Holt GR, Mattox DE, Gates GA: Decision Making in Otolaryngology. St. Louis, CV Mosby Co, 1984, pp 40–41, 88–89, 114–115.
Knight PK, Mulne AF, Vassay LE: When is lymph node biopsy indicated in children with enlarged peripheral nodes? Pediatrics 69:391–396, 1982.
Lai KK, Stottmeier KD, Sherman IH, McCabe WR: Mycobacterial cervical lympadenopathy. JAMA 251:1286–1288, 1984.
Lindberg R: Distribution of cervical lymph node metastases from squamous cell carcinoma of the upper respiratory and digestive tracts. Cancer 28:1446–1449, 1972.
Spiro RHM, DeRose G, Strong EW: Cervical node metastasis of occult origin. Am J Surg 146:441–446, 1983.
Stal S, Hamilton S, Spira M: Hemangiomas, lymphangiomas, and vascular malformations of the head and neck. Otolaryngol Clin North Am 19:769–796, 1986.

23
MALIGNANT TUMORS OF THE HEAD AND NECK

by George L. Adams, M.D.

Present concepts in the management of patients with head and neck malignancies result from advances in the fields of surgery, radiation therapy, chemotherapy, and immunology. In many circumstances, a combination of these different modalities may prove to be the most effective treatment for the patient with advanced cancer. In the 100 years since the first laryngectomy by Billroth, extensive progress has been made in treatment of head and neck malignancy. The development of the classic radical neck dissection by Crile in the early 1900's extended the surgical field to include resection of regional cervical metastases. Recent further understanding of the metastatic potential of head and neck cancer by Drs. Bocca in Italy and Byers, Schuller, Skolnik, Medina, and several others has led to modifications of the standard neck dissection as described by Dr. Crile. It has been possible to preserve the accessory (XI) cranial nerve, jugular vein, and sternocleidomastoid muscle in selected patients. Other major advances, including preservation of the mandible by methods described by Hamaker, Cunningham, and others, have led to both better cosmetic and better functional results for the patient with advanced malignancy. Endotracheal anesthesia, safe blood transfusions, improved diagnostic tests (particularly the enhanced CT scan), and perioperative antibiotics have added to the effective surgical resection of cancers. Simultaneously, advances in radiation therapy, such as cobalt-60 therapy and interstitial iridium radiation, have led to more effective treatment with greater protection of the skin, mucosa, and mandible. New surgical techniques now permit reconstructive procedures using regional rotational flaps, particularly the pectoralis major myocutaneous flap, free flap jejunal interposition with microvascular anastomoses, and more extensive procedures for the resection of tumors extending to the skull base. Chemotherapy has been employed investigationally in the initial treatment of head and neck cancer. Protocols utilizing chemotherapy preoperatively and immediately postoperatively in the adjuvant setting appear to be effective. This effect has been primarily in the reduction of the mass of both the primary and nodal metastases. The question remains, however, as to whether this size reduction and initial effectiveness of chemotherapy in producing a partial or complete response will ultimately affect survival.

The overall frequency of head and neck malignancy is rising. Currently in the metropolitan Midwest, malignant tumors of the larynx, pharynx, and oral cavity rank sixth in overall incidence, preceded only by cancer of the breast, colon and rectum, lung, uterus and cervix, and prostate and bladder. Of particular concern is the increased incidence of smoking in women. The ratio of carcinoma of the larynx to the lung has had a continuous relationship of approximately one to ten. Thus, with a rise of lung cancer in women, it is anticipated that there will be a rise in the incidence of laryngeal carcinoma.

The efforts of all physicians who deal with malignant tumors are directed toward earlier recognition, increased survival rate, prevention of distant metastases, and the early recognition of recurrent local and regional disease. In the case of head and neck cancer, the incidence of second primary malignancies ranges up to 20 per cent if the patient survives five years after treatment of the original tumor. There is also up to a 10 per cent incidence of second malignancies diagnosed at the time of recognition of the original tumor. Thus a complete physical and endoscopic evaluation of any patient with head and neck cancer is required to make certain that a second tumor does not coexist.

Patients surviving an upper airway cancer have a 20 per cent chance of developing a second primary malignancy within the next 5 years.

85 per cent of cancers of the head and neck can be detected by a complete clinical exam.

A unique circumstance exists in head and neck malignancy: in over 85 per cent of patients, the tumor can be seen or palpated by thorough head and neck examination. When patients seek early medical attention for their symptoms or when examination of the head and neck is included as part of a routine physical examination, an early tumor can be recognized in the office. A small lesion may have a cure rate as high as 90 per cent and be treated by a limited surgical resection or radiation directed to a smaller field. The use of the fiberoptic laryngoscope for examining the nasopharynx, pharynx, and larynx has added a new dimension to early detection of small tumors. Unfortunately, there are still factors that exclude early recognition and diagnosis. These include the following:

1. Failure of the patient to seek medical advice early
2. Failure of the physician to obtain an immediate biopsy of a suspicious lesion
3. Similarity of presenting signs and symptoms to more common benign disease
4. Failure to thoroughly examine the upper respiratory and digestive tracts for the source of the primary tumor before biopsy or excision of a neck mass
5. Misdiagnosis made when the presenting symptom misdirects the examination (e.g., otalgia in the case of small tongue, tonsil, or laryngeal tumor)

Hoarseness is the earliest sign of laryngeal cancer.

Persistent hoarseness requires a mirror or fiberoptic exam of the larynx.

In spite of the lay media's constant urging of the public to seek medical care early, it is not infrequent for a patient to present with laryngeal obstruction from a large cancer rather than the early symptom of hoarseness. Similarly, a patient with a pharyngeal tumor may ignore the early symptoms of pain and dysphagia only to present when pharyngeal or esophageal obstruction has developed. Thus, a great advancement in the control of head and neck malignancy would be education of the public to obtain early examination. (The physician is obligated to ensure a thorough evaluation of the patient's symptoms, including indirect mirror or flexible fiberoptic scope examination—see Chapter 1.)

ETIOLOGY

Squamous cell carcinoma comprises 90 per cent of head and neck malignancies. Adenocarcinoma, which usually develops in a major or minor salivary gland, is the next most common type. All other pathologic varieties comprise less than 1 per cent. Tobacco is the etiologic agent most frequently cited in development of squamous cell carcinoma. However, heavy alcohol ingestion is often associated with heavy smoking and is incriminated as an etiologic factor, particularly in tumors of the oral cavity, tonsillar area, and piriform sinus. Poor oral hygiene has also been implicated. On rare occasions, an elderly individual without any of these habits develops floor of mouth or tongue cancer without explanation. While most head and neck malignancy develops in the 50- to 70-year-old age group, carcinoma of the oral cavity has been recognized in individuals in their twenties. Alcohol and tobacco use does not seem to be implicated in many of these younger individuals.

Squamous cell carcinoma comprises 90 per cent of head and neck cancer.

A viral etiology, specifically the Epstein-Barr virus, has been associated with the development of nasopharyngeal carcinoma. Cantonese Chinese have a high incidence of nasopharyngeal cancer, suggesting a racial predilection. Although the incidence is extremely high in Chinese living in their homeland, the incidence remains high in Chinese born and raised in the United States. Adenocarcinoma arising high in the nasal vault and ethmoid sinuses is prevalent among hardwood furniture workers in certain areas of Great Britain, suggesting environmental factors. Workers exposed to chromium and nickel have also been demonstrated to have a higher incidence of paranasal sinus malignancies (Table 23–1).

Epstein-Barr virus has been associated with nasopharyngeal carcinoma.

Patients with head and neck malignancies are prone to develop a second tumor at an incidence rate of approximately 4 per cent per year for the first five years after discovery of the original cancer. Most of these second primary malignancies are in the upper aerodigestive tract. A second primary tumor in the lung is particularly common. Thus, the patient ostensibly cured of his original cancer should remain under constant surveillance for the rest of his life, not only for the development of metastases from that tumor but also for detection of a new malignancy.

PATHOLOGY

Squamous cell carcinoma develops as an ulcerative lesion with necrotic edges, usually surrounded by some inflammatory response. While the tumor may remain an ulcerative lesion, it is often surrounded by areas of leukoplakia of the premalignant type. The tumor initially spreads along the mucosal surface, eventually extending into the underlying soft tissue. Pathologically, these tumors are graded on the basis of histologic appearance related to the clinical course. Simply put, all classifications range from well-

Squamous cell carcinoma is far more common in men. Adenocarcinoma occurs equally in men and women.

TABLE 23–1. AGENTS ASSOCIATED WITH CARCINOMA OF THE NOSE AND PARANASAL SINUSES

Oak, beechwood	woodworkers
Radium	dial painters
Chromium	manufacturers
Nickel	manufacturers
Isopropyl oil	manufacturers

differentiated (low malignancy) to poorly differentiated (highly malignant). Tumors that are less well differentiated tend to respond well to radiation therapy; however, their long-term prognosis may be poorer than that for well-differentiated types.

Adenocarcinoma occurs in the major or minor salivary glands located in the mucosal lining or in the immediately submucosal areas. Classification of common tumors of salivary glands include:

1. Acinic cell carcinoma
2. Adenoid cystic carcinoma (cylindroma)
3. Adenocarcinoma
4. Mucoepidermoid carcinoma (high and low grade)
5. Carcinoma arising in pleomorphic adenoma
6. Malignant mixed tumor

Adenocarcinoma may occur at any age.

Adenocarcinoma appears to occur equally in men and women. It may occur in a younger age group than the more common squamous cell carcinoma. It may metastasize by both lymphogenous and hematogenous routes. The adenoid cystic carcinoma is a particular type of salivary gland malignancy that has a high propensity to spread along the neural sheaths. It is particularly known to recur after a disease-free interval of five to ten years. As opposed to squamous cell carcinomas, which are usually ulcerative, adenocarcinoma is generally submucosal, presenting as a smooth, firm, rounded mass that becomes ulcerated only late in the course of the disease or after biopsy. There appears to be no correlation with tobacco or alcohol use. Adenocarcinoma can occur in virtually any of the places squamous cell carcinoma occurs, but it occurs more commonly in the major salivary glands, at the junction of the hard and soft palate, or in the paranasal sinuses or mobile tongue.

Malignant lymphoma (Table 23–2) may present as a primary malignancy in the head and neck. Lymphomas are usually classified according to whether they are Hodgkin's disease or a non-Hodgkin's lymphoma. The latter group is then divided into reticulum cell sarcoma and lymphosarcoma. The 1965 Conference on Hodgkin's disease in Rye, New York, further classified Hodgkin's lymphoma into four types:

1. Lymphocyte predominance
2. Nodular sclerosis
3. Mixed cellularity
4. Lymphocyte depletion

TABLE 23–2. STAGING CLASSIFICATION OF LYMPHOMA

Stage I	Involvement of a single lymph node region (I) or of a single extralymphatic organ or site (I_E)
Stage II	Involvement of two or more lymph node regions (number to be stated) on the same side of the diaphragm (II) or localized involvement of an extralymphatic organ or site of one or more lymph node regions on the same side of the diaphragm (II_E)
Stage III	Involvement of lymph node regions on both sides of the diaphragm (III), which may also be accompanied by localized involvement of extralymphatic organ or site (III_E), by involvement of the spleen (III_S), or both (III_{E+S})
Stage IV	Diffuse or disseminated involvement of one or more extralymphatic organs or tissues with or without associated lymph node enlargement

Each stage is subdivided into "A" and "B" categories, "B" for those with defined general symptoms and "A" for those without.

From Beahrs OH, Myers MH (eds): Manual for Staging of Cancer. 2nd ed. Philadelphia, JB Lippincott Co, 1983, p 228.

Lymphocyte-predominant and nodular sclerosing types have been reported to have the most favorable five-year survival rates. The nodular sclerosing type is commonly localized to the cervical lymph nodes and upper mediastinum. In addition to classifying Hodgkin's lymphoma into these types, further clinical, radiologic, and surgical evaluation permits dividing the disease into stages I through IV, depending upon the extent of the disease.

Categorization of non-Hodgkin's lymphoma is more complex and is dependent upon both morphologic and immunologic characteristics. Three systems have developed. There is that of Rappaport, which divides the tumors into well-differentiated lymphocytic, poorly differentiated lymphocytic, mixed histiocytic-lymphocytic, and diffuse poorly differentiated. The Lukes-Collins system is more dependent on immunologic identification. In the European countries the Lennert classification is used.

Lymphomas may arise in any of the primary lymphatic regions of the head and neck. Thus, they are most commonly found along the anterior cervical and deep jugular nodes or arising in Waldeyer's ring. In addition, lymphoma may be found as a primary tumor within the parotid or submandibular gland as well as within the thyroid gland. The unilaterally hypertrophied tonsil, with or without pain, in an adult should be suspected of harboring a malignancy, possibly a lymphoma, especially if accompanied by involvement of several cervical nodes. If extranodal lymphoma is suspected, for example, in the palatine tonsil, then the entire tonsil should be submitted for pathologic examination. Similarly, when a lymph node biopsy is necessary, the entire node, without destruction of its architecture, should be submitted for pathologic examination, and the pathologist should be informed at the time that a diagnosis of lymphoma is being considered. This allows for "Touch" preparations to be made. Next the patient's disease process is staged to help in determining the treatment plan. This may require lymphangiography as well as special CT scanning, exploratory laparotomy, splenectomy, or mediastinoscopy. Treatment depends on the stage of the disease and usually consists of irradiation, chemotherapy, or a combination of both.

A unilateral enlarged tonsil in an adult is suspicious of lymphoma.

Connective tissue malignant tumors or sarcomas are not common in the head and neck. Among those most frequently seen are rhabdomyosarcoma in children, fibrosarcoma, liposarcoma, osteogenic sarcoma (again usually in young adults), and chondrosarcoma. The most common sarcoma, however, is malignant fibrous histiocytoma (MFH). Although it is most common in the elderly and extremely rare in children, it can occur at any age. It can be difficult pathologically to differentiate from other entities such as fibrosarcoma. It can occur in the soft tissues of the neck or involving bone of the maxilla or mandible. It has been associated with previous radiation therapy. An unusual circumstance occurs when this tumor develops in a patient who has undergone previous radiation therapy for bilateral retinoblastoma. However, the tumor may occur within or outside of the previous radiation port.

Rhabdomyosarcoma is the most common sarcoma in children. It usually occurs in the posterior nares, ethmoid, orbital, and nasopharyngeal regions.

Malignant fibrous histiocytoma (MFH) is the most common sarcoma of the head and neck in adults.

Treatment of MFH is wide surgical resection. Postoperative radiation therapy has been shown to be of value when malignant fibrous histiocytoma occurs in the extremities but has not proven to be effective for head and neck MFH. Chemotherapy regimens based on doxorubicin (Adriamycin) or high-dose methotrexate are currently being used in a prospective evaluation. MFH has a tendency to recur locally and to metastasize to the lung. Survival is better with isolated soft tissue lesions than when it occurs in the maxilla.

Rhabdomyosarcoma, usually of the embryonic form, is the most common form of sarcoma in children. It generally occurs near the orbit, nasopharynx, and paranasal sinuses. Diagnosis is confirmed by biopsy. A thorough search for distal metastases is made before initiating treatment. Treatment consists of a combination of surgical resection (when not considered mutilating), radiation therapy, and chemotherapy. A triple-drug regimen consisting of cyclophosphamide (Cytoxan), vincristine, and actinomycin has been used (VAC). Doxorubicin is often included in the treatment of rhabdomyosarcoma as well as other sarcomas.

METASTATIC TUMORS

Metastases to the head and neck from primary tumors elsewhere can occur. Hypernephroma is the most common tumor to metastasize to the paranasal sinuses. A mass in the supraclavicular fossa may represent metastases from a primary tumor of the lung, kidney (renal cell carcinoma), bladder, prostate, breast, or gastrointestinal tract. Tumors that tend to metastasize to bone can present in the mandible, maxilla, sphenoid sinus, or petrous portion of the temporal bone. Even metastatic carcinoma to the tonsil has been described.

MALIGNANT TUMORS OF THE SKIN

Basal Cell Carcinoma

Basal cell carcinoma occurs in areas of high sun exposure.

Basal cell carcinoma is the most common skin malignancy and arises in areas with a high exposure to sunlight. Thus, the cheek, nose, forehead, and ear are common sites. Basal cell carcinoma carries an excellent prognosis, since it has a metastatic rate of less than 1 per cent. However, if untreated, it can cause extensive local destruction. Basal cell carcinoma of the medial canthal area has been noted to invade the orbit, ethmoid sinus, and brain. Preauricular basal cell carcinoma can extend along the cartilage of the ear canal or into the superficial parotid gland. Treatment consists of local resection with sufficient margins. Mohs' pathologically controlled excision is commonly practiced for small and even complex tumors. The technique depends on immediate multiple-section pathologic evaluation of all margins, including the depth.

Squamous Cell Carcinoma

Squamous cell carcinoma likewise arises in areas associated with high sunlight exposure; the pinna and lower lip are the most common sites. Squamous cell carcinoma, however, can metastasize regionally and distally. These tumors must be initially excised with an adequate margin.

Malignant Melanoma

Melanoma is classified according to size, location, and depth of invasion determined histologically (Table 23–3).

TABLE 23-3. CLASSIFICATION OF MELANOMA

Clark's Classification
  Level I (epidermis to epidermal-dermal interface). Lesions involving only the epidermis have been designated level I. These lesions are considered to be "atypical melanocytic hyperplasia" and are not included in the staging of malignant melanoma, for they do not represent a malignant lesion.
  Level II (papillary dermis). Invasion of the papillary dermis; does not reach the papillary-reticular dermal interface.
  Level III (papillary-reticular dermis interface). Invasion involves the full thickness of, fills, and expands the papillary dermis; it abuts upon but does not penetrate the reticular dermis.
  Level IV (reticular dermis). Invasion occurs into the reticular dermis but not into the subcutaneous tissue.
  Level V (subcutaneous tissue). Invasion occurs through the reticular dermis into the subcutaneous tissues.

Breslow's Classification by Depth
  1. 0.75 mm or less
  2. 0.76 mm to 1.50 mm
  3. 1.51 mm to 4.0 mm
  4. More than 4.0 mm

From Beahrs OH, Myers MH (eds): Manual for Staging of Cancer. 2nd ed. Philadelphia, JB Lippincott Co, 1983, p 118.

Prognosis is related to depth of invasion, location, and size. Patients with Clark's level I or Breslow's thinnest classification have a relatively good prognosis, whereas patients with Clark's level V have a remarkably poor prognosis regardless of treatment.

Malignant melanoma may arise on mucous membranes of the nose or throat. The most common sites are intranasal or on the hard palate or buccal mucosa. Preferred treatment is wide surgical resection. Unfortunately, by the time of diagnosis the tumor has often spread beyond the resectable area. The alternative methods of treatment include radiation therapy, chemotherapy, and, more recently, immunotherapy. Occasionally, a malignant melanoma may be found in a cervical lymph node when no apparent primary tumor is evident. A history of a skin lesion should be sought. Thorough head and neck examination, particularly of the scalp, nose, oral cavities, and sinuses, should be performed. Ophthalmologic examination is required. If a thorough physical examination and radiographic studies reveal no evidence of other areas of metastases, then radical neck dissection on the involved side should be considered.

Malignant melanoma can arise on the mucous membrane of the nose.

EVALUATION OF PATIENTS WITH HEAD AND NECK CANCER

Head and neck malignancies may occur in all age groups. However, the age of the patient is useful in arousing suspicion of a particular type of tumor. For example, rhabdomyosarcoma and lymphoma would be more likely in children, whereas adenocarcinoma occurs in all ages. In the 40- to 70-year age range, tumors are most frequently the squamous cell type, with a high male predominance, and the history usually elicits heavy smoking or

Squamous cell carcinoma: male, age 60, heavy smoker, drinking history.

alcohol ingestion. Hoarseness or chronic sore throat, especially of more than three weeks' duration, requires a complete examination. The evaluation of cervical lymph nodes is discussed in Chapter 22.

Upon completion of a careful history, a thorough head and neck examination, including use of mirrors, should be performed. A suspicious ulcerative lesion in the oral cavity can be biopsied in the clinic following application of topical 4 per cent cocaine or needle infiltration of a local anesthetic. The needle track should not extend into the tumor. Use of cupped biopsy forceps requires minimal anesthesia. Biopsies of the posterior tongue, tonsil, pharynx, or larynx are usually performed under general anesthesia in the operating room to allow thorough mapping of the lesion in a relaxed patient. Laryngeal planigrams or a laryngogram may aid in determining the extent of the tumor, but the CT scan has become the preferred method. These procedures are best done prior to biopsy to avoid confusing tumor extent with edema resulting from the biopsy.

The following tests are recommended to establish the patient's general condition, the presence of metastases, and the possibility of a second primary tumor. Recall that many patients with advanced head and neck cancer have other major medical problems such as cirrhosis and chronic obstructive lung disease.

1. Complete blood count, platelet count, urinalysis
2. Chemistry studies, including complete liver function tests
3. Tests of thyroid function (T_4) or a scan if the mass is suspected to be in the thyroid
4. Chest radiographs (posteroanterior and lateral), followed by CT scan if indicated when a metastatic lesion or second primary lesion is suspected
5. Bone scan for metastasis (if history of bone pain)
6. Cardiac evaluation, including electrocardiogram
7. Blood clotting studies, including prothrombin time and partial thromboplastin time
8. CT scan of the larynx, maxilla, parotid, skull base, or neck when required in surgical planning and to determine extent and resectability; barium swallow if esophagoscopy is contemplated

The concept of "panendoscopy" developed because of the 5 to 8 per cent incidence of a second head and neck cancer.

In the operating room, thorough endoscopic evaluation is made not only of the patient's known or suspected tumor but also of other suspicious areas. Thus, leukoplakia beyond the primary tumor area must also be biopsied. The tongue and upper pharynx are carefully palpated. The nasopharynx is directly visualized and palpated. The laryngopharynx is carefully inspected using a laryngoscope, carefully lifting the arytenoid area to examine the postcricoid and hypopharyngeal regions. The tumor mass is carefully defined and outlined and an appropriate drawing made in the patient's chart. Exact knowledge of the extent of the tumor is imperative. Tattooing the margins of accessible tumors with India ink is helpful for follow-up examinations. Presence or absence of palpable neck nodes must be documented, and palpation is repeated when the patient is under anesthesia. Whether these nodes are fixed to underlying structures and whether they are present unilaterally or on the ipsilateral or contralateral side are important. Knowledge of the extent of the primary tumor and the status of regional metastases is required in order to plan definitive care and stage the tumor.

Classification

TABLE 23–4. THE TNM CLASSIFICATION SYSTEM

Three capital letters are used to describe extent of cancer:
- T   Primary tumor
- N   Regional lymph nodes
- M   Distant metastasis

This classification is extended by the following designations:

Tumor
- TX   The minimum requirements to assess the primary tumor cannot be met.
- T0   No evidence of primary tumor
- Tis   Carcinoma in situ
- T1, T2, T3, T4   Progressive increase in tumor size or involvement (see below)

Nodes
- NX   The minimum requirements to assess the regional lymph nodes cannot be met.
- N0   No evidence of regional node involvement
- N1, N2, N3, N4   Increasing degrees of demonstrable abnormality of regional lymph nodes (see below)

Metastasis
- MX   The minimum requirements to assess the presence of distant metastasis cannot be met.
- M0   No evidence of distant metastasis
- M1   Distant metastasis present
  Specify site of metastasis _____

Primary tumor (T)
- T1   Tumor confined to the antral mucosa of the infrastructure with no bone erosion or destruction
- T2   Tumor confined to the suprastructure mucosa without bone destruction or to the infrastructure, with destruction of medial or inferior bony walls only
- T3   More extensive tumor invading skin of cheek, orbit, anterior ethmoid sinuses, or pterygoid muscle
- T4   Massive tumor with invasion of cribriform plate, posterior ethmoids, sphenoid, nasopharynx, pterygoid plates, or base of skull

Nodal involvement (N)
- N1   Single clinically positive homolateral node 3 cm or less in diameter
- N2   Single clinically positive homolateral node more than 3 cm but not more than 6 cm in diameter or multiple clinically positive homolateral nodes, none more than 6 cm in diameter
- N2a   Multiple clinically positive homolateral nodes, none more than 6 cm in diameter
- N3   Massive homolateral node(s), bilateral nodes, or contralateral node(s)
- N3a   Clinically positive homolateral node(s), one more than 6 cm in diameter
- N3b   Bilateral clinically positive nodes (in this situation, each side of the neck should be staged separately; i.e., N3b: right, N2a; left, N1)
- N3c   Contralateral clinically positive node(s) only

From Beahrs OH, Myers MH (eds): Manual for Staging of Cancer. 2nd ed. Philadelphia, JB Lippincott Co, 1983, pp 44, 50.

MODALITIES OF TREATMENT

There are at present five specific methods available for treatment of head and neck malignancies:

1. Radiation therapy
2. En bloc surgical excision
3. Laser excision
4. Chemotherapy
5. Combination of modalities

In an effort to improve survival rates, it has been common in the past ten years to combine two or more of these modalities. Prior to initiation of any form of treatment, a thorough evaluation is made of the patient's general health, likelihood of responsible follow-up, and extent of the tumor and its metastases. Then, after the options are discussed with the radiation therapist, family, and others who may be involved in the patient's care, a treatment plan is derived. Although a small tumor may be treated adequately by either radiation therapy or surgery, larger tumors are usually treated by surgery, with radiation given either pre- or postoperatively. Recurrent tumors not amenable to additional surgery or irradiation are treated by chemotherapy, often as part of a research protocol. The role of each of these major modalities is discussed below.

Radiation Therapy*

Radiation plays an important part in the management of head and neck malignancies and can be employed as the sole method of treatment for certain tumors. The radiotherapist, employing x-rays and gamma-rays, must know the quantity and quality of the radiation in the particular beam being used. The quantity, or dose, of radiation designates the amount administered, and the quality, or penetration ability, determines the percentage of radiation that will reach a lesion at a given depth below the body surface. When the patient is exposed to x- or gamma-irradiation, a portion of the photons pass through unchanged, but a certain fraction is absorbed by the interaction with the atoms of the body. The absorbed photons, if sufficiently energetic, liberate photoelectrons, recoil electrons, and negatron-positron pairs that ionize other atoms nearby. In other words, the absorbed energy causes ionization that is primarily responsible for the therapeutic effects of penetrating radiation.

Definitions

In measuring radiation absorbed, the ideal method would be to calculate the number of ergs of energy absorbed in the irradiated tissue by the ionizing radiation. This method requires sophisticated apparatus. Early attempts to quantify the amounts of radiation absorbed involved exposure of photographic film to determine the degree of darkening produced by radiation exposure or observation of acute changes on the irradiated skin after a given dose of radiation was administered. This was termed *erythema dose.*

In 1908, it was suggested that radiation be quantified by measuring the ionization produced in air or some other gas by a standard radiation exposure, and hence the roentgen unit was created. The modern definition of a roentgen is very precise, but essentially it defines a certain amount of ionization occurring in a specific quantity of air under standard conditions. However, this measurement does not indicate the dose absorbed by a patient exposed to a particular beam of radiation. Therefore, an absorbed dose must also be defined. The amount of energy absorbed in tissues exposed to one roentgen depends on the type of radiation and the material irradiated. Hence, in 1953, the Seventh International Congress of Radiology adopted the rad (radiation absorbed dose) as the unit of absorbed dose. The rad is independent of the type of radiation and represents an absorbed dose of 100 ergs per gram of any material irradiated. The amount of radiation given to a patient is ordinarily expressed clinically in tissue rads.

An additional unit of interest is the rem (roentgen-equivalent-man). This

---

*The section on Radiation Therapy was contributed by Robert Haselow, M.D.

unit attempts to quantify the different biologic effects of various forms of radiation. For example, a fast neutron beam produces significantly more biologic effect than a cobalt beam for a given equal deposition of energy. The rem allows comparison of differing forms of radiation to produce a given radiobiologic effect.

Recently the Système International (SI) unit of absorbed dose has been changed to the gray (Gy), which is defined as one joule per kilogram. A subunit, centigray (cGy), is often used. The relationship between the above units is

1 Gy (gray) = 100 rad
1 rad = 10^{-2} Gy = 1 centigray (cGy)

Goals

The use of radiation therapy for treatment of head and neck carcinoma has attained greater prominence in recent years. This was made possible by technological improvements of the machines that produce ionizing radiation, greater understanding of radiobiologic principles, and increased precision in radiation measurement and delivery.

The radiotherapist employs several techniques for administering ionizing radiation. Superficial lesions such as skin carcinoma are best treated by low-voltage x-ray apparatus. More deep-seated lesions, like those of the tongue or lymph nodes, require greater penetration, such as that provided by the cobalt or electron beam. Interstitial irradiation (direct implantation) techniques utilizing radioactive materials such as radium, gold, or iridium provide additional methods of treatment. Direct implantation of radioactive materials results in high local irradiation with the least adverse effects beyond the immediate area.

The application of a particular technique to a given patient depends on many factors. It is necessary to know the site and extent of the primary tumor but also the areas of definite or suspected metastases. A careful drawing, showing the extent of tumor involvement, is made in the chart and on the patient's tumor record. The tumor should be staged according to the TNM classification system for future reference. The age and general physical condition of the patient are important factors. It should be decided initially, before treatment, whether the patient will receive full-course or only pre- or postoperative irradiation. It is important to know if the patient has had any previous radiation therapy, including the dosage and specific area.

The use of irradiation as either a preoperative or postoperative technique is designed to overcome the deficiencies of each modality when used alone. In the more advanced lesions surgery is effective in removing the bulk of the tumor in the primary site and metastatic neck nodes but may fail to cure the patient because of microscopic seeding of unresected tissues by malignant cells. Conversely, irradiation is effective in eradicating small nests of tumor cells at the periphery of the primary tumor and in metastatic neck nodes but frequently fails to control the bulky, poorly oxygenated primary tumor.

Postoperative radiation therapy is administered when there is extracapsular extension of the cancer.

It has been demonstrated that 5000 rads of gamma radiation given over five weeks can control 90 per cent of subclinical (i.e., microscopic) squamous cell carcinoma. On the other hand, 7000 to 8000 rads of gamma radiation may not control large bulky deposits of squamous carcinoma in the primary site or lymph nodes. Hence, the rationale of combination therapy is to achieve the sterilization of microscopic deposits of tumor cells in the treated volume by irradiation in conjunction with the surgical removal of the major bulk of primary and metastatic disease.

Laryngeal Lesions

Irradiation alone can be used for treatment of less advanced laryngeal lesions, thus permitting preservation of voice. With careful follow-up, surgical resection can be performed later should the carcinoma persist or recur. This approach is particularly applicable in true vocal cord lesions. Here, an 80 per cent rate of primary control is attained with irradiation alone and the surgical salvage rate for those lesions not controlled is likewise high.

In order to achieve a homogeneous dose distribution throughout the tumor volume, two or more separate beam portals are used to deliver the radiation. As an example, in treatment of an early true vocal cord lesion, both right and left lateral portals would be employed to irradiate a volume of tissue such as that seen in Figure 23–1. Here, the portal size is quite small, since these lesions are of limited extent and their potential for nodal metastasis is minimal.

Nasopharyngeal Carcinoma

In contrast, as seen in Figure 23–2, the portals used in the treatment of a nasopharyngeal carcinoma are much more extensive, as the potential for nodal metastasis in such cancers is great. Again, both right and left lateral portals would be used in order to achieve a homogeneous dose.

Lesions of the Paranasal Sinuses

For squamous cell carcinoma arising in the paranasal sinuses, radiation therapy may be employed pre- or postoperatively. In far-advanced unresectable lesions, irradiation alone is used.

For lesions that are laterally placed, such as those of the maxillary sinus, special techniques enable delivery of a homogeneous dose of radiation to the target volume without exposing uninvolved or sensitive structures, such

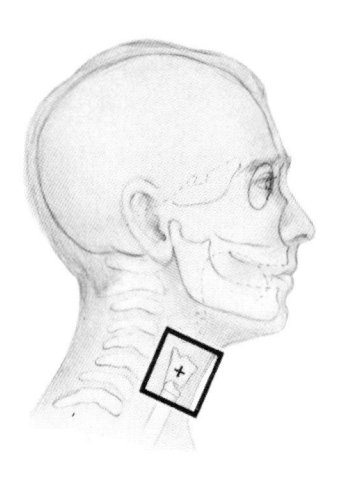

Center field 1 cm. below thyroid notch

Approx. 5 x 5 cm. field

FIGURE 23–1. Treatment portal covering larynx in T1, N0, M0 true vocal cord lesion.

TREATMENT GOALS—

Include:
1. Primary

Exclude:
1. All nodes

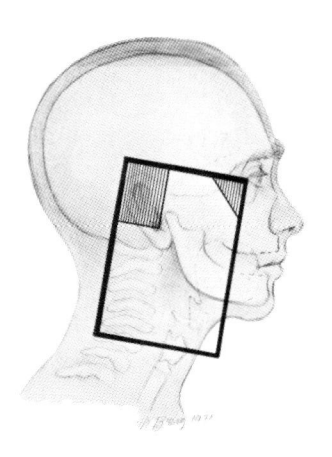

Initial 4500 rads

Borders

Superior: approx. 1cm. above upper border of zygoma
Inferior: at level of thyroid notch
Anterior: orbital margin to mandible avoiding major part of the larynx
Posterior: include spinal accessory chain

Block

1. top 2 cm. above zygoma
2. to post. margin of EAC and base of mastoid process (floor of EAC)
3. orbital contents

TREATMENT GOALS—

Include:
1. retropharyngeal nodes
2. anterior cervical chains
3. spinal accessory chains
4. posterior cervical triangles
5. supraclavicular fossae

FIGURE 23–2. Treatment portal used in treatment of nasopharyngeal carcinoma. In addition to this portal, an additional anterior beam is used to treat the lower neck (EAC = external auditory canal).

as the opposite eye. Figure 23–3 illustrates a treatment plan for a carcinoma involving the left maxillary antrum. The connecting lines drawn within the outline of a transverse section through the maxillary sinus represent isodose lines and connect points of equal dose within the treatment volume. With

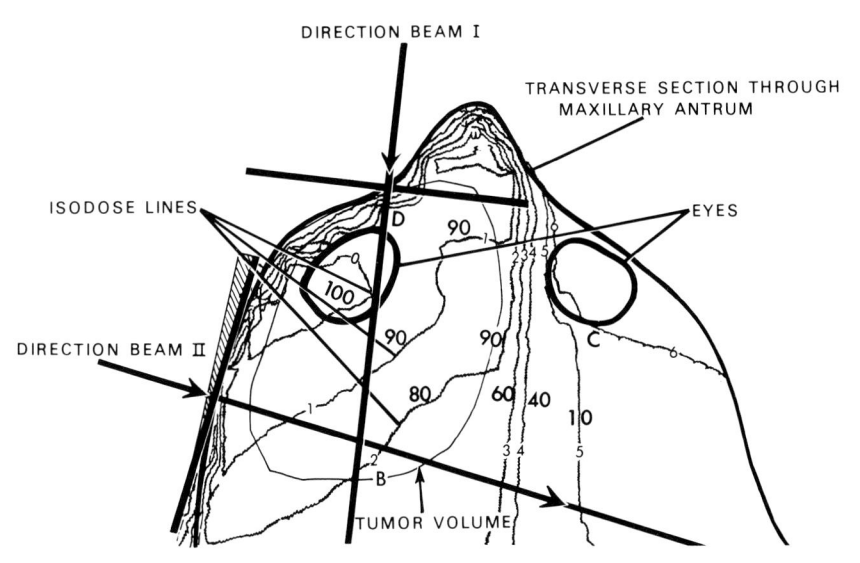

FIGURE 23–3. Contour drawn through maxillary sinus, illustrating beam directions, important anatomic structures, tumor volume, and isodose curves. Note that beam I is an open, unwedged beam but that beam II passes through a lead wedge filter in order to achieve a homogeneous dose distribution.

the proper arrangement of portals to cover the volume of the tumor and simultaneously avoid uninvolved and sensitive structures, an acceptable treatment plan may be constructed. Because of the highly complex calculations involved in designing such a plan, a computer is necessary in order to achieve precision in a reasonable period of time. Also, a radiation physicist and other ancillary personnel are required for the proper operation and application of these complex functions.

Complications

The difficulties associated with the administration of radiation therapy may be divided into early and late complications. Early problems include the following:

1. Mucositis with associated pharyngeal discomfort
2. Loss of appetite
3. Nausea
4. Dryness of mucous membranes
5. Effect on normal tissue, e.g., overlying skin
6. Hematopoietic suppression (rare in the treatment of head and neck malignancies)
7. Transverse myelitis (rare)

During therapy the patient should be examined frequently by both radiotherapist and surgeon.

Delayed complications consist of dryness of the oral cavity and the effects of radiation on underlying bone. For this reason, any patient who is about to receive radiation, particularly in the area of the mandible, should have a complete dental evaluation. All teeth of questionable durability should be extracted, and the wound must be healed prior to the onset of radiation therapy. Fluoride treatments and careful oral hygiene may prevent complications such as osteomyelitis. A young person receiving radiation therapy should be followed carefully throughout life for detection of the possible delayed development of a malignancy in the field of radiation. This problem was brought to light when a higher incidence of thyroid carcinoma was found in individuals who received radiation to the neck for benign disease as children.

Surgical Treatment

The objective of surgical treatment is total resection of the cancer with a margin or cuff of normal tissue of at least 2 cm. In addition, surgery on the primary malignancy is often combined with a cervical lymphadenectomy (radical neck dissection). The neck specimen is left attached to the primary area, for example, the larynx, so that the entire region is removed "en bloc." This basic surgical principle is applied wherever possible, with certain exceptions such as the nose, where an "en bloc" neck dissection would not be reasonable. Resection of the primary tumor combined with the neck dissection often creates a large soft tissue defect. Regional flaps consisting of the pectoralis major myocutaneous muscle flap, the forehead flap, the regional tongue flap, or flaps of cervical skin are then used to repair the defect.

The second objective of surgical resection is to restore the functional capacity of the patient. Reconstructive procedures include restoring mandibular continuity with a prosthetic graft or rib, iliac crest, or free graft. The pectoralis major myocutaneous flap is used to replace the pharynx or base of tongue, avoiding the necessity of laryngectomy to prevent chronic aspiration. Procedures are also available to create a fistula between the new pharynx and the tracheal stoma to allow voice restoration. Along with reconstructive techniques, preservation of the accessory (eleventh) cranial nerve has been possible in the majority of patients, thus avoiding the complication of a shoulder droop and the associated discomfort. Each of the more common areas of head and neck carcinoma is discussed separately below, with demonstration of how these general principles apply.

Radical neck dissection is often modified to preserve the accessory (XI) cranial nerve.

Malignant Tumors of the Internal Nose

Malignant tumors of the internal nose are uncommon. The tumor most frequently encountered is squamous cell carcinoma, which occurs at the junction of the nasal septum and the mucocutaneous margin just posterior to the columella. Male smokers predominate in the group of patients with this malignancy. Metastases to the neck are rare except in very large tumors or when the upper lip becomes involved by direct extension.

Results of treatment of early carcinomas are equal with regional resection or radiation therapy. Because of the difficult functional and cosmetic problems created by surgery, radiation therapy is often used in limited tumors. Very advanced tumors require surgical resection and radiation therapy.

An unusual tumor that arises in the superior aspect of the nose or nasal vault in the region of the middle and superior turbinate is a papillary adenocarcinoma. More frequent in males, it has been associated with certain industrial occupations.

Esthesioneuroblastoma is a rare malignant tumor of the supporting elements of the olfactory epithelium. It is slow growing and capable of pulmonary and cervical metastasis. The tumor eventually erodes into the anterior cranium through the cribriform plate. Early symptoms include epistaxis and nasal obstruction. A CT scan is essential to establish whether there is intracranial extension. While the tumor does respond initially to radiation therapy, the most favorable results are obtained by wide surgical resection, which often requires a craniotomy and then postoperative irradiation therapy.

Inverted papilloma is an unusual nasal tumor that presents as a fleshy appearing polypoid lesion. While not malignant, it has a recurrence rate of up to 40 per cent when not completely and widely excised. They occur 80 per cent of the time in the lateral nasal wall in the area of the middle meatus. While they do not undergo malignant degeneration, there may be associated areas of malignancy within the mass of tissue in 5 per cent of cases. Therefore, complete evaluation of all the specimens submitted for examination is done by the pathologist.

Nasopharyngeal Carcinoma

The nasopharynx is a primary site for squamous cell carcinoma, undifferentiated carcinoma, adenocarcinoma, and primary lymphoma. Lymphoepithelioma, which may involve the nasopharynx in younger individuals, represents a squamous cell carcinoma combined with elements of lymphatic tissue. Malignant tumors in the nasopharynx may remain silent until they involve surrounding structures. Fifth cranial nerve involvement can cause local and facial pain or numbness. When the tumor spreads superiorly it may produce diplopia by involving the sixth and then third cranial nerves. Anterior extension results in nasal obstruction. Lateral extension to involve the eustachian tube produces unilateral serous otitis media with a conductive hearing loss. Metastases are to the retropharyngeal, deep jugular, and spinal accessory nodes. A solitary enlarged lymph node located posteriorly and high in the neck is often the presenting sign.

> *Unilateral serous otitis media in an adult suggests the possibility of a nasopharyngeal neoplasm.*

> *A high posterior cervical node is often the presenting sign of a nasopharyngeal carcinoma.*

The palpable cervical metastasis does not represent the primary nodal drainage because the retropharyngeal nodes are usually involved first. Therefore, surgery is rarely indicated. Irradiation is the primary treatment for both the primary lesion and the cervical metastases. A radical neck dissection is done when the primary lesion and retropharyngeal lymph nodes have been sterilized but a cervical metastasis persists.

Malignant Tumors of the Paranasal Sinuses

Squamous cell carcinoma is the most common malignant tumor of paranasal sinuses and most frequently involves the maxillary sinus. The ethmoid sinus is the second most common site, and malignancies in the frontal and sphenoid sinuses are rare. Adenoid cystic carcinoma, the second most common sinus malignancy, is often very extensive before the patient notices any symptoms. Diagnosis of malignancy is often delayed because the symptoms of early malignant tumors of the paranasal sinuses are identical to those of the common benign chronic sinusitis. To further confuse the issue, 10 per cent of patients have a long-standing history of chronic sinusitis before the development of malignancy. The patient may first complain to his dentist because a denture no longer fits or erosion of the tumor occurs into the maxillary alveolar ridge.

> *CT or MRI scanning is required to determine the stage and extent of paranasal sinus cancer.*

Initial evaluation includes palpation of the area, examination of the nose and nasopharynx for extension, and evaluation of all cranial nerves, particularly the fifth cranial nerve. Ophthalmologic examination is essential to determine orbital invasion and the status of the eye on the opposite side. CT scan of this area is mandatory in planning the extent of surgery. Radiographic evidence of bone erosion or erosion of dental roots is highly suggestive of a malignancy. Since the tumors erode posteriorly toward the skull base, it is essential to evaluate the posterior wall of the maxillary sinus for erosion as well as the involvement of the pterygoid plates or the skull base (Fig. 23–4). Often a biopsy can be obtained of abnormal-appearing tissue where the tumor extends into the nasal cavity.

> *Paranasal sinus cancers that do not extend into the soft tissues rarely metastasize to the neck.*

> *Radiation therapy is required in sinus malignancies because of the metastases to the retropharyngeal lymph nodes.*

Treatment of sinus malignancies includes total en bloc surgical resection and pre- or postoperative irradiation therapy. To assist in the patient's postoperative phase an obturator designed by a prosthodontist is fashioned to fill the large defect created by the surgical resection. It is possible to modify a total maxillectomy to preserve the orbital floor and portions of the palate. However, these alterations in total radical resection should not be made if they could compromise total tumor resection.

Malignant Tumors of the Oral Cavity

Squamous cell carcinoma is the predominant malignancy found within the oral cavity and tongue. Other tumors are of minor salivary gland origin,

PATHWAYS OF EXTENSION OF MAXILLARY SINUS MALIGNANCIES

1) INTO NASAL CAVITY (EROSION MEDIAL WALL OF MAXILLA)
2) INTO ETHMOID AREA
3) INTO ORBIT (INFERIOR ORBITAL FISSURE)
4) INTO SOFT TISSUES OF CHEEK (EROSION ANTERIOR WALL OF MAXILLA)
5) ONTO PALATE OR ALVEOLAR RIDGE (PALATE APPEARS DEPRESSED DOWNWARD)
6) INTO BUCCAL SULCUS

DETERMINATION OF RESECTABILITY OF MAXILLARY SINUS CANCER

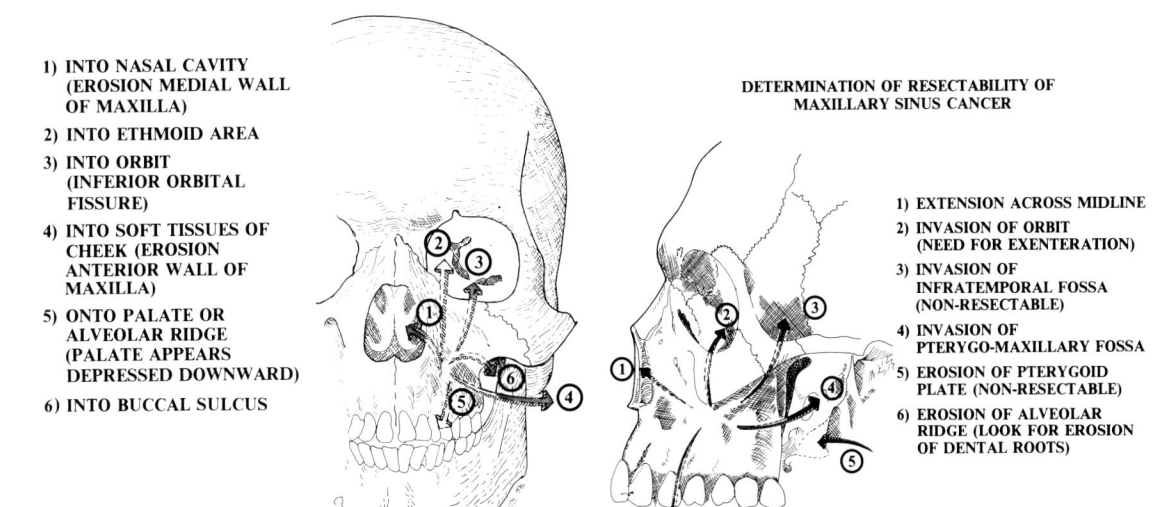

1) EXTENSION ACROSS MIDLINE
2) INVASION OF ORBIT (NEED FOR EXENTERATION)
3) INVASION OF INFRATEMPORAL FOSSA (NON-RESECTABLE)
4) INVASION OF PTERYGO-MAXILLARY FOSSA
5) EROSION OF PTERYGOID PLATE (NON-RESECTABLE)
6) EROSION OF ALVEOLAR RIDGE (LOOK FOR EROSION OF DENTAL ROOTS)

FIGURE 23–4. *A,* Frontal view of the skull showing possible pathways of extension of a maxillary sinus cancer. *B,* Side view of areas of possible extension that should be considered in determining resectability. (From McQuarrie D, Adams G, Schons A, Browne G (eds): Head and Neck Cancer: Clinical Decisions and Management Principles. Chicago, Year Book Medical Publishers, 1985, p 319.)

particularly when they arise on the hard palate. These minor salivary gland tumors are initially nonulcerating, slightly tender, submucosal masses. Squamous cell carcinoma, on the other hand, ulcerates early and is tender because of secondary surrounding inflammation.

Treatment of early oral cavity lesions is often successful with either irradiation or nonradical surgical procedures. Larger tumors are treated by a composite procedure, which includes an incontinuity neck dissection. When possible, especially in lesions originating in the anterior tongue and floor of the mouth, preservation of a rim of the mandible allows removal of the primary tumor by a "pull through" into the neck. This may avoid functional and cosmetic defects if the tongue is not bound down by the closure.

Malignant Tumors of the Base of the Tongue

Malignant tumors of the base of the tongue are the most difficult to detect by physical examination. There is often a six-month or more history of discomfort, pain on swallowing, or referred pain to the ear. The single best method of recognizing an early tumor is palpation of the base of the tongue with the finger. Biopsy in this region requires a general anesthetic and direct laryngoscopy. With the more advanced tumors the patient has difficulty and pain on swallowing and develops the so-called hot potato voice by talking and at the same time avoiding swallowing the pooled secretions.

Early tumors of the base of the tongue (T1) can be treated with radiation therapy. The neck is included in the field because of the tendency to metastasize early. When the tumor is large, a composite resection is required. Postoperative radiation therapy is often given in addition when there is cervical metastasis. Because of the high likelihood of bilateral metastases, the opposite side of the neck is always included in the radiation port.

Malignant tumors of the base of the tongue are hardest to diagnose. Physical exam requires palpation of the tongue base.

TABLE 23–5. TNM CLASSIFICATION SYSTEM APPLIED TO CANCER OF THE ORAL CAVITY

T Primary tumor
- Tis Carcinoma in situ
- T1 Greatest diameter of primary tumor 2 cm or less
- T2 Greatest diameter of primary tumor more than 2 cm but not more than 4 cm
- T3 Greatest diameter of primary tumor more than 4 cm
- T4 Massive tumor more than 4 cm in diameter with deep invasion to involve antrum, pterygoid muscles, base of tongue, skin of neck

N Regional lymph nodes
- N0 No clinically positive node
- N1 Single clinically positive homolateral node 3 cm or less in diameter
- N2 Single clinically positive homolateral node more than 3 cm but not more than 6 cm in diameter or multiple clinically positive homolateral nodes, none more than 6 cm in diameter
- N2a Single clinically positive homolateral node more than 3 cm but not more than 6 cm in diameter
- N2b Multiple clinically positive homolateral nodes, none more than 6 cm in diameter
- N3 Massive homolateral node(s), bilateral node(s), or contralateral node(s)
- N3a Clinically positive homolateral node(s), one more than 6 cm in diameter
- N3b Bilateral clinically positive nodes (in this situation, each side of the neck should be staged separately: i.e., N3b; right, N2a; left, N1)
- N3c Contralateral clinically positive node(s) only

M Distant metastasis
- M0 No evidence of distant metastasis
- M1 Distant metastasis present
    Specify _____

Prevention of aspiration is a major goal in reconstructing the base of tongue. Masssive tumors of the tongue base may even require a total laryngectomy.

Reconstruction of the posterior tongue is required to prevent continuous aspiration. The pectoralis major myocutaneous flap is ideal for this purpose. Another technique for smaller lesions involves a "push back" of the ipsilateral anterior tongue. Mandibular continuity can be maintained in certain lesions by a midline mandibulectomy, splitting the mandible and swinging it laterally to gain access. Lesions close to the margin of the tongue are approached laterally through a composite resection. Very large tumors in the base of the tongue, when treated by surgical resection, may require laryngectomy to prevent aspiration pneumonitis.

Cancer of the Tonsillar Area

Carcinoma commonly involves the tonsillar area. This region extends from the retromolar trigone to include the posterior and anterior tonsillar pillars as well as the tonsillar fossa itself. Such tumors extend inferiorly toward the base of the tongue and superiorly onto the soft palate. While small tumors (T1, T2, N0) may be treated by irradiation, larger tumors (T3, T4) require surgical resection, frequently accompanied by pre- or postoperative radiation therapy. Small lesions with palpable metastases are usually treated by surgical resection and primary closure. This resection is referred to as a composite procedure. A lateral tongue, forehead, myocutaneous, or cervical flap can close a large defect.

Carcinoma of the tonsil often metastasizes to the digastric triangle or the high jugular node known as the tonsillar node. Because of early metastases of moderate size lesions, neck dissection is usually included in the surgical procedure.

Since extranodal lymphoma can present as a unilateral enlarged tonsil, it must be included in the differential diagnosis of tonsillar tumors. Metastatic cancer from gastrointestinal sites has also been reported.

TABLE 23–6. TNM CLASSIFICATION SYSTEM APPLIED TO LARYNGEAL CANCER

Glottis
Tis	Carcinoma in situ
T1	Tumor confined to vocal cord(s) with normal mobility (includes involvement of anterior or posterior commissures)
T2	Supraglottic or subglottic extension of tumor with normal or impaired cord mobility or both
T3	Tumor confined to the larynx with cord fixation
T4	Massive tumor with thyroid cartilage destruction or extension beyond the confines of the larynx or both

From Beahrs OH, Myers MH (eds): Manual for Staging of Cancer. 2nd ed. Philadelphia, JB Lippincott Co, 1983, p 27.

Carcinoma of the Larynx

Squamous cell carcinoma is the most common laryngeal malignancy (94 per cent). Early symptoms include hoarseness and, as the involvement increases, pain, dyspnea, and eventually dysphagia. The larynx is divided into the supraglottic larynx (above the vocal cords), the glottic region (the true cord), and the subglottic area (below the level of the true cord). The lymphatic drainage of the supraglottic larynx is abundant, and consequently metastases appear early. The true cords have a poor lymphatic supply, and cervical metastases develop late and are uncommon. The lymphatics of the subglottic region leave the true larynx through the cricothyroid region and pass to the adjacent (Delphian) nodes and inferior deep cervical nodes. This division of the laryngeal lymphatic drainage is important when planning the extent of the surgical resection.

The true vocal cords have sparse lymphatic drainage; thus, tumors arising on the true cord do not metastasize to cervical nodes until late in the course of disease.

The standard supraglottic horizontal laryngectomy includes resection of the ventricle, false cord, aryepiglottic fold, and epiglottis. The tumor must not extend into the base of the tongue, to the level of the true cord, or below the petiole of the epiglottis. Extended supraglottic laryngectomy can be utilized for resection of tumors in the base of the tongue posterior to the circumvallate papillae and in the vallecula. This procedure is reserved for lesions that meet these rigid criteria in patients with good pulmonary reserve (FEV, 50 per cent of predicted). Because of a 30 per cent incidence of regional occult metastases, an ipsilateral neck dissection is generally included. The voice is preserved, but the portion of the larynx that directs food away from the airway is removed. Tracheostomy is performed at the time of surgery and is maintained until swelling subsides sufficiently to allow an adequate airway. Two to three weeks after surgery the patient will learn to swallow without aspirating, and the nasogastric tube can be removed. Postoperative, rather than preoperative, irradiation is preferred, since the wound is healed and the possibility of fistula development is reduced.

Carcinoma of the true glottic region is one of the most common head and neck malignancies. Radiation therapy or a limited surgical resection is adequate for treatment of small tumors. Slightly more advanced lesions with a mobile cord can be treated satisfactorily by a vertical hemilaryngectomy. When there is fixation of the cord (T3) there is invasion into the surrounding musculature and almost always a total laryngectomy is required. Extension of the tumor into the anterior commissure region of the larynx has a slightly poorer prognosis but, in certain instances, may still be treated by irradiation or by extending the previously described vertical hemilaryngectomy to include the anterior third of the opposite true cord as well as the anterior commissure region.

Staging of laryngeal cancer requires determination of vocal cord mobility.

If the tumor is confined entirely to one side of the larynx, it may be adequately excised by a *vertical hemilaryngectomy*. One side of the thyroid cartilage is removed, together with its medial soft tissue structures (vocal cord, false cord, aryepiglottic fold, aryepiglottic cartilage) up to or slightly across the midline. The defect is closed by a redundant mucosal flap from the adjacent ipsilateral piriform sinus. Tracheostomy is maintained until the swelling subsides and the airway is judged adequate. The nasogastric tube is removed when the patient can swallow without aspiration, generally by two weeks after surgery.

A newer alternative for select patients is *laser excision* of a T1 cordal carcinoma. Pathologic examination of margins is still necessary to assure that all tumor has been excised, so an actual specimen is resected rather than vaporizing the tumor. The advantage of this procedure is the single operative procedure, usually not requiring a tracheostomy. The disadvantage is a poorer quality voice than can be achieved by radiation therapy.

> Tumors extending into the anterior commissure are not amenable to laser excision.

Large (T3 or T4) laryngeal carcinomas are treated by surgery alone or by a combination of irradiation and laryngectomy. Carcinoma involving the subglottic region (more than 1 cm below the true cord) requires total laryngectomy and paratracheal node dissection. Approximately 40 per cent of patients who receive a laryngectomy and hemithyroidectomy followed by postoperative radiation require thyroid hormone replacement.

In a *total laryngectomy*, the larynx is removed from the anterior wall of the hypopharynx and cut off from the upper trachea. The hypopharynx is then closed upon itself and the tongue base, and the upper end of the trachea is sutured to the skin. Thus, the pharynx and airway are completely separated. If the lesion involves the adjacent hypopharynx, a partial or total *hypopharyngectomy* is additionally required. Because of the possibility of early invasion into the overlying thyroid gland, the ipsilateral lobe and isthmus of the gland are often included in the specimen. A nasogastric tube placed at the time of surgery permits food intake. It is removed about the seventh postoperative day and the patient is started on a liquid diet.

Malignant Tumors of the Hypopharynx

Carcinoma of the piriform sinus or hypopharynx is most frequently the squamous cell type. These cancers tend to metastasize early so that even a small malignancy, difficult to recognize indirectly or by direct laryngoscopy and pharyngoscopy, may present with cervical metastases. Treatment usually consists of irradiation (preoperatively or postoperatively) combined with total laryngectomy and partial pharyngectomy. Tumors in this region have a poorer prognosis than laryngeal tumors of similar size.

> Small tumors of the hypopharynx can present with advanced cervical metastatic disease.

Selected small tumors can be excised without a total laryngectomy. Such tumors are those limited to the pharyngeal side of the aryepiglottic fold and above the level of the cricoid cartilage. Another situation in which the larynx can be preserved is a limited tumor on the lateral wall of the piriform sinus. Complete or modified neck dissection is required when these tumors are treated surgically.

An unusual location for a hypopharyngeal tumor is the postcricoid area. Such tumors have been associated with the Plummer-Vinson syndrome. The prognosis is poor unless extensive surgical resection is performed, involving total laryngectomy and total pharyngectomy. Rotation flaps, jejunal interposition, colon transposition, or gastric "pull up" can be used to reconstruct the pharynx.

Cervical Lymphadenectomy (Radical Neck Dissection)

The radical cervical lymphadenectomy, or radical neck dissection, is an intrinsic part of most major head and neck surgical resections. The lymph node chains in the neck can be divided according to anatomic location into five major groups: (1) the submental nodes filling the fatty space immediately beneath the chin and superior to the hyoid bone, (2) the submandibular nodes, which occupy the region surrounding the submandibular gland and bordered by the mandible and anterior and posterior bellies of the digastric muscle, again superior to the hyoid bone (submaxillary triangle), (3) the deep jugular chain, which is closely related to the course of the internal jugular vein throughout the neck, (4) the posterior or spinal accessory chain closely associated with the spinal accessory nerve, and (5) the transverse or supraclavicular nodes, filling the supraclavicular fossa. When radical neck dissection is performed, all these nodal chains are removed.

The decision to perform radical neck dissection is based on several factors:

1. Clinically palpable nodes suspected of being metastases
2. A primary tumor in an area associated with a high incidence of occult microscopic neck metastases
3. A palpable cervical node suspected clinically of being malignant in the contralateral portion of the neck in a patient with a previous head and neck primary malignancy
4. The occult primary tumor

The occult primary condition exists when a metastatic carcinoma, usually squamous cell carcinoma or malignant melanoma, is found in a cervical lymph node other than the supraclavicular nodes. The site of the primary tumor in the upper respiratory tract or food passage is not evident, even with careful endoscopic examination including "directed" biopsies of all regions suspected of being potential sites for the primary tumor.

An occult or "unknown" primary cancer occurs when a malignant cervical lymph node is diagnosed and no primary site in the head and neck can be found.

The so-called elective radical neck dissection is performed simultaneously with resection of the primary tumor in the absence of clinically palpable cervical metastases. Regions requiring this particular procedure, which is usually done in conjunction with resection of the primary tumor, are the supraglottic larynx, base of the tongue, subglottic larynx, tonsil, and hypopharynx. The opposite or contralateral part of the neck is followed carefully for possible later metastases. Many centers prefer to irradiate the opposite side of the neck in an attempt to control possible microscopic occult metastases.

The presence of clinically palpable and obvious cervical metastases may reduce the overall survival rate by 30 to 50 per cent, regardless of the surgical procedure. The decision to undertake radical neck dissection in conjunction with resection of the primary tumor should not be made lightly. Not only does it extend the time of surgery, but it has an associated mortality of 1 per cent and increases the postoperative morbidity rate. By resecting the muscles and fascial coverings over the carotid artery, that artery is left protected only by the platysma muscle and skin. Development of a fistula from the pharynx can then cause an associated injury to the carotid artery, resulting in rupture. In an effort to reduce this disastrous complication, grafts of dermis may be obtained from the thigh to carefully cover and protect the carotid artery. Should a breakdown occur, such grafts have the ability to epithelialize, forming a protective layer over the carotid artery.

Another technique involves swinging a muscle pedicle flap from the levator scapulae muscle to protect the carotid artery. When the pectoralis major myocutaneous flap is used to reconstruct the pharynx or oral cavity, the muscle adds bulk to the site of the neck dissection and protection of the carotid artery.

An additional factor that must be recognized when planning a radical neck dissection is the associated weakness on elevation of the ipsilateral arm due to the loss of innervation of the trapezius muscle. The accessory nerve may have to be excised because of its intimate association with the spinal accessory chain in the upper neck.

A modification of the standard radical neck dissection which involves resection of the jugular, submandibular, and subdigastric nodal areas above the omohyoid is known as a *supraomohyoid neck dissection*. Indications for this procedure include tumors of the anterior oral cavity and lip. In cases of tumors of the pharynx, base of the tongue, or larynx in which bilateral nodal metastases are palpable, another option is to perform the ipsilateral neck dissection at the time of resection of the primary tumor, followed in six weeks by neck dissection on the opposite side. This two-stage, or "split," procedure is associated with considerably less morbidity than a bilateral simultaneous radical neck dissection. If it is possible to preserve one jugular vein without jeopardizing adequate tumor resection, postoperative morbidity is considerably less.

The Bocca modification of a standard neck dissection offers yet another alternative to radical neck dissection. Since the lymph nodes lie within the fascial plane of the neck, it is possible to perform a careful dissection of the layers of the superficial deep cervical fascia and its contents while preserving the sternocleidomastoid muscle, jugular vein, and accessory nerve.

This modified neck dissection is then often followed with postoperative irradiation therapy. The Bocca neck dissection is not done when (1) there are large or multiple metastases, (2) there is radiation failure, (3) there is extension into the muscles, (4) there are "fixed" metastases, or (5) there is involvement of the accessory chain or posterior group of lymph nodes. Because it is technically more difficult to perform a modified neck dissection than a classic radical neck dissection, it should be undertaken only by those doing the procedure frequently.

Supraomohyoid neck dissection can be performed for tumors of the oral cavity. Midline tumors may require bilateral supra-omohyoid neck dissections.

TABLE 23–7. REGIMENS FOR TREATMENT OF SQUAMOUS CELL CARCINOMA

Preoperative irradiation 4,000–5,000 r; 180–200/day	—4–6 weeks→	Planned surgery
Surgery	—4–8 weeks→	Postoperative radiation 6,000 r; 180–200/day

INVESTIGATIONAL PROTOCOLS

Induction chemotherapy 1–3 cycles	—3 weeks→ Surgery —4–8 weeks→	Postoperative radiation		
Surgery	—4 weeks→	Chemotherapy 3 cycles	—4 weeks→	Postoperative radiation
Induction chemotherapy	—3 weeks→ Surgery —4–8 weeks→	Postoperative radiation	—Maintenance chemotherapy × 6 months→	

TABLE 23–8. CHEMOTHERAPEUTIC AGENTS

AGENT	EFFECT	USE	ADVERSE EFFECT
Cisplatin (cis-diamminedi-chloroplatinum)	Cross-linking = DNA sensitizer	Squamous cell carcinoma; sarcoma	Nausea; nephrotoxic, ototoxic
Methotrexate	Competitive inhibition of folic acid reductase [folate inhibitor]	Squamous cell carcinoma; osteogenic sarcoma	Stomatitis; leukopenia; anemia; thrombocytopenia
Bleomycin sulfate	Inhibits DNA synthesis	Squamous cell carcinoma	Pulmonary fibrosis
Fluorouracil	Inhibits DNA synthesis	Squamous cell carcinoma in combination with cisplatin	Stomatitis; leukopenia; vomiting
Adriamycin (doxorubicin hydrochloride)	Inhibits nucleic acid synthesis	Malignant fibrous histiocytoma; sarcoma	Potentiates toxicity of other agents; mycosuppressive; cardiotoxic

Chemotherapy

Solid tumors of the head and neck area have been generally resistant to present chemotherapeutic agents. However, experimental and research protocols have demonstrated initial response rates to certain combination regimens. As exciting as these response rates have been, however, the ultimate survival rate has not been appreciably altered. Chemotherapy thus plays an adjuvant role in a research protocol setting. Some of the methods in which chemotherapy has been employed are shown in Table 23–7.

The most common chemotherapy products currently used for squamous cell carcinoma include methotrexate (MTX), 5-fluorouracil (5FU), and cisplatin (Table 23–8). These drugs (except MTX) are administered by intravenous infusion. Doxorubicin (Adriamycin) is often the control drug used for sarcoma and may be combined with methotrexate. Mithramycin has been used advantageously when hypercalcemia is associated with metastatic carcinoma.

The role of chemotherapy in the adjuvant setting is still to be defined. Some studies have demonstrated a 70 per cent response rate for advanced squamous cell carcinoma when two or three courses of chemotherapy are administered preoperatively. This has not altered surgical wound healing, but some patients have then refused surgery. Recurrence of tumor is then always the result, and this time the tumor may not be operable. Chemotherapy for recurrence of tumor in the previously operated, previously irradiated site of the surgery has been much less effective.

Chemotherapy alone or in combination with radiation therapy can produce significant response rates.

Suggested Readings

It is not possible to cover the subject of head and neck cancer in this text. Selected additional articles are suggested for more extensive reading on each of the subjects discussed in this chapter.

General

McQuarrie D, Adams G, Schons A, Browne G (eds): Head and Neck Cancer: Clinical Decisions and Management Principles. Chicago, Year Book Medical Publishers, 1985.

Million R, Cassisi NJ: Management of Head and Neck Cancer: A Multidisciplinary Approach. New York, JB Lippincott Co, 1984.

Segren SL: Recent advances in radiation therapy of head and neck cancer. Head Neck Surg 4:227–232, 1982.

Silver CE: Surgery for Cancer of the Larynx and Related Structures. London, Churchill Livingstone, 1981.

Snow JB, Belber RD, Kramer S, et al: Randomized preoperative and postoperative radiation therapy for patients with carcinoma of the head and neck: Preliminary report. Laryngoscope 90:930–945, 1980.

Suen JY, Myers EN (eds): Cancer of the Head and Neck. New York, Churchill Livingstone, 1981.

Vraebec DA, Heffron TJ: Hypothyroidism following treatment for head and neck cancer. Ann Otol Rhinol Laryngol 90:449, 1981.

Neck Dissection

Bocca E, Pignataro O: A conservation technique in radical neck dissection. Ann Otol Rhinol Laryngol 76:975–987, 1967.

Fletcher GH, Jesse RH: The place of irradiation in the management of the primary lesion in head and neck cancer. Cancer 39:862–867, 1977.

Jesse RH, Ballantyne AJ, Larson D: Radical or modified neck dissection: A therapeutic dilemma. Am J Surg 136:516–519, 1978.

Jesse RH, Fletcher GH: Treatment of the neck in patients with squamous cell carcinoma of the head and neck. Cancer 39:868–872, 1977.

Johnson JT, Barnes EL, Myers EN, et al: The extracapsular spread of tumors in cervical node metastasis. Arch Otolaryngol 107:725–729, 1981.

Medina JE, Byers RM: Supraomohyoid neck dissection. Head Neck Surg 11:111–122, 1989.

Schuller DE, et al: Analysis of disability resulting from treatment including radical neck dissection or modified radical neck dissection. Head Neck Surg 6:551–558, 1983.

White D, Byers RM: What is the preferred initial method of treatment for squamous carcinoma of the tongue? Am J Surg 140:553–555, 1980.

Second Primary Malignancies

Maisel RH, Vermeersch H: Panendoscopy for second primary tumors in head and neck cancer patients. Ann Otol Rhinol Laryngol 90:460–464, 1981.

McQuirt UF: Panendoscopy as a screening examination for simultaneous tumors in head and neck cancer. Laryngoscope 92:569–576, 1982.

Vraebec D: Multiple primary malignancies of the upper aerodigestive system. Ann Otol Rhinol Laryngol 88:846–854, 1979.

Salivary Gland Malignancies

Adams GL, Duvall AJ: Adenocarcinoma of the head and neck. Arch Otolaryngol 93:261, 1971.

Eneroth CM: Salivary gland tumors in the parotid gland, submandibular gland and the palate region. Cancer 27:1415–1418, 1971.

Frazell RL: Observations in the management of salivary gland tumors. Cancer 18:235–241, 1968.

Johns ME: Parotid cancer: A rational basis for treatment. Head Neck Surg 3:132–144, 1980.

Sarcomas

Blitzer A, et al: Clinical-pathological determination in prognosis of fibrous histiocytomas of the head and neck. Laryngoscope 91:2053–2070, 1981.

Feldman BA: Rhabdomyosarcoma of the head and neck. Laryngoscope 92:424–440, 1982.

Healy GB, et al: Rhabdomyosarcoma of the head and neck: Diagnosis and management. Head Neck Surg 1:334–339, 1979.

Malignant Tumors of the Nose and Paranasal Sinuses

Batsakis JG: The pathology of head and neck tumors: Nasal cavity and paranasal sinus. Head Neck Surg 2:410–419, 1980.

Frazell E, Lewis J: Cancer of the nasal cavity and accessory sinuses. Cancer 16:1293, 1963.

Goefert H, Guillinondequi OM, Jesse RH, et al: Squamous cell carcinoma of the nasal vestibule. Arch Otolaryngol 100:8–10, 1974.

Ketcham AS, Wilkins JM, Van Buren JM, et al: A combined intracranial facial resection for tumors of the paranasal sinuses. Am J Surg 106:698, 1963.

Mendenhall NP, Parsons JT, Cassisi NJ, Million RR: Carcinoma of the nasal vestibule treated with radiation therapy. Laryngoscope 97:626–632, 1987.
Myers EN, Schramm VL, Barnes EL: Management of inverted papilloma of the nose and paranasal sinuses. Laryngoscope 91:2071–2084, 1981.
Session GA: Symposium: Treatment of malignancies of the paranasal sinuses. Laryngoscope 80:945, 1970.
Skolnik EM, Massari FS, Tenta LT: Olfactory neuroepithelioma. Arch Otolaryngol 81:644–653, 1966.
Snow EB, Van Der Esch EP, Slotten EA: Mucosal melanomas of the head and neck. Head Neck Surg 1:24–30, 1978.

Carcinoma of the Nasopharynx

Dickson RI: Nasopharyngeal carcinoma: An evaluation of 209 patients. Laryngoscope 91:333–354, 1981.
Ho JHC: A epidemiological and clinical study of nasopharyngeal carcinoma. Int J Radiat Oncol Biol Phys 4:183–193, 1978.

Carcinoma of the Tongue, Oral Cavity, and Floor of the Mouth

Barrs DM, DeSanto LW, O'Fallon WM: Squamous cell carcinoma of the tonsil and tongue base region. Arch Otolaryngol 105:479–485, 1979.
Harold CC: Management of cancer of the floor of the mouth. Am J Surg 122:487–493, 1971.
Jesse RH, Sugarbaker EV: Squamous cell carcinoma of the oropharynx: Why we fail. Am J Surg 132:435–438, 1976.
Marks JE, Lee F, Smith PG, et al: Floor of mouth cancer: Patient selection and treatment results. Laryngoscope 93:475–480, 1983.
Matz G, Shumrick DA, Aron BS: Carcinoma of the tonsil: Results of combined treatment. Laryngoscope 84:2172–2180, 1974.
Parsons JT, Million RR, Cassisi NJ: Carcinoma of the base of the tongue: Results of radical irradiation with surgery reserved for irradiation failure. Laryngoscope 92:689–696, 1982.
Strong EW: Carcinoma of the tongue. Otolaryngol Clin North Am 12:107–114, 1979.

Carcinoma of the Larynx

DeSanto LW: The options in early laryngeal carcinomas. N Engl J Med 306:910, 1982.
Ogura JH, Bell JA: Laryngectomy and radical neck dissection for carcinoma of the larynx. Laryngoscope 62:1, 1952.
Kirchner J, Som ML: Clinical significance of fixed vocal cord. Laryngoscope 81:1029, 1971.
Som ML: Conservation surgery for carcinoma of the supraglottis. J Laryngol Otol 84:655, 1970.
Strong MS: Laser excision of carcinoma of the larynx. Laryngoscope 85:1286, 1975.
Wang CC: Treatment of glottic carcinoma by megavoltage radiation therapy and results. AJR 120:157, 1974.

Cancer of the Ear and Temporal Bone

Adams GL, Paparella MM, Elfiky FM: Primary and metastatic tumors of the temporal bone. Laryngoscope 82:1273–1285, 1971.
Conley JJ, Schuller D: Malignancies of the ear. Laryngoscope 86:1147–1163, 1976.
Lederman M: Malignant tumors of the ear. J Laryngol Otol 79:85, 1965.

Reconstruction

Baek S, Lawson W, Biller HF: An analysis of 133 pectoralis major myocutaneous flaps. Plast Reconstr Surg 69:460–467, 1982.
Bakamjian VY: A two stage method for pharyngoesophageal reconstruction. Plast Reconstr Surg 36:173–184, 1965.
Gluckman JL, et al: The free jejunal graft in head and neck reconstruction. Laryngoscope 91:1887–1894, 1981.
Schechter GL, Sly DE, Roger AL, et al: Set-back tongue flap for carcinoma of the tongue base. Arch Otolaryngol 106:668–674, 1980.
Panje W: Prosthetic voice rehabilitation following laryngectomy. Ann Otol Rhinol Laryngol 90:116–120, 1981.
Singer MI, Blom ED: An endoscopic technique for restoration of voice after laryngectomy. Ann Otol Rhinol Laryngol 89:52, 1980.

PART SEVEN

DISEASES OF THE TRACHEA AND CERVICAL ESOPHAGUS

24

DISEASES OF THE LOWER AIR PASSAGES, ESOPHAGUS, AND MEDIASTINUM:
Endoscopic Considerations

by Leighton G. Siegel, M.D.

THE ESOPHAGUS

Esophagoscopy is the most direct method of examining the lumen of the esophagus. It is essential for visualization and removal of foreign bodies, evaluation of mucosal and tissue changes, and biopsy for microscopic examination. It is the most reliable method of obtaining washings for cytologic studies and culture. The presence and character of strictures, deviations, and other esophageal abnormalities can be seen and often treated through the esophagoscope.

Esophageal Disorders

The most common esophageal disorders are probably related to motor function. They are generally classified as those of hypomotility or hypermotility or occasionally a combination of the two.

The most common esophageal disorders are those of dismotility.

Functional dysphagia or dysrhythmia is a disorder of hypomotility. It generally occurs in the older patient and produces the sensation of food sticking substernally. On radiography the peristaltic waves seem to end in the midportion of the esophagus, and swallowing is not completed until the second dry swallow is made. Esophageal achalasia, sometimes called cardiospasm, is a neuromuscular disorder. Failure of the esophagogastric junction to relax with deglutition results in a proximal dilatation of the esophagus with an absence of peristalsis. In achalasia the patient feels a need to force or push food down with water or other beverages to complete swallowing. There is a sensation of substernal fullness, and regurgitation is common. On radiography there is a significant retention of barium in the esophagus, with evident difficulty in passage from the esophagus into the stomach. In all cases of achalasia esophagoscopy should be performed to rule out malignant obstruction (Fig. 24–1).

Diffuse spasm of the esophagus is a disorder of hypermotility. Pain is the primary symptom. This is associated with diffuse spasm of the lower part of the esophagus and is usually precipitated by swallowing. These attacks are intermittent, and between attacks the patient may swallow without difficulty.

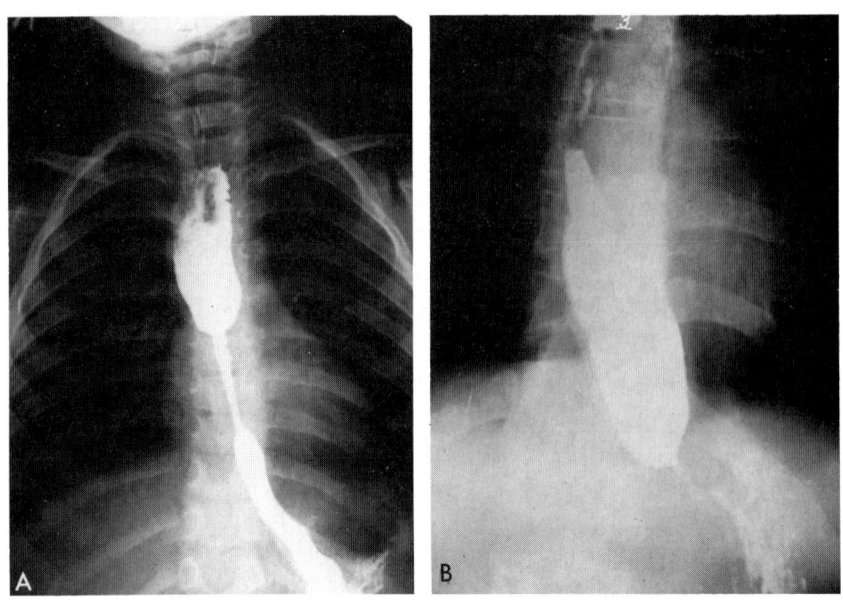

FIGURE 24–1. Barium swallow demonstrating (A) corrosive esophagitis from chemical ingestion, and (B) cardiospasm.

Cough and/or hoarseness may be the presenting symptoms of an esophageal disorder.

They may also occur without swallowing and may even awaken the patient from a sound sleep. There may be no radiographic evidence of abnormalities, but intraluminal esophageal pressure measurements may be diagnostic. Differentiation between diffuse spasm and cardiac pain is occasionally difficult.

A hiatus hernia, in which a portion of the stomach has herniated into the thoracic cavity, is common and may produce a pressure sensation or pain behind the lower sternum. Cough, dysphagia, palpitation, and tachycardia may also be present. The pain is generally relieved when the patient assumes an upright position and is aggravated when the patient is recumbent. Radiographic studies and esophagoscopy are generally diagnostic.

Schatski's contraction ring is a concentric ring-like narrowing at the level of the inferior esophageal sphincter. It produces dysphagia and discomfort with regurgitation if more than a small amount of food is swallowed at once.

Diverticuli usually arise in the cervical esophagus and may produce regurgitation of undigested food and progressive dysphagia as more food is eaten. Radiographic studies are generally diagnostic.

Many systemic diseases produce esophageal symptoms. Examples of these are scleroderma, dermatomyositis, myasthenia gravis, and cirrhosis with esophageal varices.

Inflammatory disorders of the esophagus include acute esophagitis and reflux esophagitis. Less often seen are tuberculosis and monilial inflammations. Metabolic, degenerative, and neurogenic disturbances of the esophagus may also occur. Benign and malignant neoplasia may arise from both the esophageal wall and the mucosa or may originate in the stomach or laryngopharynx and extend into the esophagus. Dysphagia, pain, and weight loss are the most common initial symptoms of malignant disease, although they may not occur early. Treatment depends upon size and location of the neoplasm and consists of surgery, irradiation, or both.

A great number of congenital anomalies of the esophagus exist. Some involve the esophagus alone. Others involve the esophagus and trachea. Still others are anomalies of adjacent structures that impinge on the esophagus. Esophageal absence is rare. A congenital duplicate esophagus may exist as either a tube or a cystlike structure adjacent to the esophagus. Simple webs are rare. Stenosis may be fibrotic or due to a failure of epithelialization of a section of the esophagus. Congenital esophageal stenosis occurring at the junction of the middle and proximal third may first become evident when the infant begins taking solid foods. Several types of tracheoesophageal fistulas exist, all of which require surgical therapy. Atresia without tracheoesophageal fistula may require repeated bronchoscopic aspirations prior to surgery. Vascular rings and other cardiovascular anomalies may produce varying degrees of obstruction because of extrinsic pressure on the lumen of the esophagus.

Anomalies that compress the esophagus commonly compress air passages also.

Caustic Ingestion

Corrosive esophagitis is most commonly produced by ingestion of household cleaning agents, usually by children. The most destructive is sodium hydroxide, or lye, which causes lysis of tissue and often deep penetration of the esophageal wall. Liquid drain cleaners may damage the esophagus or produce similar gastric lesions. Certain agents not only are caustic to the esophagus but have severe systemic effects, such as renal failure.

If there is a history of possible ingestion of caustic agents, it is imperative that the presence or absence of esophageal involvement be established. The presence or absence of oral pharyngeal ulcerations *is of no help* in deciding if there is an esophageal burn. This can be established only by esophagoscopy, which may be safely done provided that the scope is not passed beyond the first visible esophageal injury. Esophagoscopy is generally performed 24 to 48 hours after ingestion. If the caustic agent produces an early severe necrosis, perforation and resultant mediastinitis can occur. More commonly, perforation does not occur, but in the healing process a scar circumferentially constricts the esophagus, producing an esophageal stenosis (Table 24–1).

When caustic ingestion is suspected it is up to the physician to prove or disprove that it has occurred.

When large quantities of lye are ingested, as in adult suicide attempts, emergency total esophagogastrectomy may be required. If perforation is likely, steroids are not given. The use of steroids can mask a developing peritonitis or mediastinitis. In such cases all efforts are directed at the

TABLE 24–1. COMMON AGENTS PRODUCING ESOPHAGEAL BURNS

Drain cleaners (NaOH)
   Liquid Plumber
   Drano (liquid or crystal)
Oven cleaners
   Easy off
Ammonia
Clinitest tablets
Bleach
Phosphates
Acids
   Sulfuric
   Nitric
Phenol
Iodine
Potassium permanganate

treatment of the mediastinitis or peritonitis. Attention is given to the shock and toward stabilizing the patient rather than prevention of stricture.

Early diagnosis and treatment are critical.

Early diagnosis and treatment are essential if a disabling esophageal stenosis is to be avoided. By the time the patient is seen in the emergency room, the use of any substance to neutralize the lye may only cause emesis and increase the existing injury. The most common sites for burns are at the level of the cricopharyngeus and the cardia. Burns of the lower esophagus are associated with reflux. When there is significant pain with swallowing, the patient is given no food by mouth, and a small polyethylene nasogastric tube is passed and left in place until healing is complete. This tube allows feeding and maintains a lumen for future dilatation if necessary. Systemic broad-spectrum antibiotics (e.g., amoxicillin) are begun and continued throughout therapy to control infection. Steroid therapy must be initiated in the first 48 to 96 hours after the ingestion. Antibiotics and steroids may not be helpful if administration is begun after this period.

Adults may be given 80 mg of prednisone the first day, 60 mg the second day, 40 mg the third day, and then 20 mg daily until the esophagus is healed. Children may be given 1 mg prednisone per kilogram of body weight daily for two weeks; the dosage is then gradually tapered. The antibiotics, steroids, and nasogastric feedings are continued until the healing process is complete, usually for four to six weeks. Esophagoscopy or barium swallow is repeated about every two weeks until healing is completed. After complete healing is evident, the antibiotics may be discontinued and the steroid dosage gradually reduced. Follow-up should also include repeated esophagograms. In those patients who develop strictures despite therapy, dilatation is necessary. For small or short strictures, dilatation may be accomplished using esophagoscopes or mercury-filled rubber bougies. Dilatation is performed with great caution, if at all, when patients are still on steroids. If multiple strictures or severe esophageal deformities are present, a gastrotomy is performed and retrograde dilatation is accomplished by pulling the dilator from the stomach through the esophagus with a string. In the rare patient, when all measures fail to prevent obstructing stenosis, a loop of bowel may be brought up into the chest as a substitute esophagus. The incidence of carcinoma of the esophagus is increased one thousand fold in adults who experienced caustic strictures during childhood.

Foreign Body Ingestion

Ingested foreign bodies may lodge in the esophagus. The etiology of foreign body ingestion and aspiration is similar and is discussed later in the section on aspiration. The most important point in the history of ingestion of foreign bodies, as with caustic ingestion, is to believe the patient. It is up to the physician to adequately demonstrate the absence of a foreign body or caustic burn once its presence is suggested by the patient or the patient's symptoms. Whenever possible, request that the patient bring a duplicate of the foreign body so that the endoscopist may decide which type of forceps and approach will be most effective in removal. Tell the patient to take nothing to eat or drink and not to induce vomiting. This will reduce the likelihood of a peristaltic contraction inducing a perforation as it passes the foreign body and decreases the risk of vomiting and aspiration during later anesthesia induction.

The most common site for lodgment is at the entrance to the esophagus at the level of the cricopharyngeus muscle. Other common sites are where the esophagus is indented by the arch of the aorta and the left main bronchus and at the entrance to the stomach. Pathologic lesions of the esophagus may produce partial obstruction and cause the lodgment of foreign bodies that otherwise would pass through quite easily. Children account for nearly 70 per cent of foreign body ingestion. They tend to carry coins, pins, toys, and other objects in their mouths, with subsequent accidental ingestion.

A foreign body that lodges in the esophagus produces both difficulty in swallowing and discomfort. The position of a foreign body in the esophagus can often be accurately localized by the patient. If the foreign body has lodged in the cervical esophagus, pressure against the back of the larynx and trachea may produce hoarseness, cough, and dyspnea. Saliva may flow out of the esophagus and into the larynx.

Dysphagia and odynophagia are common symptoms.

Radiopaque foreign bodies may be seen easily on posteroanterior and lateral chest radiographs. Radiographs should include all areas from the nose to the anus. Often more than one foreign body has been ingested, and unless complete studies are made, additional objects, such as a needle that has passed into the colon, could be missed. More commonly, the foreign body is radiolucent and is not seen on plain roentgenogram. Thin metallic foreign bodies can be seen only if radiographed on edge. For this reason both posteroanterior and lateral films are indicated. An esophagogram and associated fluoroscopy should then be done. A large swallow of barium should not be given, as it coats the walls of the esophagus with a thick white paste that makes subsequent esophagoscopy very difficult. It is better to have the patient swallow a bit of cotton or marshmallow with contrast medium in it. Cotton fibers may catch on the foreign body for a moment or two during deglutition, thereby revealing its presence through fluoroscopy. Knowledge of the orientation of the foreign body in the esophagus is very helpful in planning endoscopic removal (Fig. 24–2).

P.A. and lateral x-rays are needed. Avoid large swallows of barium.

Symptoms associated with the ingestion of foreign bodies occur in three stages. In the first stage of initial symptoms, there is a violent paroxysm of coughing or gagging. This occurs when the foreign body is first swallowed. The second stage is a symptomless interval. The foreign body has lodged, and symptoms are no longer produced. This stage may last only a moment or two. The third stage consists of the symptoms produced by complications. There may be discomfort, dysphagia, obstruction, or perforation of the esophagus with resultant mediastinitis.

First stage
Second stage
Third stage

Unless complete airway obstruction exists, first aid during the stage of initial symptoms should consist of resisting the urge to "do something." Slapping the patient on the back, hanging the child by the heels, putting a finger down the patient's throat, or attempting blind removal may convert a simple, uncomplicated foreign body into a complicated obstructing one (Fig. 24–3). A more complete discussion on the management of acute airway obstruction is found later in this chapter under Foreign Body Aspiration.

What not to do.

Esophageal foreign bodies generally require more urgent treatment than those in the tracheobronchial tree because of the danger of perforation of the thin esophageal wall and resultant mediastinitis. Therefore, ingested foreign bodies with sharp edges or points should be removed on any emergency basis. Blunt esophageal foreign bodies, such as coins, may be trapped initially by esophageal spasm. Coins and other disc-shaped objects

Prompt removal of esophageal foreign bodies is more important than prompt removal of foreign bodies in the tracheobronchial tree.

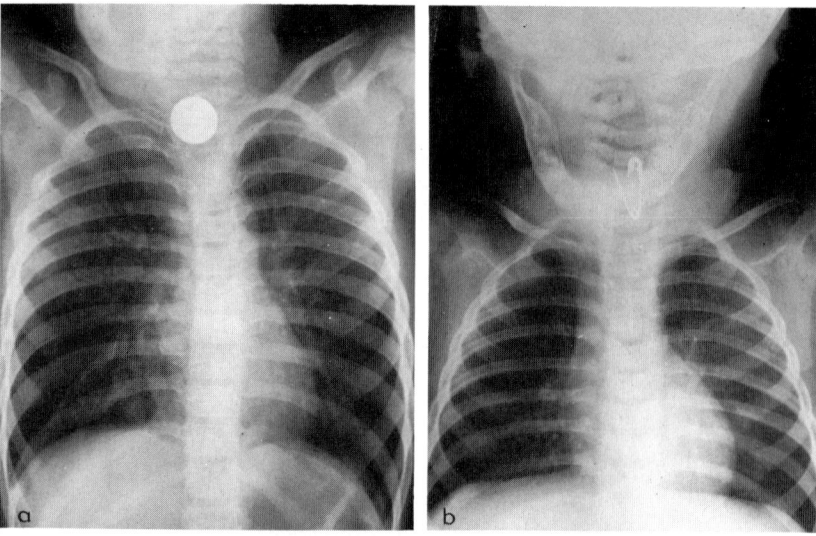

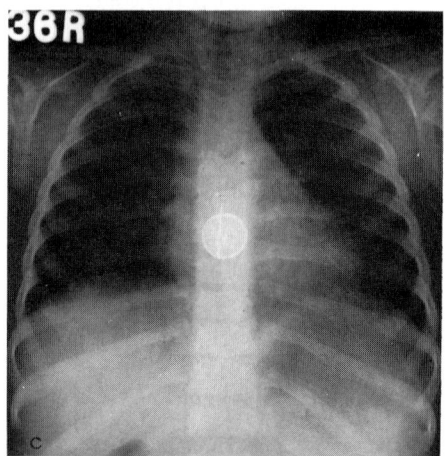

FIGURE 24–2. Common types of esophageal foreign bodies in children. *A*, Coin at the cervical narrowing ("upper pinchcock"); *B*, safety pin arrested at the same site as in *A*; *C*, campaign button arrested temporarily in the lower third of the esophagus.

generally orient in a transverse direction in the esophagus and anteroposteriorly in the trachea. They are generally trapped at the level of the cricopharyngeus muscle in children. Glucagon or a subhypnotic dose of an analgesic or sedative drug may relax the spasm, allowing the coin to pass into the stomach.

In general, foreign bodies that have reached the stomach will pass through the remainder of the gastrointestinal tract without difficulty. One important exception occurs with objects over 5 cm in length, such as bobby pins, ingested by children age two or under. At that age straight objects such as these cannot traverse the duodenal bends and may perforate in one of these locations. Patients whose foreign body has passed into the stomach should be instructed to continue a normal diet and should be given no drugs that would affect gastrointestinal motility. A low roughage diet does not provide adequate food bulk around the foreign body to protect the intestinal lumen. Similarly, a high roughage diet may increase peristaltic contractions so that the foreign body may perforate. The stool should be carefully examined to

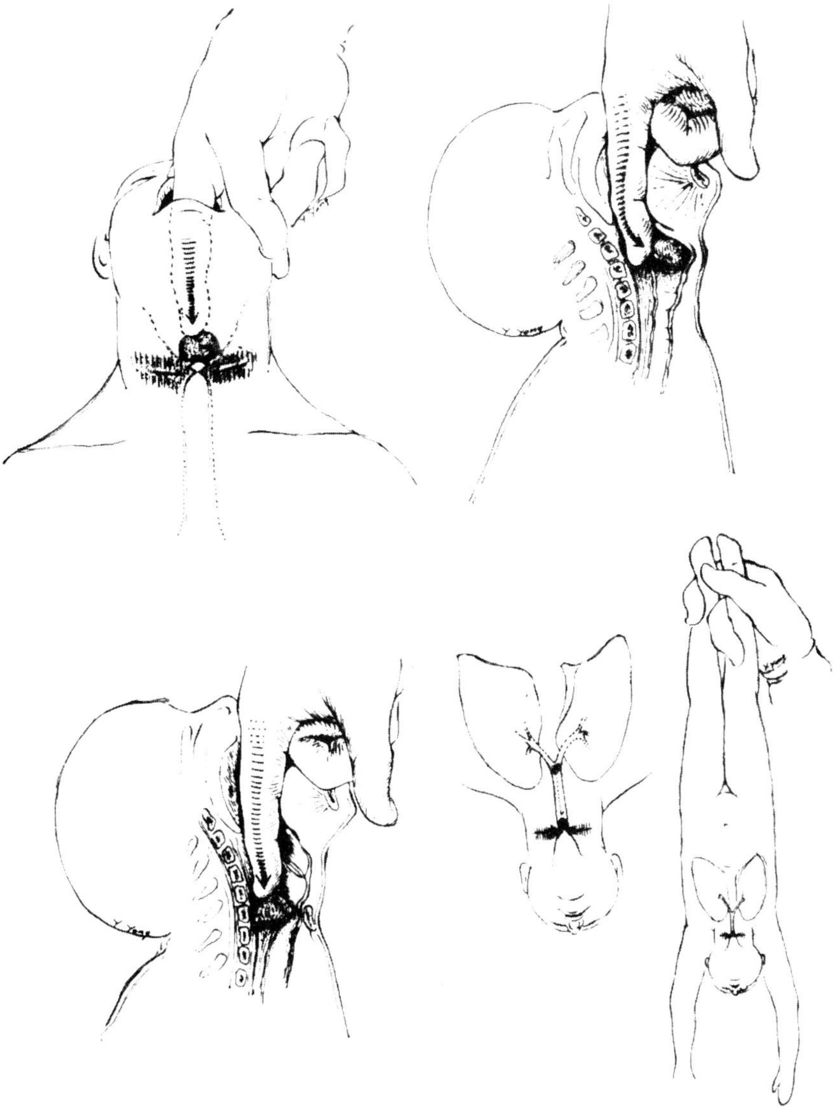

FIGURE 24–3. Possible methods of impaction of a foreign body by ill-advised first aid. (From Tucker GF Jr: Minutes Report of the Committee for the Prevention of Foreign Body Accidents. Trans Am Bronchoesophagol Assoc 49:181–183, 1969.)

prove complete passage of the foreign body. Abdominal pain in these patients may indicate that a perforation has occurred.

Evaluation of Esophageal Disease

Patient History

When a patient's presenting complaint suggests esophageal disease, the following specific history should be elicited and characterized as to location, onset, duration, frequency, relation to eating, and factors that seem to minimize or increase associated symptoms.

1. Difficulty in swallowing (dysphagia) solids or liquids
2. Complete obstruction (inability to swallow)

3. Discomfort in swallowing (odynophagia)
4. Regurgitation of undigested food
5. Hematemesis (vomiting of blood)
6. Sensation of foreign body
7. Lump in throat
8. Heartburn
9. Weight loss
10. Hoarseness
11. Sensitivity to hot or cold foods

Physical Examination

Remember to examine the larynx and neck when esophageal symptoms exist.

Physical examinations for esophageal disease should begin with an assessment of the patient's voice and speech. Careful palpation of the neck may reveal evidence of metastatic malignant disease or an enlarged or abnormal thyroid gland. The larynx and trachea normally lie in the midline and should be checked for deviation. There should not be tenderness over the cricopharyngeus muscle. Intraoral examination may reveal abnormal weakness of the tongue, soft palate, or pharyngeal walls or deviation of the uvula in the presence of neurologic disease. Vagal paralysis may produce asymmetric movement of the posterior pharyngeal wall. Mirror examination of the hypopharynx and the larynx may similarly reveal a vocal cord paralysis or abnormal puddling of secretions or saliva in the piriform sinuses. This puddling is a particularly important sign that may indicate an esophageal obstruction such as a foreign body or tumor.

Radiographic and Other Studies

Avoid large quantities of barium when doing an esophagram for foreign body evaluation.

Radiographic examination of the esophagus is perhaps the most useful method for studying this organ. A preliminary chest radiograph and scout film of the neck should precede fluoroscopy with a barium or iodized oil swallow. Videoradiographic techniques may also be helpful if they are available. Barium coats the esophagus and thus should not be used as a contrast agent if esophagoscopy is planned shortly after the radiographs are taken.

Other diagnostic tests may be done in conjunction with radiography, including intraluminal pressure measurements. In this study, water-filled tubes are positioned to measure pressure changes within the esophageal lumen during the deglutition (Fig. 24–4 *A* and *B*). Disorders of motor function, whether involving hypermotility or hypomotility, can be diagnosed and the effects of therapy quantitatively measured using this technique.

Esophagoscopy

Esophagoscopy is indicated after careful history, physical examination, and radiographic studies are completed. Esophagoscopy is advised when any question remains about the diagnosis or if therapy may be instituted via esophagoscopy. A negative radiographic study does not eliminate the need for esophagoscopy, since many small mucosal lesions, nonradiopaque foreign bodies, and nonspecific inflammatory changes can be diagnosed only in this manner. Esophagoscopy is contraindicated in the presence of an aortic aneurysm (Fig. 24–5).

Two basic types of esophagoscopes exist. One type is a rigid metal tube with an oval lumen which contains a light carrier and a channel for aspiration

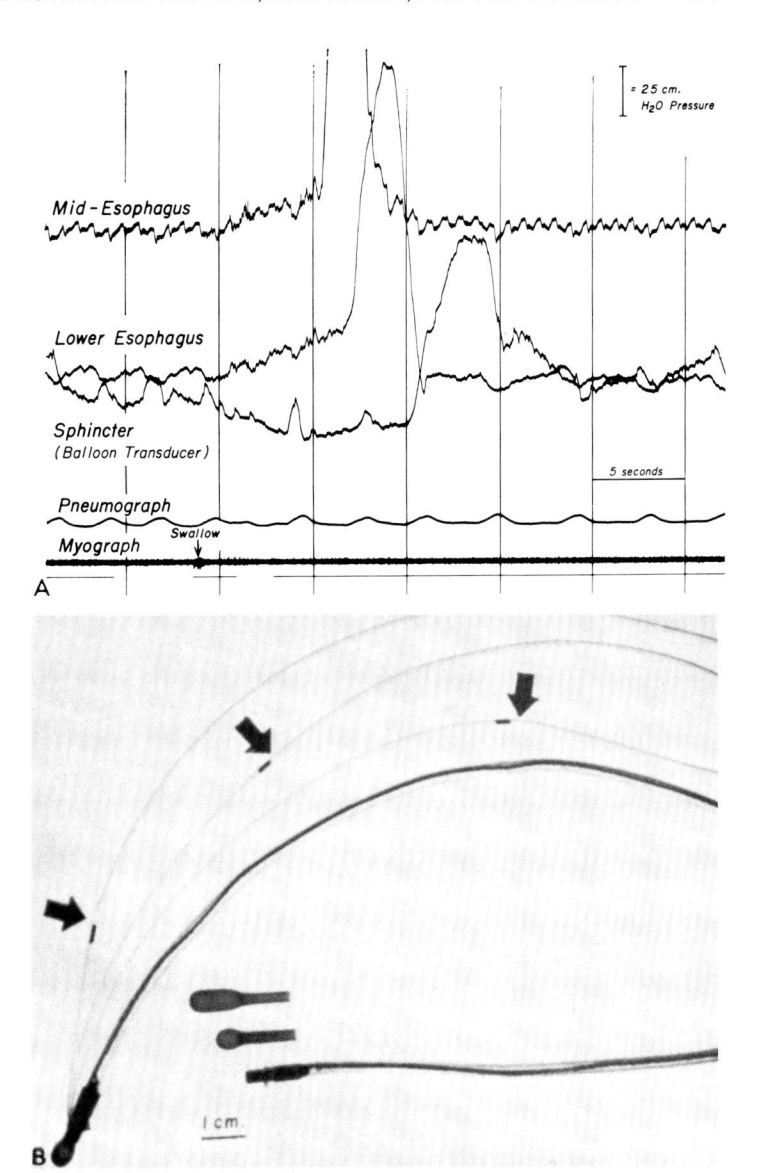

FIGURE 24–4. *A*, Esophageal motility tracing showing a normal peristaltic wave progressing down the esophagus. Note evidence of relaxation of the esophagogastric sphincter shortly after the patient swallowed. *B*, Balloon-covered transducer with associated polyethylene tubes used for detection of intraluminal pressures. (From Andersen HA: Dysfunction of the esophagus. Otolaryngol Clin North Am 1(2):197, June 1968.)

of secretions. This type of esophagoscope permits direct unobstructed visualization of the esophageal mucosa and manipulation with a variety of instruments for both biopsy and removal of foreign bodies. The second type is the flexible esophagoscope with fiberoptic illumination and fiberoptic viewing. A smaller channel exists for aspiration of secretions and insertion of a slender forceps for biopsy or foreign body removal (Table 24–2). This type provides a more magnified view of the mucosa but does not allow as wide a variety of instruments for manipulation, particularly of foreign bodies. It also will not retract and protect the esophageal wall during removal of sharp-edged foreign bodies as does the rigid esophagoscope. Esophagoscopy may be done under local or general anesthesia. The choice of anesthetic and esophagoscope usually depends upon the endoscopist, the age and general health of the patient, and the suspected disease (Fig. 24–6).

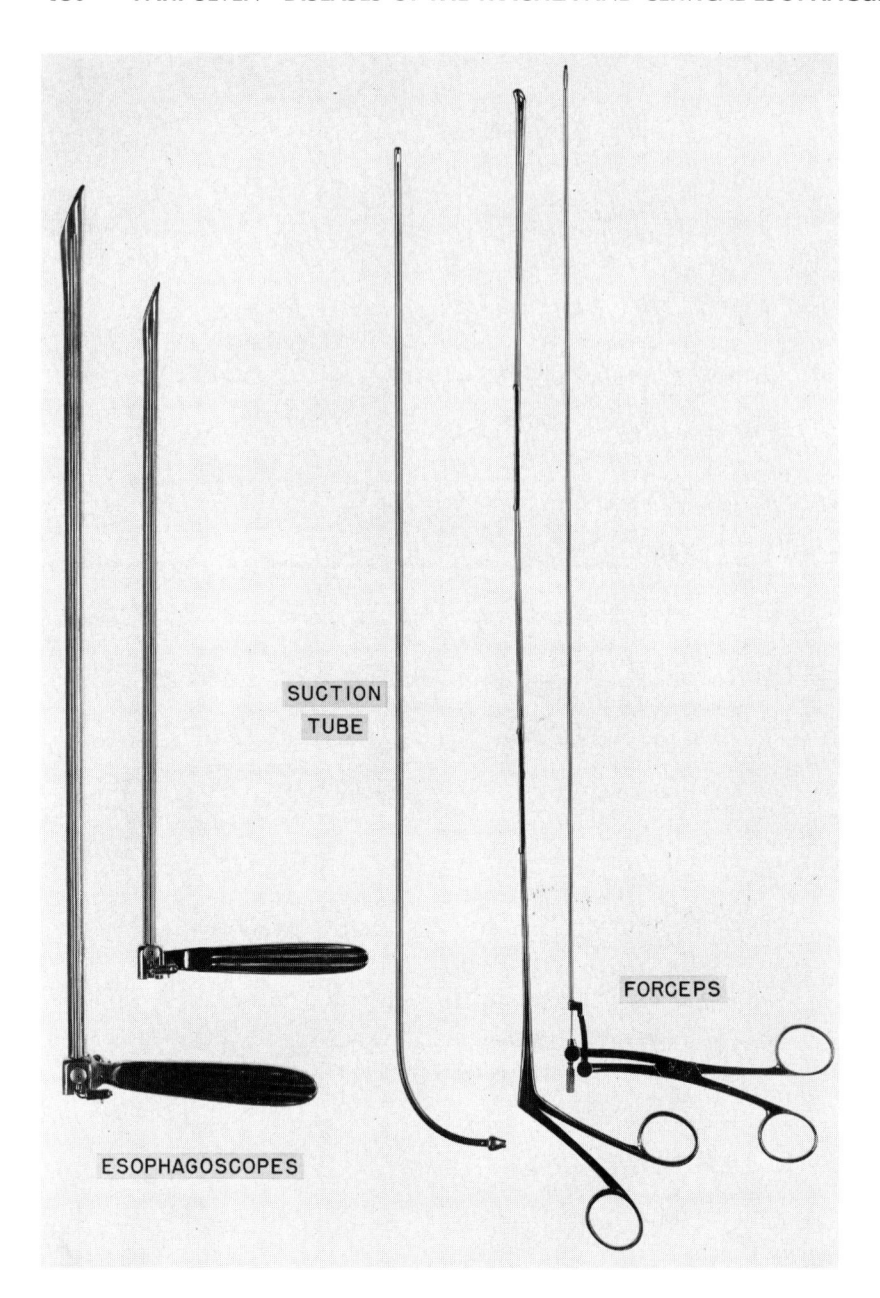

FIGURE 24–5. Adult and infant esophagoscopes (Jesberg models), grasping and biopsy forceps, and suction tube.

TABLE 24–2. ENDOSCOPE AND TRACHEOSTOMY TUBE SIZES IN INFANTS AND CHILDREN*

AGE	LARYNGOSCOPE	BRONCHOSCOPE	ESOPHAGOSCOPE	TRACHEOSTOMY TUBE
Premature	6	3.0 mm × 20 cm	3.5 mm × 25 cm	00
Newborn	6	3.5 mm × 25 cm	4.0 mm × 35 cm	0
3 to 6 months	9	3.5 mm × 30 cm	4.0 mm × 35 cm	0 or 1
1 year	9	4.0 mm × 30 cm	5.0 mm × 35 cm	1
2 years	11	4.0 mm × 30 cm	5.0 mm × 35 cm	1
4 years	11	5.0 mm × 35 cm	6.0 mm × 35 cm	2
5 to 7 years	12	5.0 mm × 35 cm	6.0 mm × 35 cm	3
8 to 12 years	16	6.0 mm × 35 cm 7.0 mm × 40 cm	6.0 mm × 35 cm	3 or 4

*The tube size for adults depends upon height and weight and usually ranges from the size used for 12-year-olds to two sizes larger.

	Birth	2 yr	3 yr	6 yr	10 yr	14 yr	Adult		
	23	27	30	33	36	43	53	cm.	Greater Curvature
	18	19	22	25	27	34	40	cm.	Cardia
	17	18	21	24	26	33	38	cm.	Hiatus
	13	15	16	18	20	24	27	cm.	Left Bronchus
	12	14	15	16	17	21	23	cm.	Aorta
	7	9	10	11	12	14	16	cm.	Cricopharyngeus

Upper Incisors

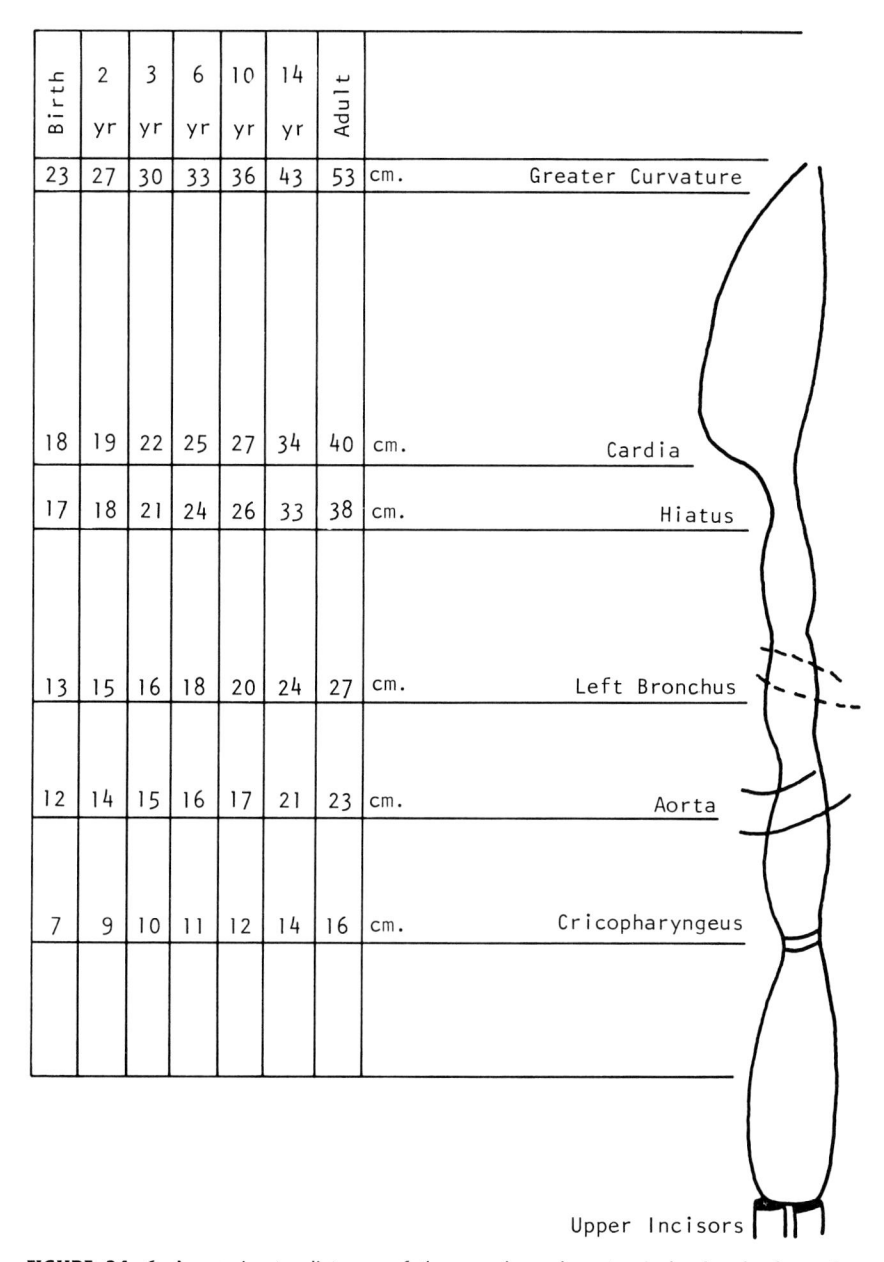

FIGURE 24–6. Approximate distance of the esophageal anatomic landmarks from the upper incisor teeth as seen by the endoscopist. (Adapted from Jackson C, Jackson CL: Bronchoesophagology. Philadelphia, WB Saunders Co, 1950, p 229.)

THE TRACHEOBRONCHIAL TREE

Bronchoscopy is the only method of directly visualizing the tracheobronchial tree and its pathology (Figs. 24–7 and 24–8). It is often the only way of confirming or making early diagnosis, for it allows direct biopsy of tumors and localized washings for cytologic studies and culture. Bronchoscopy is often needed for therapeutic reasons such as the removal of foreign bodies. Bronchoscopic cleansing is one of the most effective methods of treating obstructive or aspirated secretions.

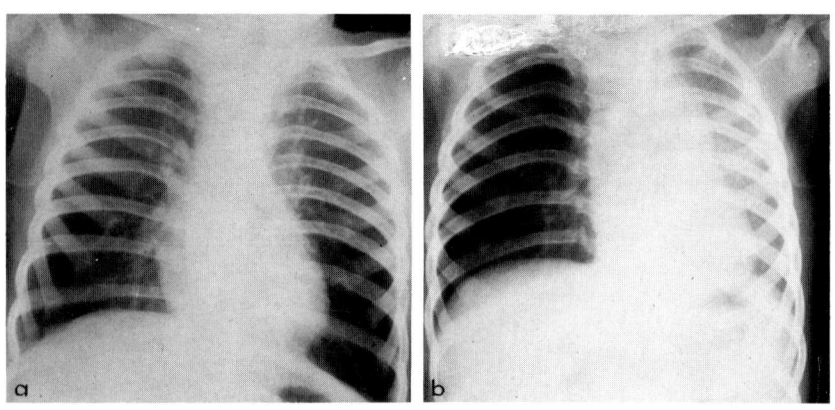

FIGURE 24–7. Obstructive emphysema in a 3½-year-old child with a foreign body (peanut) in the right main bronchus. *a*, On inspiration, the bronchus enlarges and air passes around the foreign body to inflate the right lung. *b*, On expiration, the air escapes normally from the left lung, but the right bronchus closes tightly around the foreign body, keeping the air trapped on the right side. There is a mediastinal shift to the left.

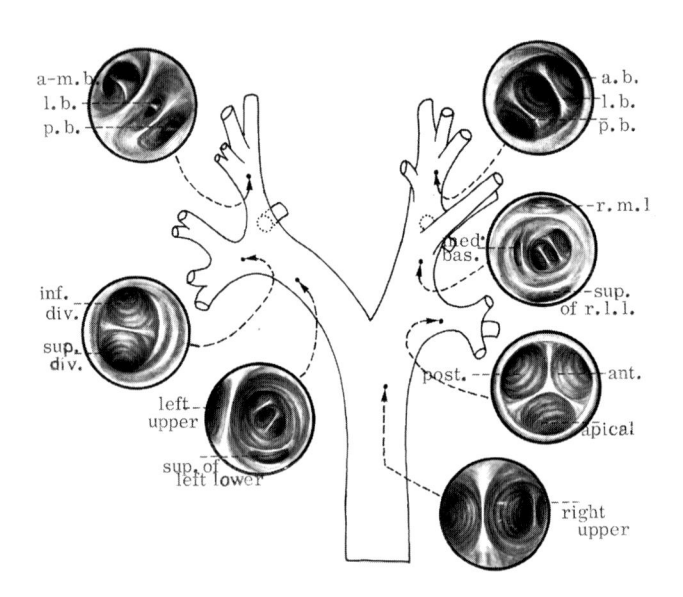

Left Lung			Right Lung		
Lobe	Bronchus	Segment	Lobe	Bronchus	Segment
Upper	Upper Division { L1&2 L3	Apical- posterior Anterior	Upper	{ R1 R2 R3	Apical Posterior Anterior
	Lower Division (lingular) { L4 L5	Superior Inferior	Middle	{ R4 R5	Lateral Medial
Lower	{ L6 L7&8 L9 L10	Superior (apical) Anterior-medial Basal Lateral Basal Posterior Basal	Lower	{ R6 R7 R8 R9 R10	Superior (apical) Medial Basal Anterior Basal Lateral Basal Posterior Basal

FIGURE 24–8. *Top,* Anatomic landmarks in the bronchial tree (inverted, as presenting to the bronchoscopist). Arrows indicate directions of bronchoscopic views. (From Norris CM: Bronchology. *In* English GM [ed]: Otolaryngology. Vol. IV. New York, Harper & Row, 1976, Ch 30.)

Bronchi are designated by simple descriptive names and numbers, according to the Jackson-Huber nomenclature. These designations are shown in the bronchoscopic report form. (Adapted from Jackson and Huber, Overholt, and Boyden.)

Tracheobronchial Disorders

Tracheobronchial congenital anomalies are not uncommon and generally produce respiratory obstruction at birth or soon after. A clear voice distinguishes tracheal from laryngeal obstruction. Tracheal atresia and agenesis are obviously incompatible with life. Membranous tracheal webs may be dilated with the tip of a bronchoscope. Longer webs may require more extensive treatment. Tracheomalacia or flaccid tracheal cartilages may be seen on videofluoroscopy and may produce symptoms of dyspnea. Tracheoesophageal fistulas are generally amenable to surgical correction. Supernumerary bronchial lobes and fissures are occasionally seen.

Metabolic, allergic, and degenerative disorders include asthma, bronchiectasis, emphysema, and chronic obstructive lung disease. Aspiration or retention of thickened secretions, especially in children and debilitated or postoperative patients, may result in atelectasis or pneumonia. This is a common problem that may be prevented or treated via bronchoscopy. Culture for identification of infection, including tuberculosis, may require bronchoscopy. The diagnosis of tracheobronchial and pulmonary malignancies requires bronchoscopic examination. Often a direct biopsy may be made or washings for cytologic study can be obtained via the bronchoscope. Benign tumors are diagnosed in a similar fashion. Blunt and penetrating trauma to the chest may involve the tracheobronchial tree, requiring endoscopic evaluation.

Foreign Body Aspiration

Aspiration of foreign bodies is most commonly encountered in children, although it is seen in patients of all ages. The most common cause of foreign body aspiration or ingestion is carelessness on the part of the patient or parent. Children age four and under are not able to adequately chew nuts, carrots, popcorn, and similar hard foods. They tend to carry such foods in their mouths as well as toys, pins, and other objects and thus often aspirate them. United States Federal Regulations specify the smallest manufactured toy size permitted for children age three and under. A large toy or other object is less likely to fit into a child's mouth, thus reducing the risk of aspiration or ingestion. Other factors leading to foreign body aspiration are intoxication, unconsciousness for any reason, and facial trauma with the aspiration of tooth fragments and dental plates. A dental plate covering the palate decreases intraoral sensation of food particle size and position and contributes to aspiration.

Symptoms of foreign body aspiration can be divided into three stages. The first stage of initial symptoms occurs while the foreign body is being aspirated. There are usually violent paroxysms of coughing and gagging. First aid at this point is identical to that for the initial stage of foreign body ingestion. It consists of resisting the urge to "do something," unless there is an obvious complete airway obstruction. Slapping the patient on the back, hanging a child by the heels, attempting to extract the foreign body with a finger, or attempting blind instrumental removal may complicate a simple nonobstructing foreign body by jamming it into the larynx and converting it into a complete obstruction. These maneuvers may also disimpact a foreign body lodged in the right main bronchus, and it can then move up into the larynx, be "caught" by the vocal cords, and produce a complete airway obstruction.

First stage: emergency management is not what your first impulse would be.

How much time do you have to dislodge a total airway obstruction?

If a complete obstruction has occurred, the foreign body must be disimpacted or an alternate airway established within four minutes. Hypoxia beyond this time limit results in permanent brain damage. Someone should immediately be sent to obtain a sharp knife so that a tracheostomy or cricothyrotomy may be attempted if measures to disimpact the foreign body fail. The measures described in the preceding paragraph may be attempted. An attempt may also be made to forcibly expel any air remaining in the lung. This is generally done by grasping the patient just below the sternum and forcibly squeezing the upper abdomen. This is the so-called Heimlich hug taught in standard cardiopulmonary resuscitation courses. If successful, the diaphragm will be elevated, compressing the lungs. The foreign body will be blown out of the airway so that the patient may breathe again. Another method that may be attempted is mouth-to-mouth resuscitation, either to force the object further down into the tracheobronchial tree so that it is not completely obstructive or to draw it out. If all these measures fail to establish an airway, an emergency tracheostomy or cricothyrotomy must be attempted. This procedure is described in Chapter 25.

The second stage is symptomless.

The second stage is the symptomless interval when the foreign body becomes lodged in one position. This stage may last only an instant or may extend over a number of years.

The third stage is complication.

The third stage is the stage of complications. Obstruction, erosion with infection, hemorrhage, or perforation may again draw attention to the foreign body. The foreign body lodged in the larynx or the cervical esophagus produces discomfort, hoarseness, cough, and perhaps dyspnea. Foreign bodies in the trachea may move back and forth between the carina and the bottom of the glottis with respiration, producing an audible slap and a palpable thud. Traumatic laryngeal edema in this situation may result in hoarseness and later airway obstruction.

Three types of bronchial obstruction exist: complete, check-valve, and nonobstructive.

If the foreign body is in the bronchus, three physiologic possibilities exist in terms of obstruction to air flow. If the object completely obstructs a bronchus, peripheral atelectasis results as air is absorbed from the distal lung into the blood. If the object is nonobstructive, allowing air to flow around it on both inspiration and expiration, all that may result is an asthma-like localized wheezing. Many foreign bodies have been thus misdiagnosed as asthma. The third possibility, and the one most commonly found, is a partial obstruction with the foreign body acting as a check-valve. The bronchus expands on inspiration, allowing air to flow past it into the distal lung. The bronchus contracts around the foreign body during expiration, trapping air in the distal lung. This produces an emphysema peripheral to the foreign body. If the foreign body is left in place, pneumonia, abscess, or hemorrhage may occur. The possibility of a foreign body is one reason for bronchoscopy in the presence of persistent or recurrent pneumonia, localized wheezing, or hemoptysis.

Physical examination should give careful attention to auscultation for findings compatible with atelectasis, emphysema, or wheezing. Mirror examination of the larynx and hypopharynx may reveal foreign bodies present in this area.

X-rays for a foreign body in the thoracic area should include the neck and abdomen.

A radiograph, particularly in children, should include the entire area from the top of the nose to the rectum. This is because children often have aspirated or ingested more than one foreign body. In such cases it is possible to be looking for a toy in the trachea and miss another object that has migrated to the colon or has been coughed into the nasopharynx. Postero-anterior and lateral chest radiographs are needed. In addition, and perhaps most important, radiographs at the height of inspiration and at the end of expiration are required. If these inspiratory and expiratory films are neglected, the presence of a foreign body may be missed. A film taken only at the height of inspiration may not show a check-valve emphysema. A film taken only on expiration will miss an obstructive atelectasis. Fluoroscopy during inspiration and expiration may also be valuable. The mediastinum moves toward the side of the foreign body on inspiration if there is a check valve and when there is a complete obstruction. A radiopaque nonobstructing foreign body may not be visible on chest radiograph (Fig. 24–7).

Inspiratory and expiratory chest x-rays are helpful.

Look for mediastinal movement.

If a foreign body is suspected, the patient should be requested to obtain a duplicate of it so that the endoscopist can more accurately determine which forceps and approach to use. The patient should be instructed to eat and drink nothing, to reduce the risk of vomiting and subsequent aspiration at the time of endoscopy. A foreign body lodged in the tracheobronchial tree, not totally occluding the airway, is not as great an emergency as one that is lodged in the esophagus unless it has sharp edges or is an uncooked or dehydrated vegetable, which can absorb fluids and swell within the lumen.

Instruct the patient/parent to bring a duplicate foreign body if possible.

Uncooked or dehydrated vegetables are a special problem.

Evaluation of Tracheobronchial Disease

Patient History

Patients with presenting symptoms suggesting disease of the tracheobronchial tree or lung should have a careful history with the following symptoms and problems characterized:

1. Cough (productive and nonproductive)
2. Hemoptysis
3. Wheeze
4. Hoarseness
5. Atelectasis or emphysema (localized and generalized)
6. Recurrent or persistent pneumonitis or lung abscess
7. Aspiration of foreign material or object
8. Unexplained radiographic shadows
9. Retention of secretions in the tracheobronchial tree
10. Dyspnea not secondary to cardiopulmonary or metabolic decompensation

Physical Examination and Laboratory Studies

Physical examination should include careful palpation of the neck for deviation of the trachea, for supraclavicular and cervical lymph nodes, and for metastasis. Inspection, percussion, and auscultation of the chest should be followed by appropriate chest radiography. Radiographic contrast study of the tracheobronchial tree, bronchography, is accomplished by instilling radiopaque liquid into the tracheobronchial tree under fluoroscopic control. Pulmonary function studies, blood gas analysis, complete blood count, sputum culture, and evaluation of the cardiovascular system are also useful.

Bronchoscopy

Bronchoscopy is indicated when the diagnosis of tracheobronchial or pulmonary symptoms is not clearly established by radiography or when therapy necessitates direct access to the tracheobronchial tree (Fig. 24–8).

Two basic types of bronchoscopes exist. One is a rigid metal tube with a light source at the distal end and the capability of ventilating the patient during the procedure. The rigid bronchoscope gives a direct view of the tracheobronchial tree and has the greatest latitude in terms of aspiration of secretions, manipulation with forceps, and removal of foreign bodies. Bronchoscopic telescopes may be placed through these to allow magnified direct and angled visualization of the more peripheral bronchi. A wide variety of foreign body and biopsy forceps are available for rigid bronchoscopes, many having a built-in telescope for magnified viewing and manipulation.

The second type is the flexible fiberoptic bronchoscope (Fig. 24–9). The larger of these bronchoscopes have small channels for aspiration of secretions and insertion of a slender forceps for biopsy or foreign body removal as well as a directable mobile tip. A small brush may be passed through the channel to obtain brushing samples, under fluoroscopic control, from peripheral lung lesions for histologic examination. The fiberoptic bronchoscope allows examination and biopsy of bronchial segments more peripheral than can be done through the rigid scope, particularly in the upper lobe branches. Although the usual flexible bronchoscopes have a smaller diameter than the comparable adult rigid scope, they are usually too large for use in infants and children. Flexible fiberoptic bronchoscopes designed for children have a smaller diameter but may lack a channel for suction or instrumentation and may not have a directable tip. They normally cannot be used for anything except diagnostic visualization and are not suitable for foreign body removal.

Bronchoscopy may be done under local or general anesthesia. The choice

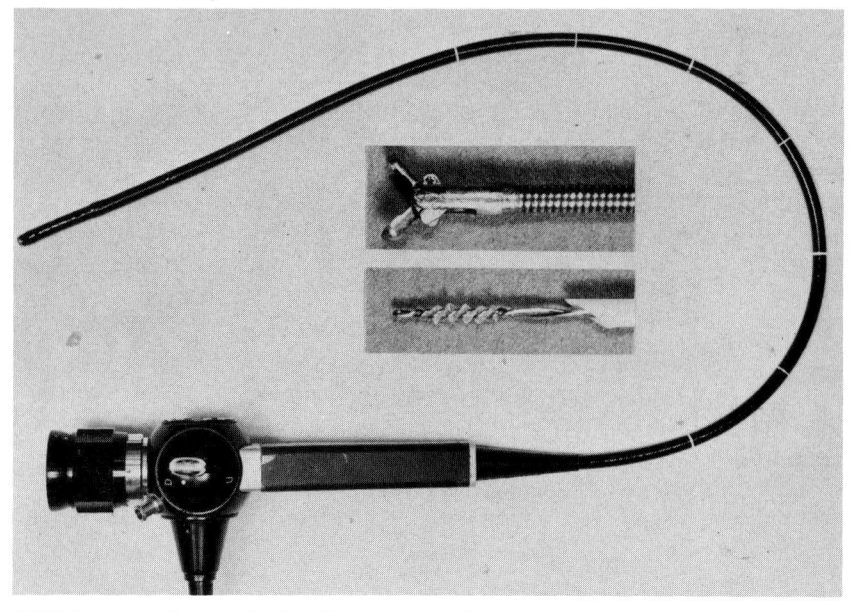

FIGURE 24–9. Olympus flexible fiberoptic bronchoscope. Inset shows closeup views of the brush (utilized for obtaining cells from peripheral lesions) and biopsy cups.

of anesthetic and the type of bronchoscope usually depends upon the endoscopist, the age and general health of the patient, and the disease suspected (Table 24–2). The procedure requires only a few minutes to perform and causes little patient discomfort.

MEDIASTINOSCOPY

Mediastinoscopy is an operative diagnostic technique for identification and biopsy of tissue in the anterior mediastinum (Fig. 24–12). Its prime uses are to determine the presence of lymph node metastases from bronchogenic carcinoma and to diagnose intrathoracic sarcoidosis. Either local or general endotracheal anesthesia is adequate. The trachea is exposed through a horizontal tracheotomy incision just above the thoracic inlet. Finger dissection is accomplished along the ventral tracheal surface into the mediastinum, after which the mediastinoscope is introduced into this tract. The procedure allows a direct examination of the paratracheal, parabronchial, and subcranial areas (Figs. 24–11 and 24–12).

Mediastinoscopy is the only means, short of thoracotomy, currently available to confirm pathologically spread to paratracheal, parabronchial, and subcarinal lymph nodes. For example, a biopsy of a small cell carcinoma may preclude the need for thoracotomy. In addition, mediastinoscopy is one means of obtaining a prethoracotomy diagnosis of bronchogenic carcinoma. It is therefore used not only to predict unresectability but also to make the

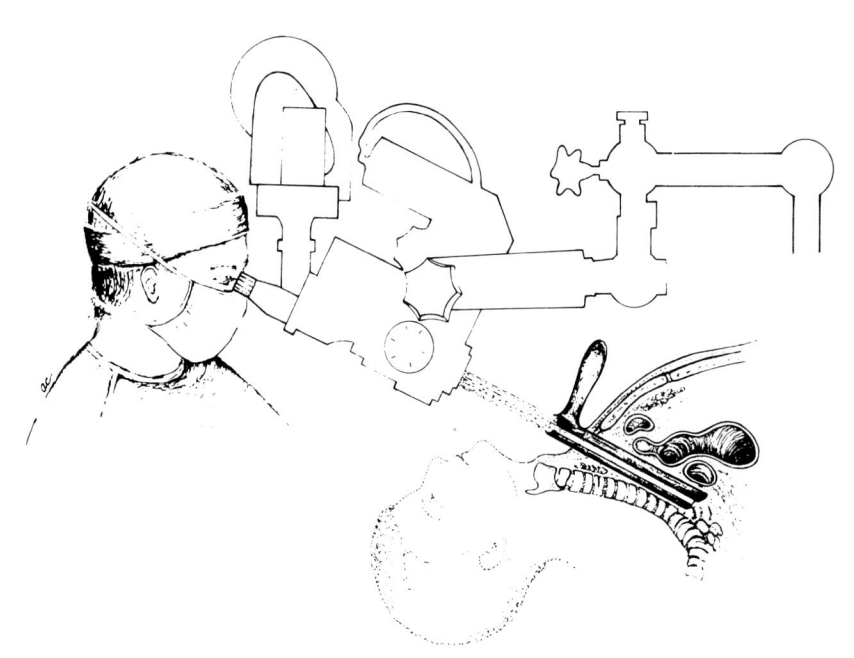

FIGURE 24–10. Access to the paratracheal and parabronchial area is direct. Arteries intervene between veins and tracheobronchial tree. The Zeiss Operating Microscope offers superior light and magnification and enables photography. (From Paparella MM, Shumrick DA [eds]: Otolaryngology. Vol. 3. Philadelphia, WB Saunders Co, 1973, p 734.)

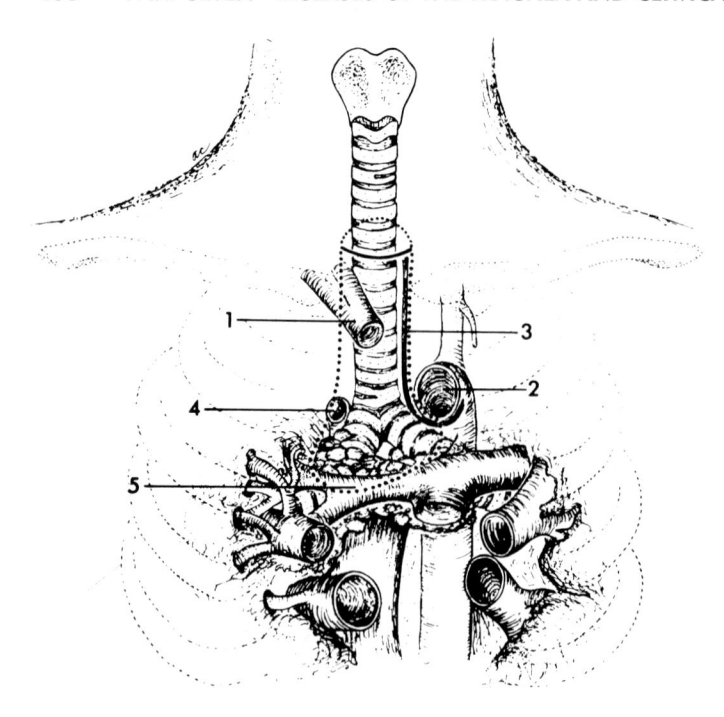

FIGURE 24–11. The area of examination is outlined by heavy dots. Vessels identified are the innominate artery (1), aortic arch (2), left recurrent laryngeal nerve (3), azygos vein (4), and right pulmonary artery (5). Biopsies should be performed to the right and left of the main bronchi and subcarinally. (From Paparella MM, Shumrick DA [eds]: Otolaryngology. Vol. 3. Philadelphia, WB Saunders Co, 1973, p 735.)

diagnosis in a significant percentage of cases. The CT scan has replaced mediastinoscopy in most situations for determining the presence or absence of hilar adenopathy.

Other diseases that have been diagnosed by mediastinoscopy include mediastinal cyst, thymomas, lymphomas, retrosternal goiter, tuberculosis, silicosis, and carcinoma of the esophagus, stomach, breast, and uterus.

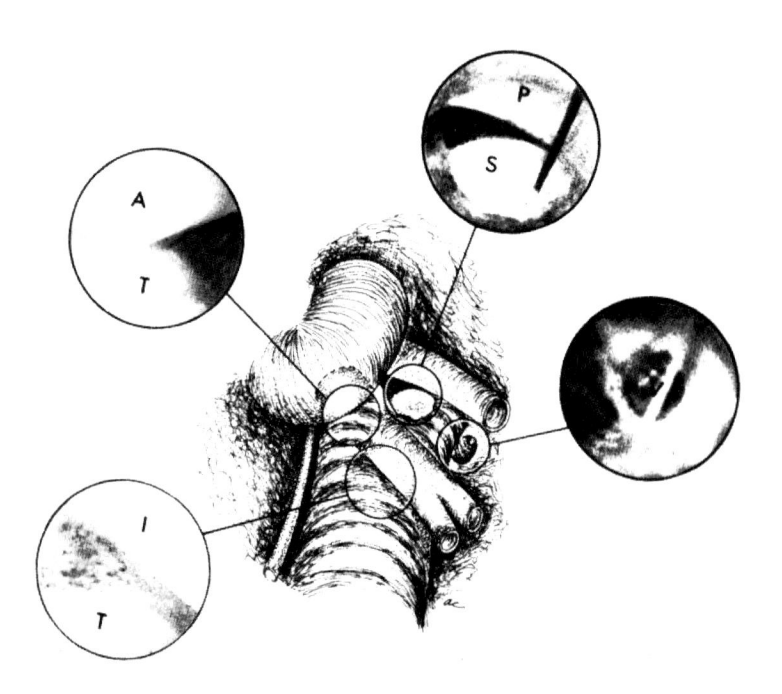

FIGURE 24–12. Composite drawing of mediastinoscopic view. Structures identified in enlarged portions are innominate artery (I), arch of aorta (A), trachea (T), azygos vein (V), right pulmonary artery (P), and subcarinal sarcoid node (S). (From Paparella MM, Shumrick DA [eds]: Otolaryngology. Vol. 3. Philadelphia, WB Saunders Co, 1973, p 735.)

References

Becker W, Buckingham RA, Holinger PH, et al: Atlas of Ear, Nose and Throat Diseases. 2nd ed. Philadelphia, WB Saunders Co, 1984.
Heimlich HJ: A life-saving maneuver to prevent food-choking. JAMA 234:398–401, 1975.
Harris CS, Baker SP, Smith GA, Harris RM: Childhood asphyxiation by food. A national analysis and overview. JAMA 251:2231–2235, 1984.
Jackson C, Jackson CL: Bronchoesophagology. Philadelphia, WB Saunders Co, 1950.
Paparella MM, Shumrick DA (eds): Otolaryngology. Vol 3: Head and Neck. Philadelphia, WB Saunders Co, 1980.
Ritter FN: Questionable methods of foreign body treatment. Ann Otol 83:729–733, 1974.
Rothmann BF, Boeckman CR: Foreign bodies in the larynx and tracheobronchial tree in children. A review of 225 cases. Ann Otol 89:434–436, 1980.

25

TRACHEOSTOMY

by Robert H. Maisel, M.D.

Tracheotomy and tracheostomy are words used interchangeably to mean a temporary opening in the anterior neck into the trachea. Tracheotomy, strictly defined, refers to the incision made in the trachea, while tracheostomy really defines the creation of a stoma through which air may pass to the lungs, bypassing the upper airway. The permanent stoma, after laryngectomy, achieved by suture of skin to tracheal mucosa is best described as a permanent tracheostomy.

HISTORY

This surgical procedure has a long and, until recently, maligned reputation. McClelland believed that five periods in the development and acceptance of tracheostomy were discernible. The earliest recorded tracheostomy is buried in legend. The sacred Hindu book *Rig Veda,* written between 2000 and 1000 BC, mentions "the bountiful one who can cause the windpipe to reunite when the cervical cartilages are cut across." Historians, however, consider Asclepiades, born about 124 BC, the first to carry out the operation. No surgeon's account appears before Brasavola (1500–1570) described his successful surgical management of Ludwig's angina in 1546. In the second era, from 1546 to 1833, such surgical attempts were feared, and only 28 successful tracheostomies were reported in this three-century period.

Trousseau and Bretonneau popularized the operation in France, using it for treatment of diphtheria with a 25 per cent rate of success (a high cure rate for the time). This third era of tracheostomy was highlighted in 1921 when Chevalier Jackson described the modern techniques and warned against incising the cricoid cartilage or first tracheal ring. This admonition, when followed, reduced the high complication rate from iatrogenic subglottic stenosis. During this era, the indication for such surgery was almost exclusively upper airway obstruction.

The fourth era began in 1932, with Wilson's suggestion that airway toilet could be managed in difficult cases of respiratory paralysis, specifically poliomyelitis. Galloway also led the thinking of this era, using tracheostomy for indications such as head injury, severe chest injury, barbiturate intoxication, and postsurgical airway control. This was the period of enthusiasm. During these years the aphorism "if you think about doing a tracheostomy, do it" was born, and this adage is still followed by many to prevent crisis tracheostomy.

Prolonged Intubation

Since the early 1960s the firm trend to use tracheostomy to bypass obstruction and to manage accumulated secretions or ventilatory failure has begun to be challenged. Endotracheal intubation has become more competitive, with better nursing care, including frequent suctioning of the trachea, and the use of humidified air and new tubes made of improved plastics that decrease the amount of crusting, thus no longer necessitating frequent exchange of the tube. The speed of intubation and the ease of extubation, as well as the avoidance of the complications of tracheostomy, make the technique attractive.

Careful endotracheal intubation has altered the indications for "emergency" tracheostomy.

Prolonged intubation has significant complications, with morbidity and some mortality. These include acute sinusitis; nasal, mucosal, and cartilage destruction; serous otitis media; and laryngeal and subglottic problems. The laryngeal problems can be more difficult to treat than tracheal stenosis posed by tracheostomy because the larynx is a functional muscular organ and not just a hollow tube to conduct air. Reconstruction can be difficult, and rehabilitation is occasionally unsatisfactory.

At present, many centers intubate patients in emergency situations or if removal of the tube is expected within one week. After 72 hours, if the tube is still needed, the tracheostomy is done. Few complications at the laryngeal and subglottic regions have occurred following this protocol. Prolonged adult intubation does increase the risks and severity of complications.

In children and infants more prolonged intubation has been successful. It may be maintained for up to six days, as shown by clinical studies. Infants have been managed for longer periods because of the great difficulty in performing and caring for tracheostomies in these patients. In neonates, intubation up to six months has been reported with success. However, occasional laryngeal complications have been seen after prolonged intubation in children.

Prolonged intubation is better tolerated in infants and newborns than in adults.

The frequency of subglottic stenosis may increase as more infants with various respiratory distress syndromes are managed this way, and caution is urged before yielding to the temptation to insert a tube. The more recent adage, "if you think of doing a tracheostomy, intubate and think again," has some merit but must be tempered by the realization that intubation is a temporary measure and must be either discontinued or replaced by a tracheostomy tube.

The argument over intubation versus tracheostomy is still unsettled. However, if intubation is elected, conversion to tracheostomy after six days in children and after 72 to 96 hours in adults at present appears to be most satisfactory.

PRESENT INDICATIONS

Indications for tracheostomy involve mechanical obstruction of the airway and nonobstructive problems that alter ventilation. Any lesion that does or may occlude the upper airway must be bypassed. Congenital laryngeal lesions such as subglottic stenosis, vocal cord paralysis, inflammatory disease that obstructs the airway (e.g., Ludwig's angina, which elevates the floor of the mouth and tongue, occluding the pharyngeal airway), epiglottitis, and vascular, neoplastic, or traumatic lesions that act by similar mechanical means are firm indications for tracheostomy.

The symptoms of upper airway obstruction are frightening to both patient and physician. Dyspnea may occur, and *stridor,* which is usually inspiratory (crowing) for lesions at or above the level of the true vocal cords, is noted. Expiratory stridor, typical of obstruction at or below the glottic aperture, is high-pitched and wheezing. *Retraction* at the suprasternal notch and supraclavicular and intercostal spaces represents an attempt to create negative intrathoracic pressure to draw air into the lungs. The patient's color may be ashen or cyanotic, while *dysphagia* or drooling saliva suggests that there is mechanical obstruction to swallowing. *Restlessness* with these signs is typical in children and must alert the physician to the urgent need to gain control of the airway. Heavy sedation for restless children with respiratory distress is absolutely contraindicated until the obstructed airway is bypassed, except during surgery. In respiratory mechanical obstruction, a restless child who becomes quiet without signs of relief is dangerously near death, and urgent measures are needed.

> *Restlessness in children with airway obstruction should not be treated by heavy sedation.*

Patients in the second category have no upper airway obstruction but have decreased ability to clear secretions, ineffective ventilation, or both. Patients with secretional obstruction due to loss of cilia, unwillingness to cough because of pain (fractured ribs), or inability to cough due to CNS injury may actually drown in their own secretions. Failure to continue to clear secretions produces mucous plugs that shunt pulmonary artery blood. This shunt produces hypoxia, since the ventilated alveoli cannot transfer sufficient oxygen. Arterial sampling shows low Po_2, minimally low Pco_2 (because of 20:1 ratio of diffusibility of carbon dioxide as opposed to oxygen), and a rise in pH. Supplemental oxygen as well as correction of the pathophysiology by tracheostomy, which allows suctioning of secretions to overcome the absent cough reflex, is sufficient treatment.

The alveolar hypoventilation syndrome or alveolar-capillary block can be due to respiratory paresis (poliomyelitis), chronic pulmonary emphysema, or mechanical chest wall problems (flail chest). These conditions often require assisted ventilation as well as control of secretions.

The pathophysiology of chronic ventilation problems is different from that described above, in that CO_2 retention occurs, reducing respiratory drive. These patients must be closely observed. The respiratory drive in such patients may be hypoxic due to CO_2 narcosis, which shuts off the medullary respiratory centers that usually stimulate respiration according to CO_2 levels. Tracheostomy with inspiration of enriched (oxygenated) air may precipitate a respiratory arrest because of loss of this last respiratory stimulant, and assisted ventilation may then be necessary.

ANATOMY

The trachea is a hollow tube supported by (elastic) cartilage rings that are incomplete posteriorly. It begins below the signet ring–shaped cricoid cartilage and extends directly anterior to the esophagus, descending into the thorax, where it divides into the two main bronchi at the carina. The great vessels of the neck parallel the trachea laterally and are encapsulated by the carotid sheath. The thyroid gland lies over the trachea anteriorly and laterally, and the isthmus crosses it anteriorly, usually at the level of the second to fifth tracheal ring. The recurrent laryngeal nerves lie in the tracheoesophageal groove. Deep to the subcutaneous tissues and anteriorly overlying the trachea are the suprasternal strap muscles, which attach to the thyroid and hyoid.

SURGICAL TECHNIQUE

Elective Tracheostomy in Adults

When surgery is not urgent, the tracheostomy is performed in the operating room unless the patient's medical condition requires equipment so cumbersome as to make the trip to the operating suite overly difficult. The patient is placed supine with the foot of the bed lowered 30 degrees to decrease the central venous pressure in the neck veins. A folded sheet is placed between the scapulae to extend the neck moderately, and the anterior neck is antiseptically cleaned and draped. The surgeons and assistants wear gloves and masks when operating at the bedside and surgical gowns as well in the operating suite. After adequate lighting is assured, the subcutaneous tissue is infiltrated with lidocaine and 1:100,000 epinephrine. A horizontal skin incision is preferred. It is made with a sharp scalpel at a level halfway between the cricoid prominence and the suprasternal notch. The incision is at least 2 inches long and reaches the medial border of each sternocleidomastoid muscle. Once the skin incision is through the platysma muscle, the dissection is done vertically, staying in the midline, using sharp and blunt dissection with scissors and hemostat. Two Allis clamps make excellent retractors of the strap muscles, which are split in the midline and retracted laterally until the pretracheal fascia is seen. Frequent palpation of the trachea through the incision ensures that the dissection is in the midline. The vertical midline dissection avoids most veins, and any that are encountered are cauterized or cut, ligated, and retracted. The thyroid gland, whose isthmus lies over the trachea, can usually be retracted inferiorly, gaining direct exposure to the first four tracheal rings. If the gland cannot be satisfactorily retracted, the isthmus is clamped, cut, and tied away from the midline operative field.

It is preferable to perform a tracheostomy in the operating room rather than in the patient's room.

At this juncture in the operation in the alert patient, 4 per cent lidocaine is injected transtracheally to prevent the violent cough spasm after incision and intubation. When a cuffed tracheostomy tube is to be used, the cuff is inflated now and checked under water to be sure that there is no leakage before incision is made in the tracheal wall.

Palpation of the thyroid and cricoid cartilages and their definite identification will prevent a high tracheostomy. The second and third rings are identified and after a cricoid hook is placed below the cricoid to pull the trachea up and into the wound, the incision in the trachea begins anteriorly, immediately below the second ring. A tissue plug of sufficient size to allow an adequate lumen for the tube is removed to include at least ring three and, if needed, ring four. A vertical incision, without cartilage removal, is also acceptable. Excision of three or more rings is risky, and animal experiments have shown significant tracheal stenosis after this is done. The tracheostomy tube used in the adult is the No. 7 Jackson or one comparable in internal diameter (8 mm) (Table 25–1). Absolute hemostasis is achieved

Tracheal rings are identified and counted.

TABLE 25–1. TRACHEOSTOMY TUBES

AGE	SIZE	JACKSON TUBES (METAL)		SHILEY TUBES (PVC)		LANZ TUBES			ENDOTRACHEAL TUBE
		OD (mm)	ID (mm)	OD (mm)	ID (mm)		OD	ID (mm)	Size (French)
Less than 3 months	00	4.5	2.80	4.5	3.1				15
3 to 6 months	0	5.0	3.20	5.0	3.4				
6 to 12 months	1	5.5	3.20	5.5	3.7				17
1 to 2 years	2	6.0	3.70	6.0	4.1				20
2 to 3 years	3	7.0	4.70	7.0	4.8				22
3 to 4 years	4	8.0	5.70	8.5	5.0	GT15	20F	5.0 mm	
4 to 5 years	5	9.0	6.40			GT16	24	6.0 mm	24
5 to 12 years	6	10.0	7.40	10.00	7.0	GT7	28	7.0 mm	26
Over 12 years									32
Adults									
Females	7	11.0	8.30			GT18	32F	8.0 mm	
Females and males	8	12.0	9.30	12.0	8.5	GT19	36F	9.0 mm	

Notes: In pediatric sizes, Shiley tubes offer a larger cross-section internally than metal Jackson tubes.
After six months of age, children require a tube size at least equal to their age at the next birthday (up to size 6).
3F = 1 cm.
Size identification of all intratracheal tubes is now standardized. A committee of the American Standard Institute requires all manufacturers to identify their intratracheal tubes by inside diameter in *millimeters*.
A simple rule to remember when selecting an endotracheal tube for a child in an emergency situation is to look at the little finger of the child. The size of the little finger of the child should approximate the outside diameter of the endotracheal tube selected.

at this point, and the umbilical tape that binds the tracheostomy tube around the neck is tied firmly while flexing the head. The skin incision is not sutured (Fig. 25–1).

Cuffed tubes are low pressure (compliant) to prevent scarring.

The cuff, which should be compliant, is then inflated. Cuffs that have been correctly manufactured to provide sufficient compliance are available; if these are not used, cuffs can be prestretched by the method of Geffin.

Tracheostomy in Children

When performing elective tracheostomy in children and infants, the smaller the patient, the greater the importance of controlled ventilation by a mask or tube. When the airway is controlled, a horizontal incision is cosmetically more satisfactory, and meticulous midline dissection is crucial because of the close proximity of the great vessels. Palpation of the endotracheal tube or bronchoscope facilitates this. The pleural cupulae ascend into the neck on inspiration, particularly under positive pressure respiration, and these must be avoided during dissection, since they may overlie the trachea. Nicking the cupula will cause pneumothorax. Needle aspiration of the trachea is an accepted procedure in children to ensure that a major arterial vessel is not mistaken for the airway. Silk sutures are placed anterolaterally on each side of the midline through two tracheal rings before a vertical incision in the second and third (and sometimes fourth) rings is made. Again, the cricoid and first ring are not to be violated. No tracheal tissue is excised in children. The tube size appropriate to the tracheal lumen is used.

Silk sutures placed at surgery are used as guides should accidental decannulation occur.

Emergency surgical control of the airway is gained by cricothyrotomy or tracheostomy. A vertical skin incision causes less hemorrhage, and the procedure is quickly performed, staying in the midline. No cartilage is

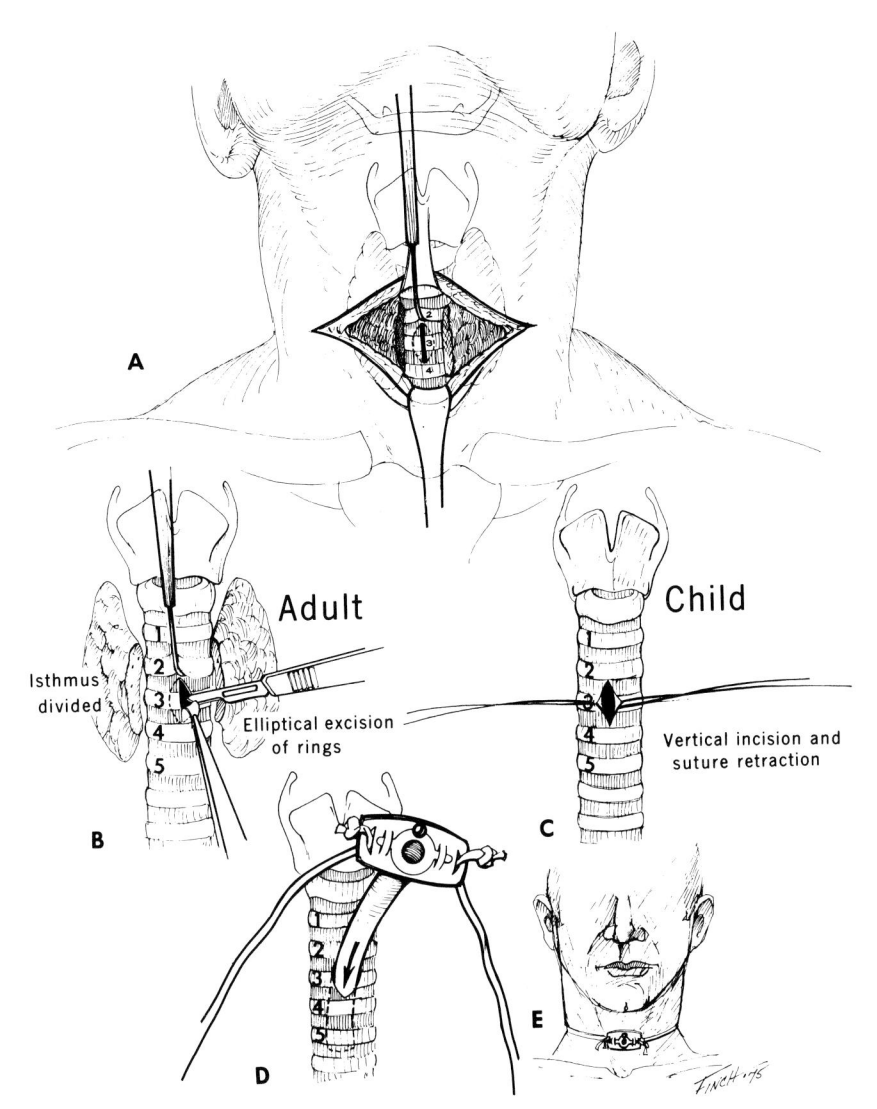

FIGURE 25–1. Technique of elective tracheostomy. *A,* After a horizontal skin incision, vertical dissection in the midline of the neck exposes the trachea. *B,* The thyroid isthmus is retracted from the field or divided in the midline and suture ligated. A vertical ellipse of the anterior tissue in interspaces 2 and 3 with the ring between them is removed. *C,* In children no ellipse is removed. Silk sutures are placed anterolaterally in each side of the midline through two tracheal rings. *D,* The metal tube is shown entering the stoma. *E,* Tracheostomy tube in place.

excised before the airway is controlled and cannulated. The cricoid and first ring should be avoided. If cricothyrotomy is urgently elected, it can be done by using a Mosher trocar or scalpel blade, extending the neck, identifying the thyroid and cricoid cartilages, and incising the cricothyroid membrane. The airway is maintained with retractors or, if available, an appropriately sized endotracheal or tracheostomy tube. The cricothyrotomy procedure allows immediate access to the airway safely below the true vocal cord in a relatively bloodless field; it is converted to a usual tracheostomy as soon as possible under controlled conditions. Similarly, an emergency tracheostomy

Cricothyrotomy is avoided in infants.

performed by cutting the cricoid and first ring is no disaster if recognized early by the surgeon. It, too, is converted by an incision at rings three and four, with removal of the initial tube; no complications should ensue if this is recognized and corrected within 24 hours.

Standard Modifications of Tracheostomy in Special Situations

Patients with severe alveolar hypoventilation and patients with severe obstructive sleep apnea (OSA) often require permanent tracheostomy. Obese patients may have difficulty maintaining a permanent stoma without bleeding, granulation, or scarring. Flap tracheostomy allows a clean, minimal-care stoma but does require use of a tracheostomy tube or stomal button.

Flap tracheostomies reduce the incidence of granulation tissue and remain patent if decannulation occurs.

Cervical skin flaps are elevated, leaving a layer of fatty tissue on the flaps, as the subdermal plexus of vessels supplying the overlying skin lies in this tissue. Undermining laterally to the sternocleidomastoid muscles, inferiorly to the manubrium, and superiorly to the hyoid bone is achieved and the adipose tissue is removed until the strap muscles are seen (Fig. 25–2). Tracheal incisions are seen in Figure 25–3, and the skin flaps are sutured to the trachea as shown in Figure 25–4. After healing is complete, a Montgomery cannula can be used as a tracheostomy stent. This is worn plugged except when needed for ventilation at night (Fig. 25–5).

The Montgomery tracheocannula as described above allows tracheal cannulation without a tracheostomy tube. The tracheal lumen is not occluded. This produces less irritation to the tracheal mucosa and permits a more widely patent upper airway at times when the airway is not obstructed.

The Communitrach tube is a new innovation of an old idea which allows patients on a ventilator to talk. The Communitrach has a separate channel for air to be instilled from an external source at 3 to 5 liters per minute. The air flows through the special channel in the tracheostomy and is sent superiorly through holes in the tube into the trachea. The airstream travels only upward (toward the larynx), since the tracheal cuff prevents downward

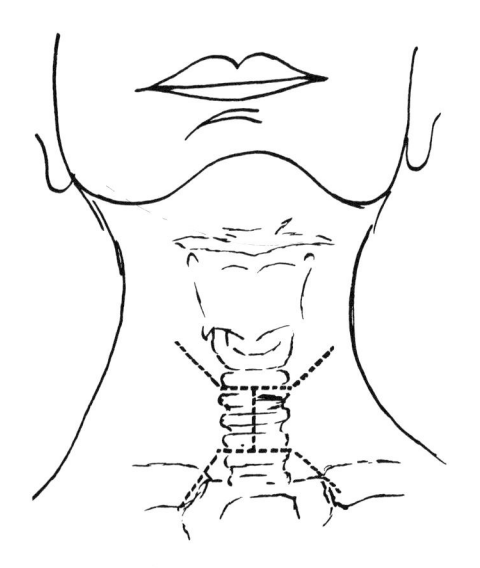

FIGURE 25–2. Anterior cervical skin incisions. (From Sahni R, Blakley B, Maisel RH: Flap tracheostomy in sleep apnea patients. Laryngoscope 95(2):221–223, 1985.)

FIGURE 25–3. *A*, Incisions over tracheal rings. *B*, Tracheal flaps. (From Sahni R, Blakley B, Maisel RH: Flap tracheostomy in sleep apnea patients. Laryngoscope 95(2):221–223, 1985.)

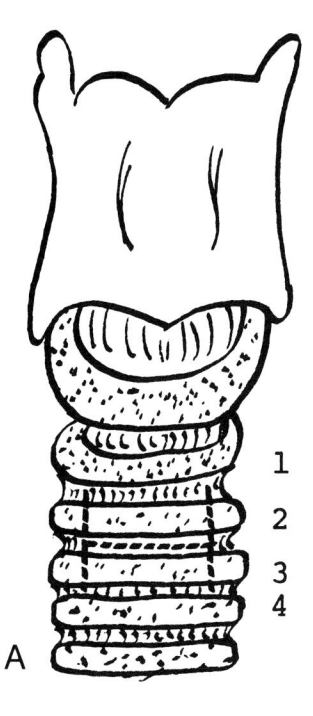

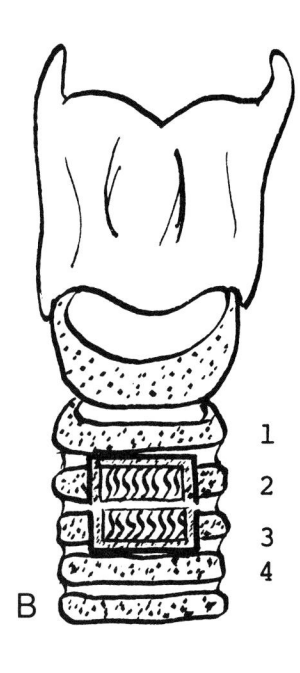

flow. This airstream goes through the larynx and creates a quiet but comprehensible voice.

An alternative to tracheostomy in the neonate who has developed acquired subglottic stenosis is the anterior cricoid split. The cricoid cartilage, the upper two tracheal rings, and the inferior portion of the thyroid cartilage are divided in the midline over an endotracheal tube. The child is placed in a pediatric intensive care unit while intubated for ten days. Precautions are taken to avoid excessive head motion, and antibiotics are administered to prevent infections with hospital-acquired *Staphylococcus* or *Pseudomonas* species. At day ten, the endotracheal tube is withdrawn.

The rationale for such a procedure is that acquired subglottic stenosis is

Anterior cricoid split offers an alternative to tracheostomy in a select group of children with subglottic stenosis.

FIGURE 25–4. Stoma after tracheocutaneous flap approximation. (From Sahni R, Blakley B, Maisel RH: Flap tracheostomy in sleep apnea patients. Laryngoscope 95(2):221–223, 1985.)

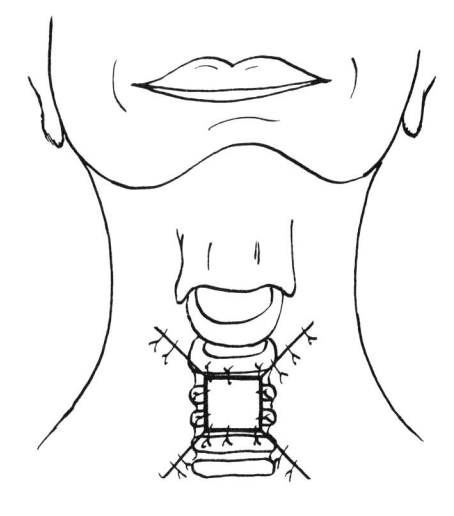

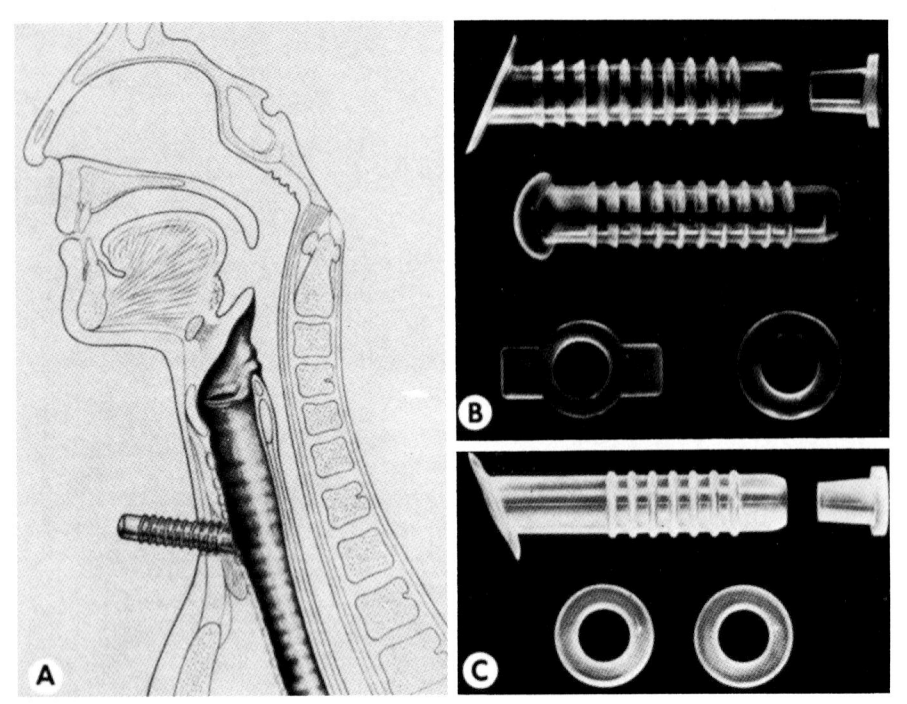

498 PART SEVEN—DISEASES OF THE TRACHEA AND CERVICAL ESOPHAGUS

FIGURE 25–5. Silicone tracheal cannula designed to be used in place of a tracheotomy tube. *A,* The cannula extends only to the inner surface of the anterior tracheal wall, eliminating foreign body projecting into trachea. *B,* Cannula, wing-shaped faceplate, plug, and ring washer. The groove along the cannula's long axis assists in drainage of secretions and serves to identify the inferior aspect of the cannula. The first three rings adjacent to flange are triangular to assist in fixing the cannula in place and make it difficult to displace anteriorly. The remaining grooves serve to secure faceplate or ring washer in place. The plug has a head to prevent introduction too far into the lumen of the cannula. *C,* Silicone tracheal cannula for long-term use shown with two washers and a plug. The surface adjacent to the intraluminal junction is smooth to permit and encourage growth of epithelium from both trachea and skin. (From Montgomery WW, Montgomery SK: Manual for use of Montgomery laryngeal, tracheal, and esophageal prostheses. Ann Otol Rhinol Laryngol (Suppl 125) 95(4):1–16, 1986.)

always soft in its initial stages. This is due to the formation of granulation tissue in the subglottic space. This granulation tissue, in large part, has an edematous component, and the anterior cricoid split is a decompressive procedure to allow the escape of edema from the otherwise intact cricoid ring. In this manner, the inexorable process of granulation tissue leading to firm cicatrix is interrupted.

Although the procedure was introduced approximately six years ago, enough experience has been gained to show that its success rate is now approximately 75 per cent. Thus, a large number of neonates with acquired subglottic stenosis are able to be extubated and not have a need for artificial airway in the form of a tracheostomy. At present, the procedure is reserved for those children who are under three years of age and whose subglottic stenosis is still in the soft granulation tissue stage. Since the procedure is a decompressive one, it would not succeed when the subglottic stenosis has progressed to a firm, dense cicatrix. The child must be otherwise extubatable by all other parameters and not have any glottic pathology that would require airway bypass (tracheostomy).

Immediate Postoperative Care

The upper airway has been bypassed, and its functions of warming of the inspired air to 36°C, humidification, and removal of particulate matter have been lost. The cilia of the trachea lose function, and the cough is ineffective. Early care of the stoma requires auscultation of the chest, and an immediate chest radiograph is necessary in all children to check tube position so it is not beyond the carina where it would enter the right bronchus and occlude the left bronchus, and to assure that no pneumothorax has occurred. The radiograph should be examined by the surgeon upon completion of the procedure. Mediastinal emphysema is frequent on chest radiograph, and repeat films at 48 hours should show no extension of the emphysema. A humidity collar passing cool water-saturated air or oxygen is placed over the stoma. A bedside tray with a tracheostomy set and a tube for replacement, scissors, and full suction apparatus should be available, as should a bell for summoning help.

The tracheostomy incision is not sutured closed.

Tracheal secretions are copious during the first 24 to 48 hours after surgery, regardless of the primary disease requiring tracheostomy. The bronchorrhea must be cleared, for these secretions will inspissate and produce atelectasis, pneumonia, and pulmonary vascular shunting. The cough is insufficient, and aspiration of the secretions through the tube is necessary. This is done as frequently as needed and at least every 15 minutes for the first several hours. The frequency thereafter is individually determined, based on the amount of secretions, auscultation of the chest, and listening to the patient. A gurgling patient with a tracheostomy is at great risk and must be suctioned. The technique is performed under sterile conditions, using a new disposable catheter every time, with the operator wearing gloves and washing hands between patients.

A loose gauze dressing is placed around the tracheal stoma.

Secretions tend to accumulate in the trachea often just below the tube. Bronchial aspiration is also necessary and is achieved by this suctioning technique. The catheter is attached by a V connector (Fig. 25–6) to a vacuum line. No negative pressure is supplied to the line unless the V is occluded. The method of choice is to insert the catheter through the tracheostomy tube lumen with no negative suction pressure. In tracheostomy tubes with an inner cannula, the cannula is removed before this is done. After the suction catheter resists further penetration into the bronchus, it is withdrawn slowly and completely by rotating the wrist while a fingertip occludes the V. This is repeated for the other bronchus after a rest period. The rest is needed because vacuum suction removes air from the lung and if repeated at frequent intervals will reduce the residual lung volume. Resuctioning of the same side is continued until auscultation is clear or gurgling respiration from the tracheostomy tube has ceased.

Tubes with an inner cannula require frequent removal and cleaning of the cannula. PVC and Silastic tubes are of one piece construction and do not accumulate crusts or mucus as much as metal tubes. They should be removed and inspected 48 hours after surgery, replaced, and reinspected at weekly intervals to ensure that a circumferential bolus of mucus does not occlude the lumen. The plastic tubes are now constructed to be most malleable at body temperature. This further decreases resistance to conformity to the trachea size and direction, which is a problem of metal tubes.

Low-pressure plastic cuffs are now available for the tracheostomy tubes. These are designed to keep the pressure against the trachea at less than 25

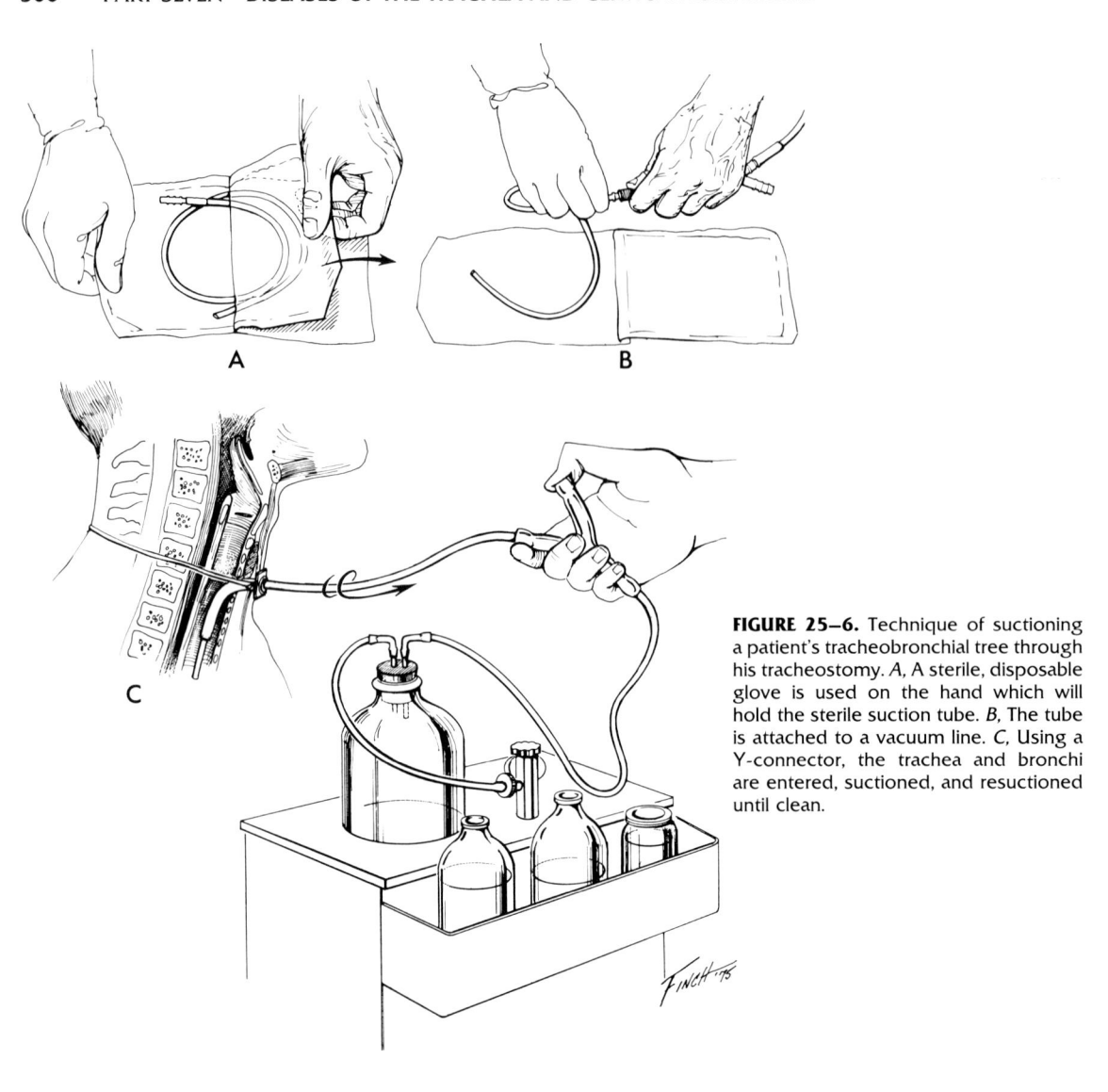

FIGURE 25–6. Technique of suctioning a patient's tracheobronchial tree through his tracheostomy. *A,* A sterile, disposable glove is used on the hand which will hold the sterile suction tube. *B,* The tube is attached to a vacuum line. *C,* Using a Y-connector, the trachea and bronchi are entered, suctioned, and resuctioned until clean.

cm H_2O. This has reduced the incidence of tracheal cuff stenosis. One of the low-pressure tubes is shown in Figure 25–7.

The alert, intelligent adult can be taught complete care of the stoma, and in children over six months old the tracheostomy can be cared for at home. Great caution and careful thought should precede discharging from the hospital a child younger than six months of age while the child is wearing a tracheostomy tube.

Complications

Surgical Complications. Complications during surgery can arise frequently, but the alert surgeon recognizes, prevents, and overcomes them. *Hemorrhage* is prevented by elective midline dissection with ligature of all vessels and careful examination of all oozing surfaces. *Pneumothorax,* a problem of tracheostomy in children due to the pleural position, is prevented as

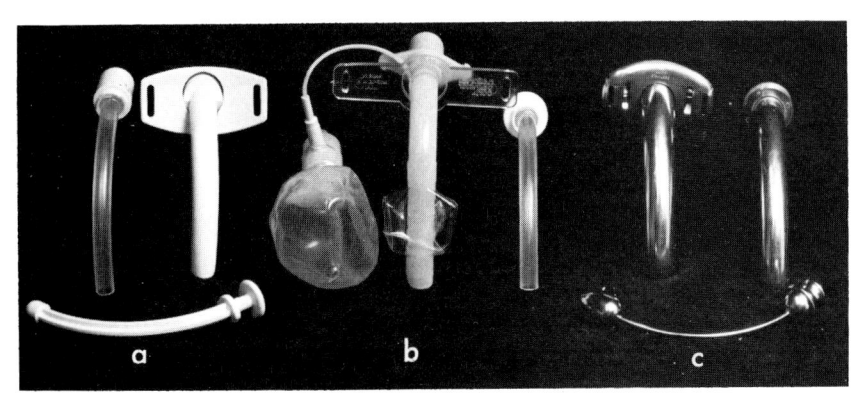

FIGURE 25–7. Three frequently used commercially available tracheostomy tubes. *A*, No. 6 Shiley tube (also available with nondetachable cuff). *B*, Lanz tube No. GT18 with controlled pressure cuff to keep pressure on tracheal wall below 26 mm Hg. *C*, Jackson metal tube. Cuff of rubber is attached by user. Not supplied by Pilling with cuff.

described above, discovered early by auscultation and chest radiograph, and treated by chest tube placement. The incidence in children is 3 per cent; it is rare in adults, in whom it is seen with increased intrathoracic pressure and rupture of emphysematous blebs. *Aspiration* should not occur, and *cardiac arrest*, which may be due to a loss of the hypoxic drive to respiration, is treated by the usual measures, including respiratory support until the CO_2 is washed out of the medulla. Pneumomediastinum is not a complication but a result. It is not unusual in children but must be followed to ensure that it does not progress or lead to pneumothorax. *Recurrent nerve paralysis* is rare and should be prevented by attention to surgical technique. The tube must be in the airway, not occluding one bronchus and not impinging on the anterior wall of the trachea. Clinical experience and radiologic evaluation will diagnose and prevent this.

A small degree of pneumomediastinum occurs in infants.

A postoperative chest radiograph is taken after a tracheostomy is performed and must be quickly reviewed by the surgeon.

Delayed Complications. These complications are significant in variety and number, and all effort must be made to prevent them. Late hemorrhage is due to erosion of the trachea into a major vessel, usually the innominate artery. (Actually counting each tracheal ring starting at the cricoid cartilage is essential.) Extending the patient's head and pulling the trachea upward with a tracheal hook can bring the ninth tracheal ring into view. A low tracheostomy (below the fifth tracheal ring) is often at fault. Prolonged cuff inflation, with necrosis of the tracheal wall, contributes to vessel erosion. Mathog recommends that soft plastic tubes are safer. Treatment of the major hemorrhage is emergent and requires the use of a cuffed tube that is long enough to pass distal to the vessel erosion with the cuff expanded. This prevents aspiration of blood into the lungs. Surgical division and suture of the vessel at fault may require a partial sternotomy.

Infections are controlled by sterile techniques and humidification. Prophylactic antibiotics are to be condemned because they allow opportunistic bacterial overgrowth. *Pseudomonas aeruginosa* is not infrequently cultured from a tracheostomy site and does not always represent systemic infection. Soaking the gauze pad with 0.5 per cent acetic acid solution may be all that is required. Patients on multiple antibiotics may have contamination of the tracheostomy site with *Candida albicans*. Before initiating systemic drugs, local wound care should be attempted.

Local wound care for **Pseudomonas** *or monilial infections often avoids systemic treatment.*

Airway obstruction due to a displaced tube or lumen occlusion is treated differently, depending on the time course since surgery. If more than 48 hours have passed since the tracheostomy was performed, a nurse can be instructed to cut the neck tie, remove the tube, and examine the lumen and tube. Mucous plugs occluding the tube lumen must be cleared. Reinsertion can be achieved when the physician arrives. Well-trained personnel can be instructed to insert the hook in the stoma and secure the airway before removing a newly placed tube for inspection. When the situation is not urgent, the physician should do this. In children, the silk tie, when gently pulled laterally, will maintain an airway and show the path back to the stoma for tube replacement.

Tracheoesophageal fistula usually occurs in patients who are hypotensive and have required prolonged intubation with cuffed tubes and controlled ventilation. These patients require nasogastric tubes but frequently die from their primary disease or from the aspiration pneumonia via the fistula. Surgical repair is complicated and involves placement of strap muscles between trachea and esophagus after primary repair of the fistula.

The most common major complication is *tracheal stenosis*. The frequency is increasing as patients require prolonged controlled ventilation with cuffed tubes. Fearon believes that stomal stenosis is not a complication but rather an expected postoperative scar and that the symptoms occur only when the lumen is 4 mm or less in diameter. When there is granulation above the stoma or cartilage in the lumen, the problem can be treated by endoscopic excision or stenting the airway. Cuffed tubes can cause circumferential mucosal obstruction within hours. The cuff should be inflated and enough air released to produce an "audible squeak." Low-pressure cuffs are also protective. Repair of tracheal stenosis becomes increasingly difficult as the length of cicatrix increases.

References

Bryant LR, Trinkle JK, Dubilier L: Reappraisal of tracheal injuries from cuffed tracheostomy tubes: Experiments in dogs. JAMA 215:625–628, 1971.
Cavo J, et al: Low resistance in tracheotomy tubes. Ann Otol Rhinol Laryngol 82:827–830, 1973.
Chew JOY, Cantrell RW: Tracheostomy: Complications and their management. Arch Otol 96:583–645, 1972.
Cotton RT, Myer CM, Bratcher GO, Fitton CM: Anterior cricoid split, 1977–1987. Arch Otolaryngol Head Neck Surg 114:1300–1302, 1988.
Cotton RT, Seid AB: Management of the extubation problem in the premature child: Anterior cricoid split as an alternative to tracheotomy. Ann Otol Rhinol Laryngol 89:508–511, 1980.
Fearon B, Cotton R: Surgical correction of subglottic stenosis of the larynx in infants and children. Ann Otol Rhinol Laryngol 84:231–235, 1974.
Goodall EW: The story of tracheotomy. Br J Child Dis 31:167–252, 1934.
Grillo HC, Cooper JD, Geffin B, Pontoppian H: A low pressure cuff for tracheostomy tubes to minimize tracheal injury. J Thorac Cardiovasc Surg 62:898–907, 1971.
Jackson C: High tracheotomy and other errors: The chief causes of chronic laryngeal stenosis. Surg Gynecol Obstet 32:392–397, 1921.
Mathog RH, Kenan PD, Hudson WR: Delayed massive hemorrhage following tracheostomy. Laryngoscope 81:107–119, 1971.
McClelland RMA: Tracheostomy: Its management and alternatives. Proc R Soc Med 65:401–403, 1972.
Montgomery WW, Montgomery SK: Manual for use of Montgomery laryngeal, tracheal, and esophageal prostheses. [Supplement 125] 95(4):1–16, 1986.
Sahni R, Blakley BW, Maisel RH: Flap tracheostomy in sleep apnea patients. Laryngoscope 95(2):221–223, 1985.
Schuller DE, Birck HG: The safety of intubation in croup and epiglottitis: An eight year follow up. Laryngoscope 85:33–46, 1975.
Snow JB, Preston WJ: Dry, aseptic method of tracheotomy care. Arch Otol 92:191–194, 1970.
Szachowicz E, Walsh J, Maisel RH: *TALC* tracheostomy tube: Normal laryngeal speech while on a ventilator. Otolaryngol Head Neck Surg 89:221, 1981.

PART EIGHT

PLASTIC AND RECONSTRUCTIVE SURGERY

26

FACIAL PLASTIC SURGERY

by Peter A. Hilger, M.D.

Plastic surgery is a surgical method for reconstructing or improving the function and appearance of various parts of the body; its principles and techniques are shared by many disciplines. In the broad field of otolaryngology there is a special emphasis on the management of functional, reconstructive, and cosmetic problems of the face, head, and neck areas. This chapter will focus on soft tissue facial plastic surgery and will also provide an overview of some of the more commonly performed cosmetic procedures in the head and neck region. Reconstructive surgery following trauma of the face and skeleton and tumor ablation are also discussed in the chapters on head and neck cancer (Chapter 23) and maxillofacial trauma (Chapter 27).

GENERAL PRINCIPLES

Principles of Wound Healing

A gratifying result following facial surgery, like other areas of surgery, is dependent upon favorable wound healing. A fundamental understanding of normal wound repair is therefore understandably a prerequisite to successful surgical planning and technique. The brief overview presented here will consider wound healing in three areas: collagen synthesis, epithelialization, and wound contraction.

Collagen and Collagen Synthesis

Collagen, the principal structural protein of the body, is the primary component of scar tissue and is found in wounds as early as the second postoperative day. Consisting of a group of glycoproteins, the basic structural unit of the collagen protein is composed of three separate linear polypeptide chains (alpha chains), which are woven in a helix. Glycine, proline, and hydroxyproline are the predominant amino acids.

Four different types of collagen exist; they are composed of different types of alpha chains. As a wound matures, the original collagen may be replaced by another type with consequent changes in the appearance of the wound.

Collagen formed early in wound healing is poorly organized and has a lower strength/mass ratio than the collagen of mature scars. Thus, immature scars are bulky and have a relatively low tensile strength. Collagen continues to be remodeled for six months to a year after injury. Collagen lysis occurs simultaneously with collagen formation, replacing immature forms of collagen with more compact, mature collagen, which has a greater tensile strength.

Collagen remodeling occurs for 6 to 12 months after injury.

Keloid and hypertrophic scars are due to abnormal collagen metabolism.

The processes of synthesis and lysis are in a delicate balance and, if disturbed, disorders such as keloid or hypertrophic scar formation can occur. Vitamin C and oxygen are essential cofactors for the rapid production of collagen. Collagen lysis primarily occurs as a result of digestion by collagenase, an enzyme whose activity is increased by corticosteroids. Thus, by manipulating these factors as well as others, hypertrophic scar and keloid formation can be minimized.

Epithelialization

Basal epithelial cells begin to migrate across a wound within hours of injury and produce collagen lytic enzymes that allow the cells to cleave through collagen at the junction of eschar and viable tissue. Eschar, fibrin, and old cellular debris impede epithelialization. If a wound is kept moist and protected so that no eschar forms, optimal epithelialization occurs if there is sufficient oxygenation.

Epithelialization occurs more rapidly if the wound surface is moist.

It is important to remember that suture tracts are microwounds and, as such, epithelial cells follow sutures into the wound to produce a cyst or a sinus tract. To minimize these disfiguring complications early suture removal and replacement or substitution by suture tape is recommended (Fig. 26–1).

Wound Contraction

Myofibroblasts cause wound contraction.

Wound contraction is not the exact equivalent of contracture. Myofibroblasts are responsible for wound contraction; causing the wound bed to contract decreases its surface area, which occasionally may be unfavorable. While a smaller wound requires less time to heal, the contraction may distort normal adjacent structures, e.g., ectropion, "trap-door" deformity. Corticosteroids inhibit this process and may be useful clinically. In an open wound this process can also be inhibited by stenting the edges during the contraction phase or by applying a full-thickness skin graft.

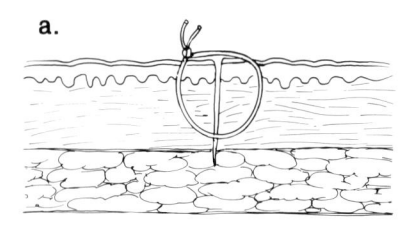

FIGURE 26–1. Suture tracts. *a,* Sutures create microwounds, and epithelial cells migrate along the suture into the depths of the wound if sutures are not removed early. *b,* Small sinus tracts and surface irregularities can develop if sutures are retained too long.

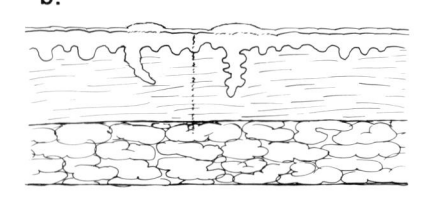

Principles of Wound Care

Anesthesia

Local anesthesia of 1 to 2 per cent lidocaine or ½ to ¾ per cent bupivacaine with 1:50,000 or 1:100,000 epinephrine decreases oozing and suffices for most regions on the face. Topical anesthesia of 4 per cent lidocaine applied with a sponge to an abrasion or open wound often allows injection of local anesthesia with less discomfort. Lidocaine is the most commonly used local anesthetic and is available with and without epinephrine. Epinephrine causes vasoconstriction, thus providing a surgical field with less oozing, and also prolongs the duration of the anesthesia. The dosage should not exceed 7 mg/kg, or a total of 500 mg, for solutions with epinephrine or 4.5 mg/kg, or 300 mg, for solutions without epinephrine. General anesthesia may be preferable for children or for adults with large or complex injuries.

Incisions

Surgery of the face requires careful planning of operative incisions. Surgical scars may be camouflaged by placing the incision along favorable lines and approximating wound edges without tension.

Incisions are less apparent if they are concealed in natural crease lines and into shadows (Fig. 26–2). Usually the crease lines* are the lines of least tension and, in such areas, the tendency for widening of the scar is minimal.

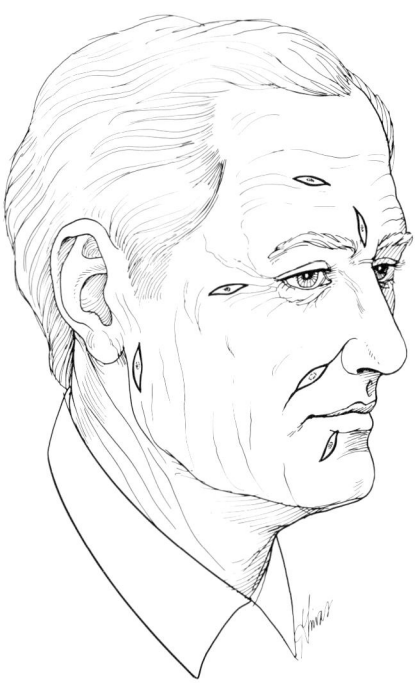

---

*Lines of least tension and crease lines should not be confused with Langer's lines, which are related to lines of least tension only in the cadaver. In the living subject these lines of least tension may change as they are affected by the adjoining dynamic forces of the tissues.

FIGURE 26–2. Favorable orientation of surgical incisions follows relaxed skin tension lines. Wounds located as shown produce the most favorable result.

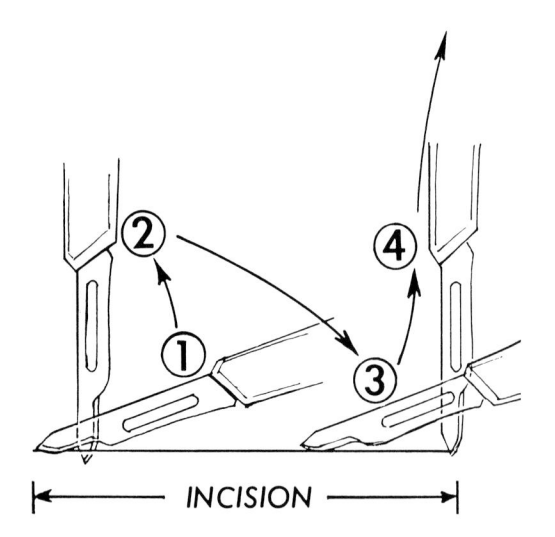

FIGURE 26–3. Technique of incision. The "belly" of the knife is introduced through the skin (1) and brought vertical to make a perpendicular cut (2). The remainder of the skin is incised with the "belly" of the knife (3), which is then brought vertical again at the end of the incision (4).

Major exceptions are noted in the glabella area, where the lines of least skin tension are horizontal rather than vertical, and in the lateral eyelid, where they are horizontal rather than slanted upward. Concealment of scars can also be achieved by placing incisions within hair-bearing areas, behind the ears, and in shadows, such as at the side of the nose and beneath the lower lip.

Incisions on the face are usually made with a small knife blade, i.e., Bard-Parker No. 15. The incision is initiated using the belly of the blade, with the physician holding tension on the skin in the direction of the incision line (Fig. 26–3). The blade is rotated through the skin and to a more vertical position to create a perpendicular cut and then rotated back to the original position so that the belly is used to create the major portion of the incision. The end of the incision is also cut in a perpendicular plane.

It is desirable to make this incision in a way that will minimize skin tension at the surface. The skin is then undermined in all directions for approximately 1 cm, a maneuver that tends to reduce the traction from underlying structures and provides for the advancement of skin during wound closure. Gentle use of sharp hooks avoids trauma to the skin edges. Hemostasis is achieved with cauterization of small vessels.

Early Care of Wounds

Although infections rarely occur on the face compared to the frequency for other areas of the body, infections that do occur may lead to conspicuous sequelae. The initial management of facial wounds requires meticulous attention to technique and a gentle concern for the tissues.

Debridement reduces the incidence of infection and traumatic tattoo.

Cleansing. Cleansing and debridement of wounds serve to decrease the bacterial count and remove devitalized tissue and any foreign material that would tend to increase the chance of infection or of tattooing the tissues.

Methods of cleansing/debridement include irrigation, removal with solvents, mechanical abrasion (by means of a brush or dermabrasion), or excision. The initial excisional debridement on the face should be conservative, as the excellent blood supply allows the repair of severely damaged tissue.

All traumatic facial wounds should be washed thoroughly with an isotonic saline solution. In the case of abrasions, embedded material should be removed with a scrub brush or by dermabrasion. All viable tissue should be salvaged and debridement applied only to those tissues that clearly cannot survive.

Patients who have had active immunization and boosters against tetanus within the last ten years should be given another booster injection. Those individuals who have not received adequate immunization during this period or have never been immunized should receive human antiserum and undergo a program of active immunization (Table 26–1). The use of antibiotics depends upon the nature of the injury and the duration of time tissue was exposed to infection.

Almost all wounds of the face should be closed primarily with sutures. If tissue has been lost, local flaps or skin graft is required. Following appropriate irrigation, lacerations should be undermined, relieved of tension at skin surfaces, and closed in layers. Areas of "dead space" are drained to prevent hematoma formation.

Dressings may be an asset in wound healing; however, they are not essential. Wounds may be managed by a "wet technique" in which an ointment-based coating is topically applied to the incision. The ointment prevents wound desiccation, and epithelialization occurs more rapidly.

Sutures. The purpose of sutures is to hold the wound in a stable position for rapid repair and healing. Ideally, sutures should not interfere with the reparative process and should maintain immobilization while relieving tension at the wound surface. Different types of suture material are classified as absorbable or nonabsorbable, based on their degree of inertness. Common

TABLE 26–1. PROPHYLACTIC TREATMENT OF TETANUS

TYPE OF WOUND	PATIENT NOT IMMUNIZED	PATIENT COMPLETELY IMMUNIZED—TIME SINCE LAST BOOSTER DOSE		
		1* to 5 Years	5 to 10 Years	10 Years or More
Clean minor	Begin or complete immunization per schedule; tetanus toxoid, 0.5 ml	None	Tetanus toxoid, 0.5 ml	Tetanus toxoid, 0.5 ml
Clean major or tetanus-prone	In one arm: human tetanus immune globulin, 250 mg In other arm: tetanus toxoid, 0.5 ml; complete immunization per schedule	Tetanus toxoid, 0.5 ml	Tetanus toxoid, 0.5 ml	In one arm: tetanus toxoid, 0.5 ml In other arm; human tetanus immune globulin, 250 mg
Tetanus-prone, delayed or incomplete debridement	In one arm: human tetanus immune globulin, 500 mg In other arm: tetanus toxoid, 0.5 ml; complete immunization per schedule thereafter Antibiotic therapy	Tetanus toxoid, 0.5 ml	Tetanus toxoid, 0.5 ml Antibiotic therapy	In one arm: tetanus toxoid, 0.5 ml In other arm: human tetanus immune globulin, 500 mg Antibiotic therapy

*No prophylactic immunization is required if the patient has had a booster within the previous year.
Note: With different preparations of toxoid, the volume of a single booster dose should be modified as stated on the package label.
Source: American College of Physicians and Surgeons. Committee on Trauma: Early Care of the Injured Patient. Philadelphia, WB Saunders Co, 1972, p. 39.

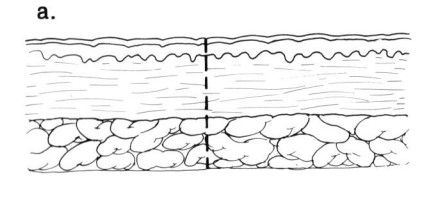

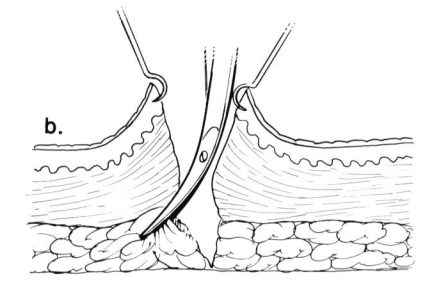

FIGURE 26–4. Technique for layered closure. *a,* An incision that penetrates several different tissues should be closed in layers. *b,* The tissues should be handled gently. Skin hooks cause less injury than forceps. Reduced tension of the closure is facilitated by undermining. *c,* Each layer should be closed separately with buried knots except for surface sutures.

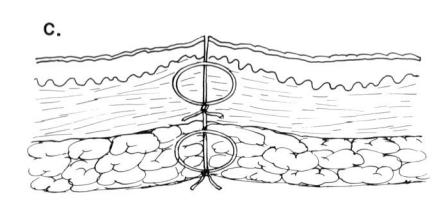

Absorbable sutures are used to close deep layers.

Fine sutures (5-0 or 6-0) are best for surface closure.

absorbable sutures include catgut or chromatized catgut, and nonabsorbable types may be made of silk, plastic, or steel.

In general, absorbable sutures are used in deep layers of contaminated wounds while, occasionally, nonabsorbable sutures such as polyester may be used in the deeper layers of clean wounds. Appropriately matched deep layers of the wound and subcutaneous tissues should be sutured with the knots buried (Fig. 26–4).

The surface epithelial layer is often closed with a fine cutting needle and nonabsorbable, nonreactive materials such as monofilament nylon or polypropylene. These skin sutures should approximate only the wound edges and should be carefully spaced. Skin sutures should be removed early (5 to 7 days) and antitension tapes (Steri-strips) should be applied; these tapes can be continued for up to six months. In general, the suturing of the deeper layers should begin at the center of the wound and the wound "halved" in sequence to avoid inequality of length of the sides. The choice of interrupted or continuous sutures is usually based on experience and personal preference.

By penetrating the dermis several millimeters away from the incision, the suture can evert the skin edges and reduce tension at the surface. The knot should be left small and "buried," as illustrated in Figure 26–4. Interrupted sutures applied to the skin surface should be loose and only approximate the skin edges. Any "tension" should be regulated primarily by the intradermal and subcutaneous sutures and not by the surface sutures.

Several different techniques are available for closure of the most superficial layer, including horizontal and vertical mattress sutures, simple interrupted or running sutures, and subcuticular sutures.

Interrupted mattress sutures require that pressure be applied to large amounts of tissue; this prevents accurate approximation and may interfere with survival of tissues at the skin edges but does sufficiently evert the wound edges (Fig. 26–5a and b). Occasionally the horizontal mattress suture may be used to attach the tip of a flap to a defect. In this case the mattress suture penetrates only the subcuticular tissues of the flap side.

A continuous or running suture is also popular for skin closure (Fig. 26–5d). When combined with an intradermal suture, the continuous stitch can accurately approximate the skin surfaces. In the eyelid, where the skin is extremely thin, a continuous, subcuticular suture line is often useful (Fig. 26–5e). Locking type stitches should be avoided, since they tend to constrict the blood supply.

Owing to the frequency of occurrence, it is worthwhile to specifically mention the treatment of lip lacerations. Careful tissue approximation and reconstruction of the orbicularis oris muscle with absorbable sutures is accomplished first. Failure to approximate this muscle may result in a depressed and widened scar with irregularities of the vermillion border. Alignment of the vermillion border is the most important step in surface layer closure and should usually be the location of the first skin suture. Mucosal closure is achieved with absorbable suture. Tongue lacerations can also be closed with absorbable sutures such as chromic catgut. Small tongue lacerations are often best managed without suture closure, substituting instead soft diet and frequent oral rinses for several days.

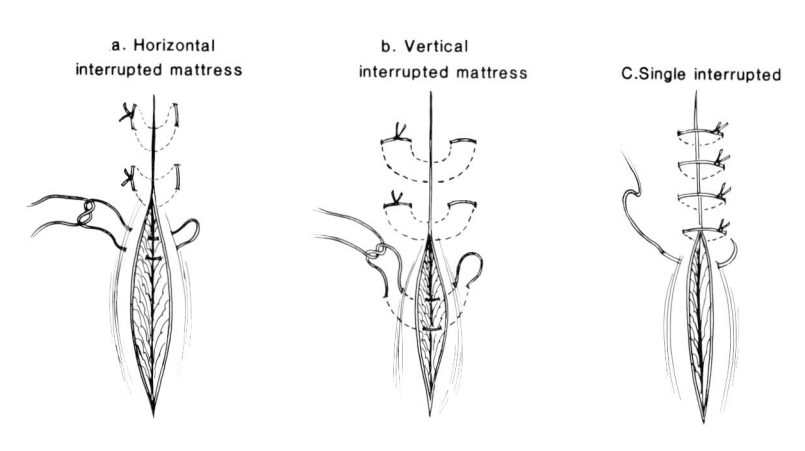

FIGURE 26–5. Surface suture techniques.

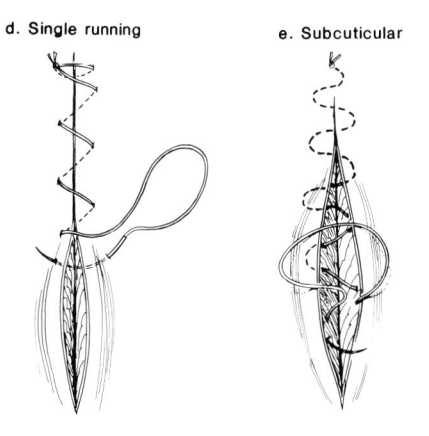

Local Flaps and Skin Grafts

The excision of larger lesions or traumatic defects can produce a tissue defect that cannot be repaired by advancement of adjoining tissues. Such cases require repair with a skin graft or skin flap. The choice of technique depends on the functional and cosmetic goals, the size of the defect, the availability of local tissues, the condition of the patient, and the experience of the physician.

Availability of local tissues is an important consideration. Size of flaps may be affected by adjoining structures such as eyelids, corner of the mouth, or nares. Skin grafts taken from the extremities, buttocks, scalp, and abdomen do not have these limitations.

Functional and cosmetic goals must also be evaluated. The thicker the transplanted tissues, the smaller the contraction and depression that may be expected with the healing process. The thicker tissues also supply a laxity that enhances the motion of adjoining structures. These are the advantages of the full-thickness grafts over split-thickness grafts and of flaps over grafts. Closure of a defect with local flaps, when feasible, usually produces a superior aesthetic result because local tissues are a better match in skin color and texture. Moreover, the use of a local flap avoids creating a second wound at the donor site of a skin graft.

Small facial defects are best closed with local flaps.

The condition of the recipient site and the general condition of the patient may also affect decisions on technique. Poor recipient areas, such as bone, or areas of tissue previously exposed to radiation or chronic infection may have an inadequate vascular supply. In these cases, flaps with their own blood vessels have a definite advantage over grafts. On the other hand, split-thickness grafts are more suitable for patients who are too incapacitated to undergo multiple procedures, and in cases in which there is a need for immediate replacement of larger areas of skin.

Local Flaps

Rotation, transposition, and advancement flaps are used primarily in the repair of facial defects. A rotation flap rotates on a pivot point (Fig. 26–8), a transposition flap is transposed over adjacent skin (Fig. 26–9), and advancement flaps are advanced in a straight line. Local flaps can be safely designed with up to a 4:1 length:width ratio (Figs. 26–6 and 26–7).

Advancement flap

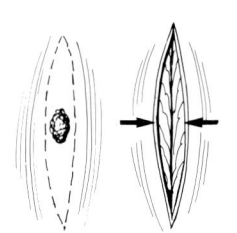

FIGURE 26–6. Simple advancement flap.

FIGURE 26–7. Advancement flap. *a,* Advancement of tissue to close an adjacent defect may cause bunching of tissues at the base of the flap that is corrected by excising Burow's triangles. *b,* Result after advancement.

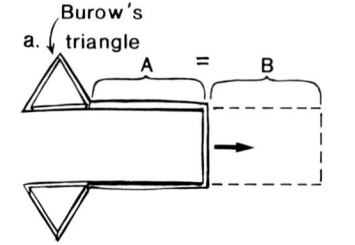

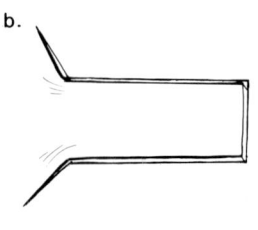

FIGURE 26–8. Rotation flap. *a*, Tissue is rotated about a pivot point to close a wedge-shaped defect. *b*, Result after closure.

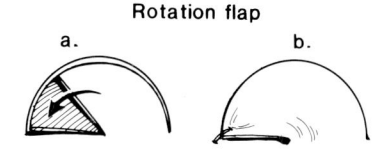

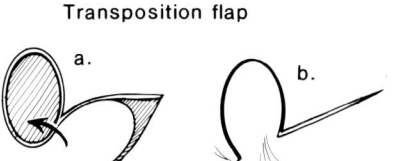

FIGURE 26–9. Transposition flap. *a*, Tissue to close a defect can be incised, elevated, and then transposed over skin adjacent to the defect to close a defect. *b*, Result after transposition and direct closure of the donor defect.

The rhomboid flap is a transposition flap that deserves further mention. This versatile flap is used for a defect designed as an equilateral parallelogram. The shape of the defect is the equivalent of placing two equilateral triangles base to base. The flap is cut identical in size and shape and rotated 60 degrees from the defect (Fig. 26–10). Four potential donor sites are available for each rhombic defect; the choice of the optimum donor area is dependent upon such factors as (1) which area provides the most skin, (2) the area's lines of maximal extensibility, (3) the presence of any anatomic structures, e.g., nose, eye, mouth, (4) which areas will be under tension after transposition, and (5) what will be the direction of any resulting vectors of tension. The principles behind rhombic flat transposition may also be applied to other flap shapes (see Fig. 26–9).

When designing a skin flap, both sides of the incision must be undermined to facilitate closure and produce a more acceptable result—this reduces the lesion and avoids a "trap door" deformity (see the section on Trap Door Deformity). Excision of Burow's triangles is frequently necessary to avoid formation of "dog ears" (see Fig. 26–7*a*). As a rule of thumb, rotation and transposition flaps for a defect of less than 30 degrees close adequately without resulting dog ears; flaps that rotate more than 30 degrees, however, may be improved with an M-plasty (Fig. 26–11).

Because flap repair is often aimed at repairing defects resulting from excision of skin malignancies, it can be carried out as soon as the physician believes that the surgery is complete. However, should repair be delayed owing to concern about the adequacy of the excision or other problems, temporary split-thickness skin grafts may be used.

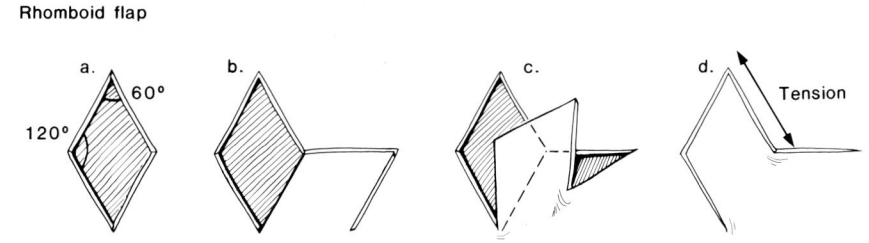

FIGURE 26–10. Rhomboid flap. *a*, The defect to be closed resembles two equilateral triangles placed base to base. *b*, A flap of similar size is created with its base at one of the two 60-degree angles. *c*, Transposition of the flap. *d*, The flap closes the recipient site, and the donor site is closed directly. The direction of tension of the wound is shown and should be oriented in a relaxed skin tension line.

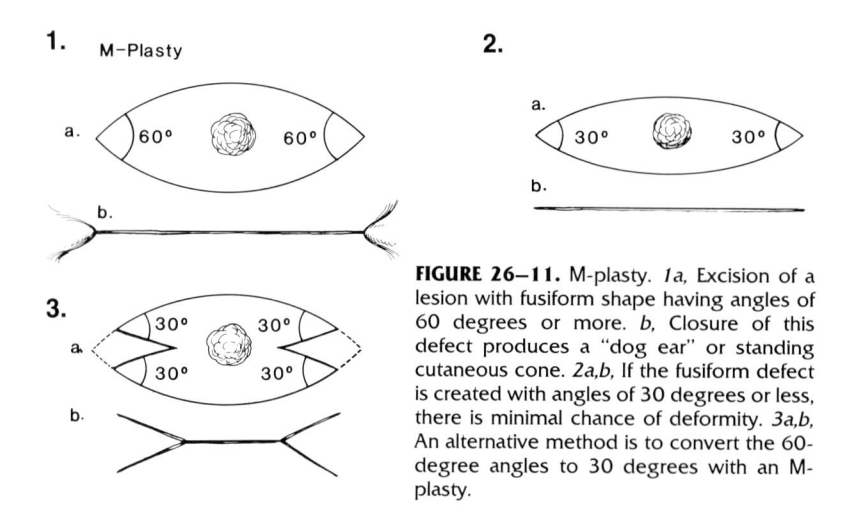

FIGURE 26–11. M-plasty. *1a*, Excision of a lesion with fusiform shape having angles of 60 degrees or more. *b*, Closure of this defect produces a "dog ear" or standing cutaneous cone. *2a,b*, If the fusiform defect is created with angles of 30 degrees or less, there is minimal chance of deformity. *3a,b*, An alternative method is to convert the 60-degree angles to 30 degrees with an M-plasty.

Tissue Expansion and Regional, Distant, and Free Flaps

Occasionally, oncologic procedures or trauma produce massive wounds that cannot be repaired with local flaps. In addition, such defects may be complex, such as through-and-through oral deficits, wounds directly over bone which will not accept a skin graft, or wounds that include the loss of essential skeletal tissues.

The introduction of tissue expanders has provided considerable help for these difficult situations. With this method, an inflatable silicone prosthesis is placed beneath the healthy soft tissues adjacent to the wound. Over several weeks, the prosthesis is gradually inflated, providing surplus soft tissue that can be mobilized to cover the wound. Expansion of hair-bearing scalp to cover areas of male pattern alopecia is a good example of this approach. This technique is not suitable for all large wounds, however, and usually requires a temporary split-thickness skin graft over the defect while the donor tissue is expanded.

Other reconstructive options for difficult situations include regional and distant flaps as well as free flaps that are transferred with microvascular anastomoses. Examples of several of these flaps can provide an understanding of the reconstructive options currently in use. Myocutaneous flaps have been used with regularity for the past 15 years. The pectoralis major myocutaneous flap is used most frequently in head and neck reconstruction. An island of skin nourished by perforating vessels from the attached pectoralis major muscle can be transferred to provide soft tissue repair and epithelial coverage for neck wounds and intraoral defects. Osteomyocutaneous flaps have the additional advantage of carrying bone into a complex wound. The trapezius osteomyocutaneous flap can be used to reconstruct both soft tissue and bony facial defects, as is necessary when a portion of the mandible and attached soft tissues have been lost. When epithelial coverage is required without a large amount of underlying bulk, an axial flap such as a deltopectoral or forehead flap is helpful. Thus, a deltopectoral flap can provide a thin epithelial flap to resurface the neck. Finally, the advent of microvascular technique allows tissue to be transferred from a distant site without the requirement of a pedicled flap or a second procedure to divide the transferred tissue from its donor site blood supply. Such free flaps can involve transfer of epithelial coverage, skeletal elements, soft tissue bulk, and/or muscle.

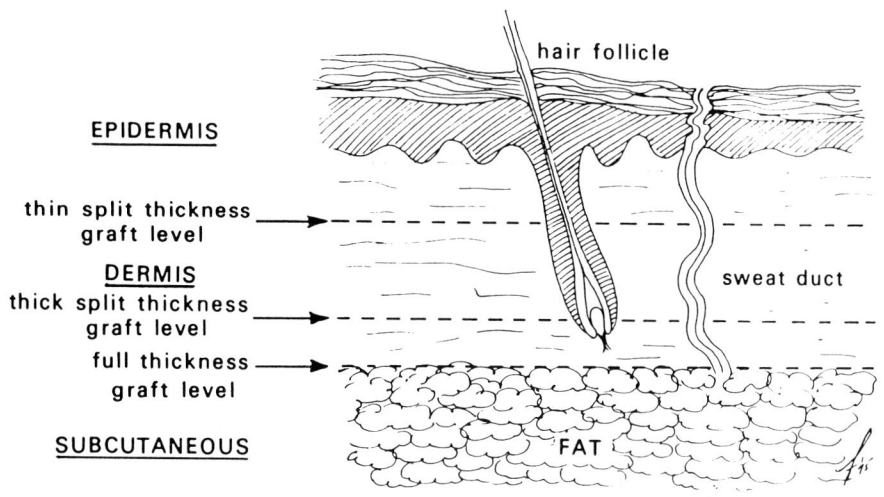

FIGURE 26–12. Graft levels in relation to thickness of skin.

The radial forearm flap is a good example of this type of flap. The lateral half of the radius and the thin overlying skin can be transferred to reconstruct a portion of the mandible and the adjacent intraoral lining or overlying skin.

Grafts

Skin grafts are classified according to the thickness of the transplanted tissue (Fig. 26–12). Thin, split-thickness grafts are taken at approximately the superficial dermis (about 0.012 inch), while the thick, split-thickness grafts are excised to a deeper level of the dermis. Preferred donor sites are the thighs, upper arms, buttocks, scalp, and abdomen.

Special instruments are available to obtain these grafts. Small grafts are probably best removed with a small battery-operated dermatome. Larger grafts may be taken with an electric, air-driven or hand-operated dermatome (Fig. 26–13).

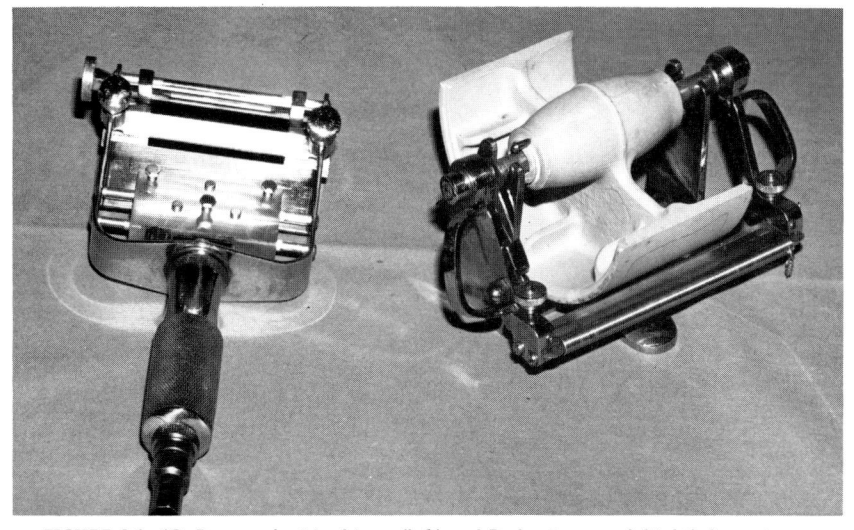

FIGURE 26–13. Brown electric driven *(left)* and Padgett manual *(right)* dermatomes.

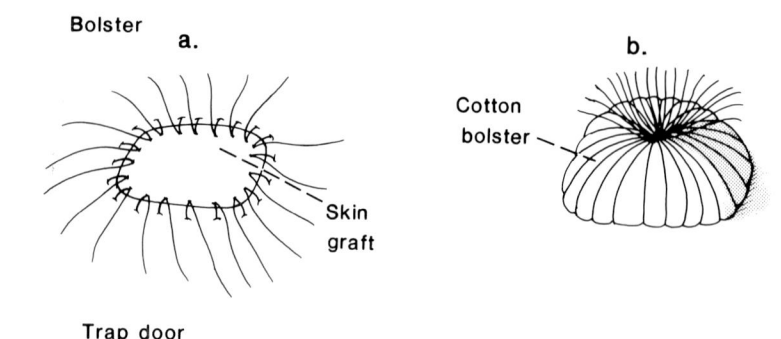

FIGURE 26–14. Bolster to secure a skin graft. *a*, A skin graft is sutured to a defect; several sutures are left long. *b*, A cotton bolster is then placed over the graft and secured with the sutures. The pressure keeps the graft stabilized on the donor site, permitting nourishment and vascular ingrowth.

Graft techniques usually require the immediate transfer of the graft to the recipient site. The graft should be immobilized by sutures and a tie-over bolus pressure dressing (Fig. 26–14). Stab wounds or "darts" within the graft may help to provide drainage of blood and serum. Donor sites are managed by occlusal dressings, open dry technique, or coverage with an adherent semipermeable membrane dressing. The donor site heals by epithelial migration from skin appendages that remain in the bed of the donor site.

Full-thickness grafts, as the name implies, involve the excision of the entire thickness of skin. The skin is usually excised in the form of an ellipse from the supraclavicular or postauricular area and cleaned of subcutaneous fat. The donor site is undermined and closed primarily. Transplanted full-thickness grafts are sutured to the recipient site and immobilized by pressure dressings similar to those used in the management of split-thickness grafts.

Complications of Wound Healing

Trap Door Deformity

This deformity is often seen when an injury leaves a flap of tissue with a relatively narrow pedicle. When the flap is sutured into its original location, not infrequently maturation of the scar results in flap elevation relative to the surrounding tissues (Fig. 26–15). Some physicians think this is due to chronic edema of the flap as a result of vascular and lymphatic compromise; others believe that contraction of the plane of scar tissue under the flap

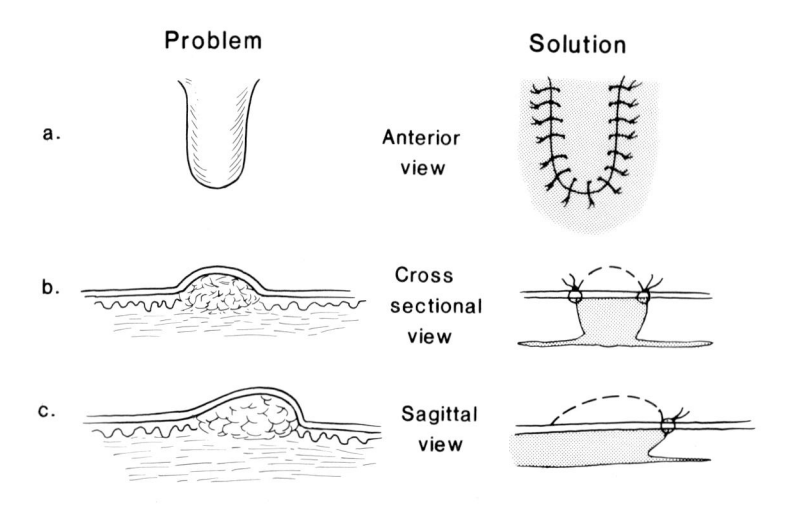

FIGURE 26–15. Trap door defect. A narrow flap of tissue may heal with an elevated contour or trap door deformity. This can be treated by undermining the tissues around the flap, which allows a sheet of scar tissue to form that matures with less flap elevation.

causes the surface to protrude. Treatment consists of undermining both sides of the incision, enlarging the plane of scar tissue. As this larger plane of scar tissue subsequently contracts, both the flap and the adjacent tissue are involved (rather than just the flap) and the resultant protrusion is decreased. Occasionally, an acceptable result can be achieved by excising the entire flap of skin and closing the defect directly.

Keloid

The incidence of keloid formation increases with increased pigmentation of the skin. Keloids occur between the ears and waist and tend to spread beyond the original wound; the overlying epithelium of the keloid is darker than the surrounding skin. The rates of both collagen synthesis and lysis in the keloid are greater than normally observed. Formation of keloids may be related to melanocyte-stimulating hormone, which is suppressed by steroids. Treatment consists of intralesional corticosteroids, subtotal excision, and/or pressure for four to six months. Rarely, low-dose radiation therapy is applicable.

Hypertrophic Scars

Hypertrophic scars, which are frequently difficult to differentiate from keloids, usually stay within the boundaries of the wound and occur more frequently in areas of motion or skin tension. Tension on wounds increases collagen formation and may explain the occurrence of this problem. Treatment consists of intralesional corticosteroids, the therapeutic application of pressure (22 mm Hg), and Z-plasty or graft if the scar is in an area of tension.

Unsightly Scars

Although most abrasions, contusions, and lacerations of the face heal with minimal scarring, a small group of individuals develop a significant deformity. Scars that are wide, red, long, or oriented in an unfavorable direction or have skin edges at different levels are more noticeable. Erythema, often seen in immature scars, usually decreases over four to six months. However, if the scar is under tension the erythema persists for a longer period of time. Treatment consists of broken line scar revision, dermabrasion, or injectable filling substances. In most cases treatment consists of revision of the scar tissue, timed to coincide with the maturation of wound healing. The techniques of scar revision are listed in Table 26–2.

Scar revision should be considered after scar maturation.

TABLE 26–2. SCAR REVISION

SCAR DEFORMITY	REQUIREMENT	TECHNIQUE
Width	Narrowing	Excision
Length (>2 cm)	Breaking the line	Z-plasty, W-plasty, zigzag-plasty
Angulation	Changing the crease line or shadow	Z-plasty
Depression	Elevation	Z-plasty or advance of subcutaneous tissues; autogenous implant
Hypertrophy and keloid	Depression and narrowing	Steroid injection or excision
Contracture	Lengthening	Transposition with Z-plasty mucosal or skin grafts

Saunders Co, 1972, p. 39.

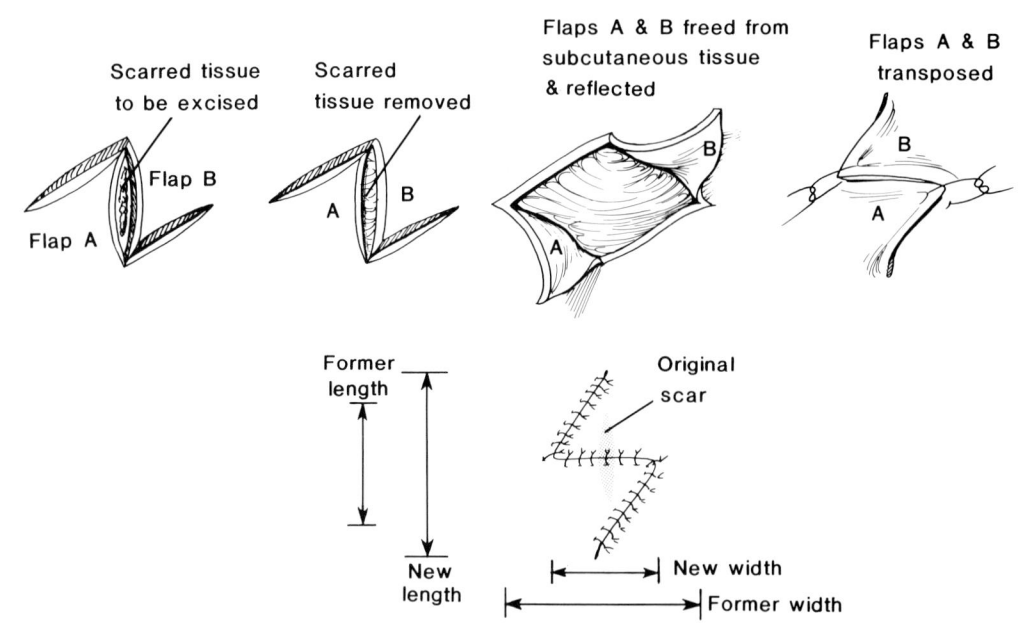

FIGURE 26–16. Z-plasty. A technique to lengthen and change the direction of a scar is shown.

When scars are contracted and angulated in an unfavorable direction, it is often necessary to lengthen the line of the scar and alter the orientation; this is best accomplished by use of the Z-plasty technique (Figs. 26–16 and 26–17). The amount of lengthening of the transposed tissues depends upon the angles of the Z. At angles of 60 degrees there is a 73 per cent increase in length of the central line of the Z; at 45 degrees there is a 50 per cent increase. The most useful angles are those from 20 to 60 degrees.

When scars of the face are longer than 2 cm they are usually conspicuous. Breaking the scar line (Fig. 26–18) with a W-plasty or zigzag-plasty often camouflages the result. These techniques are thus suitable for large scars of the face covering extensive flat areas, as in the cheek or forehead (Fig. 26–19).

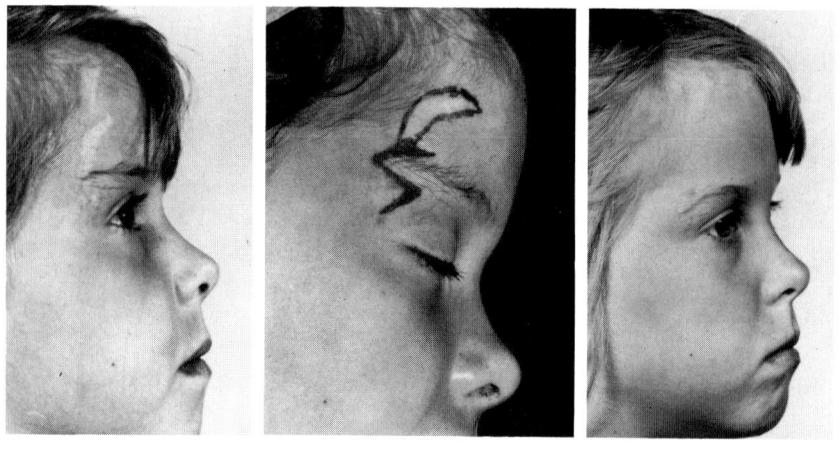

FIGURE 26–17. Large scar of temple areas, distorting the eyebrow, and appearance after excision with Z-plasty technique. (From Mathog, R. H.: Scar revision. Minnesota Med 57:31–36, 1974.)

FIGURE 26-18. Scar camouflage by W-plasty and zigzagplasty techniques. (From Mathog RH: Scar revision. Minnesota Med 57:31–36, 1974.)

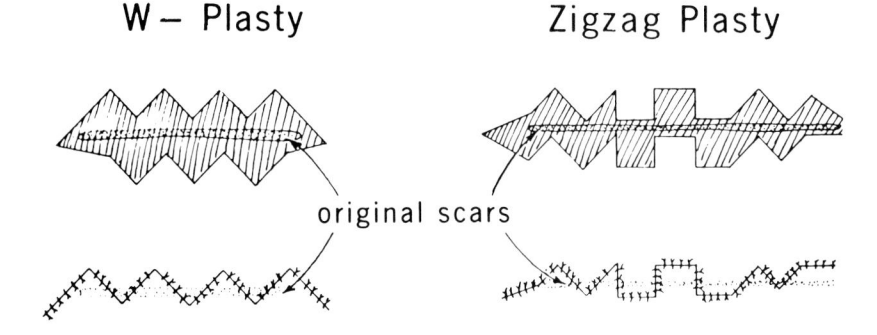

When a scar is noticeable because of a depression, simple excision is often indicated. Subcutaneous defects can be filled in with an advancement or transposition of subcutaneous tissues. A bunching of dermal layers and eversion of the skin edge can also help to obliterate the defect. Mild to moderate surface irregularities, as seen with acne scars or traumatic scars, can often be improved with dermabrasion to reduce prominent areas adjacent to a scar, or filling substances such as injectable collagen can be injected into areas of depression (Fig. 26–20).

THE AGING FACE

The desire to maintain a more youthful appearance prompts many people to seek surgical improvement of alterations that occur as a result of the aging process. It is hypothesized that the action of gravitational forces upon

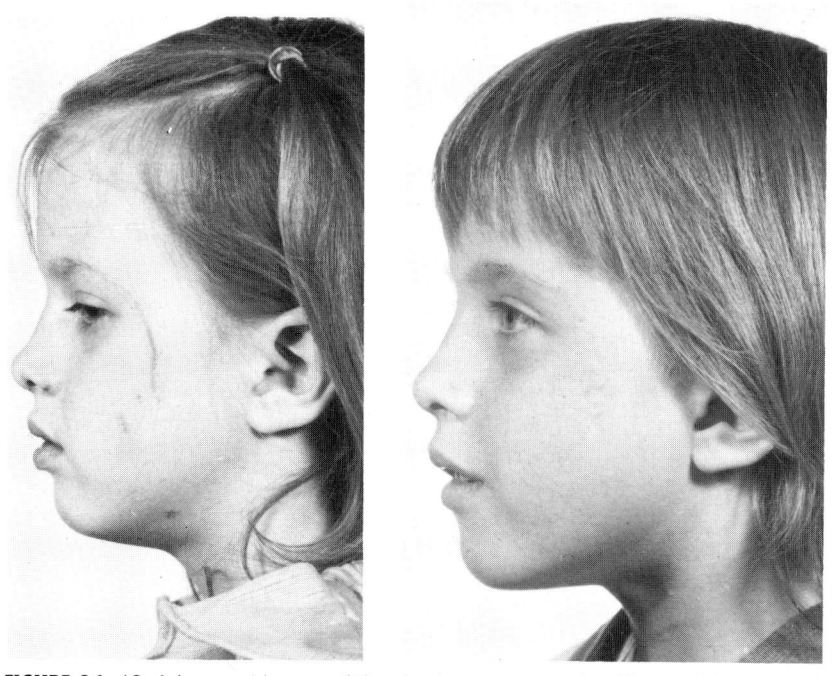

FIGURE 26–19. A large, wide scar of the cheek caused by a dog bite, and the result of treatment by zigzagplasty technique.

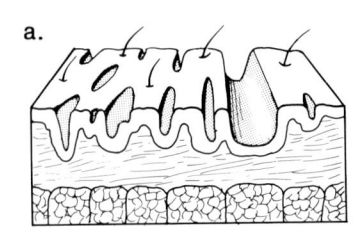

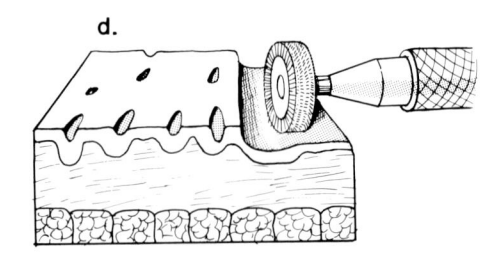

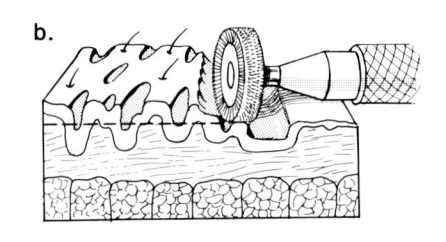

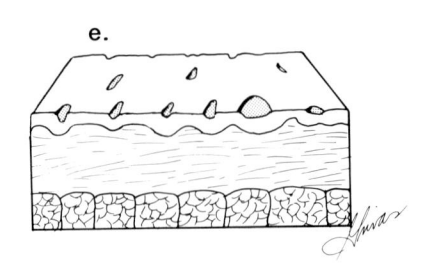

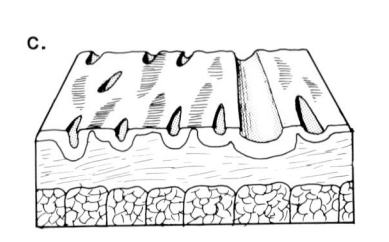

FIGURE 26–20. Dermabrasion. *a*, Skin irregularities due to trauma or acne scars. *b*, Dermabrasion planes down the surface toward the depths of the scars. *c*, After dermabrasion the surface is smoother. *d*, After the skin has healed and the epithelium thickens, the area can be dermabraded again if necessary. *e*, The final result.

the face, the repetitious pull of the facial musculature, and the loss of elasticity during degeneration of dermal collagen and elastic fibers cause the sagging of the skin and formation of wrinkles, or rhytides. Exposure to the wind and sun can accelerate degenerative skin changes. Significant weight loss also may result in excessive skin redundancy. In some cases heredity may be a factor.

A baggy appearance under the eyes denotes a laxity of skin and frequently a herniation of orbital fat associated with a weakened septum orbitale. A double chin may also be noted with the accumulation of fat in the submental area. These cosmetic problems may also appear at a younger age and are influenced by heredity.

The procedures to correct these deformities depend upon the type of cosmetic problem: Rhytidectomy (face-lift) is used for correction of facial wrinkles due to skin laxity, blepharoplasty for baggy eyelids, and submental lipectomy for double chin. Rhytidectomy, or face-lift, is especially applicable for the improvement of facial wrinkles that develop in the cheek and neck areas (Fig. 26–21). Through camouflaging incisions in the hair and behind the ears, a large area of skin is undermined and redraped; wrinkle depth is decreased but not completely abolished, and the underlying layer of facial muscles is resuspended. This procedure is not designed to correct baggy lids or finer facial wrinkles.

Blepharoplasty is the technique used to remove excessive skin and herniated fat from the lid area (Fig. 26–22), a procedure that is often performed

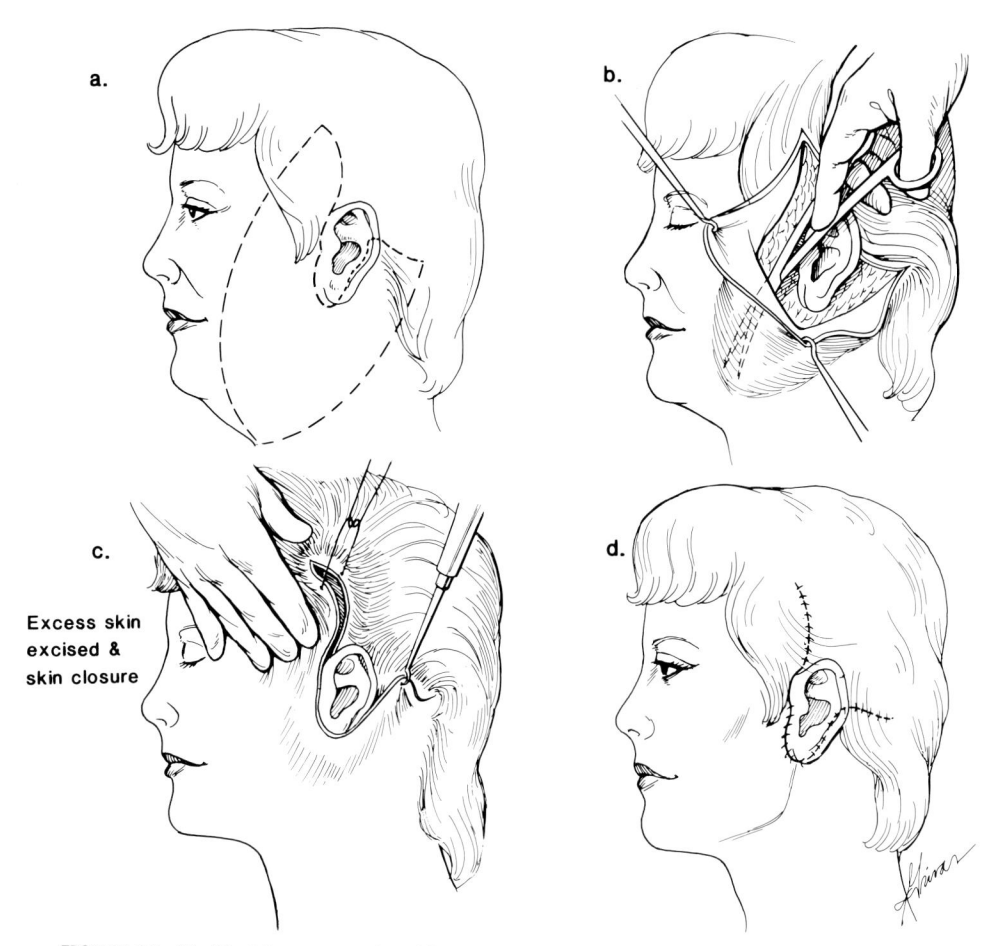

FIGURE 26–21. Rhytidectomy or face lift. *a*, Preoperative view demonstrating incisions in the hair and preauricularly as well as the area to be undermined. *b*, Skin elevation. *c*, Excision of redundant skin and skin closure. *d*, Postoperative result.

in conjunction with the face-lift. Essentially, excessive skin is removed through a crease line incision, and herniated fat is excised through the septum orbitale. Elevation of the drooping eyebrows can be accomplished by a simple excision of skin and advancement of tissues above the eyebrow area. In combination with the blepharoplasty, the brow-lift imparts a more youthful appearance to the eyes.

FIGURE 26–22. Technique of blepharoplasty. A diagram of the upper and lower lid procedure, in which the skin is undermined and excessive skin and protruding fat are removed from the area.

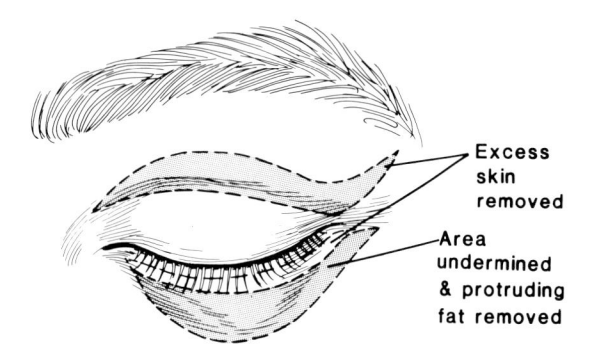

A submental lipectomy may be added to the above-mentioned procedures, depending upon the cosmetic needs of the patient. In this procedure a small incision is made beneath the chin (in the submental shadow) and the subcutaneous fat excised. The technique often provides a more graceful profile when performed with a lift of the neck skin.

Suction lipectomy has been utilized in the recent past to remove fat collections in the neck and jowl areas as well as from other areas for body sculpturing (Fig. 26–23). The technique is often performed through small incisions beneath the chin or adjacent to the ear lobe. Small diameter metal suction cannulas can be introduced through the incision and manipulated to dissect and remove excess fat and improve the facial contours. Adequate improvement of the submental and neck areas, however, requires that the relaxed and divergent anterior borders of the platysma muscles be corrected through plication, excision, and/or muscle division. This can usually be achieved through a submental incision.

Face-lift, blepharoplasty, submental lipectomy, brow-lift, and forehead-lift procedures can improve many pronounced facial rhytides or wrinkles but do not provide great improvement of the fine facial rhytides. These are often most noticeable in the perioral and periorbital areas. Chemical peel and dermabrasion are the best methods to improve these irregularities. Chemical peel is a technique in which a solution, usually containing phenol or trichloroacetic acid, is applied to the skin. The solution causes the superficial layers of skin to desquamate, and an inflammatory reaction occurs in the deeper tissues with subsequent deposition of connective tissue. As the peeled area heals, new collagen is formed and a new, smoother layer of epidermis regenerates from the remaining epidermal elements. Dermabrasion is a technique in which the surface of the skin is abraded, most commonly with a steel brush and a motorized rotary hand piece. The surface of the skin is planed down, exposing deeper areas of papillary dermis, skin appendages, and epidermis adjacent to the base of the rete pegs. As the surface is re-epithelialized, the texture of the new skin is smoother (see Fig. 26–20). This

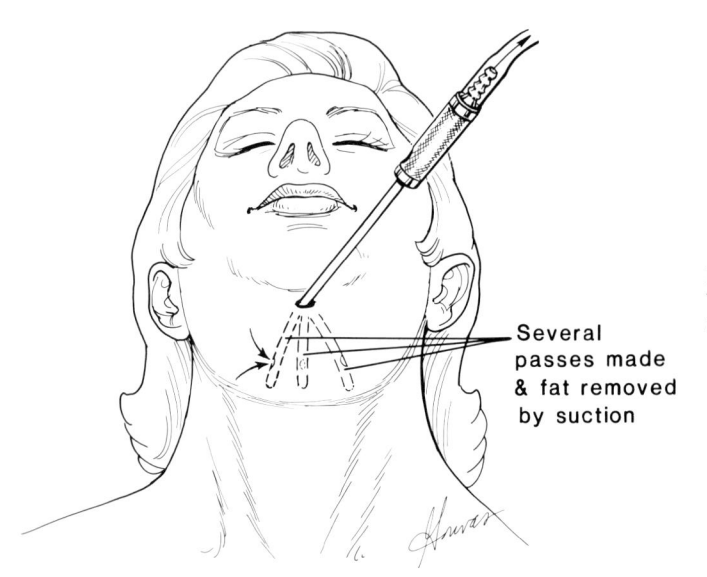

FIGURE 26–23. Submental suction lipectomy. The procedure can provide significant improvement of the neck contour.

technique is not applicable in areas where the skin is very thin, such as the eyelid.

Contour irregularities that are the result of aging or scar can also often be improved with the injection of filling substances such as injectable collagen. Recently, autologous fat injections have been advocated for this purpose, but the ability of this technique to maintain improvement is unproven. No permanent injectable filling substance is yet available with FDA approval.

DEFORMITIES OF THE NOSE

Its prominent position in the center of the face makes the nose very important to facial aesthetics. Because heredity or trauma may produce a functionally or aesthetically unacceptable appearance, rhinoplasty is one of the most commonly performed aesthetic procedures. The results of this surgery can be very gratifying to both the patient and the physician and, unlike some other cosmetic procedures such as surgery for the aging face, the improvement is influenced very little by the passage of time.

Nasal correction requires both a functional and a cosmetic evaluation; nasal obstruction is just as important as deformity of the external appearance. A detailed history, examination of the interior of the nose, and evaluation of the paranasal sinuses is essential to the diagnosis and correction of the many conditions that cause nasal obstruction (discussed in Chapter 12).

Evaluation of the external nose requires a concept of beauty. The overall proportion of the nose and general balance in relationship to the face should be considered; that is, a small chin may give the appearance of an unusually

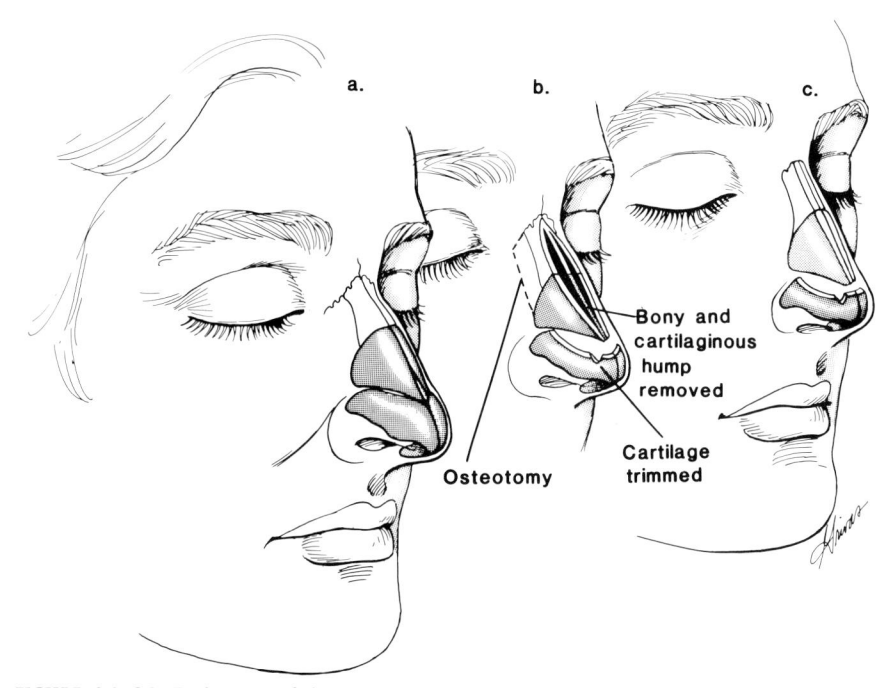

FIGURE 26–24. Technique of rhinoplasty, involving isolation of the bony and cartilaginous skeleton, trimming of appropriate portions, and repositioning under controlled conditions.

large nose. In most cases it is desirable to have a narrow and straight (or slightly curved) dorsum, a straight (nonretracted) columella, slight "supratip" depression, and accentuation of the alar rim.

Rhinoplasty is designed to correct the external appearance of the nose. Often this procedure may be combined with a septoplasty, which is used to correct internal, functional deformities (see Chapter 12). Essentially, the rhinoplasty technique requires isolation of the bony and cartilaginous skeleton and trimming and repositioning of the structures under controlled conditions (Fig. 26–24).

In cases of deformities caused by loss of skeletal support, cartilage, bone, or synthetic materials are implanted into the defect. During the healing process the nose is immobilized and protected with external and internal splints. Postoperative swelling may be observed for six months or more.

DEFORMITIES OF THE EAR

Deformities of the ear range from anotia (congenital or acquired due to trauma or neoplasms), retained auricular hillocks, skin tags, and, more commonly, the protruding auricle (cup-ear deformity). These ear malformations can be a source of embarrassment to a child, particularly in the early school years. For this reason, correction, when feasible, is usually recommended by age five or six, before the child begins school.

In the cup-ear deformity the most usual and distinctive problem is an unfurrowed antihelix with a poorly defined superior crus. The result is an ear that protrudes excessively. The repair of this defect is usually accomplished by remodeling and suturing the cartilage into position to create an antihelical fold.

Defects of the auricle from trauma or cancer resection are treated by approximation of local tissues. Most small defects can be converted to a V of the auricular rim and closed in layers of cartilage, subcutaneous tissue, and skin. Such V excisions are useful in the care of basal cell carcinoma, squamous cell carcinoma, or other neoplasms. Larger defects require more complex reconstruction procedures and some residual deformity is to be expected.

Total accidental auricular amputation is a rare and serious cosmetic injury. Replacement is worth attempting, however, because secondary plastic reconstruction is extremely difficult and the application of a prosthesis may not be satisfactory. Microvascular repair enhances the prognosis but is often not technically possible. Often the cartilage framework is salvaged and buried in a pocket behind the ear for use in later reconstruction.

MENTOPLASTY

The chin, the nose, and the forehead have a usual balancing relationship in the facial profile, and, in cases in which the chin is too large or too small, mentoplasty is performed. Aberrant maxillary, mandibular, and dental relationships may require surgical correction; it is important to evaluate the entire facial skeletal contour before planning a surgical procedure that addresses only a small chin. A better functional and cosmetic result may be produced by orthognathic surgery.

Mentoplasty can be done alone or in conjunction with rhinoplasty. Enhancement of the chin may be accompanied by sliding the lower portion of the bone of the chin forward (advancement genioplasty) or by implanting some material, usually Silastic, in front of the chin (augmentation mentoplasty).

References

American College of Surgeons. Committee on Trauma: Early Care of the Injured Patient. Philadelphia, WB Saunders Co, 1972, pp 37–41.
Bernstein L: Z-plasty in head and neck surgery. Arch Otolaryngol 89:574–584, 1969.
Borges AF: Elective Incisions and Scar Revision. Boston, Little, Brown and Co, 1973, p 1014.
Clemons JE, Connely MV: Reattachment of a totally amputated auricle. Arch Otolaryngol 97:269–272, 1973.
Converse JM, et al: The aging face. *In* Converse JM (ed): Reconstructive Plastic Surgery. 2nd ed. Vol II. Philadelphia, WB Saunders Co, 1976.
Creely JJ, Peterson JD: Carcinoma of the lip. Southern Med J 57:799–784, 1974.
Crikelair GF: Surgical approach to facial scarring. JAMA 172:160–162, 1960.
Farrior RT: A method of otoplasty. Arch Otolaryngol 69:400–408, 1959.
Fernandez AO, Ronis ML: The Treacher-Collins syndrome. Arch Otolaryngol 80:505–520, 1964.
Gillis S, Feingold M: Atlas of Mental Retardation Syndrome. Washington, DC, US Government Printing Office, 1968, p 156.
Girardi G: Principles of local skin flaps. Facial Plastic Surg 1:31–35, 1983.
Gunter JP: Rhombic flaps. Facial Plastic Surg 1:69–73, 1983.
Johnson JB, Hadley RC: The aging face. *In* Converse JM (ed): Reconstructive Plastic Surgery. Vol III. Philadelphia, WB Saunders Co, 1964, pp 1306–1342.
Lacy GM, Hemphill JE: Facial revision. Surg Clin North Am 49:1343–1350, 1969.
Mathog RH: Scar revision. Minnesota Med 57:31–36, 1974.
Mustarde JC: The correction of prominent ears using simple mattress sutures. Br J Plastic Surg 16:170–178, 1963.
Rutledge RT: The Pierre Robin syndrome. A surgical emergency in the neonatal period. Br J Plastic Surg 13:204–209, 1960.
Smith JW: Clinical experience with the vermilion bordered lip flap. Plastic Reconstr Surg 27:527–543, 1961.
Straatsma CR: Surgical technique helpful in obtaining fine scars. Plastic Reconstr Surg 2:21–24, 1947.
Tresley IJ, Arenberg JK, Polterock J: Augmentation mentoplasty; reflection. Laryngoscope 82:2092–2102, 1972.

27

MAXILLOFACIAL TRAUMA

by Kent S. Wilson, M.D.

It is essential that every physician be familiar with the basic principles involved in the care of patients who have sustained maxillofacial or laryngeal injury. Because of the increasing number of recreational vehicular accidents, the constant volume of automobile accidents, and interpersonal conflict injuries, any physician at any time may have to care for a patient who has sustained head or neck trauma. Injuries of the face and neck must be managed appropriately in both the initial and later stages, since such injuries may involve essential portions of the respiratory, vascular, central nervous, upper digestive, and visual systems as well as major portions of the face, with cosmetic implications.

Medical care of maxillofacial injuries is very much a team effort from initial evaluation to definitive therapy. Every physician should be capable of quickly assessing the severity of a maxillofacial or laryngeal injury and should be able to formulate an appropriate plan for the patient's care. The care plan for major injuries usually involves treatment by one of several members of a team that includes a maxillofacial surgeon (who may be an otolaryngologist or plastic surgeon), an ophthalmologist, a neurosurgeon, and an oral surgeon or dentist. This chapter is directed to physicians who will be responsible for initial evaluation as well as the definitive care of less severe cases.

INITIAL EVALUATION AND MANAGEMENT

Initial Care

Initial care is dependent upon the severity of injury. Maxillofacial and laryngeal injury may range from the simplest nasal fracture without significant epistaxis and only minor nasal deformity to the most massive facial crush injury with extensive involvement of the entire head and neck. The initial care involves rapid general evaluation of the patient's vital signs and the institution of basic life-support measures if appropriate.

Maintenance of the airway is the first priority and may involve suctioning of the oral or nasal cavity to remove blood or other debris. If the patient is comatose or if mandibular fracture has resulted in instability of the floor of the mouth with prolapse of the tongue into the pharynx, an oral airway may be required. If, for whatever reason, an oral airway is unsatisfactory and tracheal ventilation is necessary, endotracheal intubation is the method of choice. Emergency tracheostomy is to be avoided if at all possible, since the

Airway maintenance is the first priority.

procedure is fraught with hazard if the operator is not intimately familiar with the anatomy and experienced in the surgical technique. Emergency tracheostomy should be resorted to only if all other measures have failed or if laryngeal injury is suspected.

The second priority in the initial management of trauma patients is the *maintenance of a reasonable cardiac output.* The most common cause of inadequate cardiac output in the trauma patient is hypovolemic shock. This will usually respond to volume replacement and appropriate hemostatic measures. When stability has been obtained, following initial resuscitative measures, an orderly head and neck examination may be carried out.

Sufficient cardiac output is the second priority.

History and Physical Examination

Initial evaluation of head and neck trauma, as in injury to other organ systems, requires a thorough and accurate history and physical examination. The history of the traumatic event should include the time of injury as well as a detailed description of the circumstances surrounding the incident. Details, such as whether the patient was wearing a seat belt, approximate velocities of vehicles involved, and whether recreational vehicles such as snowmobiles were involved, may give clues as to the types of injuries which should be searched for.

The physical examination should be done as soon as possible, since swelling may obscure bony or cartilaginous deformities. The first item to be noticed is the patient's state of consciousness, since attendance to cerebral injury takes first priority in the patient's management once respiratory and cardiovascular functions have been stabilized. The soft tissue covering of the head and neck should be thoroughly inspected for lacerations, including the inner aspects of the ear, nose, and mouth. Special note should be made of facial mobility, since the presence or absence of seventh nerve paralysis may be important in the patient's later management. All wounds should be probed to their depths to determine whether bone has been injured or exposed or whether foreign bodies are present within the wound.

The examiner palpates the entire head and neck, beginning at the top of the skull and progressing inferiorly, to locate displaced fractures and abnormally mobile structures. Note should be made of the integrity of the frontozygomatic sutures, which are commonly fractured. Special attention should be paid to the frontal region, where sinus fractures may create significant intracranial complications, such as cerebrospinal fluid fistula, which may require prompt management. Frontal sinus fracture is usually characterized by a depression in the midfrontal region. Sometimes fracture fragments may be palpated through the epidermal covering or in the depths of soft tissue wounds. On palpation of the nose, special note should be made of any bony deformity or abnormal mobility, especially of the septum. Septal mobility is best ascertained by grasping the anterior septum between thumb and forefinger and applying lateral pressure. The cheeks should be palpated to determine if there is pain on compression, which usually indicates a fracture of the zygoma. The entire mandible should be palpated to determine whether tenderness suggestive of fracture is present. Abnormal mobility of portions of the mandible or displaced fractures may be identified by palpation also. The teeth should be tested for abnormal mobility or pain sensitivity because these fractures and luxations require prompt attention. The neck should be palpated for the presence of free air, which suggests rupture of the tracheobronchial tree, and for crepitation or tenderness over the larynx suggestive of fracture.

Cervical spine injury, such as fracture or dislocation, may be suggested by nuchal muscle spasm, but this not a constant finding. It is advised that severely injured patients be immobilized as though a cervical spine injury had occurred until it is radiographically and clinically demonstrated that the cervical spine is normal.

Radiographic Examination

Radiographic examinations and other tests may be helpful in arriving at an accurate diagnosis following the history and physical examination. Fractures of the nose are usually best demonstrated in lateral radiographs, while fractures of the middle third of the face and paranasal sinuses are best demonstrated in the Waters projection. Laminagraphic evaluation may be very helpful in attempting to determine whether fractures of the orbital floor or anterior cranial fossa have occurred. Fractures of the mandible are best demonstrated with oblique views of this bone or preferably with a panoramic radiograph (Fig. 27–1). Computer-assisted tomographic scanning may be extremely helpful in the diagnosis of facial bone and laryngeal injuries. Reconstructions, as demonstrated in Figure 27–2, may be quite helpful in treatment planning. Severe lacerations of the cheek may be evaluated by sialography to determine whether the parotid duct is intact. This procedure

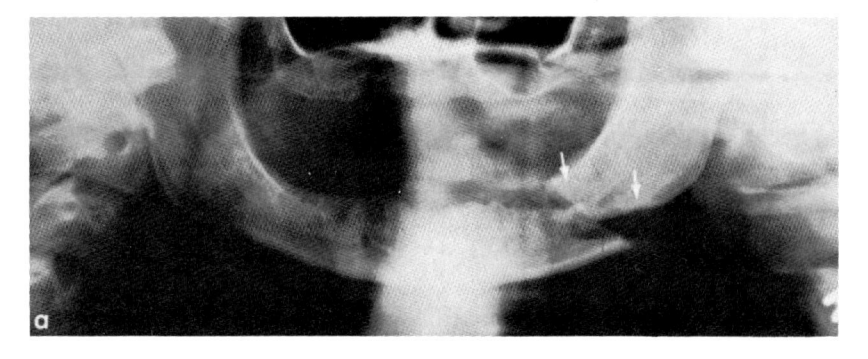

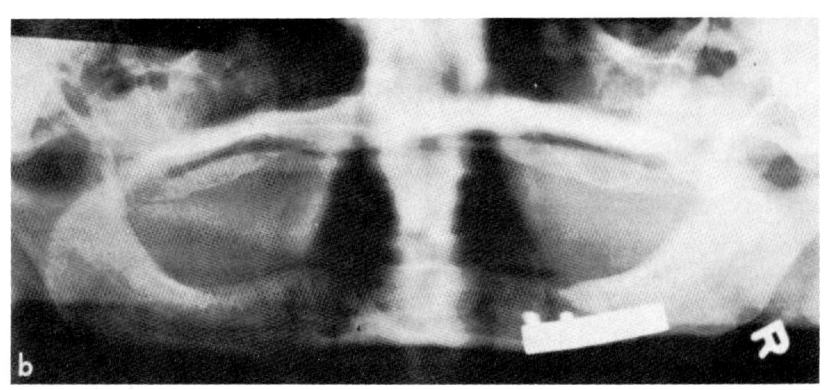

FIGURE 27–1. *a*, Fracture of the mandible demonstrated by orthopantomogram. *b*, Repair of fracture by application of metallic plate.

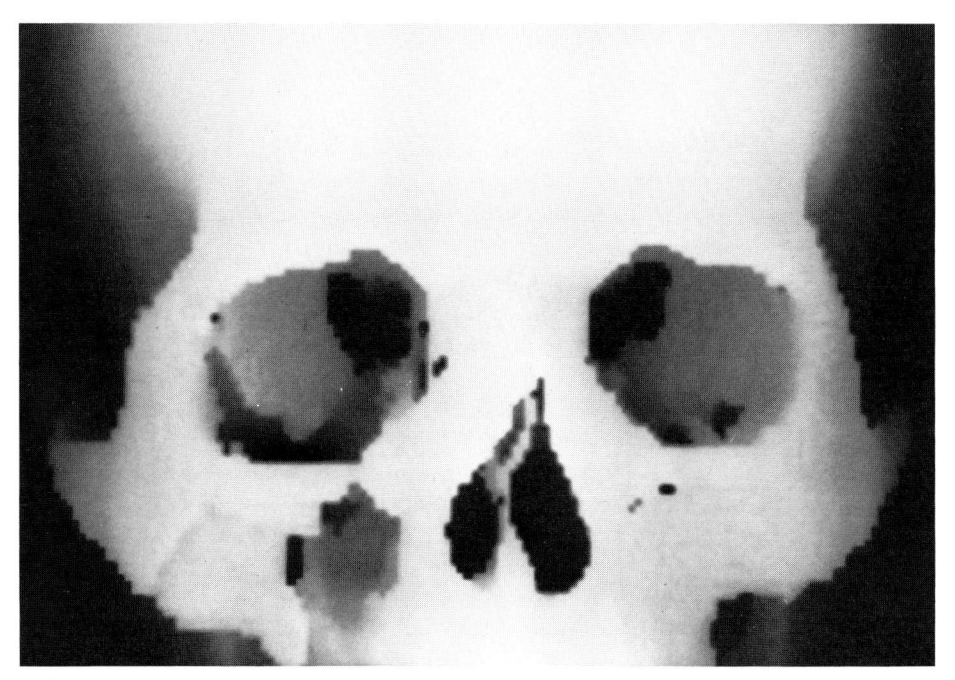

FIGURE 27–2. This CT reconstruction gives a three-dimensional view of the fractured right maxilla.

involves the retrograde instillation of radiographic contrast medium into the parotid duct orifice. If seventh nerve paralysis is present, electrical testing may be required as a guide to surgical decompression of this nerve in the fallopian canal.

Treatment Priorities

Very definite priorities have evolved in the care of the trauma patient following initial resuscitative measures that are designed to stabilize the airway and maintain cardiac output. The order of these priorities is as follows: (1) evaluation and therapy of any central nervous system injury, (2) evaluation and therapy of any abdominal or thoracic injury, (3) treatment of soft tissue, facial, and extremity trauma, and (4) reduction and fixation of both facial and extremity fractures. These guidelines, when applied to facial trauma, dictate that soft tissue wounds be closed in the first four to eight hours after injury.

The facial injury must not distract systemic evaluation.

If possible, fracture reduction should be done at that time. However, if other injuries preclude reduction and fixation of facial fractures in the early post-trauma period, this task is usually best postponed until the fourth to sixth day after trauma when facial edema has largely resolved. Under nearly all circumstances, facial fractures should be reduced within the first two weeks to avoid the problems of malunion from rapid healing or nonunion because of delayed reduction and fixation.

Soft Tissue Injury

Early evaluation and care of soft tissue injuries are absolutely critical to obtaining satisfactory functional and cosmetic results in facial reconstruction. Initial physical examination involves thorough evaluation of all wounds, even if this requires local or general anesthesia. Special care must be taken to ascertain the extent of injury in areas about the eye, in the nasolacrimal region, adjacent to or involving the facial nerve, and about the parotid duct. All tissues must be handled extremely gently, and all foreign bodies are removed by copious irrigation with sterile saline. Scrubbing with a surgical brush may be required to prevent tattooing if debris or dirt has been embedded in the skin. Debridement on the face must be kept to an absolute minimum. Because of the rich blood supply of the face, small fragments of tissue survive which would become devitalized in any other part of the body. In the treatment of facial injuries, one should follow the rule, "if in doubt, preserve tissue." Should tissue become devitalized, it can be debrided later. Lacerations should be closed in anatomic layers, beginning at the depth of the wound with absorbable sutures and progressing to the surface where subcutaneous, clear permanent sutures or absorbable sutures may be employed. Subcuticular or cutaneous permanent sutures may be employed for skin closure and require removal. Meticulous skin closure must be employed throughout to minimize scarring. After closure, facial lacerations may be supported with skin closure tape for several weeks to months to minimize scarring. The decision to use antibiotics must be based on the problems of each case, depending upon contamination, delay in closure, and similar considerations. Grossly contaminated wounds, or those that involve exposed bone, should be treated with antibiotics.

TYPES OF FRACTURES

Nasal Fracture

All nasal injuries should be evaluated for septal hematoma.

The most common bone injury involving the face is fracture of the nose. It must be remembered that the nose is composed of not only bone but also cartilage and soft tissue and that any or all of these tissues may be disrupted by an injury. The usual signs of nasal fracture are (1) depression or displacement of the nasal bones (Fig. 27–3), (2) edema of the nose, (3) epistaxis, and (4) fracture of the septal cartilage with displacement or mobility. The patient must always be examined for hematoma of the septum resulting from fracture, which, if undetected and untreated, may progress to abscess formation with resorption of the septal cartilage and severe saddle-nose deformity. Management of a septal hematoma includes incision and drainage of the hematoma, placement of a temporary drain, application of intranasal dressings to compress the septal mucosa and minimize the risk of re-formation of the hematoma, and initiation of antibiotic therapy to decrease the risk of infection.

Repair of nasal fractures can usually be carried out under local anesthesia following the resolution of edema. The topical application of 4 per cent cocaine on cotton pledgets, followed by infiltration of lidocaine, is usually satisfactory. Not more than 5 ml of 4 per cent cocaine should be used in the

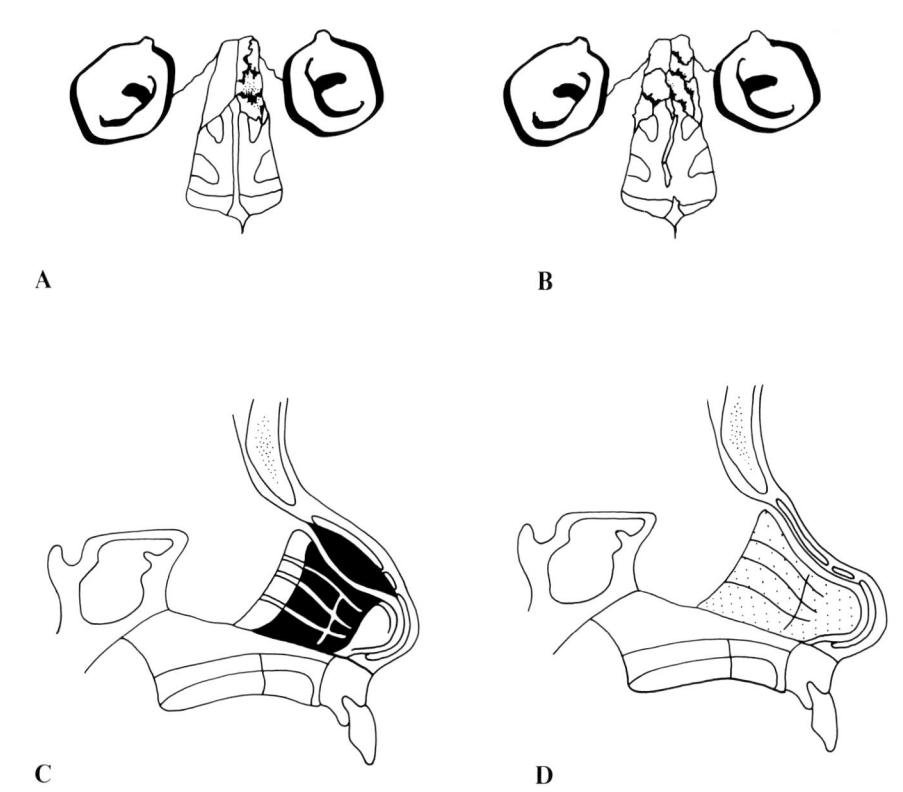

FIGURE 27–3. *A* and *B* demonstrate increasing severity of nasal fracture. *A* demonstrates depression and comminution of the left nasal bone without displacement of the dorsum or significant fracture of the septum. *B* shows more severe comminution of the nasal bones with fracture of the septal bone and cartilage. This more severe injury usually results in external deformity, and the septal fracture frequently results in obstructive deflection. *C* shows a fracture of the nasal septum with hematoma formation beneath the dorsum and throughout the central portion of the septum. This may be recognized by a "soft spot" on external palpation of the dorsum or a soft fluctuant mass to intranasal palpation with a cotton-tipped applicator. If the hematoma is unrecognized or becomes infected, then cartilage resorption may occur, resulting in collapse of the cartilaginous septum and resultant external deformity and usually nasal obstruction, as pictured in *D*.

adult, and cocaine probably should not be used in children. Children usually require general anesthesia for the reduction of nasal fractures.

The most common type of fracture involves depression of one nasal bone, with displacement of the nasal pyramid to the opposite side. Elevation of the depressed nasal bone with a flat elevator followed by displacement of the pyramid to its pre-injury position usually may be accomplished without great difficulty (Fig. 27–4). If closed reduction techniques do not yield a satisfactory configuration, then open reduction techniques involving wide exposure of the nasal septum and portions of the nasal bones may be required. Severe injuries may require not only open reduction but also a variety of fixation techniques such a direct wiring, external suspension, or even transfixation with stainless steel wire and the application of lead plates.

Internal and external nasal dressings are useful following the reduction of most nasal fractures. A satisfactory internal dressing consists of ½- to 1-inch packing gauze impregnated with antibiotic ointment. External dressings are applied to either protect the nose or maintain reduction or both. The external

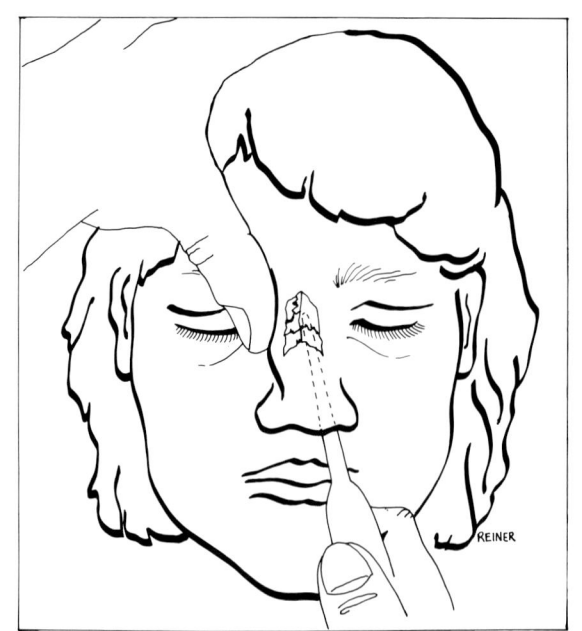

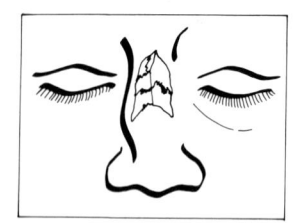

FIGURE 27–4. Reduction of a depressed and dislocated nasal bone fracture. This reduction is accomplished in two steps following anesthesia by first elevating the depressed nasal bone as illustrated and then manually displacing the pyramid to the midline.

dressing may be prefabricated of aluminum or fabricated from thermolabile plastic, plaster of paris, or dental stent material. Antibiotic therapy is indicated in most cases of nasal fracture, especially if gross soft tissue disruption has occurred, prolonged internal nasal dressing is required, or open reduction has been carried out. Internal dressings are usually left in place for three to seven days, depending upon the severity of injury.

Mandibular Fracture

Fracture of the mandible is the second most common fracture of the facial skeleton. Signs and symptoms suggestive or diagnostic of mandibular fracture include (1) malocclusion of the teeth, (2) tooth mobility, (3) intraoral lacerations, (4) pain on mastication, and (5) bone deformity. Initial evaluation includes examination for fractures of the teeth and assessment both by inquiry and by direct examination of the patient's dental occlusion. Most patients can state quite accurately whether their teeth fit normally, and examination may suggest improper alignment of the upper or lower dental arches. Intraoral examination may show lacerations over the mandible and there may be palpable or visible deformity of the mandible, both of which suggest fracture. The most frequently fractured regions of the mandible are the condyle and the angle (Fig. 27–5).

Repair of a mandibular fracture employs the general principle of splinting the mandible with its intact dentition against the maxilla with its intact dentition. The upper and lower dental arches are usually bound together by ligating arch bars to the upper and lower dental arches with wire. These arch bars have small hooks that accept either elastic or wire loops which bind the upper to the lower dental arch (Fig. 27–6). More complex types of

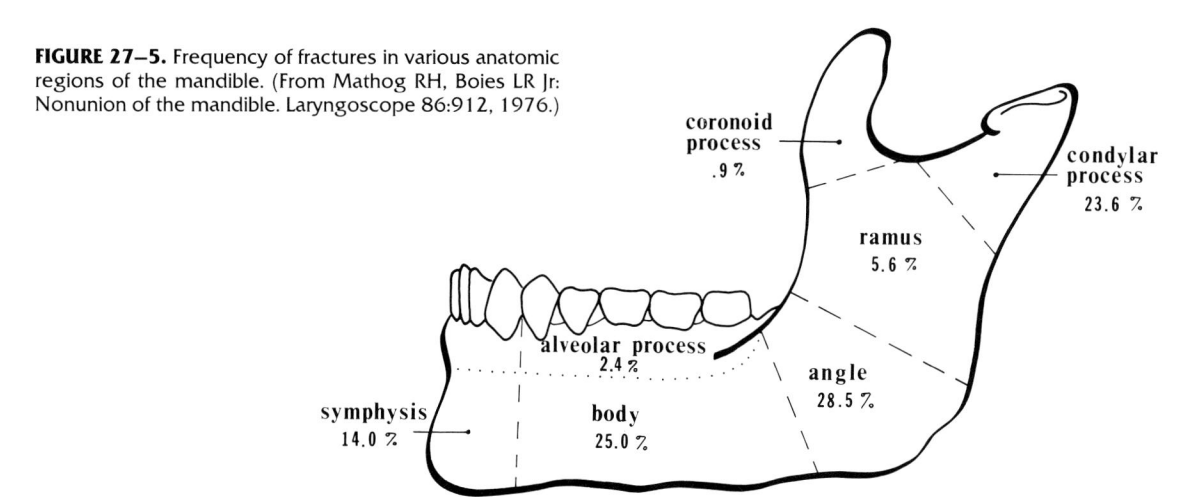

FIGURE 27–5. Frequency of fractures in various anatomic regions of the mandible. (From Mathog RH, Boies LR Jr: Nonunion of the mandible. Laryngoscope 86:912, 1976.)

- coronoid process .9 %
- condylar process 23.6 %
- ramus 5.6 %
- alveolar process 2.4 %
- angle 28.5 %
- symphysis 14.0 %
- body 25.0 %

mandibular fractures may require open reduction and the direct wiring or plating of fragments to obtain stability in addition to intermaxillary fixation with arch bars. Plating of facial fractures has become popular in the past decade and provides excellent fracture immobilization and many times eliminates the need to maintain fixation of the upper and lower dental arches. This improves patient comfort, oral hygiene, speech, airway, and alimentation. These open techniques may be required when severe comminution, gross displacement, or multiple fractures create a situation in which closed reduction and intermaxillary fixation techniques are inadequate to stabilize the fractured mandible. Antibiotics, penicillin being the drug of choice, should be given to nearly all mandibular fracture patients because the mandibular mucoperiosteum is so closely applied to the mandible that most mandibular fractures are compound. Antibiotics should be given from the time of the fracture until the mucoperiosteum has healed and the fracture has been stabilized.

Most mandibular fractures are compound.

FIGURE 27–6. Illustration of the principle of splinting one dental arch against the other, employing arch bars that are affixed to the teeth and then joined either with loops of wire or dental elastics.

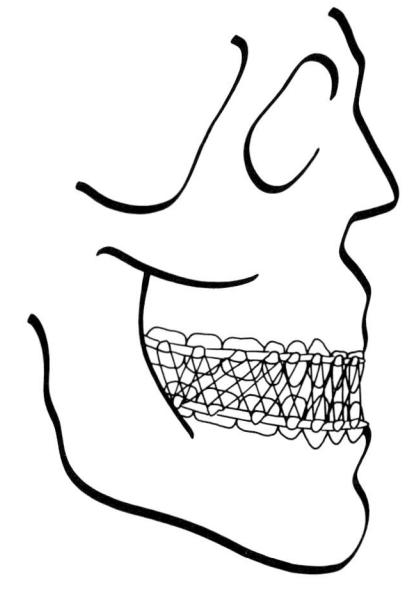

Immediate treatment following fracture of the mandible should include intraoral hygiene with suction and mouthwashes, the previously noted antibiotic therapy, and analgesia, as well as first aid type stabilization of grossly unstable fractures. Elastic figure-of-eight or Barton's bandaging about the head is commonly employed to support the mandible, stabilize the fractured fragments, and reduce pain. Clear liquids or a very soft diet may be taken by mouth, although in severe injuries tube feeding or intravenous feedings may be required. Care of the patient following reduction of the mandibular fracture requires attention to alimentation and oral hygiene. The patient's post-reduction diet should be normally nutritious and may include most foods in the diet prior to the injury. Standard dietary items may be pureed in a blender and taken through the closed jaws and teeth. Oral hygiene must be scrupulous and is best carried out with a pulsed water jet device (Water Pik). Diluted hydrogen peroxide (one-half strength) may also be employed as a mouthwash to maintain oral hygiene.

Zygoma and Orbital Floor Fractures

Recognition and treatment of a fractured zygoma or orbital floor are extremely important (Fig. 27–7). If these fractures are untreated, sequelae may include a flattened cheek and ocular complications such as enophthalmos or diplopia.

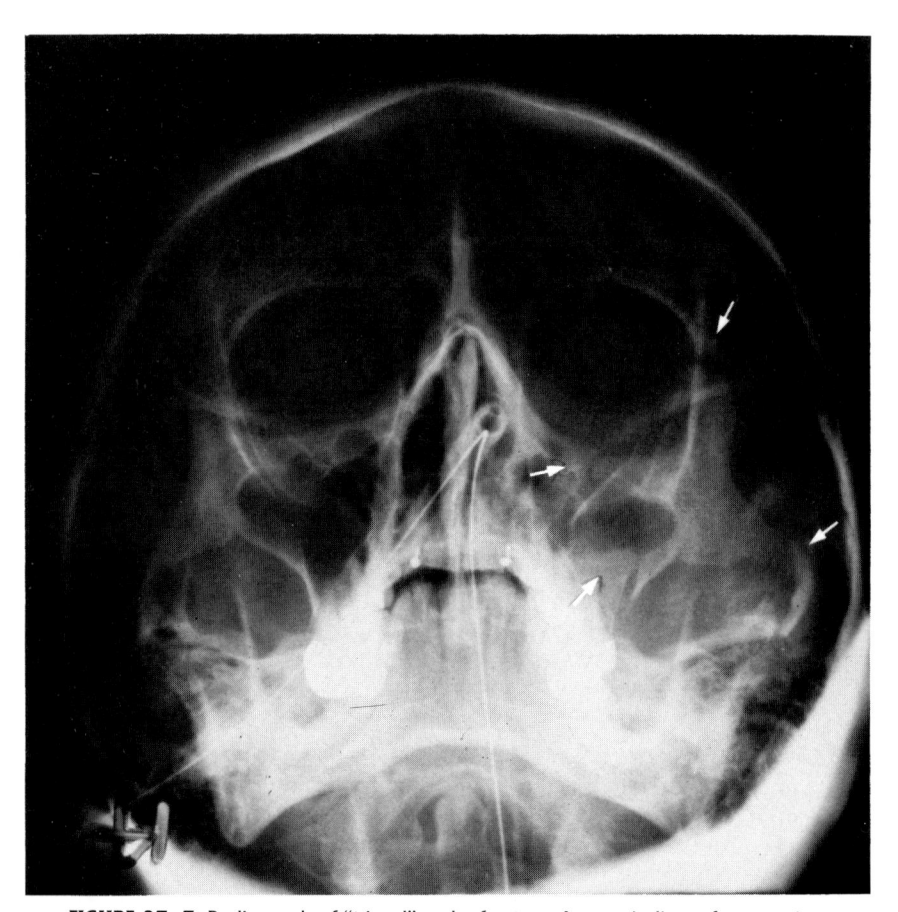

FIGURE 27–7. Radiograph of "tripod" malar fracture. Arrows indicate fracture sites.

FIGURE 27–8. *A*, The normal ocular-orbital relationship. *B*, The mechanism of orbital blow-out fracture in which external force results in increased orbital pressure and fracture-displacement into the maxillary sinus with herniation of orbital contents. If unrecognized, this may result in enophthalmos or limitation of extraocular muscle motion.

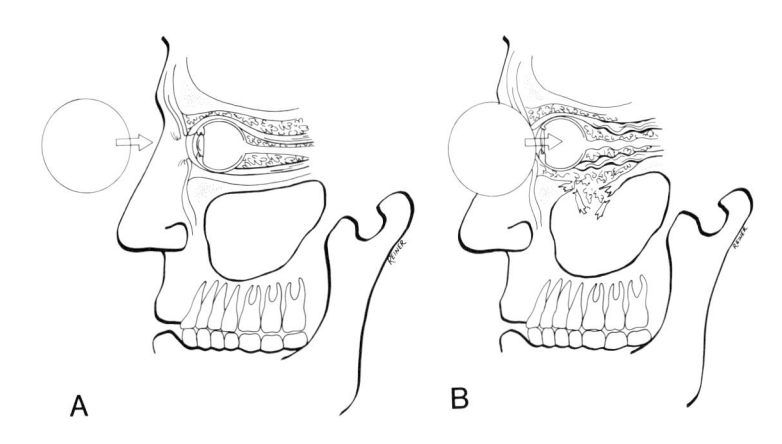

Injuries that produce zygoma fractures usually involve a blow to the body of the zygoma or "malar" prominence. The orbital floor may be fractured in this process or may be "blown out" by an object such as a baseball or tennis ball which occludes the orbit as it strikes the face (Fig. 27–8A and B). Zygoma fractures may be characterized by (1) palpable deformity (step) of the infraorbital rim, (2) diplopia on upward gaze, (3) hypesthesia of the cheek, (4) flattening of the lateral aspect of the cheek, (5) periorbital ecchymosis, or (6) inferior displacement of the ocular globe. Occasionally only the zygomatic arch is fractured with a depression of the lateral temporal region. Fractures of the orbital floor may be characterized only by restricted upward gaze due to entrapment of the inferior rectus muscle. Hypesthesia of the cheek is caused by contusion or laceration of the maxillary division of the trigeminal nerve when the maxilla fractures. If orbital floor fracture is suspected, planigraphic or CT evaluation may be very helpful in determining the degree of injury to the orbital floor.

Ophthalmologic examination should be part of the evaluation.

Repair of these fractures may occasionally be carried out by closed reduction techniques, but more often an open approach is required, especially if an orbital floor fracture is significantly displaced. An open reduction of the fractured zygoma usually involves a lateral brow incision to approach the fractured frontozygomatic suture and a medial infraorbital incision to approach the fractured zygomaticomaxillary region. Alternative approaches include an intraoral incision to expose the lower portion of the zygoma and/or subciliary, or conjunctival incisions to expose the orbital floor and orbital rim. The orbital floor may be explored and reconstructed through this infraorbital route. Orbital floor reconstruction is best done by realignment of displaced bone fragments, but when this does not yield a stable floor, an implant of transplanted bone or synthetic material may be required. When the fractured zygoma has been reduced via these approaches, it is fixed in place with stainless steel wire ligatures. Small metallic plates are also useful and may be used in place of wire ligatures. Rarely, an injury of the zygoma may be so severe that the bone must be affixed to external traction devices to maintain its position. This general technique is referred to as external fixation and usually involves a "halo" frame. When bone has been lost or when the bone is extensively comminuted, immediate grafting with hip, rib, or calvarial bone may be appropriate.

Maxillary Fractures

Fractures of the maxilla are among the most severe injuries involving the face and are characterized by (1) mobility or displacement of the palate, (2) mobility of the nose in association with the palate, (3) epistaxis, or (4) mobility or displacement of the entire middle third of the face. Le Fort's classification of maxillary fractures is satisfactory for both diagnostic and therapeutic purposes. It should be remembered, however, that any single maxillary fracture may not precisely fit the classic descriptions of Le Fort (Fig. 27–9A and B). This classification resulted from Le Fort's observation that the facial skeleton fractures in a stereotypical pattern when low-velocity blows are sustained. The Le Fort I fracture is a low transverse fracture of the maxilla involving the palate only and is characterized by mobility or

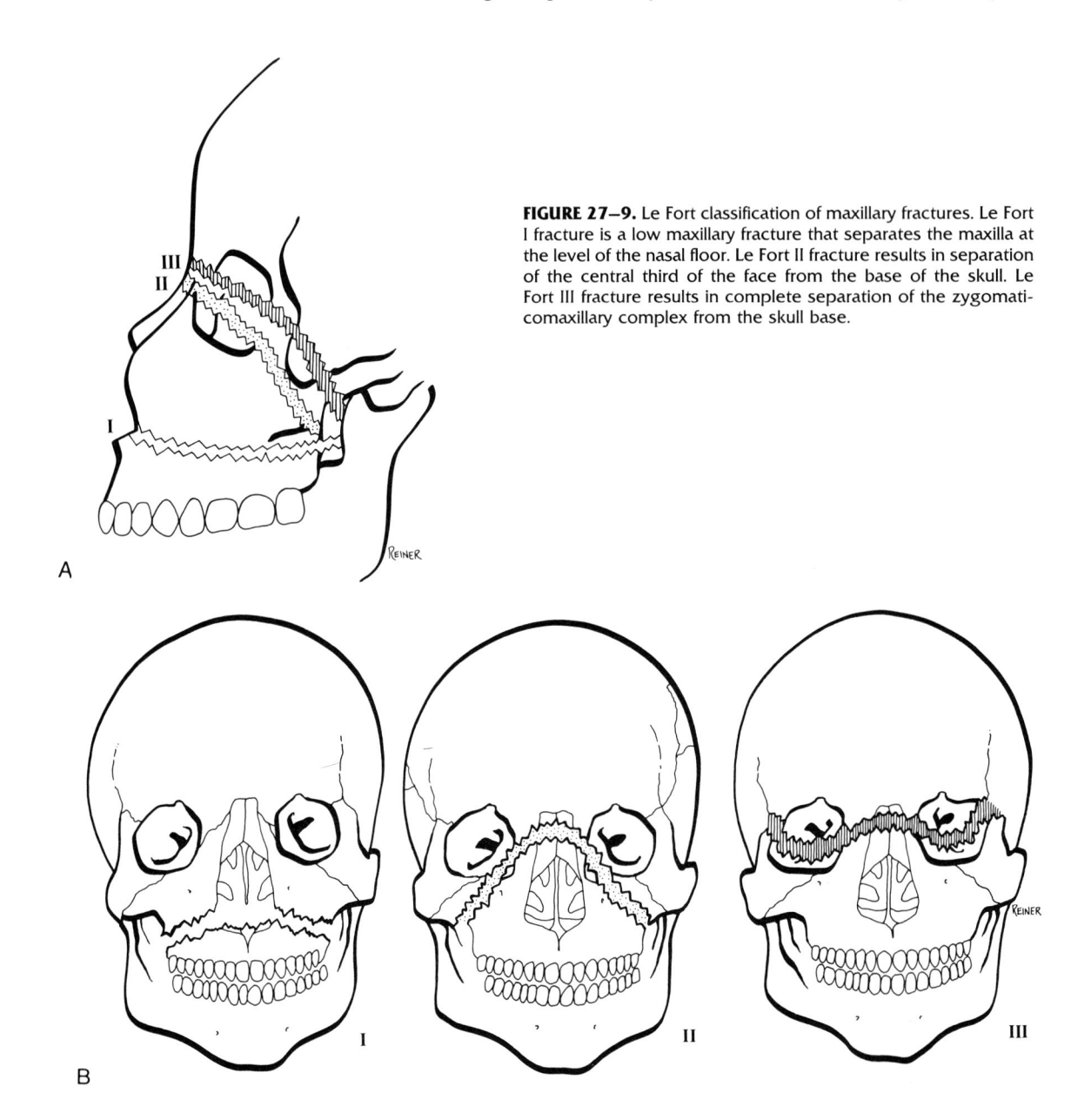

FIGURE 27–9. Le Fort classification of maxillary fractures. Le Fort I fracture is a low maxillary fracture that separates the maxilla at the level of the nasal floor. Le Fort II fracture results in separation of the central third of the face from the base of the skull. Le Fort III fracture results in complete separation of the zygomaticomaxillary complex from the skull base.

displacement of the maxillary dental arch and palate; dental malocclusion is usually present. The Le Fort II fracture, or pyramidal fracture, involves fracture en bloc of the palate and middle third of the face, including the nose. It is characterized by mobility of the palate and nose en bloc as well as significant epistaxis. Usually dental malocclusion with some retrodisplacement of the palate is present. The Le Fort III fracture is the most severe injury and involves complete disruption of the attachments of the facial skeleton to the cranium. The entire zygomaticomaxillary complex may be mobile and displaced. Open reduction techniques with direct wiring in association with intermaxillary fixation are usually required in the therapy of these injuries. The basic principle in such treatment involves firmly fixing the fractured fragments to the intact portions of the facial skeleton by employing direct wiring techniques or using internal suspension wires as illustrated in Figure 27–10A and B. Small bone plates are available to immobilize the fractured segments, replacing wire ligatures. As noted in the discussion of mandibular fractures, the use of plate stabilization may eliminate the need for fixation of the upper and lower dental arches in the postoperative period. A variety of surgical approaches may be required in treatment of these injuries. Careful incisions allow exposure of the entire facial skeleton, leaving only the most minimal postoperative scarring. When open reduction and internal fixation techniques with wire have not resulted in satisfactory reduction or fixation, external fixation devices to produce anterior or lateral traction may be required (Fig. 27–11). The previously noted "halo" frame may also be employed (Fig. 27–12).

Because most maxillary fractures are compound, involving either the oral or nasal cavity, antibiotic coverage is appropriate. Penicillin is the drug of choice in nonallergic patients.

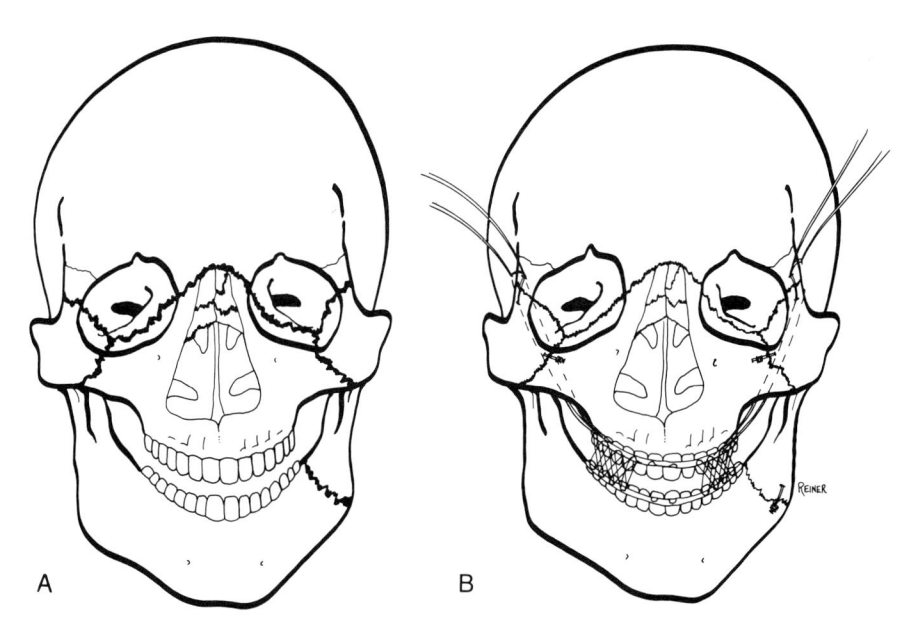

FIGURE 27–10. *A*, A severe maxillary fracture—Le Fort III, associated with a left mandibular angle fracture. *B*, Repair employing intermaxillary fixation, open reduction, and interosseous fixation with wire of the mandible and zygomaticomaxillary fractures and suspension-fixation of the maxilla from the frontal processes.

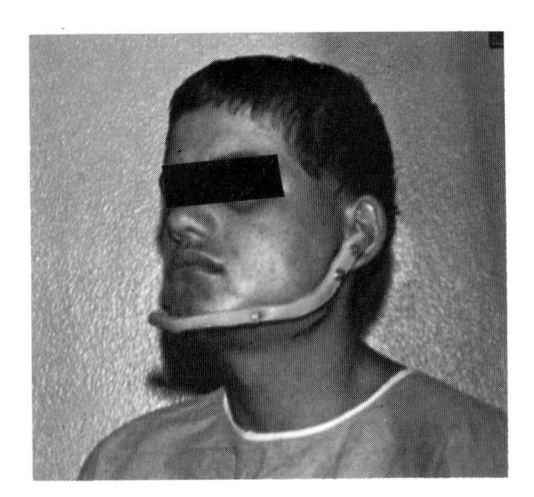

FIGURE 27–11. An acrylic splint affixed to bone screws provides three-dimensional reduction and fixation. (From Wilson KS, Christiansen TC, Quick C: External fixation in maxillofacial surgery. Otol Clin North Am 9(2):530, 1976.)

Frontal Sinus Fracture

Frontal sinus fractures, while relatively infrequent, may be extremely serious because of their cosmetic deformity and central nervous system involvement. These injuries are characterized by (1) depression of the anterior table of the frontal sinus, (2) epistaxis, and (3) occasional disruption of the posterior table of the frontal sinus with dural rupture and cerebrospinal fluid rhinorrhea. Fractures that involve only the anterior table of the frontal sinus can usually be satisfactorily treated by open reduction and internal fixation techniques. Fractures that involve the posterior table with dural rupture and cerebrospinal fluid fistula are treated neurosurgically and may require an approach either through the sinus or through the anterior cranial fossa to close the dural dehiscence.

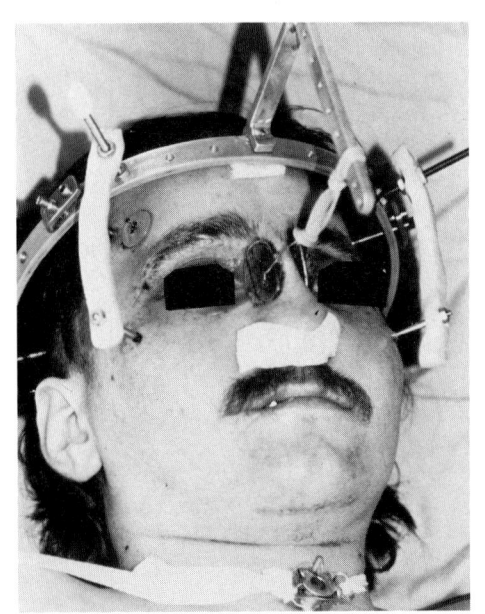

FIGURE 27–12. This figure illustrates the use of an external "halo" to stabilize a severe midfacial fracture.

Late Deformity

Late deformity of the face which results from untreated, inadequately treated, or severe trauma usually may be improved surgically. Nearly all unsightly scars may be improved by revision surgery employing camouflaging techniques in combination with instruction in the judicious use of cosmetics. Many late bone deformities may be improved by remobilization with reduction and fixation in a more natural anatomic position. This is especially applicable in the case of internal or external nasal deformity in which the airway involvement or cosmetic results are not sufficiently apparent to cause the patient to seek assistance until well after the traumatic episode. Bone deformity that does not yield to mobilization often can be camouflaged by implantation of autograft and/or homograft bone, or cartilage, or occasionally synthetic material.

References

Dingman O, Natvig P: Surgery of Facial Fractures. Philadelphia, WB Saunders Co, 1964.
Foster A, Sherman JE: Surgery of Facial Bone Fractures. New York, Churchill Livingstone, 1987.
Mathog RH: Maxillofacial Trauma. Baltimore, Williams & Wilkins, 1984.
Rowe NL, Killey HC: Fractures of the Facial Skeleton. 2nd ed. Edinburgh, E & S Livingstone, 1968.
Sisson GA, Tardy J: Plastic and Reconstructive Surgery of the Face and Neck: Proceedings of the Second International Symposium. Vol 2: Rehabilitative Surgery. New York, Grune & Stratton, 1977.
Zaydon J, Brown JB: Early Treatment of Facial Injuries. Philadelphia, Lea & Febiger, 1964.

INDEX

Note: Page numbers in *italics* refer to illustrations; page numbers followed by (t) refer to tables.

Abscess(es), alveolar, acute, 297
  dural, and sinusitis, *266*, 267
  formation of, extradural, 118
    subdural, 118
  of brain, *266*, 267
    and mastoiditis, 119
    and otitis media, 119
  of frontal lobe, *266*, 267
  of head and neck, 280
  of masticator, 360
  of nasal septum, 215, *216*
  of parapharyngeal space, *358*
  of retropharyngeal space, 360–362, *361*
    complications of, 362
    diagnosis of, 361
    etiology of, 360–361
    symptoms of, 361
    treatment of, *361*, 361–362
  orbital, 264, *264*
  peritonsillar, 345–347, 346(t), *347*
    and acute sore throat, 340(t)
    bacteriology of, 346, 346(t)
    etiology of, 345–346
    pathology of, 346
    symptoms of, 346
    treatment of, 346–347, *347*, 347(t), *348*
      immediate tonsillectomy in, 347, 347(t)
  subperiosteal, 264, *264*
  of frontal bone, 267–268
Accessory nerve, evaluation of, 21
Achalasia, esophageal, 471, *472*
Acne, scars from, dermabrasion for, 519, *520*
Acoustic immittance, 58–59, 59(t)
Acoustic neuroma, 133–134, 153
  ABR testing in, 63, *63*
  and facial nerve paralysis, 152
  computed tomographic assessment of, 108
  magnetic resonance imaging of, 133, *133*
  radiologic assessment of, 105
Acoustic reflex, and associated conditions, 60(t)
  measurement of, 59–60, 60(t)
Acousticofacial ganglion, development of, 29
Acquired immunodeficiency syndrome (AIDS), 376–377
  and cervical lymph node involvement, 437
Acrocephalosyndactyly, 290
  and micrognathia, 283
Addison's disease, and chronic nonspecific laryngitis, 401
Adenocarcinoma, 121
  classification of, 446
  etiology of, 445
  metastatic, 330–331, 438
  of parotid gland, in children, 328–329

Adenocarcinoma *(Continued)*
  pathology of, 446
  undifferentiated, of salivary gland, in adults, 329, 329(t)
Adenoid, anatomy of, 334
  hypertrophy of, 337–339, *338*
    and obstructive sleep apnea, 364
  mass of, *17*, *333*
Adenoidectomy, and nasality, 416
  for obstructive sleep apnea, 366, 368(t)
  for serous otitis media, 102
  for speech problems, 339
  indications for, 339
  instruments for, *356*
  with LaForce adenotome, *355*
  with tonsillectomy, benefits of, 350–351
Adenoiditis, and eustachian tube obstruction, 93
Adenoma, oxyphil, of salivary glands, 328
  pleomorphic, of parotid gland, in adults, 327
    in children, 325
    of salivary glands, in adults, 329
  serous cell, of salivary glands, 328
Adenopathy, cervical, examination of, *22*
Adenotonsillectomy, benefits of, 350–351
Air-bone gap, 53, 54, 55, *56*
Airway obstruction, and dysphagia, 492
  and foreign body aspiration, 483
  and foreign body ingestion, 475
  and obstructive sleep apnea, 363
  complications of, 362(t)
  emergency treatment of, 484
  in children, *482*
  in tracheostomy, 501–502
  patient history in, 11
  symptoms of, and tracheostomy, 492
Alaryngeal speech, 421–424. See also *Speech, after laryngectomy*.
Albers-Schönberg disease, *127*
Albinism, and congenital deafness, 127
Alcohol use, and laryngeal carcinoma, 445
Allergen(s), elimination of, in nasal allergy treatment, 221
  identification of, immune mechanism in, 200–202, 201(t)
    in nasal allergy, 221
    in vitro methods in, 200–202, 201(t)
    in vivo methods in, 200, 201(t)
    patient history in, 199
Allergy, cellular response in, 197
  definition of, 196
  evaluation of, in children, 12
  food, and nasal allergy, 219
  food tests for, 221
  nasal, 196–205. See also *Nasal allergy*.
Alport's disease, and congenital deafness, 129

541

Alstrom's disease, and congenital deafness, 130
Ameloblastoma, 311, *311*
American Sign Language (Ameslan), 75
Amplification, and hearing aid features, 70, *70, 71*
    binaural, advantages of, 71
Androgen therapy, laryngeal complications of, 401
    vocal changes from, in women, 401
Anesthesia, for facial plastic surgery, 507
    in examination, 22–23
Angiofibroma, juvenile, of nasopharynx, 245
    of nasopharynx, 336–337, *337*
        computed tomographic scan of, 336, *337*
Ankyloglossia, 286, *286*
Anosmia, 187
    patient history in, 12
Antibody, role of, in allergic reactions, 196–197, 197(t)
Antigen, role of, in allergic reactions, 196–197, 197(t)
Antihistamine(s), classification of, 224, 224(t)
Antihypertensive drugs, and rhinitis, 226
Antrum, anatomy of, *36*
    radiologic assessment of, *108*
Apert syndrome, 290
Aphasia, 424–425
Aphonia, psychogenic, 410
Apnea, and adenoid hypertrophy, 338
    obstructive, and sleep apnea, 364. See also *Obstructive sleep apnea.*
Applicator, selection of, 7
    use of, *9*
Apraxia, in children, 418–419
Arrhythmia(s), and obstructive sleep apnea, 362
Arteritis, temporal, and headache, 167
        diagnosis of, 167
        features of, 162(t)
Arthritis, of cricarytenoid joint, 400
Articulation, development of, in children, 418(t)
    disorders of, 418–419
Arytenoid cartilage, anatomy of, *384,* 385
Arytenoid muscle, anatomy of, 386, 388, *388*
Aspergillosis, 216
Aspergillus infection, in cancer patients, 378, *379*
    of nasal septum, in bone marrow recipient, 374
    of trachea, *374*
Asphyxia, from retropharyngeal space abscess, 362
Aspiration, in tracheostomy, 501
    laryngeal, idiopathic, 409
    of foreign body, 483–485
Aspirin sensitivity, and asthma and nasal polyps, 202, 225
Asthma, and allergic rhinitis, 218
    and aspirin sensitivity and nasal polyps, 202, 225
    and atopic eczema, 218
Atelectasis, and foreign body aspiration, 484
Atresia, choanal, congenital, 335
Audiogram, air conduction, principles of, 50
        notation for, *52*
    and aging, 65
    bone conduction, principles of, 51
        notation for, *52*
    for acute otitis media, *65*
    for serous otitis media, *64*
    in children, and speech and language disorders, *415*
    noise exposure and, *66*
Audiology, 46–76
    purposes of, 46. See also *Audiometry; Hearing test(s).*
Audiometer, pure tone, 50. See also *Pure tone audiometry.*
Audiometry, acoustic immitance in, 58–59
    brain stem evoked response. See *Auditory brain stem evoked response tests (ABR).*

Audiometry *(Continued)*
    impedance, 36, 57–58
    in facial nerve paralysis, 147
    pediatric, conditioning in, 67
    play, in children, 67
    pure tone, 50–57, *52, 55, 56* See also *Pure tone audiometry.*
    speech, 60–61. See also *Speech audiometry.*
    masking in, 54–55
Auditory brain stem evoked response tests (ABR), 61–64, *62, 63*
    clinical use of, 62–64
    for acoustic neuromas, 63, *63*
    in brain stem disorders, 63–64
    in difficult patients, 63
    in facial nerve paralysis, 147
    in Meniere's disease, 63
    in pediatrics, 63, 67
    Jewett classifications in, 62, *62*
    technique of, 62, *62*
    threshold evaluation in, 63
Auditory canal, external. See *External auditory canal.*
    internal, radiologic assessment of, 102, *104, 108*
    tumors of, 153
Auditory meatus, external, 5
Auditory training, 73
Aural rehabilitation, 73–75
    of adults, 73
    of children, 74–75
Aural speculum, use of, 6–7, *7*
Auricle, anatomy of, 5. See also *External ear.*
    gouty tophi in, 89
    infections of, 83, *83*
    laceration of, 86
    malformations of, 87
Autophony, and abnormally patent eustachian tube, 93
Axonotmesis, *145,* 146

Balance, components of, 137
Barium swallow, for dysphagia, 425–426
Barosinusitis, 268
Barotrauma, and eustachian tube function, 94
    and inner ear damage, 95
    and perilymph fistula, 140
    of middle ear, 94–95
        prevention of, 95
        symptoms of, 95
Behavioral disorder(s), in children, and speech and language disorders, 417
Bell's palsy, 152–153
    pathologic changes in, *155*
    treatment of, 154, *155,* 156
Benign lymphoepithelial disease, of salivary glands, 322
Benign paroxysmal positional vertigo, diagnosis of, 44
Benign positional vertigo, 137–138
Bing test, 49
Biopsy, directed, for metastatic disease, 438
    in head and neck examination, 23
    of cervical lymph node, 447
    of mediastinum, *487,* 487–488, *488*
Black hairy tongue, *302,* 302–303
Blast injury(ies), and middle ear damage, 98
    and sensorineural hearing loss, 135
Bleeding, in nose, patient history in, 11. See also *Epistaxis.*
Bleeding disorder(s), and epistaxis, 241
    and tonsillectomy, 353
Blepharoplasty, 520–521, *521*

Blom-Singer prosthesis, 423, *423*
Blood disorders, pharyngeal manifestations of, 345
Blow out fracture, 535, *535*
Bone marrow transplantation, 370–375, *374*
　and esophagitis, 374–375
　and immunosuppression, 370–371
　and laryngitis, 373–374, *374*
　and otitis media, 371–372
　and otomycosis, 372
　and rhinitis, 373, *374*
　and sinusitis, 372–373
　infection in, delayed, 375–376
　　early, 371
Boyle's law, 94
Brain stem, disorders of, ABR testing in, 63–64
　and aspiration, 409
　tumors of, and acoustic reflex, 59
　　and vocal cord paralysis, 406
Branchial arch apparatus, cyst of, *434*
　embryology of, 278(t), 278–279, 383, *433*
Branchial cleft, abnormalities of, *87*, 87–88
　cysts of, *433*, 433–434, *434*
　formation of, 278(t), 278–279
Branhamella catarrhalis, and tonsillitis treatment, 343
Breathiness, from adductor hypofunction, 420
Breslow's classification, of melanoma, 449(t)
Bronchoscope(s), flexible fiberoptic, 486, *486*
　rigid, 486, *486*
　selection of, 480(t)
Bronchoscopy, of tracheobronchial tree, 481, *482*, 486, 486–487
Bronchus, carcinoma of, 487
　foreign body in, 484
　obstruction of, in children, *482*
Bruxism, and temporomandibular joint dysfunction, 171
Bullous myringitis, and hearing loss, 132
Burn(s), caustic, of esophagus, 473–474
　agents in, 473(t)
　treatment of, 474
Bursitis, nasopharyngeal, 335, *336*

Cafe coronary, 410
Calculi, of salivary glands, 321
　oral, detection of, 16, *16*
Caldwell-Luc procedure, for chronic maxillary sinusitis, 258, *258*
　for sinusitis treatment, 377
Caloric stimulation, 42
　vs. rotation tests, 44
Cancer. See *Carcinoma*; *Tumor(s)*.
Candida albicans, in tracheostomy, 501
Candidiasis, of esophagus, in bone marrow recipient, 374–375
　of larynx, 373–374, 401
　of nose, 216
　of oral cavity, *309*, 309–310
　　after bone marrow transplantation, 376
　　in AIDS, 376
Carcinoma, acinic cell, metastatic, 330–331
　　of parotid gland, 329
　　of salivary gland, in adults, 329(t), 329–330
　adenocystic, 121
　　metastatic, 330–331
　　of parotid gland, 329
　　of salivary glands, in adults, 329, 329(t)
　　of sinuses, 458, *459*
　　of submandibular gland, 331
　and associated infections, 377–378

Carcinoma *(Continued)*
　and thyroid disease, 440–442
　asymptomatic, sites of, 15
　basal cell, of external ear, 89
　　of head, 448
　basal cell syndrome, 294
　bronchogenic, and mediastinoscopy, 487
　metastatic, cervical, ressection for, 463
　mucoepidermoid, metastatic, 330–331
　　of parotid gland, in children, 328, 329(t)
　　of salivary gland, in adults, 329, 329(t)
　of face, *512*, 512–513, *513*
　of larynx, classification of, 461(t)
　　treatment of, 461–462
　　　radiation in, 454, *454*
　of nasopharynx, and Epstein-Barr virus, 337
　　etiology of, 445
　　treatment of, 457–458
　　　radiation in, 454, *455*
　of neck, early detection of, 444
　　radical dissection for, 463
　of sinuses, etiologic agents of, 445, 445(t)
　　radiation therapy for, 454–456, *455*
　of thyroid, from radiation therapy, 456
　of tonsil, 460
　squamous cell, 152, 453
　　chemotherapy for, 464(t), 465(t)
　　etiology of, 445
　　metastatic, 330–331, 438
　　of external ear, 88–89
　　of head, 448
　　of larynx, treatment of, 461–462
　　of middle ear, 121
　　of nose, 457
　　of salivary gland, in adults, 329, 329(t)
　　of sinuses, 458, *459*
　　pathology of, 445–446
　　treatment of, 464(t), 465(t)
Cardiac arrest, in tracheostomy, 501
Cardiospasm, 471, *472*
Carhart notch, and otosclerosis, 57, *66*
Caries, dental, 296–297
Carotid artery, external, ligation of, for epistaxis control, 239
Carotid body tumor, 438, *439*
Carotidynia, 173
Cat scratch fever, and cervical lymph node involvement, 437
Cauliflower ear, 31, 87
Cautery, for epistaxis control, *233*, 233–234
　of nasal turbinate, *223*
Cavernous sinus thrombosis, 264, *264*, 265
Cellulitis, cervical, 375
　peritonsillar, 345–347, 346(t), *347*
　　etiology of, 345–346
　　pathology of, 346
　　symptoms of, 346
　　treatment of, 346–347, *347*, 347(t), *348*
Cementoma, 313
Central nervous system, disorders of, evaluation of, 42, 44
Cerebellopontine angle, tumors of, 152, *133*
　ABR testing in, 63
Cerebral hemisphere, right, deficits of, 425
Cerebral palsy, in children, and speech and language disorders, 417
Cerumen, accumulation of, 78–79
　removal of, 7, *7*, *9*, *10*, 79
Cervical spine, injury of, and laryngeal fracture, 397
　in maxillofacial trauma, 528

Chausse III projection, in middle ear evaluation, 104
Cheek, lacerations of, evaluation of, 528–529
Chemical peel, for rhytide obliteration, 522–523
Chemicals, ingestion of, 473–474
Chemodectoma, 438, *439*
Chemotherapy, agents for, 465, 465(t)
  and associated infection, 378, *379*
  for head and neck tumors, 464(t), 465, 465(t)
  for squamous cell carcinoma, 464(t), 465(t)
  immune system effects of, 377–378
Childbirth, trauma in, and facial nerve paralysis, 151
Chin, deformities of, plastic surgery for, 524–525
Choanal atresia, in neonates, 209
Cholesteatoma, computed tomographic assessment of, 109
  in chronic middle ear infection, 111, 112, *112*
  of external auditory canal, 80
  of mastoid, 107
Cholesterol granuloma, 112, *112*
Chondritis, in helix, 89
Chondroma, of larynx, 403
Chorda tympani nerve, anatomy of, 32
Chromosome(s), abnormalities of, and congenital deafness, 128
Cilia, respiratory, anatomy of, 183, *183*
  compromise of, 192
  function of, 191–193
  histology of, 182–183
Clark's classification, of melanoma, 449(t)
Cleft(s), laryngotracheoesophageal, 395
  of face, 289–290
  of lips, 286–291, *287*
    and associated developmental anomalies, 289–290
    formation of, 286, *287*
    treatment of, 288–289
      and speech development, 288
  of palate, 286–291, *287*
    and associated developmental anomalies, 289–290
    and eustachian tube dysfunction, 93–94
    formation of, 286, *287*
    in children, and speech and language disorders, 416
    incidence of, 287–288
    treatment of, 288–289
      and speech development, 288
Cleft lip. See *Cleft(s), of lips*.
Cleft palate. See *Cleft(s), of palate*.
Cochlea, blood supply to, 34
  computed tomographic assessment of, 109
  evaluation of, 47
    ABR testing in, 63
  function of, 37–38
  hair cells of, innervation of, 37–38, *38*
  osseous, anatomy of, *34*, 34–35, *35*
Cochlear duct, anatomy of, 35
Cochlear implants, 72–73
Cochlear microphonic, role in sound transmission, 36–37
Cochlear nerve, 38, *38*
Cochleovestibular nerve, evaluation of, 21
Collagen, synthesis of, in wound healing, 505–506
Collagen injection, in facial plastic surgery, 523
Common cold, 212–215
  clinical features of, 212–213
  treatment of, 213–214
Communication. See *Speech*; *Language*.
Communitrach tube, 496–497
Compliance, in tympanometry, 57–58, *58*
Computed tomography, of inner ear, 108–109, *109*
  of mastoid, 108–109, *109*
  of middle ear, 108–109, *109*
Conditioning, instrumental, in pediatric audiometry, 67

Conduction, air, audiogram notation for, 51, *52*
  interaural attenuation in, and masking, 54
  principles of, in audiometry, 50–51
  test models for, 47
  thresholds in, in audiogram interpretation, 55–57, *56*
    validity of 53, 54
  versus bone conduction, 47
  bone, audiogram notation for, 51, *52*
  interaural attenuation in, 53–54
  principles of, in audiometry, 50–51
  test models for, 47
  thresholds in, validity of, 53, 54
  versus air conduction, 47
  vibrator placement in, in pure tone audiometry, 51, 53
Congenital anomalies, of lips, 286–291, *287*
  of palate, 286–291, *287*
Congenital epulis, 314
Continuous positive airway pressure (CPAP), for obstructive sleep apnea, 366, 368
Contraction, in wound healing, 506
Corniculate cartilage, anatomy of, 385
Cough, in laryngeal disease, 392
  patient history in, 19
Cranial nerve(s), and herpes zoster, 305–306
  eighth, acoustic reflex of, 59
  evaluation of, 21
  seventh, dysfunction of, 85. See also *Facial nerve, paralysis of*.
Craniofacial dysostosis, 290–291
  and micrognathia, 283
Cretinism, and congenital deafness, 129
Cricoid cartilage, anatomy of, *384*, 384–385
  split of, for subglottic stenosis, 497–498
Cricothyroid membrane, anatomy of, 389
Cricothyroid muscle, anatomy of, 386, *386*
Cricothyrotomy, emergency, in children, 494–496
  for foreign body aspiration, 410–411, 484
Cross hearing, in pure tone audiometry, 53
Croup, clinical features of, 398, 399(t)
  in laryngeal disease, 392
  treatment of, 398–399
Crouzon syndrome, 290–291
  and congenital deafness, 131
Cyst(s), congenital, of branchial cleft, *433*, 433–434, *434*
  of larynx, 394, 395
  dentigerous, 292, *292*
  dermoid, of nose, 210, *211*
    of oral cavity, 295–296
  epidermoid, 295–296
  eruption, 292
  fissural, 294–296, *295*
  gingival, in newborns, 292–293
  incisive, 294, *295*
  nasoalveolar, 295
  nasopalatine, 294, *295*
  nonodontogenic, 294–296, *295*
  odontogenic, *292*, 292–294, *293*
  of branchial cleft, 22
  of hyoid bone, 434, *435*
  of jaw, 291(t), 291–296, *292*, *293*, *295*
  of nose, 210, *211*
  of oral cavity, 291(t), 291–296, *292*, *293*, *295*
  of thyroglossal duct, 22
  palatal, of newborns, 292–293
  radicular, of oral cavity, *293*, 293–294
  retention type, 296
  sebaceous, of external ear, 89

Cystic fibrosis, and sinusitis, 269
  versus sinusitis, 204
Cytology, in head and neck examination, 23
Cytomegalovirus, and infectious mononucleosis, 345

Deafness. See also *Hearing impairment; Hearing loss.*
  congenital, *125*, 125–131, 126(t), 127(t)
    delayed, genetic, 129–131, *130*
      and associated abnormalities, 129–131, *130*
    genetic, 126–128
      and associated abnormalities, 127–128
      chromosomal abnormalities in, 128
    nongenetic, 128–129
  sensorineural, and otitis media, 113, *116*
    cochlear implants for, 72
    familial progressive, 129
  unilateral, evaluation of, 68
Debridement, of facial wounds, 508–509
Decongestant(s), complications from, 226, *227*
Deglutition, 280, 390
  muscles of, 384
Dental caries, 296–297
Dental disorders, 296–301
Dental evaluation, in radiation therapy, 456
Dental replantation, in tooth trauma, 316
Dental splinting, for mandibular fractures, 532–533, *533*
Dermabrasion, for acne scars, 519, *520*
  for rhytide obliteration, *520*, 522–523
Dermatitis, eczematous, of external ear, 84
Dermatomes, *515*, 515–516
Dermoplasty, septal, and epistaxis control, 241
  and Osler-Weber-Rendu syndrome treatment, 231, *231*
Diabetes, and gingivitis, 298
  and necrotizing external otitis, 85
Diffuse otitis externa, 81–82
  treatment of, 81(t), 82
Dilantin, and gingival enlargement, 299, *300*
Diphtheria, and acute sore throat, 340(t)
  in laryngitis, 400
  treatment of, 344–345
Diplacusis, evaluation of, 68
Diplopia, from zygoma fracture, 534
Discharge, from ear, in chronic otitis media, 110
  patient history in, 5
  from nose, 11
  in throat, 13–14
Diverticuli, and dysphagia, 472
Dizziness, 4–5. See also *Vertigo.*
  differential diagnosis of, 124(t)
  origin of, vestibular versus central, 124
  patient history in, 124
Doerfler Stewart test, 69
Down's syndrome, and micrognathia, 283
  and premature periodontal destruction, 301
  and scrotal tongue, 302
Drooling, treatment of, 322
Drug(s), ototoxic, 132(t), 132–133
Drumhead, anatomy of, *32*, 36
  examination of, 7. See also *Tympanic membrane.*
Dysarthria, 425
  in children, 418–419
Dysfluency, in children, 416–417
Dysphagia, 471, 472
  and airway obstruction, 492
  and croup, 398
  and foreign body ingestion, 475
  and speech and language disorders, 425–426
  patient history in, 13, 13–14, 18

Dysphonia, plicae ventricularis, 410
  spastic, 409
    treatment of, 420
Dyspnea, in laryngeal disease, 392

Ear, anatomy of, 30–36
  deformities of, plastic surgery for, 524
  embryology of, 27–30
  examination of, 4–10
    patient history in, 4–5
  external. See *External ear.*
  function of, 36–38
  inner. See *Inner ear.*
  middle. See *Middle ear.*
Ear wax. See *Cerumen.*
Earache, patient history in, 5
Eardrum. See *Tympanic membrane.*
Electromyography, for facial nerve evaluation, 149
Electroneuronography, 149
  for facial nerve evaluation, 153, *154*
Electronystagmography, for vestibular function evaluation, 42, *43*, 125
Ellis-van Creveld syndrome, 300
Emotional disorder(s), in children, and speech and language disorders, 417
Emphysema, mediastinal, after tracheostomy, 499
  obstructive, in children, 482
Encephalocele, of nose, 210–211, *211*
Endolymphatic hydrops, audiometric findings in, *66*
Endoscopy, for head and neck tumors, 450
  for laryngeal tumor, 404
  in chronic sinusitis treatment, 259, *259*
  in nasopharyngeal examination, 17
  of nose, *207*, 209
Endotracheal intubation, 491. See also *Tracheostomy.*
Enophthalmos, from orbital floor fracture, 534, *535*
Eosinophilia, interpretation of, 198, 198(t)
Epiglottis, anatomy of, 385, 388, *388*
  function of, 390
Epiglottitis, in children, 398
Epistaxis, 231–241, *232, 233, 235–237, 239, 240*
  and frontal sinus fracture, 538
  and juvenile nasopharyngeal angiofibroma, 336
  and leukemia, 241
  and maxillary fracture, 536
  and nasal trauma, 240–241
  anterior, treatment of, 234–235, *235–237*
  evaluation of, 232
  posterior, treatment of, 236–240, *237, 239, 240*
    complications of, 238
    hospitalization in, 238
    nasal packing in, 236–238, *237*
    sphenopalatine ganglion block in, 236
  recurrent, and Osler-Weber-Rendu syndrome, 231, 241
    cautery for, *233*, 233–234
  treatment of, cautery in, *233*, 233–234
    patient history in, 233
    principles of, 231–232
    vessel ligation in, 238–240, *239, 240*
Epithelialization, in wound healing, 506, *506*
Epstein-Barr virus, and infectious mononucleosis, 345
  and nasopharyngeal carcinoma, 337, 445
Erythema dose, definition of, 452
Erythema multiforme, of oral cavity, *307*, 307–308
Erythroblastosis fetalis, and congenital deafness, 128–129
Erythroplakia, of larynx, 403–404
Esophagitis, 472
  corrosive, *472*, 473(t), 473–474
    treatment of, 474

Esophagitis *(Continued)*
   esophagoscopy for, 375
   in bone marrow recipient, 374–375
Esophagogastrectomy, for caustic ingestion, 473
Esophagoscope(s), selection of, 478–479, *480*, 480(t), *481*
Esophagoscopy, 478–479, *480*, 480(t), *481*
   anatomic landmarks for, *481*
   for achalasia, 471, *472*
   for caustic burns, 473
   for foreign body removal, 479, 480(t)
   in esophagitis diagnosis, 375
   indications for, 478
Esophagus, anatomy of, 277
   and otalgia, 169(t)
   burns of, 473–474
      agents in, 473(t)
      treatment of, 474
   discharge from, 13–14
   disorders of, 471–477, *472*, 473(t), *476*, *477*
      congenital, 473
      evaluation of, 477–481, *479*, *480*, 480(t), *481*
         diagnostic studies in, 478, *479*
         esophagoscopy in, 478–479, *480*, 480(t), *481*
         patient history in, 477–478
      inflammatory, 472
   embryology of, 273–274
   foreign body in, 474–477, *476*
      in children, *476*
      location of, 475, *476*
      patient history in, 474
      treatment for, 475–476, *477*
   herpesvirus infection of, 375
   intraluminal pressures of, 478, *479*
   spasm of, 471–472
Esthesioneuroblastoma, of nose, 457
Estrogen therapy, and nasal congestion, 227
Ethmoid artery, anterior, ligation of, for epistaxis control, 240, *240*
Ethmoidectomy, for chronic ethmoid sinusitis, 259, *260*
   for acute ethmoid sinusitis, 254
Eustachian tube, patent, 93
   anatomy of, 32, *33*, 34, *34*
   assessment of, 92
   disorders of, 92–95
      and serous otitis media, 100
   embryology of, 92
   obstruction of, 93
      and acute otitis media, 98–99
      and adenoid hypertrophy, 338
   ventilation dysfunction of, and tympanic membrane, 90
Exostosis, of external ear, 88
External auditory canal, anatomy of, 31, *77*, 77–78
   and cholesteatoma, 80
   and furuncle, *81*, *481*
   and keratosis obturans, 79
   cleansing of, 9, *9*, *19*
   foreign body in, 96, 98
   function of, 36, 77–78
   infection of, chronic, 84, *85*
      fungal, and bone marrow transplantation, 372
   radiologic assessment of, *104*
   tumors of, 88–89
External auditory meatus, embryology of, *28*
External ear, anatomy of, *5*, 30–31
   basal cell carcinoma of, 89
   dermatitis of, 84
   diseases of, 79–89. See also names of specific disorders.
   examination of, 5–9, 78
   frostbite of, 86

External ear *(Continued)*
   hematoma of, 87
   infections of, *87*
      acute, 80–84, *81*, 81(t), *83*
      chronic, 84–86, *85*
      fungal, 82–83
   inflammation of, 80–84, *81*, 81(t), *83*
      chronic, 84–86, *85*
   injuries to, 30–31
   keloid of, *88*
   lacerations of, 83, 86
   malformations of, *87*, 87–88
   neoplasms of, *88*, 88–89
   pain in, 169(t)
   trauma to, 83, 86–87
External nose, anatomy of, 177–178, *178*, 242, *242*
External otitis, 80–86, *81*
   and dermatitis, versus infection, 80, 84
   causes of, 80
   drug therapy for, 81(t)
   management of, 80
   necrotizing, 85
      antimicrobial treatment of, 85

Face, aging of, plastic surgery for, 519–523, *520–522*
   carcinoma of, *512*, 512–513, *513*
   clefts of, 289–290
   deformity of, 539
   developmental anomalies of, *282*, 282–286, *283*, *285*, *286*
   examination of, 20–22, *22*
   fractures of, 528, *529*, 529. See also *Maxillofacial trauma.*
   and sinusitis, 269–270
Face lift, 520, *521*
   and facial nerve paralysis, *155*, 155–156
Facial bone(s), fibrous dysplasia of, *245*, 245
   fracture of, 528, *529*
   reduction in, 529
Facial cleft, 289–290
Facial nerve, anatomy of, 31, 32–33, *33*, *34*, 142–143, *143*, *144*, 317
   disorders of, 85, 142–156
   evaluation of, 21
      acoustic reflex in, 59
      audiologic tests in, 147
      diagnostic tests in, 147
      nerve function tests in, *149*, 149–150, *150*
      reflex tests in, 147, 148(t)
      taste tests in, 148, 148(t)
      salivation tests in, 148(t), 149
      tear tests in, 147, *148*, 148(t)
   injury to, classification of, *145*, 145
   lesions of, and topognostic testing, 153
      site determination of, *143*, 153
   paralysis of, and acute otitis media, 147
      and Bell's palsy, 152–153
      and childbirth trauma, 151
      and face lift, *155*, 155–156
      and infections, 151
      and neoplasms, 152
      and skull fracture, 152
      and vascular lesions, 152
      causes of, congenital, 151, *151*
         idiopathic, 152–153
      complications of, 153–154
      differential diagnosis of, 150
      electromyography for, 149, *149*

Facial nerve (Continued)
  paralysis of, from otomycosis, 372
    treatment of, 153–156, 155
    prognosis for, 153, 154
  physiology of, 143–144
  repair of, 146–147
    nerve grafting in, 154
Facial plastic surgery, 505–525
  anesthesia in, 507
  complications of, 516, 516–519, 517(t), 518
  general principles of, 505–519, 506–508, 509(t), 510–516, 517(t), 518
  incisions for, 507, 507–508, 508
  wound care in, 507, 507–512, 508, 509(t), 510, 511
  wound healing in, 505–506, 506
Facial wound(s), care of, anesthesia in, 507
  incisions in, 507, 507–508, 508
  cleansing and debridement of, 508–509
  collagen synthesis in, 505–506
  contraction in, 506
  epithelialization in, 506, 506
  healing of, complications of 516, 516–519, 517(t), 518
  principles of, 505–506, 506
  suture techniques for, 509–511, 510, 511
  tetanus prophylaxis for, 509, 509(t)
Fascial space(s), of head and neck, anatomy of, 280–281, 281
Fat injection, in facial plastic surgery, 523
Fibroma, ameloblastic, 312
Fibromatosis, gingival, 299, 299
Fibromyalgia, and headache, 165
Fibrositis, and headache, 165
Fibrous dysplasia, 314, 315
  of facial bones, 245, 245
Fistula, oroantral, and maxillary sinusitis, 253
  tracheoesophageal, in tracheostomy, 502
Fistula test, for chronic middle ear infection, 111, 111
  for labyrinthitis, 117
Fixation, external, for maxillary fracture, 537, 538
  for orbital floor fracture, 535
  internal, for maxillary fracture, 537, 537, 538
Flap(s), distant, 514
  free, 514–515
  local, for facial wounds, 512–513, 512–514. See also Skin flap(s).
  regional, 514
Flouride, and dental caries prevention, 296
Flu, 214–215. See also Rhinitis.
Folliculitis, evaluation of, 13
Foreign body(ies), aspiration of, 483–485
  complications of, 484
  in children, 482
  location of, 484–485
  symptoms of, 483–484
  in esophagus, 474–477, 476, 477
    esophagoscopy for, 479, 480(t)
    in children, 476
    location of, 475, 476
    possible impaction of, 477
    symptoms of, 475
    treatment of, 475–476, 477
  in external auditory canal, 96, 98
  in nose, 246–247
    removal of, 246–247, 247
  of larynx, 410–411
Fracture(s), of facial bones, 528, 529. See also Maxillofacial trauma.
  of frontal sinus, 527–528, 538
  of hyoid bone, 396

Fracture(s) (Continued)
  of mandible, 532–534, 533
  of maxilla, 536–537, 536–538
    computed tomographic assessment of, 528, 529
  of nose, 241–243, 242, 528, 530–532, 531, 532
  of orbital floor, 534, 534–535, 535
  of skull, and facial nerve paralysis, 152
  of teeth, 316
  of temporal bone, 134, 134
  of zygoma, 534, 534–535, 535
Frontal bone, osteomyelitis of, and sinusitis, 267–268
  subperiosteal abscess of, and sinusitis, 267–268
Frontal lobe, abscess of, 266, 267
Frontoethmoidectomy, for chronic frontal sinusitis, 261, 261–262
Frontonasal duct, repair of, in chronic frontal sinusitis, 261, 261–262, 262
Frostbite, of auricle, 86
Fungal infections. See Infection(s), fungal.
Furuncle, of external auditory canal, 81
  of nose, 215, 215
  sequelae of, 83
Furunculosis, 80, 81, 215, 215
  drug therapy for, 81(t)

Gag reflex, management of, 22–23
Gargles, in tonsillitis treatment, 342–343
Genioplasty, for obstructive sleep apnea treatment, 366
Geographic tongue, 301, 301
Gingiva, enlargement of, and Dilantin use, 299, 300
Gingivitis, 297–299, 298
  and diabetes mellitus, 298
  and pregnancy, 298
  ulcerative, necrotizing, 298, 298–299
Glioma, of nose, 210–211, 211
Glomus jugulare tumor, 120, 152
Glomus tympanicum tumor, 120
Glossitis, rhomboid, median, 285, 285
Glossopharyngeal nerve, evaluation of, 21
Goiter, and thyroid disease, 440–442
Gouty tophi, of auricle, 89
Gradenigo's syndrome, 117–118
Graft-versus-host disease, and fungal sinusitis, 373
  in bone marrow transplantation, 370, 371, 376
Granuloma, dental, 297
  of larynx, from intubation, 397
Graves' disease, and thyroid disease, 440–442
Gray (Gy), definition of, 453
Gumma, of larynx, 401
Gunshot wound, of larynx, 397

Hair cell(s), cochlear, innervation of, 37–38, 38
  of organ of Corti, anatomy of, 35
  of otolith organs, 41
  vestibular, 39–40, 40
Halitosis, 310
Halo frame, for maxillary fracture, 537, 538
  for orbital floor fracture, 535
Hand-foot-and-mouth disease, after bone marrow transplantation, 375
Hat band headache, 164. See also Headache, muscle-contraction type.
Head, evaluation of, 3
  in maxillofacial trauma, 527–528
  fascial spaces of, 280, 280–281
  tumors of, classification of, 451(t)
    evaluation of, 449–450, 451(t)

Head (Continued)
  tumors of, malignant, early detection of, 444
    etiology of, 445
    frequency of, 444
    incidence of, 445
    pathology of, 445–448, 446(t)
    treatment of, 451–465, *454*, *455*, *459*, 460(t), 461(t), 464(t), 465(t)
      chemotherapy in, 464(t), 465, 465(t)
      principles of, 443
      radiation in, 452–456, *454*, *455*
      surgical, 456–457
  metastatic, 448
Head injury, and speech disorders, 425
Head mirror, 3
Head noises, 4. See also *Tinnitus*.
Head pain, features of, 162, 162(t). See also *Headache; Neuralgia*.
Headache, 157–168
  and fibromyalgia, 165
  and fibrositis, 165
  and head and neck diseases, 160
  classification of, 157–160
    major categories in, 158
  clinical examination of, 161–163
  combined type, 159
  definition of, 158
    versus neuralgia, 162
  differential diagnosis of, 162–163
  laboratory examination of, 162
  migraine, and vertigo, 137
  muscle-contraction type, 159
    and structural abnormalities of neck, 165
    features of, 162(t), *163*, 163–165
    misdiagnosis of, 165
  of nasal vasomotor reaction, 159
    and vasomotor rhinitis, 166. See also *Rhinitis, vasomotor*.
    features of, 162(t), 166–167
    pain mechanisms in, 166
    treatment of, 167
  patient history in, 160–161
  psychogenic, 159
  radiologic examination of, 162
  sinus, overdiagnosis of, 157
  traction type, 159–160
  vascular, cluster type, 159
    differential diagnosis of, 163
    features of, 162(t), 163
    treatment of, 163–164
  lower-half type, 159, 167
  migraine type, 158–159
  nonmigrainous type, 159
Hearing, evaluation of, 46. See also *Audiometry; Hearing test(s)*.
Hearing aids, 69–73, *70*, *71*
  amplification features of, 70, *70*, *71*
  Bi-CROS, 72
  cochlear implants and, 72–73
  CROS, 72
  for children, 72
    with speech and language disorders, 414
  indications for, 69
  multi-CROS, 72
  selection of, 70, *70*–72, *71*
    binaural versus uniaural amplification in, 71
  types of, *70*, *71*, *71*
Hearing conservation, in industry, 69

Hearing impairment, 4. See also *Hearing loss*.
  combined, 46–47
  conductive, 46–47
  evaluation of, in children, 67
  in children, with speech and language disorders, 74–75
  nonorganic, 68–69
    ABR testing in, 69
    acoustic reflex in, 69
    audiometric findings in, 68
    delayed feedback test in, 69
    Doerfler Stewart test in, 69
    Stenger test in, 68
  patient history in, 4
  rehabilitation of. See *Aural rehabilitation*.
  sensorineural, 46–47
  testing models for, 47
  types of, 46–47
Hearing loss. See also *Hearing impairment*.
  acoustic reflex in, 59–60, 60(t)
  and acoustic tumors, *133*, 133–134
  and barotrauma, 95
  and chronic otitis media, 110–111, *111*, 113
  and facial clefts, 288
  and inner ear disease, 117
  and serous otitis media, in children, 100
  audiologic evaluation of, 125
  causes of, aging, 135
    idiopathic, 135
    infectious, 131–132
  cochlear implants and, 72–73
  combined, 55, *56*
  conductive, 55, *56*
    and nasopharyngeal carcinoma, 458
    and Treacher Collins syndrome, 291
    causes of, 96
  congenital, 96, 125, *125*. See also *Deafness, congenital*.
    genetic, 126–128
      in children, 126(t)
  genetic, versus sensorineural, 129
  in children, screening tests for, 415, *415*
    with speech and language disorders, 414–415, *415*
  in elderly persons, 126
  sensorineural, 55, *56*, 92
    and myringitis, 92
    and tympanic membrane perforation, 98
    cochlear implants for, 72
    in children, 127(t)
  sudden, 136
  treatment of, 136–137
  unilateral, 60
    amplification in, 72
    CROS hearing aid and, 72
Hearing test(s), 46–76
  Bing test, 49
  Doerfler Stewart test, 69
  impedance audiometry, 57–59
  pediatric audiometry, *64–66*, 64–68
  pure tone audiometry, 50–57
  Rinne test, 9, *11*
  Schwabach test, 9
  speech audiometry, 60–61
  Stenger test, 68
  tuning fork tests, 9–10, *10*, *11*, 47–50
  Weber test, 9, *11*, 49
Hearing-impaired child, education of, 74–75
Heart failure, and obstructive sleep apnea, 362–363
Heerfordt's syndrome, 321

Heimlich maneuver, for foreign body aspiration, 484
Hemangioma, of larynx, 394–395
 of parotid gland, in children, 325
 subglottic, laser microsurgery for, 405
Hematoma, of external ear, 87
 of nasal septum, *216*, *531*
  and nasal obstruction, 242
Hemilaryngectomy, for laryngeal carcinoma, 462
Hemorrhage, in tracheostomy, 500
 of oral cavity, from trauma, 315
Hereditary hemorrhagic telangiectasia. See *Osler-Weber-Rendu syndrome.*
Herpes simplex, primary, inoculation, *303*, 304
 of oral cavity, *303*, 303–304
 secondary, *303*, 304
Herpes zoster, of oral cavity, 305–306
Herpes zoster oticus, 83, 91
 and facial nerve paralysis, 151
 and otalgia, *168*
Herpesvirus infection, after bone marrow transplantation, 375
 of esophagus, in bone marrow recipient, 375
 of larynx, 373
Hiatus hernia, 472
 and chronic nonspecific laryngitis, 401
Histiocytoma, fibrous, chemotherapy for, 465(t)
 treatment of, 447
Histiocytosis X, 152
 and premature periodontal destruction, 301
Histoplasmosis, of larynx, 400–401
Hoarseness, in laryngeal disease, 392, 444
 in polychondritis, 86
Hodgkin's lymphoma, and cervical lymph node involvement, 437
 and tonsillectomy, 351
 pathology of, 446–447
Horner's syndrome, and vocal cord paralysis, 406
Human immunodeficiency virus (HIV), 376
 in children, 377
Hurler's syndrome, and congenital deafness, 130
Hydrocephalus, 119
Hygroma, cystic, 435–436
 and macroglossia, 284
Hyoid bone, cyst of, 434, *435*
 fracture of, 396
Hyperkeratosis, of larynx, 403
Hypernasality, and speech and language disorders, 420
Hypernephroma, 448
Hyperostosis, cortical, infantile, 315
Hyperpigmentation, and congenital deafness, 127–128
Hypertension, and obstructive sleep apnea, 362, 362(t)
Hyperthyroidism, and thyroid disease, 440–442
Hyperventilation, and vertigo, 137
Hypoglossal nerve, embryology of, 274
 evaluation of, 21
Hypoglycemia, and vertigo, 137
Hyponasality, and speech and language disorders, 420
Hypopharyngectomy, for laryngeal carcinoma, 462
Hypopharynx, anatomy of, *19*, 277, *277*, 334–335
 diseases of, and obstructive sleep apnea, 364
 examination of, 18–20, *20*
 tumors of, malignant, treatment of, 462
Hypopnea, and obstructive sleep apnea, 364
Hypothyroidism, and chronic nonspecific laryngitis, 401
 and laryngeal involvement, 400

Immune response, and nasal allergy, 196–197, 197(t)
Immune system, abnormalities of, and bone marrow transplantation, 370–371

Immune system *(Continued)*
 development of, role of tonsils in, 351
 diseases of, congenital, 378–379
  evaluation of, 379
 dysfunction of, from cancer therapy, 377–378
 infections of, 370–380
Immunosuppression, for organ transplantation, and infection, 377
 from bone marrow transplantation, 370–371
Incus, anatomy of, 31, *33*
 embryology of, 28
 function of, 36
 radiologic assessment of, *106*, *107*
Infantile cortical hyperostosis, 315
Infection(s), acute, of external ear, 80–81, *81*, 81(t), *83*
 of nose, 215, *215*, *216*
 and bone marrow transplantation, 371–376, *374*
 and facial nerve paralysis, 151
 bacterial, of nose, 217
 chronic, and cervical lymph node involvement, 437
  of external ear, 84–86, *85*
  of mastoid, 110–113, *111*, *112*
  of nose, 216–217
 fungal, and cervical lymph node involvement, 437
  in bone marrow recipient, 372
  of external ear, 82–83
  of nose, 216
 in cancer patients, 377–378
 in immunocompromised patients, 370–380
 in tracheostomy, 501
 of deep neck, 356–362, *357–361*
 of middle ear, 110–113, *111*, *112*
 of nasal septum, *374*
 of parapharyngeal space, *358*, 358–359, *359*
 of trachea, *374*
 streptococcal, and tonsillectomy, 352
Inflammation, acute, of external ear, 80–84, *81*, 81(t), *83*
 chronic, of external ear, 84–86, *85*
Inner ear, anatomy of, *34*, 34–36
 computed tomographic assessment of, 108–109, *109*
 diseases of, 123–141. See also *Deafness; Hearing loss.*
 and barotrauma, 95
 ototoxic causes of, 132(t), 132–133
 embryology of, 28–29
 evaluation of, 123–125
  dizziness in, 124
  patient history in, 123
  physical examination in, 124–125
  tinnitus in, 123
 infections of, *131*, 131–132
  complications of, 117
 innervation of, 34–35
 trauma to, *134*, 134–135
 tumors of, *133*, 133–134
Internal auditory canal, radiologic assessment of, 102, *104*, *108*
 tumors of, 153
Internal nose, anatomy of, 178–180, *179*
 blood supply of, *185*
Intranasal balloon, for epistaxis control, 234, *235*, 236–237
Intubation, endotracheal, 491. See also *Tracheostomy.*
Irrigation, antral, for maxillary sinusitis, 252, *252*, *253*
 in cerumen removal, 79
 of external ear canal, 9, *10*
 saline, for pharyngitis, *348*

Jaw, bone disorders of, 314–315, *315*
 cysts of, 291–296, 291(t), *292*, *293*, *295*
 developmental anomalies of, *282*, 282–286, *283*, *285*, *286*

Kartagener's syndrome, and bronchiectasis, 269
    and sinusitis, 262, 269
Keloid, formation of, 517
    of ear lobule, 88
Keratosis obturans, of external auditory canal, 79
Kidney transplantation, and associated infections, 377
Klestadt's cyst, 295
Klippel-Feil syndrome, and congenital deafness, 130

Labyrinth. See also *Inner ear.*
    fistula formation in, 117
    membranous, anatomy of, 34–35, *35*
        development of, 29
    radiologic assessment of, 102, *108*
Labyrinthitis, and chronic otitis media, 117
    fistula test for, *111*, 117
    and meningitis, *131*
    and vertigo, 138–139, *139*
    suppurative, 117
Laceration(s), of cheek, evaluation of, 528–529
    of face, treatment of, 530
    of lips, 511
    of tongue, 511
LaForce adenotome, *355*
Language, definition of, 412
    development of, disorders of, 412–426
        definition of, 412
        in adults, 419–425, *422*, *423*
        in children, 414–419, *415*, 418(t)
        screening tests for, 415
    expressive, 413, 413(t)
    linguistic, 413, 413(t)
    prelinguistic, 412–413
    receptive, 413, 413(t)
    screening tests for, 414
Laryngeal nerve, anatomy of, 386, *386*
    paralysis of, 406
Laryngectomy, for hypopharyngeal tumors, 462
    for laryngeal carcinoma, 461
    mechanistic effects of, 421
    speech rehabilitation in, 423–424
Laryngitis, acute, 400
    in bone marrow recipient, 373–374, *374*
    nonspecific, chronic, 401–402
    subglottic, acute, in children, 398
Laryngocele, 389, 395
Laryngomalacia, 384, 393–394
Laryngopharynx, anatomy of, *388*
Laryngoscope(s), selection of, 480(t)
Laryngoscopy, 392–393, *393*
    for head and neck tumors, 404, 444, 450
    indirect, *19*, 19–20
Laryngotracheobronchitis, clinical features of, 399(t)
Larynx, anatomy of, *384–388*, 384–389
    and aspiration, 409
    and otalgia, 169(t)
    artificial, *422*, 422–424
    blood supply of, 388
    candidiasis of, 373–374, 401
    carcinoma of, classification of, 461(t)
        treatment of, 461–462
            laser microsurgery in, 404–406, 405(t), 462
            radiation in, 454, *454*
    contusions of, 396
    cysts of, 394, 395
    disorders of, allergic, 397–398
        and systemic disease, 400–401
        benign, 392–411
        congenital, 384, 393–396

Larynx *(Continued)*
    disorders of, functional, 410
        infectious, 398–400, 399(t)
        neurogenic, 406–409, *407*, 407(t), *408*
        symptoms of, 392
    embryology of, *383*, 383–384
    examination of, 18–20, *20*, 392–393, *393*
        endoscopy for, 404
        equipment and technique in, *19*, 19–20, *20*
        in vocal cord paralysis, 407, 407(t)
        patient history in, 18–19
    foreign bodies of, 410–411
    fractures of, 396–397
    functions of, 389–390
    infections of, granulomatous, 401
        herpesviral, 373
    innervation of, 387–388, *388*
    internal structure of, *388*, 388–389
    lymphatic drainage of, 388
    musculature of, extrinsic, 385–386, *386*
        in voice production, 390–391
        intrinsic, *386*, 386–387
    paralysis of, 406–409, *407*, 407(t), *408*
        pathology of, 407, 407(t)
    physiology of, 389–391, *390*
    skeletal structure of, *384*, 384–385
    stenosis of, 397
    trauma to, 396–397
    tumors of, benign, 402–406, *404*, *405*, 405(t)
        surgical treatment of, *404*, 404–406, *405*, 405(t)
        malignant, and otalgia, 170
Laser microsurgery, mechanism of, *404*, 405, *405*, 405(t)
    for laryngeal carcinoma, 404–406, 405(t), 462
Law position, in middle ear evaluation, 102–104, *104*
Le Fort's classification, of maxillary fractures, *536*, 536–537
Learning disability, in children, with speech and language disorders, 417–418
Lennert classification, for non-Hodgkin's lymphoma, 447
Leprosy, of larynx, 401
    of nose, 217
Leukemia, acute, 345
    and acute sore throat, 340(t)
    and mastoid infection, *379*
    and tonsillectomy, 351
    and epistaxis, 241
    versus retropharyngeal space abscess, 362
Leukoplakia, of larynx, 403–404
Lichen planus, of oral cavity, *308*, 308–309
Ligation, arterial, for epistaxis control, 238–240, *239*, *240*
Lingual thyroid, *285*, 285–286
Lip(s), anatomy of, 275
    clefts of, 286–291, *287*. See also *Cleft(s), of lips.*
    and encephalocele, 211
    and nasal deformities, 209–210, *210*
Lipectomy, of neck, 522
    submental, 522, *522*
Lipreading, 73
Ludwig's angina, 359, *360*
Lukes-Collins classification, for non-Hodgkin's lymphoma, 447
Lyme disease, and facial nerve paralysis, 151
Lymph node(s), cervical, and infection, 437
    biopsy of, 447
    evaluation of, *436*, 436–437
    location of, in metastatic disease, 438
    surgical anatomy of, 463
Lymphadenectomy, cervical. See also *Radical neck dissection.*
    for head and neck carcinoma, 456–457, 463–464

Lymphangioma, of neck, 435
  of parotid gland, in children, 325
Lymphoma, and lymph node enlargement, 437
  and tonsillar hypertrophy, *349*
  extranodal, versus tonsillar carcinoma, 460
  Hodgkin's, and cervical lymph node involvement, 437
  malignant, 437
    of head and neck, pathology of, 446(t), 446–447
  non-Hodgkin's, and cervical lymph node involvement, 437
  versus retropharyngeal space infection, 362

Macroglossia, 284
Mainstreaming, for hearing-impaired child, 74–75
Major aphthae, 305
Malformation(s), of external ear, *87,* 87–88
Malleus, anatomy of, 31, *33*
  embryology of, 28
  function of, 36
  radiologic assessment of, *105–107*
Malnutrition, in cancer patients, 378
Malocclusion, 284
  in maxillary fracture, 537
Mandible, fracture of, 532–534, *533*
    repair of, 532–533, *533*
    signs of, 532
    supportive care in, 534
Mandibulofacial dysostosis, 291
Mass(es), benign, of neck, 429–442
  of adenoid, *333*
  of hypopharynx, patient history in, 18
  of larynx, 18
  of throat, patient history in, 13
  of thyroid, 439–442, *440, 441*
Mastoid, anatomy of, 33, *33, 37, 115*
  computed tomographic assessment of, 108–109, *109*
  development of, 30, *31,* 106–107
  diseases of, 90–122
  infections of, 84, *379*
    chronic, 107, 110–113, *111, 112*
      signs of, 110–111, *111*
      treatment of, 112–113
        medical, 111–112
        surgical, 112–113
      complications of, extradural, 117–118
  pneumatization of, 106–107
  radiologic assessment of, 102, 104–108, *104-108*
  tumors of, 120–122
Mastoidectomy, for chronic middle ear infection, 112–113, *114–115*
Mastoiditis, coalescent, acute, 109–110
  and cholesteatoma, 112, *112*
  chronic, 110–113, *111, 112*
  complications of, 113, *116,* 117–120
Maxilla, fractures of, 536–537, *536-538*
  classification of, *536,* 536–537
  computed tomographic assessment of, 528, *529*
  treatment of, 537, *537, 538*
Maxillary artery, internal, ligation of, for epistaxis control, 239–240, *241*
Maxillofacial trauma, 526–539
  evaluation of, 526–530, *528, 529*
    patient history in, 527
    physical examination in, 527–528
    radiographic studies in, *528,* 528–529, *529*
  fracture reduction in, 529
  fracture types in, 530–539, *531–538*
  initial care in, 526–527
  soft tissue involvement in, 530

Maxillofacial trauma *(Continued)*
  treatment priorities in, 529–530
Maximal nerve stimulation test, and facial nerve evaluation, 149–150, *150*
Mayer position, in middle ear evaluation, 104, *106*
Median rhomboid glossitis, 285, *285*
Mediastinoscopy, *487,* 487–489, *488*
Mediastinum, examination of, *487,* 487–489, *488*
Melanoma, malignant, of head and neck, 448–449
  classification of, 449(t)
Melkersson-Rosenthal syndrome, 152
  and scrotal tongue, 302
Meniere's disease, 135
  ABR testing in, 63
  and vertigo, 139–140, *140*
Meningioma, 152
Meningitis, 118
  acute, and sinusitis, 266, *266*
  and facial nerve paralysis, 151
  and hearing loss, 131, *131*
Mental retardation, in children, with speech and language disorders, 418
Mentoplasty, 524–525
Metastases, cervical, 22
Michel's deafness, 126
Micrognathia, 283
Microtia, 96
Middle ear, anatomy of, 31–33, *33, 36*
  barotrauma to, 94–95
  computed tomographic assessment of, 108–109, *109*
  congenital stenosis of, 96
  diseases of, 90–122
    adenotonsillectomy for, 350
  embryology of, 27–28, *28*
  fluid in, 8–9
  function of, 36
  infections of, and sensorineural hearing loss, 131
    chronic, 110–113, *111, 112*
      and cholesteatoma, 112, *112*
      fistula test in, 111, *111*
      signs of, 110–111, *111*
      treatment of, medical, 111–112
        surgical, 112–113
    complications of, 113, *116,* 117–120
      extradural, 117–118
      in central nervous system, 118–120
  innervation of, 28
  pain in, 169(t)
  radiologic assessment of, 102, 104–108, *104-108*
  trauma to, 96–98
  tumors of, 120–122
Mirror, head, 3
  nasopharyngeal, 16, *17, 18, 333*
Möbius' syndrome, 151
Mondini's deafness, 126
Mononucleosis, infectious, 345
  and acute sore throat, 340(t)
  and cervical lymph node enlargement, 437
Montgomery tracheocannula, 496, *497*
Mouth, developmental anomalies of, *282, 282–286, 283, 285, 286*
  examination of, 13–16
    equipment and technique in, *15,* 15–16
    patient history in, 13–14
Mucocele, 296
Mucormycosis, 216
Mucosa, nasal, changes in, and medication misuse, 227
  respiratory, 192
    function of, *191,* 191–193
      in disease prevention, 193

Mucosa *(Continued)*
    respiratory, histology of, 181–182, *183*
Multiple sclerosis, and hearing loss, 135
    and vocal cord paralysis, 406
    assessment of, acoustic reflex in, 59
    diagnosis of, ABR testing in, 63–64
Mumps, 318
Myalgia, and headache, 165
Myasthenia gravis, 409
Mycosis, of larynx, 401
Myoblastoma, granular cell, of larynx, 403
Myofascitis, and headache, 165
Myringitis, 91
Myringotomy, *116*, 119–120
    and otitis media complications, 119–120
    for serous otitis media, 102, *103*
    indications for, 120
Myxoma, 313

Nasal allergy, 217–225. See also *Rhinitis, allergic*.
    and associated conditions, 224–225
    and chronic nonspecific laryngitis, 401
    and sinusitis, 256
    diagnosis of, 197–202, 198(t), 199(t), 201(t), 218–221
        allergen identification in, 199
        allergen-immune mechanism in, 200
        dietary tests in, 199, 221
        histamine-release assay in, 201–202, 202(t)
        immune response in, 198(t), 198–199, 199(t)
        in vitro tests in, 221
            versus in vivo tests, 201–202, 202(t)
        nasal smear in, 220
        patient history in, 198, 219
        physical examination in, 198, 219, *219*
        radioallergosorbent test (RAST) in, 200–202, 201(t)
        radiologic studies in, 219, *220*
        skin tests in, 200–202, 201(t)
    differential diagnosis of, 218
    treatment of, 221–224
        allergen elimination in, 221
        medical, 221–222
        surgical, 221–223
        systemic, 223–224, 224(t)
Nasal cavity, blood supply of, 185, *185*
    mass of, *337*
Nasal congestion, 225–228, 226(t), *227*
Nasal deformity(ies), in maxillofacial trauma, 527
Nasal filtration, 190–191
Nasal fracture(s), 241–243, *242*, 530–532, *531*, *532*
    reduction of, 530–531, *533*
    signs of, 530, *531*
Nasal infection, acute, bacterial, 215, *215*, *216*
    chronic, 216–217
Nasal obstruction, and hypernasality, 194
    and juvenile nasopharyngeal angiofibroma, 336
    and nasal fractures, 241–243, *242*
    and obstructive sleep apnea, 363
    and septal hematoma, 242
    causes of, 207
    from foreign bodies, 246–247, *247*
    paradoxical, 228
Nasal packing, anterior, for epistaxis control, 234–235, *235*, *236*
    posterior, complications of, 238
        for epistaxis control, 236–238, *237*
Nasal pain, causes of, 166
Nasal septum, abscess of, 215, *216*,
    anatomy of, 180, *180*
    blood supply of, 185, *185*, *232*

Nasal septum *(Continued)*
    deformities of, 180
        septoplasty for, *242*
    deviation of, and airway resistance, 189
        and compensatory hypertrophic rhinitis, 228
        and maxillary sinusitis, *251*
        and obstructive sleep apnea, 364
        and paradoxical nasal obstruction, 228
        evaluation of, 12
    infections of, in bone marrow recipient, 374
    hematoma of, 530, *531*
    perforation of, 246, *246*
    trauma to, 241–243, *242*
Nasal speculum, 12
Nasal tampons, for epistaxis control, 234, *236*
Nasal turbinate, cautery of, *223*
    hypertrophy of, and obstructive sleep apnea, 364
Nasal vestibule, examination of, 207
Nasal vestibulitis, 215
Nasality, after adenoidectomy, 416
Nasoantrostomy, for chronic maxillary sinusitis, *257*, 257–258, *258*
Nasopharyngeal mirror, 16, *17*, *18*, *333*
Nasopharyngitis, and eustachian tube obstruction, 93
Nasopharyngoscopy, 333–334, *334*
Nasopharynx, anatomy of, 275–276, *276*, 332–334, *333*, *334*
    carcinoma of. See *Carcinoma, of nasopharynx*.
    disorders of, 335–339, *336–337*
        and obstructive sleep apnea, 364
    examination of, *333*, 333–334, *334*
        equipment and technique in, *15*, 15–17, *17*, *18*
        patient history in, 14
    obstruction of, and adenoid hypertrophy, *338*
    tumors of, 335–337, *337*
        and Epstein-Barr virus, 337
        and eustachian tube obstruction, 93
        versus epistaxis, 234
Neck, anatomy of, 278(t), 278–280, 429, *430*
    carcinoma of, early detection of, 444
        radical dissection for, 463
    deep, infection of, 356–362, *357–361*
    examination of, 3, 20–22
        in maxillofacial trauma, 527–528
    fascial spaces of, *280*, 280–281
        infection of, 358
    lipectomy of, 522
    lymph nodes of, evaluation of, *436*, 436–437
    masses of, 431–432, *432*
        benign, 429–442. See also specific types.
        biopsy of, open, 437
        classification of, 432, 433(t)
        cystic, congenital, 433(t), *433–435*, 433–436
        evaluation of, 429–432, 431(t), *432*
            computed tomography in, 431, *432*, 432(t)
            diagnostic tests in, 431–432, *432*, 432(t)
            MRI scans in, 431, *432*, 432(t)
            patient history in, 429–431, 431(t)
            ultrasonography in, 431, 432(t)
        location of, 429, *430*
    metastatic disease of, 438–439
    palpation of, 22, *22*
    tumors of, classification of, 451(t)
        evaluation of, 449–450, 450(t)
        malignant, early detection of, 444
            etiology of, 445
            pathology of, 445–448, 446(t)
            treatment of, 451–465, *454*, *455*, *459*, 460(t), 461(t), 464(t), 465(t)
                chemotherapy in, 464(t), 465, 465(t)

Neck *(Continued)*
   tumors of, malignant, treatment of, principles of, 443
      radiation in, 452–456, *454, 455*
         surgical, 456–457
      metastatic, 448
Necrotizing external otitis, 85
Neuralgia, 160, 167
   definition of, 162
   glossopharyngeal, 162(t), 172–173
   trigeminal, 162(t), 172
Neurapraxia, 145, *145*
   diagnosis of, 153
Neurilemmoma, of neck, 439
Neurofibroma, of neck, 439
Neuroma, acoustic. See *Acoustic neuroma.*
Neutropenia, from bone marrow transplantation, 371
Nevoid basal cell carcinoma syndrome, 294
Nocturnal polysomnography, in obstructive sleep apnea diagnosis, 365, *365*
Nodule, in helix, 89
Non-Hodgkin's lymphoma, and cervical lymph node involvement, 437
   pathology of, 446–447
Nose, airflow through, filtration of, 190–191, *191*
      temperature regulation of, 189–190, *190*
   airway resistance in, function of, *188,* 188–189
   anatomy of, 12, *12,* 177–181, *178–181,* 183–188
   and pulmonary physiology, 193
   and speech production, 194
   blood supply of, 185, *185,* 232, *232*
   candidiasis of, 216
   carcinoma of, squamous cell, etiologic agents of, 445, 445(t)
   cysts of, 210, *211*
   deformities of, congenital, 209–212, *210, 211*
      plastic surgery for, *523,* 523–524
   discharge from, 11
   diseases of, 206–248
      and obstructive sleep apnea, 364
      and systemic disorders, 229–231
      inflammatory, 212–217
      symptoms of, 206–207
   examination of, 10–13
      anesthesia in, 209
      instruments for, 12, 206, *208*
      patient history in, 11–12
      radiography in, 13
      techniques for, 206–209, *207*
   external, anatomy of, 177–178, *178,* 242, *242*
   fractures of, 241–243, *242,* 528, 530–532, *531, 532*
   histology of, 181–187, *182–187*
   infections of, acute, bacterial, 215, *215, 216*
      chronic, 216–217
   innervation of, 186, *187*
   internal, anatomy of, 178–180, *179*
   lymphatic system of, 186, *186*
   mucociliary function in, *191,* 191–193
   mucosa of, histology of, 181–182, *183*
   obstruction of. See *Nasal obstruction.*
   olfactory area of, function of, 187–188
      histology of, 184–185, *185*
   physiology of, 187–193, *188, 190, 191*
   trauma to, 24–241
   tumors of, 243–246, *245*
      evaluation of, 244
      malignant, 457
   turbinates of, 12, *12*
Nosebleed. See *Epistaxis.*

Obesity, and obstructive sleep apnea, 363
Obliteration procedure, for chronic frontal sinusitis, 261, *262*
Obstructive sleep apnea. See *Sleep apnea, obstructive.*
Odontoma, ameloblastic, 312, *313*
Odynophagia, and foreign body ingestion, 475
Olfaction, 187–188
   histologic basis of, *184,* 184–185
   laboratory measurements of, 188
Oncocytoma, of salivary glands, 328
Onychodystrophy, and congenital deafness, 128
Optic nerve, evaluation of, 21
Oral cavity, anatomy of, 274–275
   and otalgia, 169(t)
   candidiasis of, *309,* 309–310
   diseases of, 282–316
   embryology of, 273–274
   erythema multiforme of, *307*
   hemorrhage of, from trauma, 315
   tumors of, malignant, 458–459
Oral mucosa, disorders of, *301–303,* 301–310, *308, 309*
   herpes zoster of, 305–306
   white lesions in, 308
Oral tori, *282,* 282–283, *283*
Orbital cellulitis, 263, *264*
   and ethmoid sinusitis, 254, *254*
Orbital complications, of sinusitis, 263–265, *264, 265*
Orbital floor, fractures of, *534,* 534–535, *535*
   repair of, 535
   signs of, 535
Organ of Corti, anatomy of, 35, *35*
   embryology of, 29
   function of, 36–37
Organ transplantation, and associated infections, 377
Oropharynx, anatomy of, 276, 334, *355*
   diseases of, *340,* 340–350, *341,* 346(t), *347–349*
   and obstructive sleep apnea, 364
Osler-Weber-Rendu syndrome, and epistaxis, 241
   treatment of, 231, *231*
Ossicles, anatomy of, *34*
   embryology of, 27–28, *28*
Ossicular chain, and tympanic membrane perforation, 98
   disorders of, 95–98
      congenital, 95–96
Ossicular disarticulation, audiometric findings in, 65
Ossicular system, audiologic evaluation of, 57–58
Osteoma, of external auditory canal, 88
   of sinuses, 270
Osteomyelitis, from radiation therapy, 456
   of frontal bone, and sinusitis, 267–268
Otalgia, *168,* 168–170, 169(t)
   and herpes zoster oticus, *168*
   and temporomandibular joint dysfunction, 171
   causes of, 169, 169(t)
   referred, 170, *170*
Otic capsule, anatomy of, 34, *34*
   development of, 28–29, *29*
Otitis, external, 80–86, *81, 83*
   drug therapy for, 81(t)
   necrotizing, 85
Otitis externa, circumscripta, 80, *81*
   drug therapy for, 81(t)
   diffuse. See *Diffuse otitis externa.*
Otitis media, acute, 6, 98–110, *99*
   audiometric findings in, 65
   bacteria in, 99(t)
   eustachian tube obstruction and, 98–99
   purulent, symptoms of, 99, *99*
      treatment of, 99–100
   treatment of, 113, *117*

Otitis media *(Continued)*
    after bone marrow transplantation, 376
    and cleft palate, 288
    and facial nerve paralysis, 147
    and meningitis, 118
    and subdural abscess, 118
    chronic, 91, 110–113, *111, 112*
        and labyrinthitis, 117
        fistula test in, 111, *111*
        treatment of, medical, 111–112
            surgical, 112–113
    complications of, 113, *116*, 117–120
    from bone marrow transplantation, 371–372
    in children, 100
    recurrent, in HIV-positive children, 377
    serous, *6*, 100–102, *101*
        and adenoid hypertrophy, 338
        and chronic allergic rhinitis, 224
        and cleft palate, 94
        and hearing loss, in children, 100
        and nasopharyngeal tumors, 336, 337, 458
        audiometric findings in, *64*
        chronic, adenoidectomy for, 339
        etiology of, 100
        examination of, 101, *101*
        in children, 100
        treatment of, medical, 101
            surgical, 102, *103*
Otocyst, development of, 29
Otolaryngology, anesthesia in, 22–23
    biopsy in, 22–23
    equipment for, 3
    examination in, 3–23
        and headache, 161
        and temporomandibular joint, 171
    neurologic evaluation in, 21
    restraint in, 22–23
Otolith organs, evaluation of, 44
Otologic examination, in otosclerosis, *97*
Otomycosis, 82–83
    in bone marrow recipient, 372
Otosclerosis, 96
    and congenital deafness, 129
    assessment of, 96, *97*
    audiometric findings in, *66*
    Carhart notch in, *57, 66*
Otoscope(s), battery powered, 7, *8*
    pneumatic, 8, *8*
    Siegle, 8, *8*
Ototoxicity, causative agents of, 132(t), 132–133
Owens view, in middle ear evaluation, 104, *107*
Ozena, 226(t), 228–229

Paget's disease, and congenital deafness, *130*, 130
Palatal myoclonus, 93
Palate, anatomy of, 275
    clefts of, 286–291, *287.* See also *Cleft(s), of palate.*
        and encephalocele, 211
        and nasal deformities, 209–210, *210*
    embryology of, 274
    fractures of. See *Maxilla, fractures of.*
    soft, evaluation of, 13
Palpation, in oral and pharyngeal examinations, 16, *16*
Papillary adenocystoma lymphomatosum, 327
Papilloma, inverted, of nose, 244, 457
    juvenile, 402–403
        laser microsurgery for, 405
        treatment of, 403

Papilloma *(Continued)*
    squamous, of nose, 244
Papillon-Lefèvre syndrome, and premature periodontal destruction, 301
Paralysis, congenital, of vocal cord, 395–396
    of cranial nerve, and nasopharyngeal tumors, 336, 337
    of facial nerve. See also *Facial nerve, paralysis of.*
        and herpes zoster oticus, 83, *168*
        and otitis media, 113–117
        and temporal bone malignancy, 121
    of recurrent nerve, in tracheostomy, 501
Parapharyngeal space, infections of, *358*, 358–359, *359*
    complications of, 359
    treatment of, 358–359, *359*
    tumors of, 328
Parotid gland, anatomy of, 317
    computed tomographic assessment of, *320*
    hemangioma of, in children, 325
    tumors of, benign, in adults, 327–328
        in children, 325
        malignant, in children, 328–329, 329(t)
            treatment of, 327
    ultrasonographic assessment of, *320*
Parotitis, acute, 318–319
    chronic, 322
    suppurative, acute, 319
Pectus excavatum, 393
Pediatric audiometry, *64–66*, 64–68
Pemphigoid, of mucous membrane, 306–307
Pemphigus, of oral cavity, 306
Pemphigus vulgaris, of larynx, 401
Pendred's disease, and congenital deafness, 128
Perichondritis, *83*, 83–84
Perilymph fistula, and vertigo, 140
Periodontal disorders, 296–301
    destruction in, premature, 301
Periodontitis, 297–299
Peripheral nervous system, disorders of, evaluation of, 42
Petrositis, 117–118
Pharyngectomy, for hypopharyngeal tumors, 462
Pharyngitis, acute, *340*, 340–342, *341*
    and acute sore throat, 340(t)
    diagnosis of, 342
    etiology of, 340–341, *341*, 341(t)
    pathology of, 340–341
    symptoms of, 341
    treatment of, 342
    and tobacco use, 349
    atrophic, 347–348
        treatment of, 348–349
    lateral, 341, *341*
    membranous, 344–345
    recurrent, adenotonsillectomy for, 350
    viral, etiology of, 340–341, 341(t)
Pharynx, anatomy of, *274*, 274–277, *276, 277*
    and otalgia, 169(t)
    blood supply of, 279
    embryology of, 273–274
    examination of, 13–16
        and otalgia, 161
        equipment and technique in, *15*, 15–16
        patient history in, 13–14
    function of, in voice production, 391
    innervation of, 279–280
    physiology of, 280
Pierre Robin syndrome, 283–284
Piriform sinus, anatomy of, 389
Plasmacytoma, extramedullary, of nose, 244–245
Plastic surgery, facial, 505–525. See also *Facial plastic surgery.*

Plate stabilization, for mandibular fractures, 533, *533*
  for maxillary fractures, 537
  for zygomatic fractures, 535
Plaut's angina, 344
  and acute sore throat, 340(t)
Play audiometry, 67
Plummer-Vinson syndrome, and hypopharyngeal tumors, 462
Pneumomediastinum, in tracheostomy, 501
Pneumothorax, in tracheostomy, 501–502
Poliomyelitis, incidence of, after tonsillectomy, 351
Polychondritis, relapsing, nasal manifestations of, 230
  of external ear, 86
Polycythemia, and obstructive sleep apnea, 362
Polyp(s), antrochoanal, 256, 257
  nasal, 202–204
    and aspirin sensitivity and asthma, 202, 225
    and chronic ethmoid sinusitis, 259
    and obstructive sleep apnea, 364
    and sinusitis, 256
    clinical features of, 202
    differential diagnosis of, 222
    treatment of, 203–204
      complications of, 204
      surgical, 222, *223*
      with hyposensitization, 204
    versus inverted papilloma, 244
  of sinuses, 268–269
Polypectomy, nasal, 222, *223*
Polyposis, nasal. See *Polyp(s), nasal.*
Positional tests, 44
Posturography, 44–45
Pregnancy, and gingivitis, 298
Presbycusis, audiometric findings in, 65
Prognathism, 284
Pseudomonas aeruginosa, in tracheostomy, 501
Pulmonary disease, detection of, 22
Pulpitis, 297
Pure tone audiometry, air conduction in, 50–51
  audiogram in, and air-bone gap, 55, *56*
    classic interpretation of, 55, *56,* 57
    notation for, 51, *52*
  audiometric zero, and intensity range, 51
  bone conduction in, 50–51
  cross hearing in, 53–54
  interaural attenuation in, 53–54
  masking in, 54–55, *55*
  threshold determination in, 51–53
    patient preparation in, 51–52
    procedures for, 52–53
    validity of, 53
  versus speech audiometry, 60
Pyocele, and sinusitis, 265–266

Rad (radiation absorbed dose), definition of, 452
Radiation therapy, after neck dissection, 463
  complications of, 456
  for base of tongue tumors, 459
  for head and neck carcinoma, 452–456, *454, 455*
    dosage definitions in, 452–453
  for laryngeal carcinoma, 454, *454,* 461
  for nasal tumors, 457
  for nasopharyngeal carcinoma, 454, *455*
  for sinus carcinoma, 454–456, *455*
  for squamous cell carcinoma, 464(t)
  for tonsillar tumors, 460
  immune system effects of, 377–378

Radiation therapy *(Continued)*
  preoperative versus postoperative, 453
  techniques of, 453–454
    and tumor stage, 453
Radical neck dissection, for head and neck carcinoma, 456–457, 463–464
  for occult tumors, 463
  indications for, 463
  modifications of, 464
Radiculopathy, cervical, and headache, 165
Radioallergosorbent test (RAST), 200–201, 201(t)
Radiosialographic scanning, 323
Ramsay Hunt syndrome, 83, 91, 305
  after bone marrow transplantation, 375
  and facial nerve paralysis, 151, *151*
Rappaport classification, for non-Hodgkin's lymphoma, 447
Refsum's disease, and congenital deafness, 130
Rem (roentgen-equivalent-man), definition of, 452–453
Renal dysfunction, and hearing loss, 129
Respiratory tract, obstruction of, and associated disease, 193
Restlessness, in children, and airway obstruction, 492
Restraint, in otolaryngologic examination, 22–23
Reticulosis, polymorphic, nasal manifestations of, 230
Retraction, and airway obstruction, 492
Rhabdomyosarcoma, 121, 152
  in children, 447–448
Rheumatoid arthritis, and laryngeal disease, 400
Rhinitis, 212–217. See also *Nasal allergy.*
  allergic, 196, 202–204, 217–225, *219*
    and hyperplastic sinusitis, 224
    chronic, and nasal polyps and aspirin sensitivity, 225
      and serous otitis media, 224
    diagnosis of, 202–203, 218–221
    differential diagnosis of, 204
    incidence of, 202
    pathogenesis of, 202
    treatment of, 203–204
      allergen elimination in, 203
      medical, 203
      surgical, 204
      systemic, 223–224, 224(t)
      with hyposensitization, 204
  and temperature change, 227
  and viral exanthemas, 215
  atrophic, 226(t), 228–229
    and atrophic pharyngitis, 348
    treatment of, 229
  hypertrophic, 226(t), 228
    and decongestant use, 226
  in bone marrow recipient, 373, *374*
  infectious, versus nasal allergy, 218
  influenzal, 214–215
  nonallergic, chronic, 225–229, 226(t)
  suppurative, 215
  vasomotor, 225–228, 226(t), *227*
    and drug usage, 226, 226(t), *227*
    etiologic factors of, 226–228
Rhinoliths, 247
Rhinophyma, 247
Rhinoplasty, 523, *523*
Rhinoscleroma, 217
Rhinoscopy, *207,* 209
  for headache, 161
  for nasal allergy, 219
Rhytidectomy, 520, *521*
Rhytides, formation of, 520
  obliteration of, 522–523

Richards-Rundle syndrome, and congenital deafness, 131
Rinne test, 9, *11*, 48
  interpretation of, 49(t)
  validity of, 50
Roentgen, definition of, 452
Rollover, in speech discrimination, 61
Rotation test(s), 42–44
  versus caloric stimulation, 44
Rubella, and congenital sensorineural hearing loss, 128

Salicylate, ototoxicity and, 132
Salivary gland(s), anatomy of, 317–318
  computed tomographic assessment of, 325
  disorders of, 317–331
    inflammatory, 318–321, *320*
    symptoms of, 14
    systemic, 321–322
  embryology of, 274
  examination of, 13–16
    equipment and technique in, *15*, 15–16
    patient history in, 13–14
  innervation of, 318
  radiologic assessment of, *323*, 323(t), 323–325, *324*
  tumors of, benign, in adults, 327–328
      in children, 325
    differentiation of, 328(t)
    malignant, in adults, 329(t), 329–331
      classification of, 330, 330(t)
      treatment of, 330
      in children, 328–329, 329(t)
    TNM classification of, 330(t)
Sarcoid, of larynx, 400
Sarcoidosis, and cervical lymph node involvement, 437
  nasal manifestations of, 230–231
  of parotid gland, 321
  thoracic, and mediastinoscopy, 488
Sarcoma, 447–448
Scar(s), acne, dermabrasion for, 519, *520*
  hypertrophic, 517
  of face, concealment of, *507*, 507–508, *508*, 539
  revision of, 517(t), 517–519, *518*, *519*
  traumatic, dermabrasion for, 519, *520*
Scheibe's disease, 127, *127*
Schirmer test, 147, *148*, 148(t)
Schüller view, in middle ear evaluation, 104, *105*
Schwabach test, 9, 48
  interpretation of, 48(t)
  validity of, 50
Sclerosis, amyotrophic, 409
  and vocal cord paralysis, 406
Scrotal tongue, 302, *302*
Sedation, in examination, 22–23
Seeing Essential English (SEE), 75
Semicircular canals, anatomy of, *34*, 36
  physiology of, 39–40
Septoplasty, 524
  for septal deformity, *242*
  for obstructive sleep apnea, 366, 368(t)
Shadow curve, in pure tone audiometry, 53
Sialadenitis, acute, of submandibular gland, 319
  and sialography, 325
  chronic, of parotid gland, 319–321, *320*
    treatment of, 320–321
  recurrent, 318–319
  of submandibular gland, 321
Sialodochiectasis, 319–321, *320*
Sialography, *320*, *323*, 323–325, *324*, *326*
  for cheek lacerations, 528–529

Sialolithiasis, 321
Sialorrhea, 322
Sinus(es), anatomy of, 179, *179*, 180–181, *181*
  carcinoma of, squamous cell, 458, *459*
      etiologic agents of, 445, 445(t)
      radiation therapy for, 454–456, *455*
  cysts of, 210, *211*
  diseases of, 209, 247, 249–270
    and trauma, 269–270
    congenital, 269
  examination of, 10–13
    instruments in, 12
    patient history in, 11
    radiography in, 13
  frontal, fracture of, 538
    obliteration of, *262*
  infections of, after bone marrow transplantation, 376
    and nasal polyps, 222
  polyps of, 268–269
  radiologic assessment of, 219, *220*
  tumors of, 243–246, *245*, 270
    malignant, 458
      extension of, *459*
    versus epistaxis, 234
Sinusitis, 167–168, 202–204
  acute, 250–255, *251–255*
    features of, 162(t)
  allergic, 268–269
  and asthma, 224
  and headache, 167
  and nasal polyps, 222
  and vascular atony, 228
  bacterial, 250
  chronic, 255–262, *256–262*
    and tumors, 168, 458
    computed tomographic assessment of, 259, *260*
    features of, 162(t)
    in HIV-positive children, 377
    predisposing factors of, 255–256, *256*
    symptoms of, 256–257
    treatment of, 257
      endoscopy in, 259, *259*
    versus acute sinusitis, 255
    versus epistaxis, 234
  complications of, 263–268, *264–266*
    computed tomographic assessment of, 263
    intracranial, *266*, 266–267
    orbital, 263–265, *264*, *265*
  differential diagnosis of, 204
  ethmoid, acute, 254, *254*
    chronic, 259
  frontal, acute, 254–255, *255*
    chronic, 259, *261*, 261–262, *262*
    complications of, *266*, 267
  fungal, in bone marrow recipient, 372–373
  hyperplastic, and allergic rhinitis, 224
  in AIDS, 376–377
  in cancer patients, 378, *379*
  in children, 262–263
  in organ transplantation, 377
  infectious, etiologic agents in, 250
    general considerations in, 249–250
  maxillary, acute, 250–253, *251–253*
    causes of, 250–251, 253
    evaluation of, *251*, 251–252
    of dental origin, 253, *253*
    treatment of, 252, *252*, *253*
  chronic, 257, 257–258, *258*
  noninfectious, 268–269

Sinusitis *(Continued)*
  sphenoid, acute, 255
    chronic, treatment of, 262
  treatment of, 203–204, *204*
  versus impaired ciliary physiology, 192
  viral, 250
Situs inversus, and Kartagener's syndrome, 269
Sjögren's syndrome, 322
  and chronic parotitis, 322
  and sialography, 325
  nasal manifestations of, 231
Skin tumors, malignant, 448–449, 449(t)
Skin flap(s). See also *Flap(s)*.
  advancement, 512, *512*
  in tracheostomy, 496, *496*, *497*
  local, general considerations in, 512, 513
    of face, 512–513, *512*–*514*
  rhomboid, 513, *513*
  transposition, 512, *513*
Skin grafts, classification of, 515, *515*
  general considerations in, 512
  harvesting of, *515*, 515–516, *516*
Sleep apnea, obstructive, 362–368
  and cardiopulmonary syndrome, 362, 362(t)
  clinical presentation of, 362–363
  diagnosis of, 364–365, *365*
  mechanisms of, 363–364
  psychosocial effects of, 364–365
  treatment of, 365–368, *366*, *367*, 367(t), 368(t)
    continuous positive airway pressure (CPAP) in, 368
    genioplasty in, 366
    medical, 367(t), 368
    surgical, 368(t)
    tracheostomy in, 366, *366*
    uvulopalatopharyngoplasty in, 366–367, *367*, 368(t)
Smell. See *Olfaction*.
Snoring, 362–368. See also *Sleep apnea, obstructive*.
Soft tissue, injury of, in maxillofacial trauma, 530
Sore throat. See also *Pharyngitis*; *Tonsillitis*.
  acute, and associated diseases, *340*, 340–350, *341*, 346(t), *347*–*349*
  patient history in, 13, *13*–14
Sound, transmission of, 36
  air conduction in, 47
Speculum, aural, 6–7, *7*
  nasal, 12
Speech, after laryngectomy, 421–424
    and artificial larynx, *422*, 422–423
    and voice prosthesis, 423, *423*
    methods for, 421–422
    rehabilitation in, 423–424
    support groups for, 424
  definition of, 412
  disorders of, 412–426
    adenoidectomy in, 339
    definition of, 412
    in adults, 419–425, *422*, *423*
    in children, 414–419, *415*, 418(t)
    screening tests for, 415
  hypernasal, 194
  hyponasal, 194
  rehabilitation services in, 426
Speech audiometry, in children, 67–68
  masking in, 54–55
  speech discrimination tests in, 61
  speech reception threshold (SRT) test in, 60–61
  versus pure tone audiometry, 60
Speech discrimination, 61
Speech pathology services, 426

Speech reception threshold (SRT), 60–61
Speechreading, 73
Splinting, for mandibular fractures, 532–533, *533*
Spondylosis, cervical, and headache, 165
Squamous cell carcinoma. See *Carcinoma, squamous cell*.
Stapes, anatomy of, 33, *33*
  embryology of, 28
  function of, 36
Stenger test, 68
Stenosis, esophageal, 473, 473(t)
    prevention of, 474
  laryngeal, 397
  of external auditory canal, 84, *85*
  subglottic, 397
    congenital, 394
    from intubation, 385
    in children, 491
    treatment of, in neonates, 497–498
      laser microsurgery for, 405
  tracheal, in tracheostomy, 502
Stensen's duct, dilatation of, *323*
  sialographic assessment of, *326*
Stenvers position, in middle ear evaluation, 104, *108*
Stomatitis, aphthous, recurrent, 304–305
Stridor, and airway obstruction, 492
  in laryngeal disease, 392
Stuttering, in children, 416–417
Sublingual glands, anatomy of, 318
Submandibular glands, anatomy of, 317–318
  sialographic assessment of, 323–325, *324*, *326*
  tumors of, 327
    malignant, 331
Suctioning, in tracheostomy care, 499, *500*
Supraclavicular fossa, mass of, 448
Supraglottitis, clinical features of, 399(t)
Sutton's disease, 305
Suture(s), absorbable, versus nonabsorbable, 510
  interrupted mattress, 510–511, *511*
  running, 511, *511*
  technique for, in facial plastic surgery, 509–511, *510*, *511*
  tracts of, 506, *506*
Swallowing, stages of, 280
Swimmer's ear, 81–82. See also *Diffuse otitis externa*.
Syphilis, and cervical lymph node involvement, 437
  and hearing loss, 131–132
  laryngeal involvement in, 401
Syringe, irrigating, *10*

Taste, innervation for, 275
Teeth, anatomy of, 275
  embryology of, 273–274
  eruption of, disorders in, 300
  fractures of, 316
Teflon, injection of, for vocal cord paralysis, *408*
Temporal bone, anatomy of, *144*
  embryology of, 29–30, *30*
  fractures of, 134, *134*
  radiologic assessment of, 102, 104–108, *104*-*108*
  trauma to, and facial nerve paralysis, 152
Temporomandibular joint, dysfunction of, 171–172
  differential diagnosis of, 171
  features of, 162(t)
  treatment of, 171–172
  examination of, and headache, 161
Tetanus, prophylaxis for, 509, 509(t)
Tetracycline, dental side effects of, 300
Thornwaldt's disease, 335, *336*

Thrombophlebitis, and brain abscess formation, 266, 267
　of lateral sinus, 118
　septic, and parapharyngeal space infection, 359
Thrombosis, of cavernous sinus, 264, 264, 265
Thyroglossal duct, anatomy of, 435
　cysts of, 434, 434, 435
　embryology of, 278–279
Thyroid gland, anatomy of, 389, 440
　carcinoma of, from radiation therapy, 456
　cysts of, 434, 435
　diseases of, 439
　　diffuse, 440–442
　examination of, 22, 22
　masses of, 439–442, 440, 441
　　diagnosis of, 439–440
　　　thyroid scans in, 440, 440, 441
　nodules of, evaluation of, 440, 441, 442
Thyroid cartilage, anatomy of, 384–386, 384
　fracture of, 396
Thyroiditis, and diffuse thyroid disease, 440–442
　diagnosis of, 441
Thyrotoxicosis, 197
Tic douloureux, 172. See also *Neuralgia*.
Tinnitus, audiologic evaluation of, 125
　etiology of, 123–124
　in polychondritis, 86
　treatment of, 136–137
Tissue expansion, in facial plastic surgery, 514
TNM classification, for head and neck tumors, 451(t)
　for laryngeal carcinoma, 461(t)
　for oral cavity tumors, 460(t)
Tobacco use, and chronic nonspecific laryngitis, 401
　and pharyngitis, 349
　and squamous cell carcinoma, 445
Tongue, anatomy of, 275
　base of, malignant tumors of, treatment of, 459–460
　embryology of, 274
Tongue depressor, in oral and pharyngeal examination, 15, 15–16
Tongue tie, in children, 418
Tonsil(s), anatomy of, 276, 276–277, 334, 354, 355
　and immune system development, in children, 351
　carcinoma of, 460
　hypertrophied, and lymphoma, 447
Tonsillectomy, 350–356, 355, 356
　and otalgia, 170
　and poliomyelitis, 351
　anesthesia for, 354, 357
　contraindications to, 353
　dissection technique in, 357
　for obstructive sleep apnea, 366, 368(t)
　hemostasis control in, 354–355, 357
　immediate, indications for, 347, 347(t)
　indications for, 351–353
　instruments for, 356
　outpatient versus inpatient, 356
　patient preparation in, 353–354
　postoperative bleeding in, 354–355
　surgical anatomy for, 354, 355
　technical considerations in, 354–356, 355
　with adenoidectomy, benefits of, 350–351
Tonsillitis, acute, 342–343
　　and acute sore throat, 340(t)
　　pathology of, 342
　　treatment of, 342–343
　chronic, diagnosis of, 349–350, 350
　　treatment of, 350
　etiology of, 352
　lingual, 343–344
　　and acute sore throat, 340(t)

Torus mandibularis, 283, 283
Torus palatinus, 282, 282
Total communication, 75
Towne view, in middle ear evaluation, 104
Toxic shock syndrome, and nasal packing, 215
Trachea, anatomy of, 386, 492–493
　Aspergillus infection of, 374
Tracheal atresia, 483
Tracheal cannula, 498
Tracheitis, bacterial, 399(t)
Tracheobronchial tree, anatomy of, 482
　disorders of, 483–485
　　congenital, 483
　　evaluation of, 481, 482, 485–487
　　　bronchoscopy in, 486, 486–487
　　foreign bodies in, location of, 484–485
　　symptoms of, 483–484
Tracheomalacia, 394, 483
Tracheostomy, 389, 490–502
　alternatives to, in neonates, 497–498
　complications of, delayed, 501–502
　　surgical, 500–501
　definition of, 490
　elective, in adults, 493–494, 494(t), 495
　　in children, 494
　emergency, 494–496
　　in maxillofacial trauma, 526–527
　for bilateral vocal cord paralysis, 408, 408–409
　for foreign body aspiration, 484
　for laryngeal fracture, 396
　for laryngitis, 373–374
　for Ludwig's angina, 360
　for obstructive sleep apnea, 365–366, 366
　history of, 490–491
　incisions for, 496, 497
　indications for, 491–492
　modifications of, 496–498, 496–498
　postoperative care in, 499–500, 500
　surgical technique for, 493–502, 494(t), 495–498, 500, 501
　tubes, postoperative care of, 499–500, 500
　　sizes of, for adults, 493, 494(t)
　　　for children, 494(t)
　　types of, 496–497, 501
　versus endotracheal intubation, 491
Tracheotomy, and laryngeal stenosis, 397
　definition of, 490
Transplantation, bone marrow. See *Bone marrow transplantation*.
　organ, and associated infections, 377
Trap door deformity, 513, 516, 516–517
Trauma, acoustic, 36
　auricular defects from, 524
　during childbirth, and facial nerve paralysis, 151
　to external ear, 86–87
　to maxillofacial area, treatment of, 526–539. See also *Maxillofacial trauma*.
　to nose, and epistaxis, 240–241
　to oral cavity, 315–316
Treacher Collins syndrome, 95, 279, 291
Trephination, for frontal sinusitis, 255
Trigeminal nerve, evaluation of, 21
Trismus, and deep neck infection, 358
Trisomy 13–15 (D), and congenital deafness, 128
Trisomy 18 (E), and congenital deafness, 128
Tuberculosis, and cervical lymph node involvement, 437
　of esophagus, 472
　of larynx, 401
　of middle ear, 111
　of nose, 217

Tubotympanic recess, formation of, 27, *28*
Tumor(s), acoustic, *133*, 133–134
  benign, of salivary glands, in adults, 327–328
    in children, 325
  carotid body, 438, *439*
  malignant, connective tissue, 447–448
    of head and neck, 443–467
      treatment of, 451–465, *454*, *455*, *459*, 460(t), 461(t), 464(t), 465(t)
        chemotherapy in, 464(t), 465, 465(t)
        radiation in, 452–456, *454*, *455*
        surgical, 456–457
    of middle ear, 121
    of nose, 457
    of oral cavity, 458–459
    of salivary glands, 329(t), 329–331
    of sinuses, 458, *459*
    of skin, 448–449, 449(t)
  metastatic, to head, 448
    to middle ear region, 121–122
  neuroectodermal, of neural crest origin, 314
  neurogenic, 439
  nonodontogenic, 314
  occult, and cervical metastasis, 463
  odontogenic, 310(t), 310–313, *311*, *313*
    adenomatoid, 311
    epithelial, calcifying, 312
  of cerebellopontine angle, *133*, 152
  of middle ear and mastoid, 120–122
  of oral cavity, 310(t), 310–314, *311*, *313*
  of parotid gland, 327
  of salivary glands, differentiation of, 328(t)
    TNM classification of, 330(t)
  of skull base, and vocal cord paralysis, 406
  of submandibular gland, 327
    malignant, 331
  of tongue base, 459–460
Tuning fork, Riverbank 512 cycle, 9
Tuning fork test(s), 9–10, *10*, *11*, 47–50. See also *Hearing test(s)*.
  Bing test, 49
  reliability of, 49–50
  Rinne test, 9, *11*, 48, 49(t)
  Schwabach test, 9, 48, 48(t)
  threshold determination in, 47–48
  validity of, 49–50
  Weber test, 9, *11*, 49
Tympanic cavity, radiologic assessment of, *104*
Tympanic membrane, anatomy of, *6*, 31, *32*, *33*
  appearance of, in acute otitis media, 99, *99*
    in disease, 90–91
  audiologic evaluation of, 57–58. See also *Tympanometry*.
  diseases of, 90–92, *91*
  examination of, 5, *7*, 7–8, *8*
  inflammation of, 91–92
  perforation of, 8–9, 91, *91*, 96, 98, 111
    and ossicular chain damage, 98
    treatment of, 98
Tympanocentesis, for otitis media, in bone marrow transplantation, 371
Tympanogram, classification of, 57–58, *58*
  of tympano-ossicular system, 57
Tympanometry, 57–58
  acoustic immittance in, 58–59, 59(t)
Tympano-ossicular system, tympanometry and, 57–58
Tympanoplasty, for chronic middle ear infection, 112–113, *115*
Tympanosclerosis, 110
  audiometric findings in, *65*

Ulcers, contact, of vocal cord, 402
Usher's disease, and congenital deafness, 128
Uveoparotid fever, 321
Uvulopalatopharyngoplasty, for obstructive sleep apnea, 366–367, *367*, 368(t)

Vagus nerve, evaluation of, 21
Varicella-zoster virus infection, after bone marrow transplantation, 375
Vasoconstrictor(s), topical, in examination, 13
Venous system, and sinusitis complications, *266*, 266–267
Ventilation problems, chronic, versus airway obstruction, 492
Ventilation tube(s), placement of, for serous otitis media, 102, *103*
  indications for, 120
Vertigo, 137–141
  and chronic otitis media, 111
  and inner ear disease, 117
  and tympanic membrane perforation, 98
  assessment of, fistula test in, 111, *111*
  benign paroxysmal positional, 137–138
    diagnosis of, 44
  benign positional, 137–138
  causes of, nonvestibular, 137
    vascular, 137
    vestibular, 137–140, 138(t), *139*, *140*
  cervical, 137
  differential diagnosis of, 124(t)
  evaluation of, 41–42
  in polychondritis, 86
  treatment of, 141
Vestibular function, disorders of, 21
  evaluation of, 41–45, *43*
    caloric stimulation in, 42, 44
    electronystagmography in, 42, *43*
    positional tests in, 44
    posturography in, 44–45
    rotation tests in, 42–44
    vestibulo-ocular reflex in, 42
Vestibular nerve, pathways of, 38
Vestibular neuronitis, and vertigo, 138
Vestibular reflex, pathways of, 41
Vestibular system, disorders of, 138(t)
  physiology of, 39–41
Vestibule, of inner ear, anatomy of, *34*, 35–36
  radiologic assessment of, *104*
Vestibulo-ocular reflex, evaluation of, 42
  pathways of, 41
Vincent's angina, 344
  and acute sore throat, 340(t)
Vincent's infection, *298*, 298–299
Virus(es), and hearing loss, 131
  respiratory, 213–215
Vocal abuse, adductor hyperfunction and, 420
Vocal cord(s), anatomy of, *388*, 389
  contact ulcer of, in men, 402
  examination of, in chronic laryngitis, 402
  function of, 390, *390*
  leukoplakia of, 403
  musculature of, 386–387
  nodules of, 400, 402
  paralysis of, 406–409, *407*, 407(t), *408*
    bilateral, 406, 407(t), *408*, 408–409
    causes of, 406–407
    congenital, 395–396
    cord designation in, 406, 406(t), *407*

Vocal cord(s) *(Continued)*
  paralysis of, unilateral, 406, *407*, 407(t)
    in children, 407–408
      treatment of, 408, *408*
Vocal weakness, 410
Voice, artificial larynx for, *422*, 422–423
  disorders of, and loudness, 419–420
    and pitch, 419
    and vocal quality, 420
    functional versus organic, 419
    in adults, 419–421
    in children, 415–416
    incidence of, 419
    psychologic factors in, 419
    therapy for, 421
  esophageal, and artificial larynx, 422–423
    methods for, 421–422
    outcome factors in, 424
  production of, 390
  prosthesis for, 423, *423*
Von Recklinghausen's disease, and acoustic neuroma, 133
  and congenital deafness, 130

W-plasty, 517(t), 518, *519*
Waardenburg's disease, and congenital deafness, 127

Waldeyer's ring, lymph nodes of, and non-Hodgkin's lymphoma, 437
  lymphoma in, 447
Warthin's tumor, 327
Waters' view, *220*
Weber test, 9, *11*, 49
Web(s), congenital, of larynx, 394
Wegener's granulomatosis, nasal manifestations of, 229–230
Wharton's duct, dilatation of, *323*
  sialographic assessment of, *326*
Wheezing, and foreign body aspiration, 484
Wire stabilization, for mandibular fractures, 533, *533*
  for maxillary fractures, 537, *537*
Wound care, principles of, 503–512, *507*, *508*, 509(t), *510*, *511*. See also *Facial plastic surgery; Facial wound(s)*.
Wrinkles, formation of, 520
  obliteration of, 522–523

Z-plasty, 517(t), 518, *518*
Zenker's diverticulum, 277
  and chronic nonspecific laryngitis, 401
Zigzag-plasty, 517(t), 518, *519*
Zygoma, fractures of, *534*, 534–535, *535*
  repair of, 535